Design and Analysis of Bioavailability and Bioequivalence Studies

Third Edition

Chapman & Hall/CRC Biostatistics Series

Chapman & Hall/CRC Biostatistics Series

Published Titles

1. *Design and Analysis of Animal Studies in Pharmaceutical Development,* Shein-Chung Chow and Jen-pei Liu
2. *Basic Statistics and Pharmaceutical Statistical Applications,* James E. De Muth
3. *Design and Analysis of Bioavailability and Bioequivalence Studies, Second Edition, Revised and Expanded,* Shein-Chung Chow and Jen-pei Liu
4. *Meta-Analysis in Medicine and Health Policy,* Dalene K. Stangl and Donald A. Berry
5. *Generalized Linear Models: A Bayesian Perspective,* Dipak K. Dey, Sujit K. Ghosh, and Bani K. Mallick
6. *Difference Equations with Public Health Applications,* Lemuel A. Moyé and Asha Seth Kapadia
7. *Medical Biostatistics,* Abhaya Indrayan and Sanjeev B. Sarmukaddam
8. *Statistical Methods for Clinical Trials,* Mark X. Norleans
9. *Causal Analysis in Biomedicine and Epidemiology: Based on Minimal Sufficient Causation,* Mikel Aickin
10. *Statistics in Drug Research: Methodologies and Recent Developments,* Shein-Chung Chow and Jun Shao
11. *Sample Size Calculations in Clinical Research,* Shein-Chung Chow, Jun Shao, and Hansheng Wang
12. *Applied Statistical Design for the Researcher,* Daryl S. Paulson
13. *Advances in Clinical Trial Biostatistics,* Nancy L. Geller
14. *Statistics in the Pharmaceutical Industry, Third Edition,* Ralph Buncher and Jia-Yeong Tsay
15. *DNA Microarrays and Related Genomics Techniques: Design, Analysis, and Interpretation of Experiments,* David B. Allsion, Grier P. Page, T. Mark Beasley, and Jode W. Edwards
16. *Basic Statistics and Pharmaceutical Statistical Applications, Second Edition,* James E. De Muth
17. *Adaptive Design Methods in Clinical Trials,* Shein-Chung Chow and Mark Chang
18. *Handbook of Regression and Modeling: Applications for the Clinical and Pharmaceutical Industries,* Daryl S. Paulson
19. *Statistical Design and Analysis of Stability Studies,* Shein-Chung Chow
20. *Sample Size Calculations in Clinical Research, Second Edition,* Shein-Chung Chow, Jun Shao, and Hansheng Wang
21. *Elementary Bayesian Biostatistics,* Lemuel A. Moyé
22. *Adaptive Design Theory and Implementation Using SAS and R,* Mark Chang
23. *Computational Pharmacokinetics,* Anders Källén
24. *Computational Methods in Biomedical Research,* Ravindra Khattree and Dayanand N. Naik
25. *Medical Biostatistics, Second Edition,* A. Indrayan
26. *DNA Methylation Microarrays: Experimental Design and Statistical Analysis,* Sun-Chong Wang and Arturas Petronis
27. *Design and Analysis of Bioavailability and Bioequivalence Studies, Third Edition,* Shein-Chung Chow and Jen-pei Liu

Chapman & Hall/CRC Biostatistics Series

Design and Analysis of Bioavailability and Bioequivalence Studies

Third Edition

Shein-Chung Chow

Jen-pei Liu

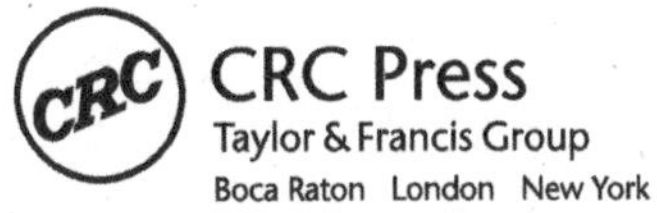

CRC Press
Taylor & Francis Group
Boca Raton London New York

CRC Press is an imprint of the
Taylor & Francis Group, an **informa** business
A CHAPMAN & HALL BOOK

CRC Press
Taylor & Francis Group
6000 Broken Sound Parkway NW, Suite 300
Boca Raton, FL 33487-2742

First issued in paperback 2022

ISBN 13: 978-1-03-247777-0 (pbk)
ISBN 13: 978-1-58488-668-6 (hbk)
ISBN 13: 978-0-429-14036-5 (ebk)

DOI: 10.1201/9781420011678

Publisher's Note
The publisher has gone to great lengths to ensure the quality of this reprint but points out that some imperfections in the original copies may be apparent.

Visit the Taylor & Francis Web site at
http://www.taylorandfrancis.com

and the CRC Press Web site at
http://www.crcpress.com

Contents

Preface

As the first decade of the twenty-first century draws to an end, the arena of bioavailability and bioequivalence has generated a lot of scientific, statistical, and regulatory activities and issues from the pharmaceutical industry, health authorities, as well as academia, since the publication of the second edition of our book in 2000. In particular, a series of regulatory guidelines or guidances were issued by different health authorities in the world. In January 2001, the U.S. Food and Drug Administration (FDA) issued the guidance on *Statistical Approaches to Establishing Bioequivalence*. Six months later, in July 2001, the European Agency for the Evaluation of Medicinal Products (EMEA) issued the *Note for Guidance on the Investigation of Bioavailability and Bioequivalence*. In March 2003, the U.S. FDA released the guidance on *Bioavailability and Bioequivalence Studies for Orally Administrated Drug Products—General Considerations*. Later, the World Health Organization, in 2005, issued the draft revision of the guidelines on *Multisource (Generic) Pharmaceutical Products: Registration Requirements to Establish Interchangeability*. On the other hand, tremendous opportunities as well as challenges still lie ahead for bioavailability and bioequivalence in the twenty-first century because of breakthroughs in biotechnology and methodological research in medicine, pharmacokinetics, and statistics. In response to the challenges, upon the invitation of Professor R.B.D'Agostino, one of the co-editors of *Statistics in Medicine*, we were invited as guest editors for a special issue of 13 papers on individual bioequivalence that was published on October 30, 2000. In addition, the U.S. FDA issued a document on *Critical Path Opportunities for Generic Products* on May 1, 2007 to address emerging challenges and opportunities for generic drug products. The issues on the regulations and scientific issues of biosimilar products or follow-on biologics still remain unresolved. Consequently, there is an urgent need for the third edition of this book to provide a complete and overall presentation of the latest development of activities and results in bioavailability and bioequivalence on regulatory requirements, scientific and practical issues, and statistical methodology.

The third edition is different from the first and second editions in four aspects. First, we have revised and updated each section to reflect recent developments in statistical methodology in the design and analysis of bioavailability and bioequivalence studies. For example, the third edition provides a complete update of the status of regulations on bioavailability and bioequivalence, especially, the guidelines issued by the U.S. FDA, EMEA, and WHO. Second, the third edition is expanded to 20 chapters, 4 chapters more than the second edition and 8 chapters more than the first. The third edition includes four new chapters as well as some new sections to present a complete account of the new developments in bioavailability and bioequivalence studies. The four new chapters include "Population Pharmacokinetics" (Chapter 17), "Other Pharmacokinetic Studies" (Chapter 18), "Review of Regulatory Guidances on Bioequivalence" (Chapter 19), and "Frequently Asked Questions and Future Challenges" (Chapter 20). Third, to deliver an effective presentation of the material, we modified the configurations of the 20 chapters into 5 parts: "Preliminaries," "Average Bioequivalence," "Population and Individual Bioequivalence," "*In Vitro* and Alternative Evaluation of Bioequivalence," and "Other Bioequivalence Studies." Part I, "Preliminaries", describes the regulatory history of bioavailability and bioequivalence, design of bioavailability studies, and statistical inference for the standard 2×2 crossover design. Part II, "Average Bioequivalence," reviews the methods for evaluation of average bioequivalence, power and sample size determination, transformation and assessment of intra- and inter-subject variabilities, outlier detection, and higher-order designs for evaluation of average bioequivalence. Part III, "Population and Individual Bioequivalence," gives an update of the methods for the design and analysis of population and individual bioequivalence. Part IV, "*In Vitro* and Alternative Evaluation of Bioequivalence," includes assessment of average bioequivalence with negligible plasma levels, *in vitro* bioequivalence studies, and *in vitro* dissolution profile comparison. Part V, "Other Bioequivalence Studies," consists of meta-analysis for bioequivalence review, population pharmacokinetics, other pharmacokinetic studies, review of regulatory guidance, and future challenges. Finally, the third edition has 120 new references from the bioavailability and bioequivalence literature.

Similar to the first two editions, the third edition is also entirely devoted to the design and analysis of bioavailability and bioequivalence studies. It covers all of the statistical issues that may occur in the various stages of design and data analysis in bioavailability and bioequivalence studies. We strongly believe that this new, updated and much expanded third edition not only is an extremely useful reference book for pharmaceutical scientists and researchers, regulatory reviewers, clinicians, and biostatisticians in the academia, regulatory agencies, and pharmaceutical industry but also serves as an advanced textbook for graduate courses dealing with the topics of bioavailability and bioequivalence in the areas of pharmacokinetics, clinical pharmacology, and biostatistics. It is also our intent that this book will serve as a bridge among the pharmaceutical industry, government regulatory agencies, and academia.

Although the information, material, and presentation configuration of the third edition are different from the first two editions, the third edition still focuses on concepts rather than technical details. The mathematics and statistics dealt in the book are still fundamental. We have received many positive and constructive feedbacks and comments from scientists and researchers in academia, regulatory agencies, including the FDA, and pharmaceutical industry. Therefore, we have maintained our intuitive writing style as well as the emphasis on concepts through numerous examples and illustrations.

We would like to thank Jessica Vakili and David Grubbs of Taylor & Francis for their administrative assistance and support. We are deeply indebted to the Duke

University School of Medicine (especially, Rob Califf, MD, Robert Harrington, MD, Ralph Corey, MD, John McHutchison, MD, and Wesley Burks, MD) and the National Taiwan University for their encouragement and support. We also want to express our sincere gratitude to many pharmaceutical scientists, researchers, and biostatisticians for their feedbacks, support, and encouragement. Chow wishes to thank his fiancée Annpey Pong, PhD, for her constant encouragement and support during the preparation of this edition. Liu wishes to express his appreciation to his wife, Professor Wei-Chu Chie, MD, PhD, and daughter, Angela, for their patience, endurance, understanding, and support during the preparation of this edition.

Finally, we are fully responsible for any errors remaining in the book. The views expressed in this book are those of the authors and are not necessarily those of the Duke University School of Medicine, the National Taiwan University, or the National Health Research Institutes of Taiwan.

Shein-Chung Chow
Jen-pei Liu

Authors

Shein-Chung Chow, PhD is currently a professor in the Department of Biostatistics and Bioinformatics, Duke University School of Medicine, Durham, North Carolina. Before joining Duke University, he was the director of the Taiwan Cooperative Oncology Group Statistical Center and the executive director of National Clinical Trial Network Coordination Center of Taiwan. Dr. Chow has also held various positions in the pharmaceutical industry including vice president. He has worked in the areas of biostatistics and data management, and as a medical writer at Millennium Pharmaceuticals, Inc., Cambridge, Massachusetts. He had also been executive director, statistics and clinical programming, at Covance, Inc. Princeton, New Jersey; director and department head at Bristol-Myers Squibb, Plainsboro, New Jersey; senior statistician at Parke-Davis Pharmaceutical Division, Warner-Lambert Company, Ann Arbor, Michigan; and research statistician at Wyeth-Ayerst Laboratories, Rouses Point, New York. Through these positions, Dr. Chow provided technical supervision and guidance to project teams on statistical issues and made presentations for partners, regulatory agencies, or scientific bodies, defending the appropriateness of statistical methods used in clinical trial design, data analyses, and the validity of reported statistical inferences. Dr. Chow has identified best statistical and data management practices, organized and led working parties for the development of statistical design, analyses, and presentation applications, and has participated on many data safety monitoring boards.

Dr. Chow's professional activities include playing key roles in many professional organizations such as officer, board of directors member, advisory committee member, and executive committee member. He has served as program chair, session chair/moderator, panelist, and instructor/faculty at many professional conferences, symposia, workshops, tutorials, and short courses. He is the editor-in-chief of the *Journal of Biopharmaceutical Statistics*. Dr. Chow is also the editor-in-chief of the CRC Press biostatistics series. He was elected fellow of the American Statistical Association in 1995 and was elected member of the International Statistical Institute in 1999. He was the recipient of the DIA Outstanding Service Award (1996), the ICSA Extraordinary Achievement Award (1996), and the Chapter Service Recognition Award of the American Statistical Association (1998). Dr. Chow was scientific advisor to the Department of Health, Taiwan, Republic of China during 1999–2001 and from 2006 till date. Dr. Chow was president of the International Chinese Statistical Association, chair of the advisory committee on Chinese pharmaceutical affairs, and a member of the advisory committee on statistics of the DIA.

Dr. Chow has authored/co-authored over 170 methodology papers and 14 books, which include *Advanced Linear Models*, *Design and Analysis of Bioavailability and Bioequivalence Studies* (first and second editions), *Statistical Design and Analysis in Pharmaceutical Science*, *Design and Analysis of Clinical Trials* (first and second editions), *Design and Analysis of Animal Studies in Pharmaceutical Development*, *Encyclopedia of Biopharmaceutical Statistics* (first and second editions), *Sample Size Calculations in Clinical Research*, *Adaptive Design Methods in Clinical Trials*, and *Statistical Design and Analysis of Stability Studies*.

Dr. Chow received a BS in mathematics from the National Taiwan University, Taipei, Taiwan and a PhD in Statistics from the University of Wisconsin, Madison.

Jen-pei Liu, PhD is currently the director of Statistical Education Center, Nationa Taiwan University, the director of Consulting Center for Statistics and Bioinformatics, National Taiwan University, and a Professor of Statistics, Division of Biometry, Department of Agronomy, National Taiwan University, Taipei, Taiwan. Professor Liu is a clinical biostatistician with more than 20 years experience, and has been involved with all phases of clinical trials in a wide spectrum of therapeutic areas. He also has extensive publications. His publication includes five reference books in statistical methods for the biopharmaceutical industry (Marcel Dekker) and *Design and Analysis of Clinical Trials* (co-authored with S.C. Chow; John Wiley & Sons), over 120 articles in peer-reviewed statistical journals, and over 20 invited book chapters in the *Encyclopedia of Biostatistics* and *Encyclopedia of Biopharmaceutical Statistics*. His papers were cited in the 2001 FDA guidance on *Statistical Approach to Establishing Bioequivalence* and in the 2005 WHO guideline on multisource drug products. He is an associate editor for the *Journal of Biopharmaceutical Statistics*, an associate editor for the *Taiwan Journal of Public Health* (since January 2002), and a member of the advisory committee on *Statistics in Biosciences* (since January 2008). He is one of the editors for the CRC Press biostatistics series. He serves as a referee for many international statistics journals. Currently, he is on the Drug Consultation Committee, the Committee for Medical Devices, and the Committee for the Chinese Drug and Pharmacy, all for the Department of Health, Taiwan. Dr. Liu received his BS in agronomy and MS in biometry from the National Taiwan University, Taipei, Taiwan and his MS and PhD in Statistics from the University of Kentucky, Lexington.

Part I

Preliminaries

Chapter 1

Introduction

1.1 History of Bioavailability Studies

The term *bioavailability* is a contraction for biological availability (Metzler and Huang, 1983). The definition of bioavailability has evolved over time with different meanings by different individuals and organizations. For example, differences are evident in the definitions by Academy of Pharmaceutical Sciences, the Office of Technology Assessment (OTA, 1974) of the Congress of the United States (1974), Wagner (1975), and the 1984 Drug Price Competition and Patent Restoration amendments to the Food, Drug, and Cosmetic Act. Throughout this book, however, the definitions and some related terms regarding bioavailability provided in the Act, which are adopted by the United States Food and Drug Administration (FDA), will be used (21 CFR, Part 320.1, 1983).

The bioavailability of a drug is defined as the rate and extent to which the active drug ingredient or active moiety from a drug product is absorbed and becomes available at the site of drug action. For drug products that are not intended to be absorbed into bloodstream, bioavailability may be assessed by measurements intended to reflect the rate and extent to which the active ingredient or active moiety is absorbed and becomes available at the site of action. A comparative bioavailability study refers to the comparison of bioavailabilities of different formulations of the same drug or different drug products. When two formulations of the same drug or two drug products are claimed *bioequivalent*, it is assumed that they will provide the same therapeutic effect or that they are therapeutically equivalent and they can be used interchangeably. Two drug products are considered pharmaceutical equivalents if they contain identical amounts of the same active ingredient. Two drugs are identified as pharmaceutical alternatives to each other if both contain an identical therapeutic moiety, but not necessarily in the same amount or dosage form or as the same salt or ester. Two drug products are said to be bioequivalent if they are pharmaceutical equivalents (i.e., similar dosage forms made, perhaps, by different manufacturers) or pharmaceutical alternatives (i.e., different dosage forms) and if their rates and extents of absorption do not show a significant difference to which the active ingredient or active moiety in pharmaceutical equivalents or pharmaceutical alternatives become available at the site of action when administered at the same molar dose under similar conditions in an appropriately designed study. For more discussion regarding the definition of bioavailability, see Balant (1991) and Chen et al. (2001a,b).

The study of absorption of an exogenously administered compound (sodium iodide) can be traced back to 1912 (Wagner, 1971). The concept of bioavailability, however, was not introduced until some 30 years later. Oser et al. (1945) studied the relative absorption of vitamins from pharmaceutical products and referred to such relative absorption as physiological bioavailability. In recent years, generic drug products, which are those manufactured by generic drug companies or the innovator companies themselves, have become very popular. Bioavailability/bioequivalence studies are of particular interest to the innovator and the generic drug companies in the following ways. First, for the approval of a generic drug product, the FDA usually does not require a regular new drug application (NDA) submission, which demonstrates the efficacy, safety, and benefit–risk of the drug product, if the generic drug companies can provide the evidence of bioequivalence between the generic drug products and the innovator drug product through bioavailability and bioequivalence studies in a so-called abbreviated new drug application (ANDA). Second, when a new formulation of a drug product is developed, the FDA requires that a bioavailability study be conducted to assess its bioequivalence to the standard (or reference) marketed formulation of the drug product. Thus, bioavailability studies are important because an NDA submission includes the results from phases 1–3 clinical trials, which are very time consuming and costly to obtain. Finally, under the Food and Drug Administration Modernization Act (FDAMA) passed by the U.S. Congress in 1997, after the approval, depending on the magnitudes of changes in components and composition or method of manufacture, the FDA may require the evidence of bioequivalence between the pre- and postchange products under NDA or postchange generic product with the reference list product under ANDA. For details, see the FDA guidance on scale-up and postapproval changes (FDA, 1995a; FDA, 1997a).

The concept of bioavailability and bioequivalence became a public issue in the late 1960s because of the concern that a generic drug product might not be as bioavailable as that manufactured by the innovator. These concerns rose from clinical observations in humans together with the ability to quantify minute quantities of drug in biological fluids. This initiated not only a period of four decades of extremely active scientific research and development in bioavailability and bioequivalence, but also started the process and formulation of the current regulatory requirements for approval of generic drug products. Spanning from the early 1970s to date, the research and development of bioavailability and bioequivalence can be roughly divided into four phases. The first phase is from early 1970s to 1984 when the U.S. Congress passed the Drug Price Competition and Patent Term Restoration Act that authorized the to approve generic drug products through bioavailability and bioequivalence studies. The second phase begins from 1984 to 1992 after the issue of the U.S. FDA guidance entitled *Statistical Procedures for Bioequivalence Studies Using a Standard Two-Treatment Crossover Design in 1992*, which provides the sponsors a guidance as to how the data should be analyzed and presented in an ANDA submission for bioequivalence review. The concept of population and individual bioequivalence for addressing drug interchangeability in terms of drug prescribability and drug switchability and their corresponding statistical methods has been discussed in the third phase since 1992. The fourth phase starts at the dawn of the twenty-first century when based on the fruit of research conducted in the last 30 years of the twentieth century, the FDA issued and implemented the new guidance on general considerations and statistical approaches to bioavailability and bioequivalence studies.

In 1970, the FDA began to ask for evidence of biological availability in applications submitted for approval of certain new drugs. In 1971, a drug bioequivalence study panel was formed by the OTA to examine the relationship between the chemical and therapeutic equivalence of drug products. On the basis of the recommendations in the OTA report, the FDA published a set of regulations for the submission of bioavailability data in certain new drug applications. These regulations became effective on July 1, 1977 and are currently codified in 21 CFR, Part 320. In 1971, by the time the FDA began to require evidence of bioavailability for NDA of some drug products, the Biopharmaceutical Subsection of the American Statistical Association simultaneously formed a Bioavailability Committee to investigate the statistical components for the assessment of bioequivalence. Metzler (1974) summarized the efforts by the Committee and addressed several concerns about some statistical issues in bioavailability studies. During the decade of the early 1980s, the search for statistical methods for the assessment of bioequivalence received tremendous attention. Several methods that met the FDA requirements for statistical evidence of bioequivalence were proposed. These methods included an a posteriori power approach, reformation of bioequivalence hypotheses (Schuirmann, 1981; Anderson and Hauck, 1983), a confidence interval approach (Westlake, 1972, 1976, 1979; Metzler, 1974), and a Bayesian approach (Rodda and Davis, 1980; Mandallaz and Mau, 1981). A detailed discussion of these statistical developments during this period can be found in Metzler and Huang (1983).

In 1984, the FDA was authorized to approve generic drug products under the Drug Price Competition and Patent Term Restoration Act. However, as more generic products become available, the following concerns were raised:

1. Whether generic drug products are comparable in quality to the innovator drug product.

2. Whether the generic copies of innovator drug products have comparable therapeutic effect.

To address these concerns, a hearing on bioequivalence of solid oral dosage forms was conducted by the FDA during September 29–October 1, 1986 in Washington, DC. As a consequence of the hearing, a bioequivalence task force was formed to examine the current procedures adapted by the FDA for the assessment of bioequivalence between immediate solid oral dosage forms. Some efforts were also directed at investigating the statistical issues that often occur in various stages of design and data analysis in bioavailability and bioequivalence studies. A report from the bioequivalence task force was released in January 1988. Several statistical issues related to the assessment of bioequivalence are summarized below:

1. Lot-to-lot uniformity
2. Alternative statistical designs for intra-subject variability
3. Statistical methodology in decisional criteria for bioequivalence
4. Product-to-product variability
5. Detection and treatment of outlying data.

Relative to these issues, several statistical methods have been developed that provide some answers to the above statistical questions. For example, for the evaluation of lot-to-lot (or batch-to-batch) uniformity, Chow and Shao (1989) proposed several statistical tests for batch-to-batch variability. To account for the heterogeneity of intra-subject variability, an estimation procedure for the assessment of intra-subject variability, assuming that the coefficient of variation (CV) is the same from subject to subject, was proposed by Chow and Tse (1990b) under a conditional random effects model. Chow (1989) and Chow and Shao (1991) compared the decision rules under lognormality assumption. Chow and Shao (1990) also proposed an alternative approach for assessing bioequivalence using the idea of a confidence region. The proposed procedure was shown to rigorously meet the FDA's requirements for average bioequivalence. For outlier detection, Chow and Tse (1990a) proposed two tests using the idea of likelihood distance and estimates distance for detection of a possible outlying subject. The same problem was also examined by Liu and Weng (1991).

In June, 1992, the first edition of this book was published, which provides a comprehensive and unified summarization of literature on statistical design and analysis of bioavailability and bioequivalence up to 1991. Two weeks after the first edition of this book was published, the FDA guidance on *Statistical Procedures for Bioequivalence Studies Using a Standard Two-Treatment Crossover Design* was issued. Chow and Liu were invited by the Division of Biometrics and Division of Bioequivalence of the FDA to give a presentation on the review of the guidance from the pharmaceutical perspectives in April, 1983 (Chow and Liu, 1994a,b). As a follow-up, Chow and Liu also organized a special invited paper session on the FDA guidance at the 1993 American Statistical Association (ASA) Joint Statistical Meetings held in San Francisco, California on August 9, 1993. At the invited paper session, various issues concerning the 1992 guidance were discussed. Other details on the discussion of the issue of bioequivalence during the second phase can be found in a supplement entitled *Bioequivalence Assessment: Methods and Applications of* the *International Journal of Clinical Pharmacology Therapy and Toxicology* edited by V.W. Steinijans and H.U. Shulz (Vol. 30, Suppl. 1, 1992).

As the century closes to the end, generic drug products have played more important role in health care than before because of the necessity for reduction of health cost by all countries. As a result, in the third phase after 1992, different concepts of bioequivalence, such as drug interchangeability including drug prescribability and drug switchability (Hauck and Anderson, 1992; Chow and Liu, 1995a), have evolved, with suggestions of different requirements for approval of generic drugs: for example, population bioequivalence (Liu and Chow, 1992b) and individual bioequivalence (Hauck and Anderson, 1992). At the same time, several important symposia and workshops were held to discuss and exchange ideas and views in definition and procedures of population and individual bioequivalence between drug products. To enhance communications and to exchange information of the state-of-the-art scientific developments and advancements among regulatory agencies, academia, and the pharmaceutical industry, on September 19–20, 1994, the authors of this book, along with the experts from the FDA organized a major symposium on Bioavailability and Bioequivalence, which was sponsored by the Drug Information Association (DIA) held in Rockville, Maryland. The papers presented in this symposium were published in a special issue of the *Drug Information Journal*, edited by S.C. Chow (Vol. 29, No. 3) (see, Chow, 1995). In addition, L. Endrenyi of the University of Toronto, J. Mau of the Heinrich Heine University, Düsseldorf Medical Institutions, and R. Williams of the FDA held an international workshop on statistical and regulatory issues on the assessment of bioequivalence in Düsseldorf, Germany, October 19–20, 1995, to address current regulatory viewpoints and unsolved scientific issues on bioequivalence. The papers presented at this workshop were published in a special issue of the *Journal of Biopharmaceutical Statistics*, edited by S.C. Chow (Vol. 7, No. 1). Furthermore, Fédération Internationale Pharmaceutique (FIP) held its Bio-International'96 Conference in Tokyo, Japan, April 22–24, 1996 to address various issues of bioequivalence including highly variable drug products, individual bioequivalence, alternative metrics and approaches, and the role of *in vitro* dissolution test. The papers presented at this conference were published in the proceedings of FIP Bio-International, 1996 *Bioavailability, Bioequivalence and Pharmacokinetics Studies*, edited by K.K. Midha and T. Nagai, Tokyo, Japan.

In late October 1997, the FDA circulated a draft guidance entitled *In Vivo Bioequivalence Studies Based on Population and Individual Bioequivalence Approaches* for comments. According to the FDA, the draft guidance is not for implementation at that time. However, when it is finalized, it will replace the 1992 guidance for bioequivalence assessment. This new draft guidance requires the sponsors to provide evidence of individual bioequivalence for approval of generic drugs as well as innovator drug products for which postapproval changes are required in bioequivalence testing as specified in the scale-up and postapproval change (SUPAC) guidelines.

Note that since this new draft guidance will have a great influence on the design and analysis of bioequivalence studies, several professional (statistical) meetings were organized to (1) review the guidance, (2) evaluate the feasibility and scientific merits of individual bioequivalence for approval of generic products, (3) exchange ideas for improvement of the recommended statistical procedures, and (4) discuss the strategy for future implementation of the guidance from the perspectives of the academia, the pharmaceutical industry, and regulatory agencies around the world. Just to name a few, professional meetings held in 1998 including Midwest Biopharmaceutical Statistics Workshop (MBSW), Muncie, Indiana; Drug Information Association (DIA) annual meeting, Boston, Massachusetts; the American Statistical

Association (ASA) annual Joint Statistical Meetings, Dallas, Texas; Statisticians in the Pharmaceutical Industry (PSI) annual meeting, Horragate, the United Kingdom; and the International Biometric Conference (IBC), Cape Town, South Africa. Most comments from these professional meetings indicated that the draft guidance in its current content and format lacks clinical and statistical considerations (Chow, 1999). In addition, since many important scientific and methodological issues still remain unresolved, Chow and Liu assembled a special issue on individual bioequivalence for *Statistics in Medicine*, which was published on October 30, 2000. In this special issue, 13 papers by the authors from academia, government as well as industry were published for various opinions and comments and different scientific approaches to individual bioequivalence. On the basis of this issue and other research on the merits, feasibility, methodology of population and individual bioequivalence, on February 2, 2001, the FDA issued the guidance entitled *Statistical Approaches to Establishing Bioequivalence*. Six months later, the European Agency for the Evaluation of Medicinal Products (EMEA) issued the *Note for Guidance on the Investigation of Bioavailability and Bioequivalence*. On March 19, 2003, the FDA issued the current guidance entitled *Bioavailability and Bioequivalence Studies for Orally Administrated Drug Product–General Considerations*. Recently, the World Health Organization (WHO) recognizes that the quality and supply of generic drugs is a critical issue of global health and are vital to developing countries. As a result, after a series of meetings among the members of FIP/WHO BCS Task, for multisource (generic) pharmaceutical products, in 2005, the WHO issued the draft revision of the guidelines on *Registration Requirements to Establish Interchangeability*. Research on methodological development for bioequivalence assessment is still very active in the twenty-first century. More details will be provided in later chapters of this book.

1.2 Formulations and Routes of Administration

When a drug is administered to a human subject, the drug generally passes through an absorption phase, distribution phase, metabolism phase, and finally an elimination phase within the body. As mentioned in Section 1.1, the bioavailability of a drug is defined as the rate and extent to which the active ingredient of the drug is absorbed and becomes available to the body. Because clinical effects may be associated with blood or plasma levels of the drug, the information of bioavailability is useful for the assessment of a drug's efficacy and safety. Bioavailability is usually determined by some pharmacokinetic measurements that can be estimated from the blood or plasma concentration–time curve obtained following drug administration. The blood or plasma concentration–time curve, however, is dependent, in part, on the dosage form and the route of administration.

In the pharmaceutical industry, when a new drug is discovered, it is important to design an appropriate dosage form for the drug so that it can be delivered to the body efficiently for optimal therapeutic effect. The dosage form, however, should also account for the acceptability to the patients. Dosage forms, such as tablet, capsule, solution, powder, and liquid suspension, are usually considered. For a given drug product, several dosage forms may be designed for different purposes. For example, solution and liquid suspension dosage forms may be more appropriate than solid dosage forms for children and elderly patients. However, in practice, most drugs are taken orally in solid dosage forms (e.g., tablet and capsule). Generally, solid dosage forms have to dissolve to be absorbed. The dissolution of the drug depends on the particle size. The reduction of particle size may increase the bioavailability of the drug. Examples of drugs for which bioavailability has been increased as a result of particle size reduction are aspirin and estradiol (Dare, 1964).

The route of administration can certainly affect the bioavailability of a drug. Different routes of administration may result in a significant difference in bioavailability. For example, a study of kanamycin (Kunin, 1966) demonstrated that the oral administration has extremely low bioavailability (about 0.7%). In contrast, the bioavailability of intramuscularly administered kanamycin is much greater (about 40%–80%). Basically, there are several routes by which drugs are commonly administered. These routes may be classified as either intravascular or extravascular. Intravascular administration refers to giving the drug directly into the blood, either intravenously or intra-arterially. Extravascular administration includes the oral, intramuscular, subcutaneous, sublingual, buccal, pulmonary, rectal, vaginal, and transdermal routes. Drugs administered extravascularly must be absorbed to enter the blood.

Because different dosage forms may affect the bioavailability of the drug, they may exhibit market variability in their absorption. Thus, before a drug can be released for medical use, the FDA requires that the drug be tested *in vitro* in compliance with United States Pharmacopeia and National Formulary (USP/NF) specifications to ensure that the drug contains the labeled active ingredient within an acceptable variation. The USP/NF standards for the evaluation of the drug include potency testing, content uniformity testing, dissolution testing, disintegration testing, and weight variation testing (Chow and Liu, 1995b). In addition, a bioavailability study is also required by the FDA. The assay method used for the active ingredients to quantify the drug must be validated in terms of the closeness of the test results obtained from the assay method to the true values (accuracy) and the degree of closeness of the test results to the true values (precision).

Note that since different dosage forms or routes of administration may affect the bioavailability of the drug, a comparative bioavailability (bioequivalence) study may involve the comparison of different dosage forms (or formulations) of the same drug, generic drug product, and the marketed (innovator) drug product of the same active ingredient, and different routes of administration.

1.3 Pharmacokinetic Parameters

In a comparative bioavailability study in humans, following the administration of a drug, the blood, serum, or plasma concentration–time curve is often used to study the rate of absorption and elimination of the drug which can be characterized by taking blood samples immediately before and at various time points after drug administration. However, instead of direct and indirect pharmacokinetic measures, the 2003 FDA guidance recommends that reliance on systemic exposure measures reflects comparable rate and extent of absorption. These exposure measures are defined relative to early, peak, and total portion of the plasma, serum, or blood concentration–time curve. The pharmacokinetic parameters representing different exposure measures involve the area under the plasma or blood concentration–time curve (AUC) for total exposure, partial AUC for early exposure, maximum or peak concentration (C_{max}), and time to achieve maximum concentration (t_{max}) for peak exposure, respectively. The measurements of these pharmacokinetic parameters can be derived either directly from the observed blood or plasma concentration–time curve, which is independent of a model, or is obtained by fitting the observed concentrations to a one- or a multicompartment pharmacokinetic model. In the following case, the determination of some pharmacokinetic parameters assumes first-order absorption and elimination.

One of the primary pharmacokinetic parameters for total exposure in a bioavailability study is the AUC. The AUC is often used to measure the extent of absorption or total amount of drug absorbed in the body. Several methods exist for estimating the AUC from zero time until time t, at which the last blood sample is taken. These methods include the interpolation using the trapezoidal rule, the Lagrange and spline methods, the use of a planimeter, the use of digital computers, and the physical method that compares the weight of a paper corresponding to the area under the experimental curve to the weight of a paper of known area. Among these methods, the method of interpolation appears to be the one most commonly used. Yeh and Kwan (1978) discussed the advantages and disadvantages of using the Lagrange and spline methods relative to the trapezoidal rule in the method of interpolation. For simplicity, we introduce only the method of linear interpolation using the trapezoidal rule. Let $C_0, C_1, \ldots, C_k$ be the plasma or blood concentrations obtained at time $0, t_1, \ldots, t_k$, respectively. The AUC from zero to t_k, denoted by AUC($0 - t_k$), is obtained by

$$\text{AUC}(0 - t_k) = \sum_{i=2}^{k} \left(\frac{C_{i-1} + C_i}{2} \right) (t_i - t_{i-1}). \tag{1.3.1}$$

The AUC, however, should be calculated from zero to infinity, not just to the time of the last blood sample, as is so often done. The portion of the remaining area from t_k to infinity could be large if the blood level at t_k is substantial (Martinez and Jackson, 1991). The AUC from zero to infinity, denoted by AUC($0 - \infty$), can be estimated as follows (Rowland and Tozer, 1980):

$$\text{AUC}(0 - \infty) = \text{AUC}(0 - t_k) + \frac{C_k}{\lambda}, \tag{1.3.2}$$

where

C_k is the concentration at the last measured sample after drug administration

λ is the terminal or elimination rate constant, which can be estimated as the slope of the terminal portion of the log concentration–time curve multiplied by -2.303

The FDA regulation requires that sampling be continued through at least three more terminal half-lives of the active drug ingredient or therapeutic moiety, or its metabolites, measured in the blood or the decay of the acute pharmacological effect so that the elimination would have been completed and any remaining area beyond time t_k is negligible. Therefore, the FDA recommends that at least three to four samples should be obtained during the terminal log–linear phase to get an accurate estimate of λ from linear regression. Note that a few missing values or unexpected observations in the plasma concentration–time curve within (t_1, t_k) will generally have little effect on the calculations of AUC$(0 - t_k)$ and AUC$(0 - \infty)$. However, if there are many missing values or unexpected observations in the plasma concentration–time curve, especially at endpoints (i.e., t_1 and t_k), the bias of the estimate of AUC could be substantial.

In addition of the AUC, the absorption rate constant is usually studied during the absorption phase. Under the single-compartment model, the absorption rate constant can be estimated based on the following equation using the method of residuals (Gibaldi and Perrier, 1982).

$$C_t = \frac{k_a F D_0}{V(k_a - k_e)}(e^{-k_e t} - e^{-k_a t}), \tag{1.3.3}$$

where

k_a and k_e are the absorption and elimination rate constants, respectively
D_0 is the dose administered
V is the volume of distribution
F is the fraction of the dose that reaches the systemic circulation

Given Equation 1.3.3, C_{max} and t_{max} can similarly be obtained as follows:

$$t_{max} = \frac{2.303}{k_a - k_e} \log\left(\frac{k_a}{k_e}\right), \tag{1.3.4}$$

and

$$C_{max} = \frac{k_a F D_0}{V(k_a - k_e)}(e^{k_e t_{max}} - e^{k_a t_{max}}). \tag{1.3.5}$$

In practice, however, the estimates from a pharmacokinetic model usually are not used for the comparison of formulations. Thus, C_{max} is estimated directly from the observed concentrations. That is, $C_{max} = \max\{C_0, C_1, \ldots, C_k\}$. Similarly, t_{max} is estimated as the corresponding time point at which the C_{max} occurs. Because the partial AUC is an early exposure measure, the FDA suggests that the partial AUC be truncated at the population median of t_{max} and at least two quantifiable samples be collected before the expected C_{max} to allow estimation of the partial AUC.

During the elimination phase, the pharmacokinetic parameters that are often studied are the elimination half-life ($t_{1/2}$) and rate constant (k_e) (Chen and Pelsor, 1991). The plasma elimination half-life is the time taken for the plasma concentration to fall by one-half. Assume that the decline in plasma concentration is of first order, the $t_{1/2}$ can be obtained by considering

$$\log D = \log D_0 - \frac{k_e t}{2.303}, \tag{1.3.6}$$

where D is the amount of drug in the body. Thus, at $D = D_0/2$ (i.e., $t = t_{1/2}$) we have

$$\log\left(\frac{1}{2}\right) = -\frac{k_e t_{1/2}}{2.303}.$$

Hence,

$$t_{1/2} = \frac{0.693}{k_e},$$

where k_e is given by

$$k_e = (-2.303)\left(\frac{d \log D}{dt}\right).$$

The first order elimination half-life is independent of the amount of drug in the body. In practice, all the drug may be regarded as having been eliminated (about 97%) by five half-lives.

The above pharmacokinetic parameters are usually considered in a single dose trial. In practice, drugs are most commonly prescribed to be taken on fixed time interval basis (i.e., multiple doses such as b.i.d., t.i.d., or q.i.d.). Dosing a drug several times a day can result in a different drug concentration profile than that produced by a single dose. If the dosing interval is less than the time required to eliminate the entire dose, the peak plasma level following the second and succeeding doses of a drug is always higher than the peak level after the first dose. This leads to drug accumulation in the body relative to the initial dose. For a multiple dose regimen, the amount of drug in the body is said to have reached a steady-state level if the amount or average concentration of the drug in the body remains stable. The following pharmacokinetic parameters at steady are usually studied:

$$\begin{aligned} C_{max} &= \frac{D_0}{1 - \left(\frac{1}{2}\right)^{\varepsilon}}, \\ C_{min} &= \frac{D_0}{1 - \left(\frac{1}{2}\right)^{\varepsilon}}\left(\frac{1}{2}\right)^{\varepsilon}, \\ C_{av} &= \frac{C_{max} - C_{min}}{\log\left(\frac{C_{max}}{C_{min}}\right)}, \\ \text{Percent fluctuation} &= \left(\frac{C_{min}}{C_{max}}\right) \times 100\%, \end{aligned} \tag{1.3.7}$$

where ε is the dosing interval τ divided by elimination half-lives. Note that τC_{av} is the area under the curve within a dosing interval at steady state, which is equal to that following a single dose. In a multiple dose study, however, how to choose or combine the information of several pairs of C_{max} and C_{min} from a subject is an interesting question. This certainly has some influence on statistical analysis of the data. Wang et al. (1996) studied patient compliance and fluctuation of the serum drug concentration.

Example 1.3.1

To illustrate how to estimate AUC, C_{max}, t_{max}, $t_{1/2}$, and k_e from the observed concentrations, it is helpful to consider the following example. Table 1.3.1 lists the primidone concentrations (μg/mL) versus time points (hours) from a subject over a 32 hours period after administered a 250-mg tablet of a drug. The blood samples were drawn immediately before and at time points 0.5, 1.0, 2, 3, 4, 6, 8, 12, 16, 24, and 32 hours. The plot of primidone concentration–time curve for the subject is exhibited in Figure 1.3.1. From Table 1.3.1, AUC(0 – 32) and C_{max} can be obtained as follows.

$$\begin{aligned}
\text{AUC}(0-32) &= \sum_{i=2}^{12} \left[\frac{C_{i-1}+C_i}{2}\right](t_i - t_{i-1}) \\
&= \frac{(0+0)}{2}(0.5-0) + \frac{(0+2.8)}{2}(1-0.5) + \cdots \\
&\quad + \frac{(2+1.6)}{2}(32-24) \\
&= 85.95\ (\mu\text{g} \times \text{h/mL}), \\
C_{max} &= \max(0,0,2.8,\ldots,1.6) = 4.7\ \mu\text{g/mL}.
\end{aligned}$$

TABLE 1.3.1: Calculation of AUC using the trapezoidal rule.

Blood Sample (i)	t_i	C_i	$(C_i+C_{i-1})/2$	t_i-t_{i-1}	$(C_i+C_{i-1})(t_i-t_{i-1})/2$
1	0.0	0.0	—	—	—
2	0.5	0.0	0.00	0.5	0.00
3	1.0	2.8	1.40	0.5	0.70
4	1.5	4.4	3.60	0.5	1.80
5	2.0	4.4	4.40	0.5	2.20
6	3.0	4.7	4.55	1.0	4.55
7	4.0	4.1	4.40	1.0	4.40
8	6.0	4.0	4.05	2.0	8.10
9	8.0	3.6	3.80	2.0	7.60
10	12.0	3.0	3.30	4.0	13.20
11	16.0	2.5	2.75	4.0	11.00
12	24.0	2.0	2.25	8.0	18.00
13	32.0	1.6	1.80	8.0	14.40

Note: AUC(0 – 30) = 85.95.

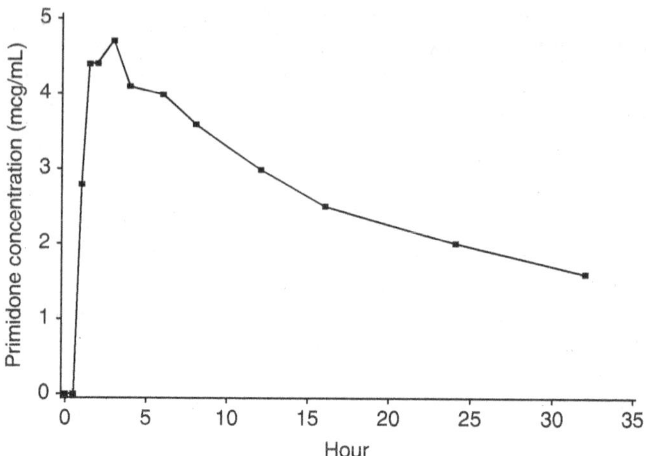

FIGURE 1.3.1: Primidone concentration–time curve.

t_{max} is estimated as the corresponding time point at which C_{max} was achieved. Thus, $t_{max} = 3.0$ hours. For the estimation of the elimination rate k_e, the last seven concentrations during the elimination phase were used to fit a linear regression based on the log concentrations with a base 10 using the least-squares method (Draper and Smith, 1981). The resultant regression line is given by

$$\log_{10}(C_i) = 0.6713 - 0.01518t_i.$$

Thus, the elimination rate is

$$k_e = (-2.303)\,(-0.01518) = 0.03496\ (\text{h}^{-1}).$$

Consequently, the elimination half-life is

$$t_{1/2} = \frac{0.693}{0.03496} = 19.8\ (\text{h}).$$

The AUC$(0 - \infty)$ can be obtained as

$$\begin{aligned}\text{AUC}(0-\infty) &= \text{AUC}(0-32) + C_{32}/0.03496\\ &= 85.95 + 1.6/0.03496\\ &= 131.72\ (\mu\text{g}\cdot\text{h/mL}).\end{aligned}$$

In the above example, we selected the last seven concentrations during the elimination phase to calculate the elimination rate. In practice, the number of concentrations used may depend on the plasma concentration–time curve for each subject. This is an interesting statistical question that needs further attention.

1.4 Clinically Important Differences

The definition of a clinically significant difference is important for the assessment of therapeutic equivalence in terms of efficacy, safety, and benefit–risk ratio. In bioavailability and bioequivalence studies, it is our intention to consider bioequivalence in terms of therapeutic equivalence. However, this ultimate assumption of bioequivalence can be verified only through rigorous prospective clinical trials that may relate bioavailability parameters with clinical endpoints through the data from blood concentrations and clinical efficacy and safety evaluations. In practice, such clinical trials are rarely carried out owing to the following difficulties:

1. Unlike healthy subjects who are often used for bioavailability–bioequivalence studies, patients cannot be well controlled.

2. Patients are more heterogeneous in a wide variety of characteristics.

However, the ultimate obstacle lies in the estimation and translation of the differences in bioavailability into the therapeutic differences of interest.

Westlake (1979) pointed out that a statistically significant difference in the comparison of bioavailability between drug products does not necessarily imply that there is a clinically significant difference between drug products. For example, the AUC for the test product may exhibit an 80% bioavailability compared with the reference product. The 20% difference in AUC, which may be statistically significant, however, may not be of clinical significance in terms of therapeutic effect. In other words, although there is a 20% difference, both test and reference products can still reach the same therapeutic effect. Thus, they should be considered therapeutically equivalent. Generally, a set of bioequivalence limits, say (a, b), is given for the evaluation of clinical difference. If the difference (usually in percentage) in AUC between the test and reference products is within the limits, then there is no clinical difference, or they are considered to be therapeutically equivalent. Bioequivalent limits for therapeutic equivalence generally depend on the nature of the drug, targeted patient population, and clinical endpoints (efficacy and safety parameters) for the assessment of therapeutic effect. For example, for some drugs, such as topical antifungals or vaginal antifungals, that may not be absorbed in blood (Huque and Dubey, 1990), the FDA proposed some equivalent limits for some clinical endpoints (binary responses), such as cure rate as in Table 14.4.1. This table indicates that if the cure rate for the reference drug is greater than 95%, then a difference in cure rate within 5% is not considered a clinically important difference (see Table 1.4.1).

TABLE 1.4.1: Equivalence limits for binary responses.

Equivalence Limits (%)	Response Rate for the Reference Drug (%)
±20	50–80
±15	80–90
±10	90–95
±5	>95

1.5 Assessment of Bioequivalence

The assessment of bioequivalence for different drug products is based on the following fundamental bioequivalence assumption: When two drug products are equivalent in the rate and extent to which the active drug ingredient or therapeutic moiety is absorbed and becomes available at the site of drug action, it is assumed that they will be therapeutically equivalent and can be used interchangeably.

Given the fundamental bioequivalence assumption, bioequivalence studies are, therefore, the surrogates for clinical trials for assessment of therapeutic equivalence in efficacy and safety between drug products. This is the reason why the title of the WHO guidelines is on the requirements for establishment of interchangeability of multisource pharmaceutical products. The purpose of bioequivalence trials, hence, is to identify pharmaceutical equivalents or pharmaceutical alternatives that are intended to be used interchangeably for the same therapeutic effect (21 CFR, 320.50). Thus, bioequivalent drug products are therapeutic equivalents and can be used interchangeably. As a result, US FDA was authorized to ask the sponsors, through an ANDA, to provide the evidence of bioequivalence for approval of generic copies of an innovator drug product after the patent has expired under the Drug Price Competition and Patent Term Restoration Act passed by the U.S. Congress in 1984.

As indicated in Hauck and Anderson (1992) and Chow and Liu (1995a), drug interchangeability can be classified as either drug *prescribability* or drug *switchability*. Drug prescribability is referred to as the physician's choice for prescribing an appropriate drug product for his or her new patients among an innovator drug product and a number of its generic copies that have been shown to be bioequivalent to the innovator drug product. Drug prescribability is usually assessed by population bioequivalence (Chow and Liu, 1992). On the other hand, drug switchability (Anderson, 1993; Liu and Chow, 1995) is related to the switch from an innovator drug product to a generic product within the same subject whose concentration of the active ingredients has been titrated to a steady, efficacious, and safe level. To assure drug switchability, it is recommended that bioequivalence be assessed within individual subjects.

Once the fundamental assumption and the purpose of bioequivalence trials are clearly defined and understood, the next question is what and how to assess bioequivalence. The essential pharmacokinetic parameters for systematic exposure in the FDA regulations for an *in vivo* bioavailability study are AUC$(0-\infty)$, $C_{\max}$, λ, and $t_{1/2}$ of the therapeutic moiety. As discussed in Section 1.3, these pharmacokinetic parameters can be derived either directly from the observe blood or plasma concentration–time curve or obtained by fitting the observed concentrations to a one- or multicompartment pharmacokinetic model. In general, the use of the observed AUC$(0-\infty)$, $C_{\max}$, or $t_{\max}$ from the blood or plasma concentration–time curve is preferred, for they provide the essential information about the pharmacokinetic characteristics in assessment of bioequivalence, and are model-independent and easy to calculate. However, there are some drawbacks in these estimates. For example, the predetermined sampling time points are often too few to have reliable estimates on $C_{\max}$ and $t_{\max}$ in most bioavailability studies. Consequently, the distribution of the estimated $t_{\max}$ is not continuous, but rather, discrete. On the other hand, when a pharmacokinetic model is considered, the goodness of fit of the model should be performed by examining the residuals. In practice, it is almost impossible to fit the same theoretical model for each subject in the study. Moreover the sampling time points are too few to provide reliable estimates for the pharmacokinetic parameters under the model, even though, theoretically, the assumed pharmacokinetic model may adequately describe the observed blood or plasma concentration–time curve. Therefore, the 2003 FDA guidance of general considerations for bioequivalence studies suggests that 12 to 18 samples, including a predose sample, be collected per subject per dose. This sampling can continue for at least three or more terminal half-lives of the drug. In addition, the sampling time should be spaced in such a way that $C_{\max}$ and λ can be estimated accurately.

The statistical concept for evaluation of bioequivalence lies with investigation of the closeness between the marginal distributions of pharmacokinetic responses of interest from the two drug products. As a result, there are three types of bioequivalence, namely, *average bioequivalence* (ABE), *population bioequivalence* (PBE), and *individual bioequivalence* (IBE). On the basis of the fact that the distribution of some random variables (e.g., normal random variable) is uniquely determined by its moments, the equivalence between two distributions can be assessed through the moments of the marginal distributions of the test and reference formulations. The first two moments of the distribution reflect the average and the variability of the distribution. The comparison of the first moments of the distributions of the pharmacokinetic parameters [say, $\text{AUC}(0 - \infty)$] for the two drug products refers to the comparison of *average bioavailability*, whereas the comparison between the second moments refers to the *variability of bioavailability*. To provide a better understanding of average bioavailability and variability in bioavailability, equivalence in averages and variabilities are illustrated in Figures 1.5.1 through 1.5.3. For example,

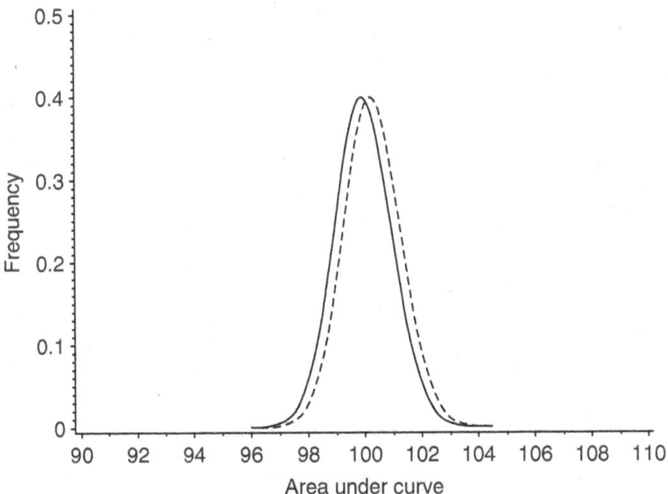

FIGURE 1.5.1: Equivalence in both means and variabilities.

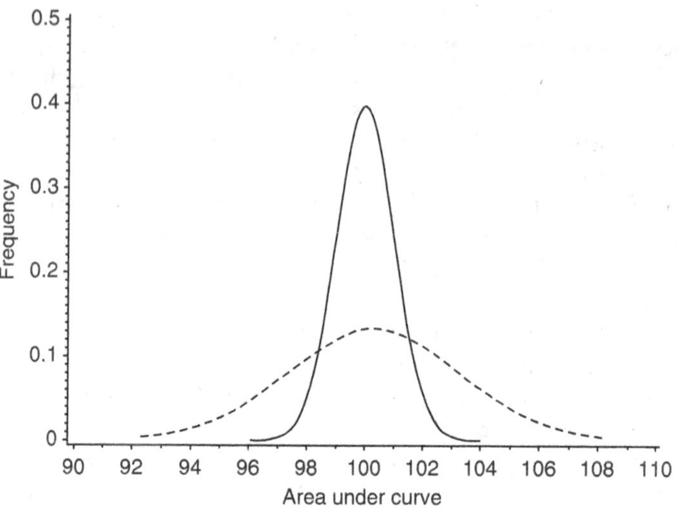

FIGURE 1.5.2: Equivalence in means, but not in variabilities.

if the distribution for AUC$(0-\infty)$ is normal and if the AUC$(0-\infty)$ of two products are equivalent in both averages and variabilities, then the two drug products are bioequivalent. As a result, to ensure drug prescribility, it is required to establish population bioequivalence which, in turn, dictates bioequivalence in both average and variability. However, in general, equivalence in the first two moments does not guarantee equivalence between formulations. Average bioequivalence, a part of population bioequivalence is referred to as equivalence in averages of the marginal distributions of the bioavailabilities between drug products. Currently, the regulations of

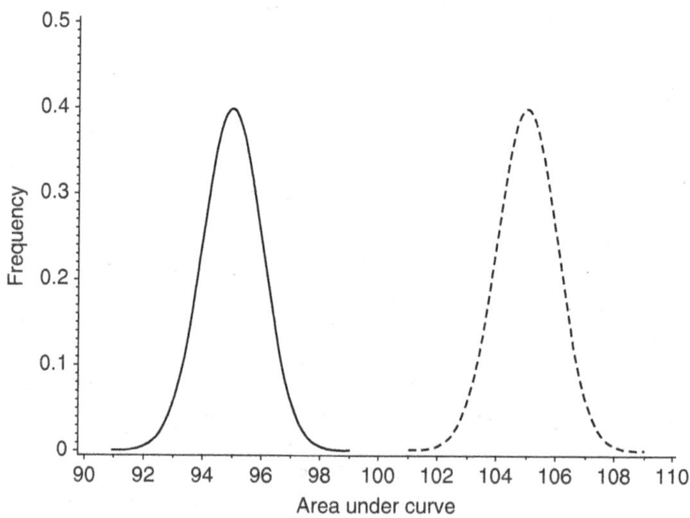

FIGURE 1.5.3: Equivalence in variabilities, but not in means.

most countries including the United States, European Union (EU), and Japan require only that evidence of average bioavailability be provided for approval of generic drug products (FDA, 2003b). However, in practice, this regulation on average bioavailability does not guarantee that two drug products can be used interchangeably in terms of drug efficacy and safety, especially the interchangeability among generic copies of the same innovator drug product. Some discussions can be found in Cornell (1980), Metzler and Huang (1983), Liu (1991), Liu and Chow (1992b), Chow and Liu (1995a), and Chow and Shao (1999).

It has been recognized that drug switchability requires individual bioequivalence (Hauck and Anderson, 1992; Anderson, 1993; Chow and Liu, 1995a). For a given individual, the statistical concept of individual bioequivalence is to examine the closeness between the two marginal distributions of the pharmacokinetic responses that are obtained under the repeated administrations of the test and reference formulations from the same subject. Under the normality assumption, it is then necessary to establish equivalence in average and variability of the two marginal distributions for a given individual. Results of comparison between the test and reference formulations for each individual over a population of subjects can then be assembled for evaluation between the test and reference formulations, as illustrated in Figure 1.5.4. Because assessment of individual bioequivalence requests the comparison of the marginal distributions of bioavailability between the two drug

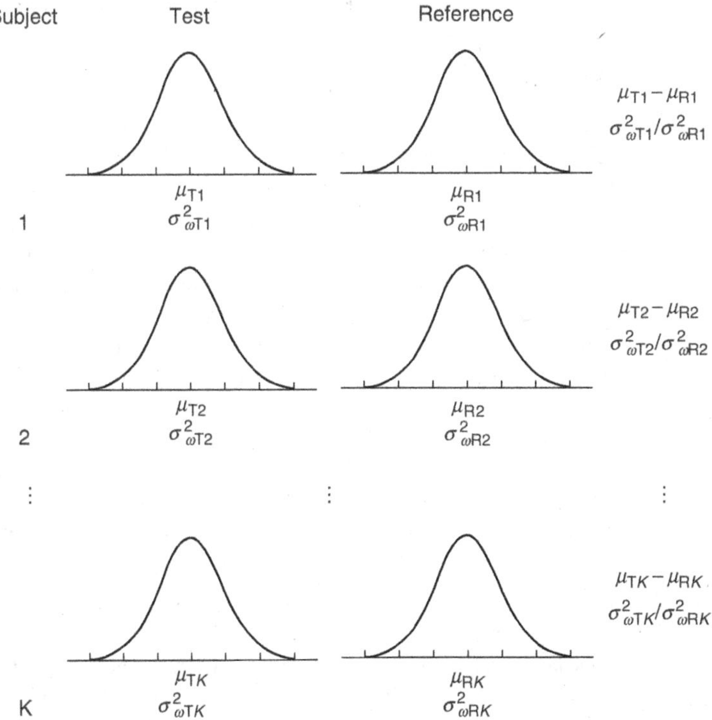

FIGURE 1.5.4: Concept of individual bioequivalence.

products within the same subject, then the replicated crossover designs are required to generate the multiple pharmacokinetic responses of the same formulations from an individual (Liu, 1995; Liu and Chow, 1995). The guidance on *Statistical Approaches to Establishing Bioequivalence* (FDA, 2001) provides the definitions and criteria for individual bioequivalence. The concept of individual bioequivalence is totally different from the usual average bioequivalence, and hence has a tremendous influence on statistical design, conduct, and analysis of bioequivalence trials. For more discussion, see Liu and Chow (1997a,b).

1.6 Decision Rules and Regulatory Aspects

1.6.1 Average Bioequivalence

The association between bioequivalence limits and clinical difference is difficult to assess in practice. The following decision rules were proposed by the FDA between 1977 and 2003 (Purich, 1980; FDA, 2003) for testing the bioequivalence in terms of average bioavailability of specific drugs, such as anticonvulsants, carbonic anhydrase inhibitors, and phenothiazines. Suppose AUC and C_{max} are the primary systematic exposure measures of the extent and rate of absorption. For each parameter, the following decision rules for assessment of average bioequivalence are applied.

1.6.1.1 75/75 Rule

Bioequivalence is claimed if at least 75% of individual subject ratios (relative individual bioavailability of the test formulation to the reference formulation) are within (75%, 125%) limits.

For the 75/75 rule, although it possesses some advantages, such as (1) it is easy to apply, (2) it compares the relative bioavailability within each subject, and (3) it removes the effect of heterogeneity of inter-subject variability from the comparison between the formulations, it is not viewed favorably by the FDA owing to some undesirable statistical properties. In a simulation study, Haynes (1981) showed that the 75/75 rule is very sensitive for drugs that have large inter- or intra-subject variabilities; even in the situation where the mean AUCs for the test and reference formulations are exactly the same. Metzler and Huang (1983), in another simulation study, also indicated that the 75/75 rule may reject as much as 56.3% of test products when the inter-subject variability is large. Thiyagarajan and Dobbins (1987) discussed the use of the 75/75 rule for assessment of bioequivalence. Chow (1989) and Chow and Shao (1991) provided an analytic evaluation of the 75/75 rule relative to the ±20 rule. The results suggest that the 75/75 rule will never be met when the intra-subject variability is large (say 20%) for any given true ratio of means. For small variability (say 10%), only 61.3% of individual subject ratios will fall within (75%, 125%) limits when the true ratio of means is within 80% and 120% limits. Anderson and Hauck (1990) discussed the 75/75 rule and considered the use of individual subject ratios for assessment of individual bioequivalence.

1.6.1.2 80/20 Rule

If the average of the test product is not statistically significantly different from that of the reference product, and if there is at least 80% power for detection of a 20% difference of the reference average, then bioequivalence is concluded.

The 80/20 rule, which often requires that a study be large enough to provide at least 80% chance of correctly detecting a 20% difference in average bioavailability, is based on the concept of testing a hypothesis of equality for a single variable rather than equivalence. In the past three decades, however, hypothesis testing for the evaluation of bioequivalence has been questioned and was not encouraged. The 80/20 rule is considered only as a prestudy power calculation for sample size determination in the planning stage of study protocol.

1.6.1.3 ±20 Rule

Bioequivalence is concluded if the average bioavailability of the test formulation is within ±20% of that of the reference formulation with a certain assurance.

The ±20 rule, which allows a test formulation to exhibit up to a 20% variation in average bioavailability in comparison with a reference formulation, is commonly employed for most drug products. Levy (1986), however, indicated that the ±20 rule does not accommodate the effect that the 20% variation could have on the safety and efficacy of a specific drug. Another concern is the interchangeability of the formulations. As more generic products become available, the generic substitution for a brand name drug may involve the substitution of one generic product for another during a patient's therapy. Under the ±20 rule, interchanging the generic products can lead to a more than 20% difference from one to another. For example, substitution of a bioequivalent product providing 120% of the reference for a bioequivalent product providing 80% of the reference would result in an increase in the relative dose of 50%. In this case, the toxicity or efficacy is significantly magnified when bioequivalent products varying by as much as 50% are interchanged one for another. Thus, it is suggested that individualized drug-by-drug bioequivalence criteria (i.e., the acceptable degree of variation in bioavailability) be developed by the FDA at the time a generic product becomes eligible for approval.

On the basis of the report by the bioequivalence task force, the 75/75 rule is not required for the assessment of bioequivalence because it is not based on rigorous statistical tests. It appears that the ±20 rule was acceptable to the FDA for evaluation of average bioequivalence in early 1980. The 80/20 rule was recommended as the secondary analysis, which is often used as a supplement to the ±20 rule. However, frequently, the ±20 rule and the 80/20 rule may result in inconsistent conclusions. That is, the average bioequivalence is concluded based on the ±20 rule, but the power for detecting a 20% difference is far below 80% or vice versa. The possible causes of the inconsistency between the two decision rules were discussed by Chow and Shao (1991).

1.6.1.4 80/125 Rule

Bioequivalence is concluded if the average bioavailability of the test formulation is within (80%, 125%) that of the reference formulation, with a certain assurance.

From a multiplicative model for pharmacokinetic responses postulated by Westlake (1973, 1986), the logarithmic transformation is suggested for AUC $(0-\infty)$ or AUC$(0-t_{last})$ and C_{max} in the guidance (FDA, 2003). As a result, the Division of Bioequivalence, the FDA suggested use of an equivalence criterion of 80%–125% for assessment of bioequivalence based on the ratio of average bioavailability. This criterion is not symmetric about 1 on the original scale where the maximum probability of concluding average bioequivalence occurs. However, on the logarithmic scale, the criterion has a range of −0.2231 to 0.2231, which the symmetric about 0 where the probability of concluding average bioequivalence is at maximum. Had the criterion of the ±20 rule been used for the logarithmic transformation, which is not linear, the maximum probability of concluding average bioequivalence would occur when the ratio of the average bioavailability is approximately about 0.98. The EMEA (2001) and WHO (2005) used the same equivalence criterion of 80%–125% for the log-transformed AUC$(0-\infty)$ or AUC$(0-t_{last})$ and C_{max}. However, for C_{max}, in certain cases, the EMEA and WHO allow a wider interval of 75%–133% for the ratio of average bioavailability to address any safety and efficacy concerns for patients switched between formulations. If a wider interval is used, it must be prespecified in the protocol.

It should be noted that bioequivalence determinations based on mean values do not account for the differences in inter- or intra-subject variabilities between formulations. Although the Pitman–Morgan test (Morgan, 1939; Pitman, 1939) is suggested for testing the equality of the variance between formulations, until recently, little or no attention in the literature has been given to address how much difference in variability, including inter- or intra-subject variabilities would be of clinical significance. In general, a much larger sample size is required for testing a difference in variances than that of testing for a difference in average. More details on the variability of bioavailability are given in Chapter 7.

1.6.2 Population and Individual Bioequivalence

Statistical evaluations for population/individual bioequivalence depend on different definitions of population/individual bioequivalence and their corresponding criteria. Basically, the criteria for evaluation of population/individual bioequivalence can be classified into the moment- and probability-based criteria, which are described below.

1.6.2.1 Moment-Based Criteria

The current moment-based criteria are based on the expected squared error loss in the form of the intra-subject difference of bioavailabilities in a subject who receives the test and reference formulations on two different occasions, and intra-subject variability which can be expressed as the expected squared error loss in the form of the intra-subject difference of bioavailabilities in a subject who receives the reference formulation of two different occasions. These moment-based criteria are then functions of difference in average bioavailability, the variability of the subject-by-formulation interaction, and the ratio of the test intra-subject variability to the reference intra-subject variability. These three components, in fact, represent the three characteristics for quality assurance of a generic drug product, as compared with the approved reference product. As a result, individual bioequivalence can be assessed either by the aggregate or disaggregate moment-based criteria. The aggregate moment-based criteria are linear combinations of the three components, such that the decision-making process for conclusion of individual bioequivalence can be made by comparing the sample observed value of the combined criterion with some prespecified upper bioequivalence limit without consideration of the contributions made by individual components. For more details about the aggregate criteria, see Sheiner (1992), Schall and Luus (1993), Holder and Hsuan (1993), Chen (1996, 1997), Chen et al. (2000), Hyslop et al. (2000), Endrenyi et al. (2000). McNally et al. (2003), Chow et al. (2002a,b), Hsuan and Reeve (2003), and FDA (2001).

Liu and Chow (1996) and Chow (1999) suggested the use of the disaggregate criterion for which individual components must meet their respective prespecified limits to conclude individual bioequivalence. The disaggregate criteria are more intuitive appealing and appreciate contributions made by individual components. Vuorinen and Turunen (1996) and Vuorinen (1997) applied disaggregate criteria in a stepwise manner for assessment of average, population, and individual bioequivalence sequentially. Carrasco and Jover (2003) suggested using the structural equation model for assessment of individual bioequivalence in a disaggregate manner. Discussion on advantages and drawbacks of aggregate and disaggregate criteria can be found in Liu and Chow (1997a).

1.6.2.2 Probability-Based Criteria

The probability-based criteria are based on the probability that the intra-subject difference of bioavailabilities in a subject receiving the test and reference formulations on two different occasions is within some prespecified limits. Anderson and Hauck (1990) first introduced the individual equivalence ratio (IER) as a probability-based criterion for assessment of individual bioequivalence and proposed a nonparametric binomial test (TIER). Under the normality assumption, Liu and Chow (1997b) showed that the usual t-statistic for evaluation of average bioequivalence can also be used for TIER, but with different critical values from noncentral t-distribution. Chinchilli and Esinhart (1994) also suggested that, under the normality assumption, the concept of tolerance interval be applied for assessment of individual bioequivalence. Schall and Luus (1993) and Schall (1995) suggest that the probability, based on the intra-subject difference between test and reference formulations, should be compared with that based on the intra-subject difference in bioavailabilities in the same subject who receives the reference formulations on two different occasions. Other probability-based criteria and their procedures can also be found in Wellek (1993) and Liu and Chow (1997a). Schall and Luus (1993) and Schall (1995) provided the discussion of the relationship between the moment- and probability-based criteria.

Note that decision rules, regulatory aspects, and statistical evaluations regarding population bioequivalence and individual bioequivalence are discussed further in Chapters 11 and 12, respectively.

1.7 Statistical Considerations

In this section, some statistical considerations that may occur in the assessment of bioequivalence are summarized.

1.7.1 AUC Calculation

As indicated in Section 1.3, among the pharmacokinetic parameters, AUC is the primary systematic exposure measure of the extent of absorption; or the amount of drug absorbed in the body, which is often used to assess bioequivalence between drug products. AUC is usually calculated using the trapezoidal rule based on the blood or plasma concentrations obtained at various sampling time points. In practice, a few missing values or unexpected observations may occur at some sampling time points owing to laboratory error, data transcription error, or other causes unrelated to bioequivalence. Generally, missing values or unexpected observations between two end sampling time points have little effect on the comparison of bioavailability (Rodda, 1986). However, if many missing values or unexpected observations occur in the plasma concentration–time curve, especially at two end sampling time points, the bias of the estimated AUC could be substantial and, consequently, may affect the comparison of bioavailability. Thus, how to justify the bias in the calculation of AUC is an important statistical issue. Furthermore, because the concentration at time zero (i.e., immediately before drug administration) may be different from subject to subject, whether or not the AUC should be adjusted from the baseline concentration is an interesting problem for both the clinician and biostatistician.

1.7.2 Model Selection and Normality Assumptions

Let μ_T and μ_R be the true averages for test and reference products, respectively. According to the 80/125 rule for assessment of average bioequivalence, the ratio of true averages (μ_T/μ_R) must be within (80%, 125%), with 90% assurance to claim bioequivalence. A typical approach is to construct a 90% confidence interval for μ_T/μ_R and compare it with (80%, 125%). If the constructed confidence interval is within (80%, 125%), then average bioequivalence is concluded. To construct a 90% confidence interval for μ_T/μ_R, two statistical models, namely, the raw data model (or additive model) and the log-transformed model (or multiplicative model), are often considered.

For the raw data model, an exact 90% confidence interval for $\mu_T - \mu_R$ is constructed based on the original data (raw data) and is converted to the confidence interval for μ_T/μ_R by dividing by the observed reference mean ($\overline{Y}_R$) (assuming that $\overline{Y}_R$ is the true μ_R). The constructed confidence interval, however, is not at the exact 90% confidence level because the method ignores the variability of $\overline{Y}_R$. Another method is to use Fieller's theorem (Locke, 1984; Schuirmann, 1989) to construct an exact 90% confidence interval for μ_T/μ_R. This method is derived based on the ratio of sample means for test and reference products. The disadvantage of this method is that the distribution of the ratio of sample means is rather complicated and its moments may not exist (Hinkley, 1969). In practice, it is important to provide a further statistical evaluation of the above confidence intervals because the decision of bioequivalence is made based on whether or not the confidence interval is within 80% and 125% (Schuirmann, 1989).

The primary assumptions of the raw data model are normality assumptions. Since the AUCs, t_{max}, and C_{max} are positive quantities, the underlying distributions are, in fact, normal distribution truncated at 0. This is a valid argument against the raw data model. In addition, the distribution of AUC is often skewed. Thus, a log transformation on AUC is usually performed to remove the skewness. The log-transformed data is then analyzed using the raw data model, which is equivalent to analyzing the raw data using the log-transformed model. Under the normality assumptions, the log-transformed model can provide an exact confidence interval for μ_T/μ_R (Mandallaz and Mau, 1981). Thus, compared with the raw data model, the FDA recommends that the log-transformed model should be used for the analysis of AUC and C_{max} in the bioequivalence studies (FDA, 2003b; see also, Attachment 5, report by the Bioequivalence Task Force, 1988).

The above methods, based on either the raw data model or the log-transformed model, are derived under the assumptions of normality or lognormality for between subject (inter-subject) and within subject (intra-subject) variabilities. One of the difficulties commonly encountered is whether or not the assumption of normality or lognormality is valid. Thus, it is suggested that the normality or lognormality assumptions be checked before an appropriate statistical model is used. The tests for normality or lognormality assumptions are critical for choosing an appropriate model. Unfortunately, thus far, there exist no convincing statistical tests for normality or lognormaltiy assumptions for inter- and intra-subject variabilities in bioequivalence studies. Jones and Kenward (2003) recommended a method using studentized residuals, which are obtained under the model (they are approximately independent) for testing normality of an intra-subject variability based on the Shapiro–Walk statistic (Shapiro and Wilk, 1965). A similar approach is also suggested for testing the normality of an inter-subject variability. Owing to the difficulty of testing normality assumptions, in the past four decades, some research efforts were directed to the search for nonparametric alternatives (see e.g., Koch, 1972; Cornell, 1980; Hauschke et al., 1990).

1.7.3 Inter- and Intra-Subject Variabilities

Because individual subjects may differ widely in their responses to the drug, the knowledge of inter- and intra-subject variabilities may provide valuable information in the assessment of bioequivalence (Wagner, 1971). To improve the intra-subject variability from the comparison of bioavailability between drug products, a crossover design, which is the design of choice by many investigators and is acceptable to the FDA (21 CFR, 320.26 and 320.27), is often considered. The advantages of using a crossover design are

1. Each subject can serve as his or her own control.
2. The assessment of bioequivalence is based on the intra-subject variability.
3. Fewer subjects are required to provide the desired degree of accuracy and power compared with other designs, such as parallel design.

However, in a crossover design, the intra-subject variability may be confoudned with some expected and unexpected variabilities, such as lot-to-lot, product-to-product, and subject-by-product variabilities. These sources of variabilities are difficult to assess based on a nonreplicated crossover design or other currently available designs (Ekbohm and Melander, 1989). Thus, appropriate replicated crossover designs or methods are necessary for assessing these variabilities (Liu and Chow, 1995; Chow, 1996b; FDA, 2001, 2003b).

1.7.4 Interval Hypothesis and Two One-Sided Tests

As early as the 1970s, statisticians became aware that the usual hypothesis testing for equality was not appropriate for bioavailability studies (Metzler, 1974). The purpose of bioequivalence is to verify that two formulations are indeed bioequivalent. Thus, from a statistical viewpoint, it may be more appropriate to reverse the null hypothesis of bioequivalence and the alternative hypothesis of bioinequivalence. Let θ_1 and θ_2 be two known bioequivalence limits and θ be the parameter of interest. The hypotheses for assessment of bioequivalence are given as follows:

$$\begin{aligned} &\mathrm{H_0}: \ \theta \le \theta_1 \text{ or } \theta \ge \theta_2 \\ \text{versus} \quad &\mathrm{H_a}: \ \theta_1 < \theta < \theta_2, \end{aligned}$$

which can be further decomposed into two one-sided hypotheses as

$$\begin{aligned} &\mathrm{H_{01}}: \ \theta \le \theta_1 \\ \text{versus} \quad &\mathrm{H_{a1}}: \ \theta_1 < \theta, \end{aligned}$$

and

$$\begin{aligned} &\mathrm{H_{02}}: \ \theta \ge \theta_2 \\ \text{versus} \quad &\mathrm{H_{a2}}: \ \theta < \theta_2. \end{aligned}$$

Since the hypothesis of bioequivalence in $\mathrm{H_a}$ is expressed as an interval, it is referred to as the interval hypothesis. The test procedures for the average bioavailability based on the interval hypothesis were proposed by Schuirmann (1981, 1987) and Anderson and Hauck (1983). The distribution of the observed test statistic proposed by Anderson and Hauck can be approximated by a central t-distribution. Schuirmann's procedure uses two one-sided tests for assessment of equivalence in average bioavailability. In this approach, two p-values are obtained to evaluate whether the bioavailability of the test product is not too low for one side (H_{01} vs. H_{a1}) and whether the bioavailability is not too high for the other side (H_{02} vs. H_{a2}). However, it is unclear what the exact p-value is for H_0 versus H_a because for any given θ_1 and θ_2 and the observed statistic for H_{01} versus H_{a1}, the p-value for H_{02} versus H_{a2} is not a random variable, but a fixed known quantity. In addition, the above two approaches suffer from the fact that under the normality assumption and unknown variances, in finite samples, there is no unconditional uniformly most powerful unbiased (UMPU) (nor invariant) test (Kendall and Stuart, 1979; Hsu et al., 1994; Lehmann and Romano, 2005). In other words, there always exist procedures with greater power for the same hypotheses under certain conditions. Alternatively, several nonparametric procedures have been proposed (Hauschke et al., 1990; Liu, 1991). However, there is little or no information available on the relative efficiency of the nonparametric procedures to the parametric methods (Liu and Weng, 1994).

1.7.5 Outlier Detection

As indicated in the report by the bioequivalence task force, the detection and treatment of outlying data in bioequivalence studies are important issues because the results and decisions of bioequivalence could be totally different by including or excluding the outlying data in the analysis. Several tests have been proposed for the detection of outlaying data (Chow and Tse, 1990a; Lin and Tsong, 1990; Liu and Weng, 1991; Wang et al. 1995, Wang and Chow, 2003). However, additional research and the development of some robust procedures are needed in this area.

1.7.6 Subject-by-Formulation Interaction

The concept of individual bioequivalence is first to investigate the closeness of the marginal distributions in bioavailabilities between the test and reference formulations in a subject, and then to assemble this information over a group of K subjects for assessment of individual bioequivalence. As a result, the individual difference in average and the individual ratio of intra-subject variabilities of the marginal distributions may be different from subject to subject. This phenomenon is referred to as the subject-by-formulation interaction. Thus, the subject-by-formulation interaction, in a general sense, should consider both average and intra-subject variability. However, the current state-of-art moment-based criteria for individual bioequivalence take into account only the difference in averages in the form of the variance of the deviations of the individual differences from the population difference. They ignore the differences (ratios) of the individual ratios of intra-subject variabilities from the population ratio. Most recently, Endrenyi and Tothfalusi (1999) and Endrenyi et al. (2000) studied statistical properties of the estimated variance component for subject by formulation in studies of individual bioequivalence. However, further research is required to understand whether this information is important in assessment of bioequivalence.

1.7.7 Meta-Analysis of Bioequivalence

The current regulations only request that bioequivalence of the generic copies to the innovator drug product be established. As a result, all development of concepts, such as prescribability and switchability, and definitions of average, population, and individual bioequivalence are concentrated only on the comparison of the test formulation with the approved innovator reference product. However, as more generic copies become available, switch between different generic copies of the same innovator product is inevitable. This situation is particularly true for developing countries when only cheaper generic copies are available. Even in the well-developed countries, such as the United States, owing to a desire to contain spiral increasing health cost, switch between generic copies is still possible under certain circumstance; for example, change of health care providers because of cheaper premium paid by employers or job changes by employees. As a result, the safety of generic copies has become a public issue not only because the number of generic copies for the same approved reference product can be as many as 160, but also they are not identical in terms of inactive ingredients that are binded and bulked, coated and colored, and may vary from one version to another. Chow and Liu (1997) and Chow and Shao (1999) showed how to apply meta-analysis to a systemic overview of independent bioequivalence trials for assessment of prescribability between generic copies. This is that one area in bioequivalence that is often ignored, but truly required for immediate attention.

1.7.8 Other Issues

Several issues concerning the assessment of bioequivalence have been discussed. See, e.g., Chow and Ju (1994), Chow and Liu (1995a), Chow (1996a), Chow (1997a), and Liu (2004). These include the determination of the bioequivalence limit for individual bioequivalence (Chen, 1996). The equivalence limit of 80%–125% has been accepted by the regulatory agencies, academia, and pharmaceutical industry of most countries for average bioequivalence. However, debates for selection of the equivalence limits for subject-by-formulation interaction and ratio of intra-subject variabilities is still going on and will last for the foreseeable future. More research is required for a procedure of determination of equivalence limits for aggregate and disaggregate moment-based criteria and probability-based criteria and their justifications. On the other hand, the sponsor needs to use more resources for assessment of individual bioequivalence. As a result, search for the optimal or nearly optimal replicated crossover designs in terms of relative efficiency is also urgently needed for individual bioequivalence. In most of developing countries, due to the cost, only the generic copies of the innovator from the original country are available.

Then how to assess bioequivalence between the generic drugs developed by the local generic sponsors with that from the original country is not only an important regulatory issue but also a critical public health issue for the developing countries.

1.8 Aims and Structure of the Book

This is intended to be the first book entirely devoted to the design and analysis of bioavailability/bioequivalence studies. It covers all of the statistical issues that may occur in the various stages of design and data analysis in bioavailability/bioequivalence studies. It is our goal to provide a useful desk reference and state-of-the-art examination of this area to scientists engaged in pharmaceutical research, those in government regulatory agencies who have to make decisions on the bioequivalence between drug products, and to biostatisticians who provide the statistical support for bioavailability/bioequivalence studies and related clinical projects. More importantly we would like to provide graduate students in pharmacokinetics, clinical pharmacology, biopharmaceutics, and biostatistics an advanced textbook in bioavailability studies. We hope that this book can serve as a bridge among the pharmaceutical industry, government regulatory agencies, and academia.

This book is configured into the following five components: preliminaries, average bioequivalence, population/individual bioequivalence, *in vitro* and alternative evaluation of bioequivalence, and other bioequivalence studies. The preliminary part covers from Chapters 1 through 3. In this chapter, the history, definition, decision rules, and some statistical considerations for bioavailability studies have been discussed. In Chapter 2, some basic considerations on the concerns of the investigator, monitor, and biostatistician for the designs of bioavailability studies are discussed. We then introduce some designs that are currently available for bioavailability studies. The relative advantages of a crossover design that is acceptable to the FDA are extensively discussed in this chapter. In Chapter 3, statistical inference for a variety of effects from a standard 2×2 crossover design is discussed. Because currently the regulatory agencies of most countries in the world require the evidence of average bioequivalence, Chapters 4 through 10 of this book are entirely devoted to the design and analysis of average bioequivalence. Statistical methods currently available for the assessment of average bioequivalence are provided in Chapter 4. The nonparametric methods including bootstrap resampling procedure will also be extensively explored in this chapter. These methods are compared in terms of power and relative efficiency in Chapter 5. Sampling size determination for average bioequivalence is also included in this chapter. The log-transformed model and the approach using individual subject ratios are given in Chapter 6. In addition to the examination of intra-subject variability and inter-subject variability, the assessment of bioequivalence using the variability of bioavailability is explored in Chapter 7. In Chapter 8, some tests for normality assumptions and procedures for detection of outliers are derived. Chapter 9 provides statistical methods for assessing average bioequivalence under a higher-order crossover design for two formulations. Assessment of average bioequivalence for more than two formulations is outlined in Chapter 10. Population and individual bioequivalence are covered in Chapters 11 and 12. In Chapter 11, the merits, desirable features of population bioequivalence and individual bioequivalence, and different criteria of individual bioequivalence, and different criteria of individual bioequivalence and their rationales and relations are discussed. In addition, different replicated crossover designs are introduced and compared for evaluation of individual bioequivalence in this chapter. Different statistical procedures for aggregated and disaggregate moment-based criteria and probability-based criteria are provided in Chapter 12. Chapters 13 through 15 discuss the topics on *in vitro* and alternative evaluation of bioequivalence. Chapter 13 gives an introduction for assessment of bioequivalence based on clinical endpoints, such as response data and time to onset of a therapeutic response when plasma concentrations are negligible. In Chapter 14, statistical methods for assessment of bioequivalence based on *in vitro* bioequivalence testing for local delivery drug products such as nasal aerosols and nasal sprays are described. Criteria and statistical procedures for assessment of similarity between dissolution profiles are given in Chapter 15. Chapters 16 through 20 review some other bioequivalence studies. Chapter 16 proposes meta-analysis approaches to bioequivalence review based on average bioequivalence. The approach can be applied to the concept of population and individual bioequivalence. Comparison between these methods and power and sample size determination are also discussed in this chapter. In Chapter 17, objectives as well as the design and procedures for population pharmacokinetics are provided. Also included in this chapter is the assessment of inter- and intra-subject variabilities in multicompartmental PK model. In Chapter 18, other pharmacokinetic studies such as drug interaction studies, dose proportionality studies, steady-state analyses for multiple doses, and food effects studies are given. Chapter 19 provides a thorough review of the FDA guidances on bioequivalence including the 2001 FDA guidance on statistical approaches (FDA, 2001), the 2003 FDA guidance on general considerations for orally administrated drug products (FDA, 2003b), and other FDA guidances such as the guidance on fed bioequivalence, Clozapine tablets, and the SUPAC guidances. Chapter 20 addresses some frequently asked questions and future challenges on bioequivalence, which include assessment of bioequivalence with genomic data, bridging bioequivalence studies, and bioequivalence for biological products (follow-on biologics or biosimilar drug products).

Chapter 2

Design of Bioavailability Studies

2.1 Introduction

Before a clinical trial is conducted, a protocol that details the conduct of the trial is usually developed. A thoughtful and well-organized protocol includes study objectives, design, patient selection criteria, dosing schedules, and statistical methods. Unlike clinical trials, bioavailability studies are often conducted with healthy volunteers. Thus, the choice of the design and the statistical methods for the analysis of data becomes two important aspects in planning a bioavailability study. These two aspects are closely related to each other because the method of analysis depends on the design employed. Generally meaningful conclusions can only be drawn based on data collected from a valid scientific design using appropriate statistical methods. General considerations that one should consider when planning a bioavailability study include

1. What is to be studied, or what are the study objectives?

2. How are the data to be collected, or what design is to be employed?

3. How are the data to be analyzed, or what statistical methods are to be used?

In this chapter, our efforts will be directed to the determination of study objectives and the selection of an appropriate design for a bioavailability study. We intend to explore and compare some basic designs that are currently available for such studies. Some specific designs that are used for different purposes under various circumstances are discussed further in Chapter 9. Unless otherwise specified, throughout this book, for the sake of convenience, we restrict our attention to the comparison of different formulations of the same drug product. The comparison of different drug products of the same active ingredient and different ways of administration can be treated similarly.

The choice of the design depends primarily on the variability in the observations. For example, as indicated in Section 1.7.3, the individual subjects may differ very widely in their responses to the drug products. Thus, one major source of variability arises from differences between subjects. As a result, a criterion for choosing an appropriate design is whether or not the selected design can identify, estimate, and isolate the inter-subject variability in data analysis. Any design that can remove this variation from the comparison in average bioavailability between formulations would be appropriate. Such a design is generally more efficient than a design that cannot account for the inter-subject variability. In this chapter, we induce several designs that are often considered for bioavailability and bioequivalence studies. These designs include the complete randomized designs (or the parallel designs), the randomized block designs, the crossover designs, the Latin square designs, and the (balanced) incomplete block designs. These designs, which may remove the expected variability from the comparison of bioavailability between formulations, may be useful, depending on the parameters to be evaluated, the characteristics of the drug, or the medical restrictions.

The remainder of this chapter is organized as follows. In Section 2.2, objectives for some studies related to bioavailability, such as bioequivalence studies, proportionality studies, and steady-state analyses are discussed. In Section 2.3, we provide some design considerations when planning a bioavailability study. In Section 2.4, a brief description of a parallel design is given. An extensive discussion on crossover designs is presented in Section 2.5. Balanced incomplete block designs are introduced in Section 2.6. Some factors for choosing an appropriate design for bioavailability studies are discussed in Section 2.7.

2.2 Study Objective

In clinical trials, a description of the general aims of the study is a useful preliminary that helps explain why the study is considered worthwhile (Pocock, 1983). The statement of study objectives is a concise and precise definition of prespecified hypotheses or parameters concerning the drug products that are to be examined or estimated. In clinical trials, a clear statement of study objectives not only ensures that the investigator adhere to the hypotheses at the time of analysis and interpretation of results, but also enables statisticians to select an appropriate design and statistical methods for data analysis.

In the following, some examples of study objectives and corresponding hypotheses or parameters of interest in bioavailability and related studies are given.

2.2.1 Bioequivalence Studies

One of the objectives of a bioequivalence study is to compare bioavailability between two formulations (a test and a reference formulation) of a drug product and to determine bioequivalence in terms of the rate and extent of absorption. The primary hypothesis may be whether the difference in average bioavailability between a test and reference product is within 80%–125% of the reference mean with certain assurance. On the other hand, individual bioequivalence might be the objective of other bioequivalence studies. To achieve this objective, a crossover design is often considered. Several statistical methods are available for the evaluation of different hypotheses.

2.2.2 Dose Proportionality Studies

For a dose proportionality (or dose linearity study), the objective is to evaluate whether the relationship between dose level and a pharmacokinetic parameter (such as AUC) is linear over a given dose range. The results may provide useful information in determining dose levels at which the minimum concentration for therapeutic effect and toxic concentration will be achieved. The hypothesis of interest is that there is a linear relation between dose level and AUC. Several statistical tests for the hypothesis of dose proportionality are available for both serial blood collection and single time-point blood collection. More details on dose proportionality studies are discussed further in Chapter 18.

2.2.3 Steady-State Studies

For a steady-state study, comparison of the blood (or plasma) concentration is made after steady state is achieved (generally, after multiple dosing). The objective of such a study is to determine whether a steady state has been reached and when it was reached. This may be evaluated by testing the hypothesis that there is no difference in concentrations at the end of each dosing interval. In Chapter 18, more details on a steady-state analysis are given.

2.2.4 Variability and Interchangeability

Because the determination of bioequivalence may not adequately characterize different types of variation that can occur both within a given individual as well as among different individuals, an appropriate design may be considered to provide information on the inter-subject and the intra-subject variabilities and the interchangeability of one formulation for another. The objective of such design is to estimate the inter-subject and intra-subject variabilities and provide statistical inference on both the variability and the interchangeability. This issue is examined in Chapters 7 and 11.

Pocock (1983) indicated that, in clinical trials, the study objectives are built on more expansive descriptions of patient selection criteria, treatment schedules, and the methods of patient evaluation. Although a precise and detailed explanation of these issues can help ensure that an unbiased assessment of the study objectives is achieved, a valid scientific design with appropriate statistical methods for the analysis of data is the key to carry out the study objectives.

2.3 Basis Design Considerations

In the *Federal Register* [Vol. 42, No. 5, Sect. 320.25(b), 1977], the U.S. Food and Drug Administration indicated that a basic design for an *in vivo* bioavailability study is determined by the following:

1. Scientific questions to be answered
2. Nature of the reference material and the dosage form to be tested
3. Availability of analytical methods
4. Benefit–risk considerations relative to human testing

Consideration of the reference dosage form is critical. For example, a suspension may not be an appropriate reference material because of high variability in bioavailability of the suspension dosage form. In many instances, a suspension of poorly soluble active drug ingredient may be more poorly absorbed than a well-formulated tablet.

The availability of the analytical method that is used to measure the immediate pharmacological effect or concentration of the active drug ingredient, therapeutic moiety, or metabolites is important. The FDA requires that the analytical method used in bioavailability studies be of sufficient accuracy, sensitivity, and reproducibility to discriminate between inequivalent products. The requirement implies that a product of known poor bioavailability must be compared against the reference product to determine whether the method can detect differences between the two products.

Finally, in practice, most bioavailability studies are conducted with healthy normal subjects. Bioavailability studies conducted on critically ill patients may not be appropriate and be contrary to the best medical practice unless there is a definitive benefit to the patients. For example, a bioavailability study with kanamycin in patients with stable renal disease would permit dosage adjustments based on renal creatinine clearance and serum kanamycin levels.

In addition to these basis design considerations, some specific considerations when planning a design for a bioavailability study are given in the following.

2.3.1 Experimental Design

The *Federal Register* [Vol. 42, No. 5, Secs. 320.26(b) and 320.27(b), 1977] indicated that a bioavailability study (single-dose or multidose) should be crossover in design, unless a parallel or other design is more appropriate for valid scientific reasons. For a parallel design, each subject receives one and only one formulation in random fashion, whereas for a crossover design each subject receives more than one formulation at different periods. In practice, subjects account for a large source of variability in plasma or blood drug concentrations. Thus, an appropriate design should allow estimation and removal of the inter-subject variability from drug comparisons. More details on the parallel, crossover, and other designs are discussed in the following sections.

2.3.2 Randomization

Valid statistical inferences are usually drawn based on the assumption that the errors in observations are independently distributed, random variables. Randomization usually ensures the validity of this assumption. The randomization schedules depend on the design selected. For example, for a parallel design comparing two formulations of a drug product, the subjects are assigned to receive each formulation at random. For a crossover design, each subject is a block that represents a restriction on complete randomization because the formulations are randomized within the subject. An example of randomization for a standard two-sequence, two-period (2×2) crossover design is given in Section 2.5.4.

2.3.3 Sampling Time Intervals

For the estimation of the rate and extent of absorption, although the sampling time intervals for both the test and reference formulations need not be the same, it is preferred that sampling time intervals are identical to assure true equivalence. It, however, should be noted that the actual sampling times may deviate from the scheduled sampling times in practice. On the other hand, blood or plasma samples should be collected at the time before dosing and over an interval of sufficient time (e.g., three to five half-lives of the drug active ingredient or therapeutic moiety) to accurately determine the individual terminal disposition curve.

2.3.4 Drug Elimination Period

For a single-dose study, the terminal drug elimination period should allow at least three or more terminal half-lives of the active drug ingredient or therapeutic moiety, or its metabolite, either measured in the blood or as the decay of the immediate pharmacological effect. For a multiple dose study, the elimination period should allow at least five half-lives.

2.3.5 Number of Subjects

For a bioavailability study, usually 18–24 healthy normal subjects are used. To detect a clinically important average difference (e.g., 20%), a prestudy power calculation is often performed to determine the number of subjects needed for detection of such difference with a desired probability (e.g., 80%). The issue of power and sample size determination is discussed further in Chapter 5.

2.4 Parallel Design

A parallel design is complete randomized design in which each subject receives one and only one formulation of a drug in a random fashion. The simplest parallel design is the two-group parallel design, which compares two formulations of a drug.

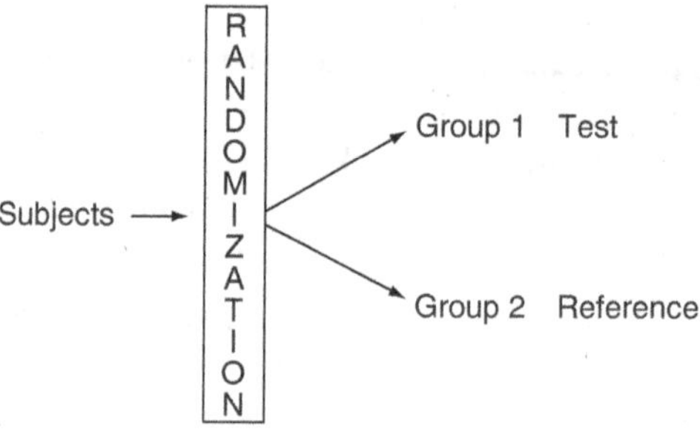

FIGURE 2.4.1: Two-group parallel design.

Each group usually contains the same number of subjects. An example of a two-group parallel design is illustrated in Figure 2.4.1.

For phase II and III clinical trials, the parallel design probably is the one most frequently used. However, it may not be an appropriate design for bioavailability and bioequivalence studies. This is because the variability in observations (e.g., AUC) consists of the inter-subject and intra-subject variabilities and the assessment of bioequivalence between formulations is usually made based on the intra-subject variability. A parallel design, however, is not able to identify and separate these two sources of variations because each subject in the parallel design usually receives the same drug during the entire course of study. Although the equivalence in average bioavailability between formulations can still be established through this design, the comparison is made based on the inter-subject and intra-subject variabilities. As a result, for a fixed number of subjects, the parallel design would, in general, provide a less precise statistical inference for the difference in average bioavailability between formulations than that of a crossover design.

Although the parallel design is not widely used for bioavailability studies owing to the incapability of identifying and removing the inter-subject variability from the comparison between formulations, there are some rare occasions in which a parallel design may be more appropriate than a crossover design. For example, for generic topical antifungals bioequivalence study, the FDA requires a three-arm parallel design (i.e., test, reference, and vehicle control). If the drug is known to have a very long half-life, it is not desirable to adapt a crossover design. In a crossover design, a sufficient length of washout is necessary to eliminate the possible carryover effects and, consequently, the study may take considerable time. This, in turn, may increase the number of dropouts and make the completion of a study difficult. In addition, if the study is to be conducted with very ill patients, a parallel design is usually recommended so that the study can be completed quickly. As a result a parallel design may be considered as an alternative to a crossover design if (1) the inter-subject variability is relatively small compared with the intra-subject variability; (2) the drug is potentially toxic or has a very long elimination half-life; (3) the population of interest consists of very ill patients; and (4) the cost for increasing the number of subjects is much less than that of adding an additional treatment period.

2.5 Crossover Design

2.5.1 Introduction

A crossover design is a modified, randomized block design in which each block receives more than one formulation of a drug at different periods. A block may be a subject or a group of subjects. Subjects in each block receive a different sequence of formulations. A crossover design is called a complete crossover design if each sequence contains each of the formulations. For a crossover design, it is not necessary that the number of formulations in each sequence be greater than or equal to the number of formulations to be compared. We shall refer to a crossover design as a $g \times p$ crossover design if there are g sequences of formulations administered at p different periods. For bioavailability and bioequivalence studies, the crossover design is viewed favorably by the FDA and other regulatory agencies such as EMEA in the world because of the following advantages:

1. Each subject serves as his or her own control. It allows a within-subject comparison between formulations.
2. It removes the inter-subject variability from the comparison between formulations.
3. With a proper randomization of subjects to the sequence of formulation administrations, it provides the best unbiased estimates for the differences (or ratios) between formulations.

The use of crossover designs for clinical trails has been extensively discussed in the literature. See, for example, Brown (1980), Huitson et al. (1982), Jones and Kenward (2003), and Senn (1993).

In the following, we introduce several different types of crossover designs that are often used in bioavailability studies. The relative advantages and drawbacks of these designs are also discussed.

2.5.2 Washout and Carryover Effects

It is helpful to introduce the concepts of washout and carryover effects (or residual effects) in a crossover design because the presence of carryover effects usually has an influence on statistical inference of bioavailability between formulations.

The washout period is defined as the rest period between two treatment periods for which the effect of one formulation administered at one treatment period does not carry over to the next. In a crossover design, the washout period should be long enough for the formulation effects to wear off so that there is no carryover effect from one treatment period to the next. The washout period depends on the nature of the drug. A suitable washout period should be long enough to return any relevant changes that influence bioavailability to baseline (usually, at least five times the blood–plasma elimination half-life of the active ingredient, therapeutic moiety or its metabolite, or the decay of the immediate pharmacological effect since the last sampling time point of the previous period).

If a drug has a long half-life or if the washout period between treatment periods is too short, the effect of the drug might persist after the end of dosing period. In this case, it is necessary to distinguish the difference between the direct drug effect and the carryover effects. The direct drug effect is the effect that a drug product has during the period in which the drug is administered, whereas the carryover effect is the drug effect that persists after the end of the dosing period. Carryover effects that last only one treatment period are called first-order carryover effects. A drug is said to have c-order carryover effects if the carryover effects last up to c treatment periods. In bioavailability and bioequivalence studies, however, it is unlikely that a drug effect will carry over more than one treatment period because a sufficient length of washout is usually considered. In this book, therefore, we consider only the first-order carryover effects if they are present.

2.5.3 Statistical Model and Linear Contrast

In a crossover design, because the direct drug effect may be confounded with any carryover effects, it is important to remove the carryover effects from the comparison if possible. To account for these effects, the following statistical model is usually considered. Let Y_{ijk} be the response (e.g., AUC) of the ith subject in the kth sequence at the jth period.

$$Y_{ijk} = \mu + S_{ik} + P_j + F_{(j,k)} + C_{(j-1,k)} + e_{ijk}, \tag{2.5.1}$$

where

μ is the overall mean

S_{ik} is the random effect of the ith subject in the kth sequence, where $i=1, 2, \ldots, g$

P_j is the fixed effect of the jth period, where $j=1, \ldots, p$ and $\Sigma_j P_j=0$

$F_{(j,k)}$ is the direct fixed effect of the formulation in the kth sequence which is administered at the jth period, and $\Sigma F_{(j,k)}=0$

$C_{(j-1,k)}$ is the fixed first-order carryover effect of the formulation in the kth sequence which is administered at the $(j-1)$th period, where $C_{(0,k)}=0$; and $\Sigma C_{(j-1,k)}=0$

e_{ijk} is the (within-subject) random error in observing Y_{ijk}.

It is assumed that $\{S_{ik}\}$ are independently and identically distributed (i.i.d.) with mean 0 and variance σ_S^2, and $\{e_{ijk}\}$ are independently distributed with mean 0 and variance σ_t^2, where $t=1, 2, \ldots, L$ (the number of formulations to be compared). $\{S_{ik}\}$ and $\{e_{ijk}\}$ are assumed mutually independent. The estimate of σ_S^2 is usually used to explain the inter-subject variability, and the estimates of σ_t^2 are used to assess the intra-subject variabilities for the tth formulation.

Let $\bar{Y}_{\cdot 1k}, \bar{Y}_{\cdot 2k}, \ldots, \bar{Y}_{\cdot pk}$ be the observed means for periods in the kth sequence. That is,

$$\bar{Y}_{\cdot jk} = \frac{1}{n_k}\sum_{i=1}^{n_k} Y_{ijk}, \quad j = 1, \ldots, p \quad \text{and} \quad k = 1, \ldots, g. \tag{2.5.2}$$

Under the normality assumptions, the carryover effects and other fixed effects, such as the direct drug effect and the period effect, can be estimated based on these gp means because there are $(gp-1)$ degrees of freedom (df) among these gp means, which can be decomposed as follows:

$$(gp-1)=(p-1)+(g-1)+(p-1)(g-1),$$

where $(p-1)$ df are attributed to the period effect, $(g-1)$ df are assigned to the sequence effect, and $(p-1)(g-1)$ are associated with the sequence-by-period interaction. The $(p-1)(g-1)$ df are of particular interest because they preserve the information related to the direct drug effect and the carryover effects. For example, for a standard 2×2 crossover design, there are 3 df associated with four sequence-by period means: 1 for the sequence effect, 1 for the period effect, and 1 for the sequence-by-period interaction which is, in fact, the direct drug effect when there are no carryover effects.

A within-subject linear contrast for the kth sequence is defined as a linear combination of $\overline{Y}_{\cdot 1k}$, $\overline{Y}_{\cdot 2k}, \ldots,$ and $\overline{Y}_{\cdot pk}$. That is,

$$l=c_1\overline{Y}_{\cdot 1k}+c_2\overline{Y}_{\cdot 2k}+\cdots+c_p\overline{Y}_{\cdot pk},$$

where $\Sigma_j c_j=0$.

Two linear combinations of $\overline{Y}_{\cdot jk}, j=1,2,\ldots,p$ are said to be orthogonal if the sum of the cross-products of the coefficients of the two contrasts is 0. In other words, let

$$l_1=\sum_{j=1}^{p}c_{1j}\overline{Y}_{\cdot jk} \quad \text{and} \quad l_2=\sum_{j=1}^{p}c_{2j}\overline{Y}_{\cdot jk}$$

be two linear contrasts, then l_1 and l_2 are orthogonal if

$$\sum_{j=1}^{p}c_{1j}c_{2j}=0.$$

It can be seen that the variance of l involves only the intra-subject variabilities $\sigma_t^2, t=1,2,\ldots,L$. Thus, statistical inferences for the fixed effects, such as the period effects, the direct drug effects, and the carryover effects, can be made based on within-subject variabilities using appropriate linear contrasts of these gp means.

2.5.4 Crossover Designs for Two Formulations

In this section, we focus on the assessment of bioequivalence between test formulation (T) and a reference (or standard) formulation (R) of a drug product. The most commonly used statistical design for comparing average bioavailability between two formulations of a drug probably is a two-sequence, two-period, crossover design, we shall refer to this design as the standard 2×2 crossover design. For the standard 2×2 crossover design, each subject is randomly assigned to either

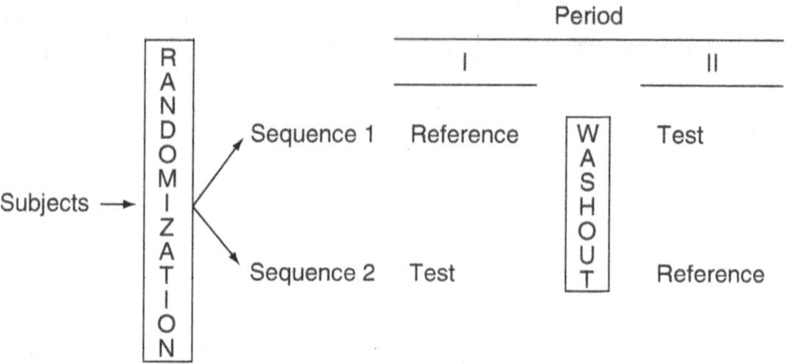

FIGURE 2.5.1: 2 × 2 crossover designs.

sequence RT or sequence TR at two dosing periods. In other words, subjects within RT (RT) receive for mulation R(T) at the first dosing period and formulation T(R) at the second dosing period. The dosing periods are separated by a washout period of sufficient length for the drug received in the first period to be completely metabolized or excreted from the body. An example of a 2 × 2 crossover design is illustrated in Figure 2.5.1. Although the crossover design is a variant of the Latin square design, the number of the formulations in a crossover design does not necessarily have to be equal to the number of periods. One example is a 2 × 3 crossover design for comparing two formulations as illustrated in Figure 2.5.2. In this design, there are two formulations, but three periods. Subjects in each sequence receive one of the formulations twice at two different dosing periods. The design of this kind is known as a higher-order crossover design which is discussed in detail in Chapter 9.

Randomization for the standard 2 × 2 crossover design can be carried out by using either a table of random numbers or an SAS procedure, PROC PLAN (SAS®*, 2005). For example, suppose the standard 2 × 2 crossover design is to be conducted with 24 healthy volunteers to assess bioequivalence between a test formulation and a

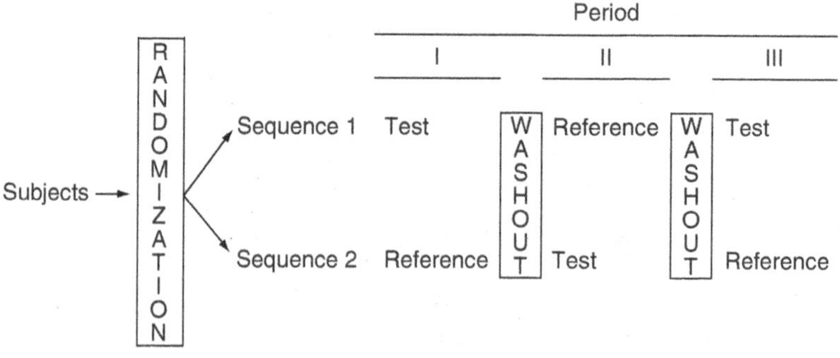

FIGURE 2.5.2: 2 × 3 crossover designs.

* Registered trademark SAS Institute, Cary, North Carolina.

reference formulation of a drug product. Because there are two sequences of formulations (RT and TR), 12 subjects are to be assigned to each of the two sequences. In other words, one group will receive the first sequence of formulations (RT) and the other group will receive the second sequence of formulations (TR). Thus, we first generate a set of random permutations from 1 to 24 using PROC PLAN, which follows

16, 19, 20, 11, 4, 24, 1, 12, 5, 23, 15, 6,
17, 2, 10, 14, 18, 13, 21, 3, 7, 8, 22, 9

Then, subjects are sequentially assigned a number from 1 through 24. Subjects with numbers in the first half of the above random order are assigned to the first sequence (RT) and the rest are assigned to the second sequence (TR) (see Table 2.5.1). In practice, a set of randomization code for more than the total number of subjects planed is usually prepared to account for the possible replacement of dropouts.

TABLE 2.5.1: Randomization codes for the standard 2×2 crossover design with 24 subjects.

Subject	Sequence	Formulations
1	1	RT
2	2	TR
3	2	TR
4	1	RT
5	1	RT
6	1	RT
7	2	TR
8	2	TR
9	2	TR
10	2	TR
11	1	RT
12	1	RT
13	2	TR
14	2	TR
15	1	RT
16	1	RT
17	2	TR
18	2	TR
19	1	RT
20	1	RT
21	2	TR
22	2	TR
23	1	RT
24	1	RT

For the standard 2×2 crossover design, from Equation 2.5.1, the two responses for the ith subject in each sequence are given as

$$\begin{aligned} \text{Sequence 1} \quad & Y_{i11} = \mu + S_{i1} + P_1 + F_1 + e_{i11} \\ & Y_{i21} = \mu + S_{i1} + P_2 + F_2 + C_1 + e_{i21} \\ \text{Sequence 2} \quad & Y_{i12} = \mu + S_{i2} + P_1 + F_2 + e_{i12} \\ & Y_{i22} = \mu + S_{i2} + P_2 + F_1 + C_2 + e_{i22} \end{aligned} \tag{2.5.3}$$

where

$P_1 + P_2 = 0$
$F_1 + F_2 = 0$
$C_1 + C_2 = 0.$

For each subject, a pair of observations is observed at periods 1 and 2. Thus, we may consider a bivariate random vector (i.e., [period 1, period 2]) as follows:

$$\mathbf{Y}_{ik} = (Y_{i1k}, Y_{i2k})', \quad i = 1, 2, \ldots, n_k \quad \text{and} \quad k = 1, 2. \tag{2.5.4}$$

Then, $\mathbf{Y}_{ik}$ values are independently distributed with the following mean vector and covariance matrix

$$\begin{aligned} \text{Sequence 1} \quad & \boldsymbol{\alpha}_1 = \begin{bmatrix} \mu + P_1 + F_1 \\ \mu + P_2 + F_2 + C_1 \end{bmatrix} \\ & \boldsymbol{\Sigma}_1 = \begin{bmatrix} \sigma_1^2 + \sigma_S^2 & \sigma_S^2 \\ \sigma_S^2 & \sigma_2^2 + \sigma_S^2 \end{bmatrix} \\ \text{Sequence 2} \quad & \boldsymbol{\alpha}_2 = \begin{bmatrix} \mu + P_1 + F_2 \\ \mu + P_2 + F_1 + C_2 \end{bmatrix} \\ & \boldsymbol{\Sigma}_2 = \begin{bmatrix} \sigma_2^2 + \sigma_S^2 & \sigma_S^2 \\ \sigma_S^2 & \sigma_1^2 + \sigma_S^2 \end{bmatrix} \end{aligned} \tag{2.5.5}$$

It can be seen that the intra-subject variabilities are different between formulations. If, however, $\sigma_1^2 = \sigma_2^2 = \sigma_e^2$, then $\boldsymbol{\Sigma}_1 = \boldsymbol{\Sigma}_2 = \boldsymbol{\Sigma}$, where

$$\boldsymbol{\Sigma} = \begin{bmatrix} \sigma_e^2 + \sigma_S^2 & \sigma_S^2 \\ \sigma_S^2 & \sigma_e^2 + \sigma_S^2 \end{bmatrix} \tag{2.5.6}$$

When the carryover effects are present (i.e., $C_1 \neq 0$ and $C_2 \neq 0$), the standard 2×2 crossover design may not be desirable, for it may not provide estimates for some fixed effects. For example, as indicated in the Subsection 2.5.3, there is only 1 degree of freedom, which is attributed to the sequence effect. The sequence effect, which cannot be estimated separately, is confounded (or aliased) with any carryover effects. If the carryover effects are unequal (i.e., $C_1 \neq C_2 \neq 0$), then there exists no unbiased estimated for the direct drug effect from both periods. In addition, the carryover effects cannot be precisely estimated because it can be evaluated based on only the between subject comparison. Furthermore, the intra-subject variabilities σ_1^2 and σ_2^2 cannot be estimated independently and directly from the observed data because each subject receives either the test formulation or the reference formulation only once during the study. In other words, there are no replicates for each formulation within each subject.

To overcome these undesirable properties, a higher-order crossover design may be useful. A higher-order crossover design is defined as a crossover design in which either the number of periods is greater than the number of formulations to be compared, or the number of sequences is greater than the number of formulations to be compared. There are several higher-order crossover designs available in the literature (Kershner and Federer, 1981; Laska et al., 1983; Laska and Meinser, 1985; Jones and Kenward, 2003). These designs, however, have their own advantages and disadvantages. An in-depth discussion can be found in Jones and Kenward (2003).

In the following, we discuss three commonly used higher-order crossover designs, which possess some optimal statistical properties, for comparing average bioavailability between two formulations. We shall refer to these three designs as design A, B, and C, respectively. Designs A, B, and C are given in Table 2.5.2. In each of the

TABLE 2.5.2: Optimal crossover designs for two formulations.

Design A

	Period	
Sequence	**I**	**II**
1	T	T
2	R	R
3	R	T
4	T	R

Design B

		Period	
Sequence	**I**	**II**	**II**
1	T	R	R
2	R	T	T

Design C

		Period		
Sequence	**I**	**II**	**III**	**IV**
1	T	T	R	R
2	R	R	T	T
3	T	R	R	T
4	R	T	T	R

TABLE 2.5.3: Variances for designs A, B, and C in multiples of $\hat{\sigma}_e^2/n$.

Design	$V(\hat{C}\|F)^a$	$V(\hat{F}\|C)$	$V(\hat{F})$
S[b]	—	—[c]	1.0000
A	4.0000	2.0000	1.0000
B	1.0000	0.7500	0.7500
C	0.3636	0.2500	0.2500

[a] $V(\hat{C}|F)=4\,(2\hat{\sigma}_s^2+\hat{\sigma}_e^2)/n$.
[b] S is the standard 2×2 crossover design.
[c] The direct drug effect is not estimable in the presence of the carryover effects.

three designs, the estimates of the direct drug effect and carryover effects are obtained based on the within-subject linear contrasts. As a result, statistical inferences for direct drug effect and carryover effects are mainly based on the intra-subject variability. For the comparisons of these three designs with the standard 2×2 crossover design, it is helpful to use the following notations. The direct drug effect after adjustment for the carryover effects is denoted by $F|C$. Then, F simply refers to the unadjusted direct drug effect. Also the variance of the estimator of $F|C$ (i.e., $\hat{F}|C$) is denoted by V $(\hat{F}|C)$. Table 2.5.3 gives the variances (in the multiples of σ_e^2/n) of the direct drug effect and carryover effects for the three designs and the standard 2×2 crossover designs (Senn, 1993; Jones and Kenward, 2003). The variances of designs A, B, and C are derived under the assumptions that (1) $n_k = n$ for all k; (2) $\sigma_1^2 = \sigma_2^2 = \sigma_e^2$; and (3) there is no direct drug-by-carryover interaction. For designs B and C, the direct drug effect adjusted for the carryover effects is the same as the unadjusted direct drug effect (i.e., no carryover effects). This is because the direct drug effect and carryover effects for designs B and C are estimated by the linear contrasts which are orthogonal to each other. Note that an orthogonality of linear contrasts for the direct drug effect and carryover effects implies that their covariance is zero. In other words, the estimators of the direct drug effect and carryover effects in designs B and C are not correlated (or independent).

Design A is also known as Balaam's design (Balaam, 1968). It is an optimal design in the class of the crossover designs with two periods and two formulations. This design is formed by adding two more sequences (sequences 1 and 2) to the standard 2×2 crossover design (sequences 3 and 4). These two augmented sequences are TT and RR. With additional information provided by the two augmented sequences, not only can the carryover effects be estimated using the within-subject contrasts, but the intra-subject variability for both test and reference formulations can also be obtained because there are replicates for each formulation each subject.

Design B is an optimal design in the class of the crossover designs with two sequences, three periods, and two formulations. It can be obtained by adding an additional period to the standard 2×2 crossover designs. The treatments administered in the third period are the same as those in the second period. This type of designs is also known as the extended-period or extraperiod designs. Note that this design is made of a pair of dual sequences TRR and RTT. Two sequences, the treatments of which are mirror images of each other, are said to be a pair of dual sequences. As pointed out by Jones and Kenward (2003), the only crossover designs worth considering are those that are made up of dual sequences. Compared with the standard 2×2 crossover design, the variance for the direct drug effect is reduced by 25%.

For the carryover effects, the variance is reduced by about 75% as compared with the Balaam's design. In addition, the intra-subject variability can be estimated based on the data collected from periods 2 and 3.

Design C is an optimal design in the class of the crossover designs with four sequences, four periods, and two formulations. It is also made up of two pairs of dual sequences (TTRR, RRTT) and (TRRT, RTTR). Note that the first two periods of design C are the same as those in Balaam's design and the last two periods are the mirror image of the first two periods. The design is much more complicated than designs A and B, although it produces the maximum in variance reduction for both the direct drug effect and the carryover effects among the designs considered.

2.5.5 Crossover Designs for Three or More Formulations

The crossover designs for comparing three or more formulations are much more complicated than those for comparing two formulations. For simplicity, in this section, we restrict our attention to those designs in which the number of periods equals the number of formulations to be compared. In Section 2.6, the designs for comparing a large number of formulations with a small number of treatment periods are discussed.

For comparing three formulations of a drug, there are a total of three possible pairwise comparisons between formulations: formulation 1 versus formulation 2, formulation 1 versus formulation 3, and formulation 2 versus formulation 3. It is desirable to estimate these pairwise differences in average bioavailability between formulations with the same degree of precision. In other words, it is desirable to have equal variances for each pairwise differences in average bioavailability between formulations (i.e., $V(\hat{F}_i - \hat{F}_j) = \nu\sigma_e^2$) where ν is a constant and σ_e^2 is the intra-subject variability. Designs with this property are known as variance-balanced designs. It should be noted that, in practice, ν may vary from design to design. Thus, and ideal design is one with the smallest ν, such that all pairwise differences between formulations can be estimated with the same and possibly best precision. However, to achieve this goal, the design must be balanced. A design is said to be balanced if it satisfies the following conditions (Jones and Kenward, 1989, 2003):

1. Each formulation occurs only once with each subject.
2. Each formulation occurs the same number of times in each period.
3. The number of subjects who receive formulation i in some period followed by formulation j in the next period is the same for all $i \neq j$.

Under the constraint of the number of periods (p) being equal to the number of formulations (t), balance can be achieved by using a complete set of "orthogonal Latin squares" (John, 1971; Jones and Kenward, 2003). However, if $p = t$, a complete set of orthogonal Latin squares consists of $t(t-1)$ sequences except for $t = 6$. Some

TABLE 2.5.4: Orthogonal latin squares for $t=3$ and 4.

Three Formulations ($t=3$)

	Period		
Sequence	**I**	**II**	**III**
1	R[a]	T_1	T_2
2	T_1	T_2	R
3	T_2	R	T_1
4	R	T_2	T_1
5	T_1	R	T_2
6	T_2	T_1	R

Four Formulations ($t=4$)

	Period			
Sequence	**I**	**II**	**III**	**IV**
1	R[a]	T_1	T_2	T_3
2	T_1	R	T_3	T_2
3	T_2	T_3	R	T_1
4	T_3	T_2	T_1	R
5	R	T_3	T_1	T_2
6	T_1	T_2	R	T_3
7	T_2	T_1	T_3	R
8	T_3	R	T_2	T_1
9	R	T_2	T_3	T_1
10	T_1	T_3	T_2	R
11	T_2	R	T_1	T_3
12	T_3	T_1	R	T_2

[a] R is the reference formulation and T_1, T_2, and T_3 are the test formulations 1, 2, 3, respectively.

examples of orthogonal Latin squares with $t=3$ and $t=4$ are presented in Table 2.5.4. As a result, when the number of formulations to be compared is large, more sequences and consequently more subjects are required. This, however, may not be of practical use.

A more practical design has been proposed by Williams (1949). We shall refer to this as a Williams design. A Williams design possesses balance property and requires fewer sequences and periods. The algorithm for constructing a Williams design with t periods and t formulations is summarized in the following numerical steps (Jones and Kenward, 2003):

1. Number of formulations from $1, 2, \ldots, t$.
2. Start with the $t \times t$ standard Latin square. In this square, the formulations in the ith row are given by $i, i+1, \ldots, t, 1, 2, \ldots, i-1$.
3. Obtain a mirror image of the standard Latin square.

4. Interlace each row of the standard Latin square with the corresponding mirror image to obtain a $t \times 2t$ arrangement.

5. Slice the $t \times 2t$ arrangement down to the middle to yield two $t \times t$ squares. The columns of each $t \times t$ squares correspond to the periods and the rows are the sequences. The numbers within the square are the formulations.

6. If t is even, choose any one of the two $t \times t$ squares. If t is odd, use both squares.

In the following, to illustrate the use of this algorithm as an example, we will construct a Williams design with $t = 4$ (one reference and three test formulations) by following the above steps.

1. Denote the reference formulations by 1, and test formulations 1, 2, and 3 by 2, 3, and 4.

2. The 4×4 standard Latin square is given as

$$\begin{matrix} 1 & 2 & 3 & 4 \\ 2 & 3 & 4 & 1 \\ 3 & 4 & 1 & 2 \\ 4 & 1 & 2 & 3 \end{matrix}$$

3. The minor image of the 4×4 standard Latin square is then given by

$$\begin{matrix} 4 & 3 & 2 & 1 \\ 1 & 4 & 3 & 2 \\ 2 & 1 & 4 & 3 \\ 3 & 2 & 1 & 4 \end{matrix}$$

4. The 4×8 arrangement after interlacing the 4×4 standard Latin square with its mirror image is

$$\begin{array}{cccc|cccc} 1 & 4 & 2 & 3 & 3 & 2 & 4 & 1 \\ 2 & 1 & 3 & 4 & 4 & 3 & 1 & 2 \\ 3 & 2 & 4 & 1 & 1 & 4 & 2 & 3 \\ 4 & 3 & 1 & 2 & 2 & 1 & 3 & 4 \end{array}$$

5. The 4×4 squares obtained by slicing the above 4×8 arrangement are

		Period			
Square	**Sequence**	**I**	**II**	**III**	**IV**
1	1	1	4	2	3
	2	2	1	3	4
	3	3	2	4	1
	4	4	3	1	2
2	1	3	2	4	1
	2	4	3	1	2
	3	1	4	2	3
	4	2	1	3	4

6. Because $t = 4$, we can choose either square 1 or square 2. The resultant Williams design from square 1 is given in Table 2.5.5 by replacing 1, 2, 3, 4, with R, T_1, T_2, and T_3.

From the above example, it can be seen that a Williams design requires only 4 sequences to achieve the property of "variance-balanced," whereas a complete set of 4×4 orthogonal Latin squares requires 12 sequences. The Williams designs with $t = 3$ and 5 using the above algorithm are also given in Table 2.5.5.

TABLE 2.5.5: Williams designs for $t = 3$, 4, and 5.

Three Formulations ($t = 3$)

	Period		
Sequence	**I**	**II**	**III**
1	R[a]	T_2	T_1
2	T_1	R	T_2
3	T_2	T_1	R
4	T_1	T_2	R
5	T_2	R	T_1
6	R	T_1	T_2

Four Formulations ($t = 4$)

	Period			
Sequence	**I**	**II**	**III**	**IV**
1	R	T_3	T_1	T_2
2	T_1	R	T_2	T_3
3	T_2	T_1	T_3	R
4	T_3	T_2	R	T_1

Five Formulations ($t = 5$)

	Period				
Sequence	**I**	**II**	**III**	**IV**	**V**
1	R	T_4	T_1	T_3	T_2
2	T_1	R	T_2	T_4	T_3
3	T_2	T_1	T_3	R	T_4
4	T_3	T_2	T_4	T_1	R
5	T_4	T_3	R	T_2	T_1
6	T_2	T_3	T_1	T_4	R
7	T_3	T_4	T_2	R	T_1
8	T_4	R	T_3	T_1	T_2
9	R	T_1	T_4	T_2	T_3
10	T_1	T_2	R	T_3	T_4

[a] R is the reference formulation, and T_1, T_2, T_3, and T_4 are test formulations 1, 2, 3, and 4, respectively.

2.6 Balanced Incomplete Block Design

When comparing three or more formulations of a drug product, a complete crossover design may not be of practical interest for the following reasons (Westlake, 1973):

1. If the number of formulations to be compared is large, the study may be too time consuming, since t formulations require $t-1$ washout periods.

2. It may not be desirable to draw many blood samples for each subject owing to medical concerns.

3. Moreover, a subject is more likely to drop out when he or she is required to return frequently for tests.

These considerations suggest that one should keep the number of formulations that a subject receives as small as possible when planning a bioavailability study. For this, a randomized incomplete block design may be useful. An incomplete block design is a randomized block design in which not all formulations are present in every block. A block is called incomplete if the number of formulations in the block is less than the number of formulations to be compared. For an incomplete block design the blocks and formulations are not orthogonal to each other; that is, the block effects and formulation effects may not be estimated separately.

When an incomplete block design is used, it is recommended that the formulations in each block be randomly assigned in a balanced way so that the design will possess some optimal statistical properties. We shall refer to such a design as a balanced incomplete block design. A balanced incomplete block design is an incomplete block design in which any two formulations appear together an equal number of times. The advantages of using a balanced incomplete block design, rather than an incomplete design, are given as follows:

1. Difference in average bioavailability between the effects of any two formulations can always be estimated with the same degree of precision.

2. Analysis is simple in spite of the nonorthogonality provided that the balance is preserved.

3. Unbiased estimates of formulation effects are available.

Suppose that there are t formulations to be compared and each subject can only receive exactly p formulations ($t > p$). A balanced incomplete block design may be constructed by taking $C(t,p)$, the combinations of p out of t formulations, and assigning a different combination of formulations to each subject. However, to minimize the period effect, it is preferable to assign the formulations in such a way that the design is balanced over period (i.e., each formulation appears the same number of times in each period). In general, if the number of formulations is even (i.e., $t = 2n$) and $p = 2$, the number of blocks (sequences) required is $g = 2n(2n-1)$. On the other hand, if the number of formulations is odd (i.e., $t = 2n+1$) and $p = 2$, then $g = (2n+1)n$. Some examples for balanced incomplete block design are

TABLE 2.6.1: Balanced incomplete block designs for $t = 4$ with $p = 2$ and 3.

I. Each Sequence Receives Two Formulations ($p = 2$)

	Period	
Sequence[a]	**I**	**II**
1	R[b]	T_1
2	T_1	T_2
3	T_2	T_3
4	T_3	R
5	R	T_2
6	T_1	T_3
7	T_3	T_1
8	T_2	R
9	R	T_3
10	T_3	T_2
11	T_2	T_1
12	T_1	R

II. Each Sequence Receives Three Formulations ($p = 3$)

	Period		
Sequence	**I**	**II**	**III**
1	T_1	T_2	T_3
2	T_2	T_3	R
3	T_3	R	T_1
4	R	T_1	T_2

[a] A sequence (or block) may represent a subject or a group of homogeneous subjects.

[b] R is the reference formulation, and T_1, T_2, and T_3 are test formulations 1, 2, and 3, respectively.

given in Tables 2.6.1 and 2.6.2. Table 2.6.1 gives examples for $p = 2$ and 3 when four formulations ($t = 4$) are to be compared. For $p = 2$, the first six blocks are required for a balanced incomplete block design. However, to ensure the balance over period, an additional six blocks (7 through 12) are needed. For $t = 5$, Table 2.6.2 lists examples for a balanced incomplete block design with $p = 2$, 3, and 4. A balanced incomplete block design for $p = 3$ is the complementary part of that balanced incomplete block design for $p = 2$. The design for $p = 4$ can be constructed by deleting each formulation in turn to obtain five blocks successively.

For $t > 5$, several methods for constructing balanced incomplete block designs are available. Among these, the easiest way is probably the method of cyclic substitution. For this method to work, we first choose an appropriate initial block. The other blocks can be obtained successively by changing formulations A to B, B to C, ..., and so on in each block. For example, for $t = 6$ and $p = 3$, if we start with (A, B, D), then the second block is (B, C, E), and the third block is (C, D, F), and so on.

TABLE 2.6.2: Balanced incomplete block designs for $t=5$ with $p=2$, 3, and 4.

I. Each Sequence Receives Two and Three Formulations

$p=2$			$p=3$			
	Period			**Period**		
Sequence[a]	**I**	**II**	**Sequence**	**I**	**II**	**III**
1	R[b]	T_1	1	T_2	T_3	T_4
2	T_1	T_2	2	T_3	T_4	R
3	T_2	T_3	3	T_4	R	T_1
4	T_3	T_4	4	R	T_1	T_2
5	T_4	R	5	T_1	T_2	T_3
6	R	T_2	6	T_1	T_3	T_4
7	T_2	T_4	7	T_3	R	T_1
8	T_4	T_1	8	R	T_2	T_3
9	T_1	T_3	9	T_2	T_4	R
10	T_3	R	10	T_4	T_1	T_2

II. Each Sequence Receives Four Formulations ($p=4$)

	Period			
Sequence	**I**	**II**	**III**	**IV**
1	T_1	T_2	T_3	T_4
2	T_2	T_3	T_4	R
3	T_3	T_4	R	T_1
4	T_4	R	T_1	T_2
5	R	T_1	T_2	T_3

[a] A sequence (or block) may represent a subject or a group of homogeneous subjects.

[b] R is the reference formulation, and T_1, T_2, T_3, and T_4 are test formulations 1, 2, 3, and 4, respectively.

Note that a balanced incomplete block design is, in fact, a special case of variance-balanced design, which are discussed in Chapter 10. For an incomplete block design, balance may be achieved with fewer than $C(t,p)$ blocks. Such designs are known as partially balanced incomplete block designs. The analysis of these designs, however, is complicated, and hence, of little practical interest. More details on balanced incomplete black designs and partially balanced incomplete block designs can be found in Fisher ad Yates (1953), Bose et al. (1954), Cochran and Cox (1957), John (1971), and Cox and Reid (2000).

2.7 Selection of Design

In Sections 2.4 through 2.6, we briefly discussed three basic statistical designs, the parallel design, the crossover design, and the balanced incomplete block design for bioavailability and bioequivalence studies. Each of these has its own advantages and drawbacks under different circumstances. How to select an appropriate design when planning a bioavailability study is an important question. The answer to this question depends on many factors that are summarized as follows:

1. Number of formulations to be compared
2. Characteristics of the drug and its disposition
3. Study objectives
4. Availability of subjects
5. Inter- and intra-subject variabilities
6. Duration of the study or the number of periods allowed
7. Cost of adding a subject relative to that of adding one period
8. Dropout rates

For example, if the intra-subject variability is the same as or larger than the inter-subject variability, the inference on the difference in average bioavailability would be the same regardless of which design is used. Actually, a crossover design in this situation would be a poor choice, because blocking results in the loss of some degrees of freedom and will actually lead to a wider confidence interval on the difference between formulations.

If a bioavailability and bioequivalence study compares more than three formulations, a crossover design may not be appropriate. The reasons, as indicated in Section 2.6, are (1) it may be too time consuming to complete the study because a washout is required between treatment periods; (2) it may not be desirable to draw many blood samples for each subject owing to medical concerns; and (3) too many periods may increase the number of dropouts. Here, a balanced incomplete block design is preferred. However, if we compare several test formulations with a reference formulation, the within-subject comparison is not reliable, as subjects in some sequences may not receive the reference formulation.

If the drug has a very long half-life, or it possesses a potential toxicity, or bioequivalence must be established by clinical endpoint because some drugs do not work through systemic absorption, then a parallel design may be a possible choice. With this design, the study avoids a possible cumulative toxicity from the carryover effects from one treatment period to the next. In addition, the study can be completed quickly. However, the drawback is that the comparison of average bioavailability is made based on the inter-subject variability. If the inter-subject variability is large relative to the inter-subject variability, the statistical inference on the difference in average bioavailability between formulations is unreliable. Even if the inter-subject variability is relatively small, a parallel design may still require more subjects to reach the same degree of precision achieved by a crossover design.

In practice, a crossover design, which can remove the inter-subject variability from the comparison of average bioavailability between formulations, is often considered to be the design of choice if the number of formulations to be compared is small, say no more than three. If the drug has a very short half-life (i.e., there may not be carryover effects if the length of washout is long enough to eliminate the residual effects), a crossover design may be useful for the assessment of the intra-subject variability, provided that the cost for adding one period is comparable with that of adding a subject.

In summary, to choose an appropriate design for a bioavailability/bioequivalence study is an important issue in the development of a study protocol. The selected design may affect the data analysis, the interpretation of the results, and the determination of bioequivalence between formulations. Thus, all factors listed in the above should be carefully evaluated before an appropriate design is chosen.

Chapter 3

Statistical Inferences for Effects from a Standard 2 × 2 Crossover Design

3.1 Introduction

In Chapter 2, several useful designs for assessing bioequivalence in a variety of situations were discussed. Among these designs, the standard 2×2 crossover design, as outlined in the following, appears to be the most common design for assessing average bioequivalence between two formulations (a test formulation T and a reference formulation R) of a drug product or two drug products (a test drug T and a reference drug R).

Sequence	Period I	Period II
1 (RT)	Reference formulation Data: Y_{i11}	Test formulation Data: Y_{i21}
2 (TR)	Test formulation Data: Y_{i12}	Reference formulation Data: Y_{i22}

Each subject is randomly assigned to either sequence 1 (RT) or sequence 2 (TR). Subjects within sequence RT (TR) receive formulation or drug product R (T) during the first dosing period and formulation or drug product T (R) during the second period. Dosing periods are usually separated by a washout period of at least five times of the half-life of the active drug ingredient or therapeutic moiety.

The general model 2.5.1 can be used to describe the above standard 2×2 crossover design as follows:

$$Y_{ijk} = \mu + S_{ik} + P_j + F_{(j,k)} + C_{(j-1,k)} + e_{ijk}, \tag{3.1.1}$$

where

i (subject) $= 1, 2, \ldots, n_k$
j (period), k (sequence) $= 1, 2.$

$F_{(j,k)}$ is the direct fixed effect of the formulation or drug product administered at period j in sequence k. In the standard 2×2 crossover design, there are only two formulations. Thus, because the formulation administered at the first period in the first sequence is the reference formulation, then

$$F_{(j,k)} = \begin{cases} F_R & \text{if} \quad k = j \\ F_T & \text{if} \quad k \neq j \end{cases} \quad k = 1, 2; \quad j = 1, 2. \tag{3.1.2}$$

$C_{(j-1,k)}$ is the residual effect carried over from the $(j-1)$th period to the jth period in sequence k. For the standard 2×2 crossover design, the carryover effects can occur only at the second period. We will denote the carryover effect of the reference formulation from the first period to the second period at sequence 1 by C_R. Thus,

$$C_{(j-1,k)} = \begin{cases} C_R & \text{if} \quad k = 1, \quad j = 2 \\ C_T & \text{if} \quad k = 2, \quad j = 2. \end{cases} \tag{3.1.3}$$

It can be seen that this model includes fixed effects such as the period effects, the direct drug effects, and the carryover effects. For each subject, those fixed effects that occur at each period in each sequence are summarized as follows.

Sequence	**Period I**	**Period II**
1 (RT)	$\mu_{11} = \mu + P_1 + F_R$	$\mu_{21} = \mu + P_2 + F_T + C_R$
2 (TR)	$\mu_{12} = \mu + P_1 + F_T$	$\mu_{22} = \mu + P_2 + F_R + C_T$

where

$\mu_{jk} = E(Y_{ijk})$
$P_1 + P_2 = 0$
$F_R + F_T = 0$
$C_R + C_T = 0.$

For the comparison of average bioavailability between formulations or drug products, it is desirable to estimate and separate these effects from the direct drug effect (or formulation effect). In practice, for a bioavailability and bioequivalence study, it is usually assumed that (1) there are no period effects and (2) there are no carryover effects. This is because (1) a well-conducted study can eliminate the possible period effects and (2) the washout period of sufficient length can be chosen to ensure that there are no residual effects from previous dosing period to the next dosing period. Frequently, however, the period effects or carryover effects may still be present. The presence of the carryover effects can certainly increase the complexity of statistical analyses for the assessment of average bioequivalence between formulations. Thus, it is of interest to perform some preliminary tests for the presence of the period effects or the carryover effects before the comparison of average bioavailability between formulations is made.

In this chapter, statistical inferences on these effects are reviewed under model 3.1.1 with the following assumptions:

1. $\{S_{ik}\}$ are i.i.d. normal with mean 0 and variance σ_S^2.
2. $\{e_{ijk}\}$ are i.i.d. normal with mean 0 and variance σ_e^2. (3.1.4)
3. $\{S_{ik}\}$ and $\{e_{ijk}\}$ are mutually independent.

These assumptions are much stronger than those specified in model 2.5.1, which does not impose normality assumptions on $\{S_{ik}\}$ and $\{e_{ijk}\}$ and which allows the intra-subject variability to vary from formulation to formulation. Under these assumptions, statistical inferences such as estimation, confidence interval, and hypothesis testing for the fixed effects can be derived based on two-sample t statistics (Hills and Armitage, 1979; Jones and Kenward, 1989, 2003).

In Sections 3.2 through 3.4, statistical inferences for the carryover effects, the direct drug effect, and the period effect are obtained based on two-sample t statistics. The method of the analysis of variance for a general crossover design is presented in Section 3.5. In Section 3.6, an example is given to illustrate the use of the derived statistical methods.

3.2 Carryover Effects

For the assessment of carryover effects, it is helpful to consider the following subject totals for each sequence.

$$U_{ik} = Y_{i1k} + Y_{i2k}, \quad i = 1, 2, \ldots, n_k; \quad k = 1, 2. \tag{3.2.1}$$

The expected value and variance for U_{ik} are given, respectively, by

$$E(U_{ik}) = \begin{cases} 2\mu + C_R & \text{for subjects in sequence 1} \\ 2\mu + C_T & \text{for subjects in sequence 2,} \end{cases} \tag{3.2.2}$$

and

$$\sigma_u^2 = V(U_{ik}) = 2\left(2\sigma_S^2 + \sigma_e^2\right) \quad \text{for all subjects.} \tag{3.2.3}$$

Let $C = C_T - C_R$. Then, C can be used to assess the carryover effects. Under the constraint of $C_R + C_T = 0$, carryover effects are equal for the two formulations (i.e., $C = 0$) if and only if $C_R = C_T = 0$. Therefore, a test for no carryover effects is equivalent to a test for equal carryover effects. When there are no carryover effects, the direct drug effect (i.e., $F = F_T - F_R$) can be estimated based on the data from both periods. However, there is no unbiased estimator for the direct drug effect if unequal carryover effects are present. Thus, it is of interest to examine whether or not the unequal carryover effects are present. The unequal carryover effects can be determined by testing the following hypotheses:

$$\begin{aligned} &\text{H}_0\colon\ C = 0 \text{ (or } C_\text{R} = C_\text{T}) \\ \text{versus}\quad &\text{H}_\text{a}\colon\ C \neq 0 \text{ (or } C_\text{R} \neq C_\text{T}). \end{aligned} \tag{3.2.4}$$

The rejection of the null hypothesis leads to the conclusion of the presence of unequal carryover effects between formulations. To draw a statistical inference on C, it is useful to consider the following sample mean of the subject totals for each sequence:

$$\overline{U}_{\cdot k} = \frac{1}{n_k} \sum_{i=1}^{n_k} U_{ik}, \quad k = 1, 2. \tag{3.2.5}$$

$\overline{U}_{\cdot 1}$ and $\overline{U}_{\cdot 2}$ are the sample means of two independent random samples from normal populations with equal variances. Thus, statistical inference on C can be made based on an unpaired two-sample t statistic.

First, C can be estimated by the difference in sample means of the subject totals for the two sequences. That is,

$$\begin{aligned} \widehat{C} &= \overline{U}_{\cdot 2} - \overline{U}_{\cdot 1} \\ &= (\overline{Y}_{\cdot 12} + \overline{Y}_{\cdot 22}) - (\overline{Y}_{\cdot 11} + \overline{Y}_{\cdot 21}). \end{aligned} \tag{3.2.6}$$

Under the assumptions 1–3, as specified in Section 3.1, $\widehat{C}$ is normally distributed with mean C and variance $V(\widehat{C})$, which is given by

$$\begin{aligned} V(\widehat{C}) &= 2\left(2\sigma_\text{S}^2 + \sigma_\text{e}^2\right)\left(\frac{1}{n_1} + \frac{1}{n_2}\right) \\ &= \sigma_\text{u}^2\left(\frac{1}{n_1} + \frac{1}{n_2}\right). \end{aligned} \tag{3.2.7}$$

The variance $V(\widehat{C})$, can be estimated by replacing σ_u^2 with $\widehat{\sigma}_\text{u}^2$, the pooled sample variance of the subject totals from the two sequences. That is,

$$\widehat{V}(\widehat{C}) = \widehat{\sigma}_\text{u}^2\left(\frac{1}{n_1} + \frac{1}{n_2}\right), \tag{3.2.8}$$

where

$$\widehat{\sigma}_\text{u}^2 = \frac{1}{(n_1 + n_2 - 2)} \sum_{k=1}^{2} \sum_{i=1}^{n_k} (U_{ik} - \overline{U}_{\times k})^2.$$

Note that $\widehat{C}$ is the minimum variance unbiased estimator (MVUE) for C and $\widehat{\sigma}_\text{u}^2$ is an unbiased estimator for σ_u^2. The MVUE is the unbiased estimator with the smallest variance among all unbiased estimators. Furthermore, $(n_1 + n_2 - 2)\,\widehat{\sigma}_\text{u}^2$ is distributed as

$$\sigma_\text{u}^2 \chi^2(n_1 + n_2 - 2),$$

where $\chi^2(n_1+n_2-2)$ is a chi-square random variable with (n_1+n_2-2) degrees of freedom, which is independent of $\widehat{C}$. Thus, under H_0 in Equation 3.2.4,

$$T_c = \frac{\widehat{C}}{\widehat{\sigma}_u\sqrt{\dfrac{1}{n_1}+\dfrac{1}{n_2}}} \tag{3.2.9}$$

has a Student central t distribution with (n_1+n_2-2) degrees of freedom. As a result, we would reject the null hypothesis of H_0: $C_R = C_T$ and in favor of H_a: $C_R \neq C_T$ at the α level of significance if

$$|T_c| > t(\alpha/2,\ n_1+n_2-2), \tag{3.2.10}$$

where $t(\alpha/2,\ n_1+n_2-2)$ is the upper $\alpha/2$ critical value of a t distribution with (n_1+n_2-2) degrees of freedom. In other words, we reject the hypothesis of no carryover effects or equal carryover effects and conclude that there are unequal carryover effects if $|T_c| > t(\alpha/2,\ n_1+n_2-2)$.

As the test statistic T_c involves the estimate of $\sigma_u^2 = 2(2\sigma_S^2 + \sigma_e^2)$, which includes the inter-subject and the intra-subject variabilities, it may have little power when the inter-subject variability is relatively larger than the intra-subject variability. This is because in most bioavailability and bioequivalence studies, the sample size is chosen based on a prestudy power calculation on the direct drug effect that involves only the intra-subject variability. To increase the test power, however, Grizzle (1965) suggested testing the null hypothesis at the $\alpha = 10\%$ level, instead of the traditional 5% level.

On the basis of the t statistic, a $(1-\alpha)\times 100\%$ confidence interval for C can be obtained as follows:

$$\widehat{C} \pm t(\alpha/2,\ n_1+n_2-2)\ \widehat{\sigma}_u\sqrt{\frac{1}{n_1}+\frac{1}{n_2}}. \tag{3.2.11}$$

If the confidence interval contains 0, then we are in favor of (or fail to reject) the null hypothesis of no or equal carryover effects for the two formulations. If the confidence interval does not include 0, we conclude that there are unequal carryover effects between the two formulations.

3.3 Direct Drug Effect

It is helpful to start with the period differences for each subject within each sequence, which are defined as follows:

$$d_{ik} = \tfrac{1}{2}(Y_{i2k} - Y_{i1k}), \quad i = 1, 2, \ldots, n_k; \quad k = 1, 2. \tag{3.3.1}$$

The expected value and variance of the period differences are given respectively by

$$E(d_{ik}) = \begin{cases} \frac{1}{2}[(P_2 - P_1) + (F_T - F_R) + C_R] & \text{for subjects in sequence 1} \\ \frac{1}{2}[(P_2 - P_1) + (F_R - F_T) + C_T] & \text{for subjects in sequence 2,} \end{cases} \tag{3.3.2}$$

and

$$V(d_{ik}) = \sigma_d^2 = \sigma_e^2/2. \tag{3.3.3}$$

It can be seen that the variance of the period differences involves only the intra-subject variability, which reflects the usefulness of the crossover design in comparing the direct drug effects. However, the expected value of d_{ik} consists of the period effects and the carryover effects.

Denote the period effect and the direct drug effect by $P = P_2 - P_1$ and $F = F_T - F_R$, respectively. To draw statistical inference on F, consider the sample means of the period differences for each sequence. That is,

$$\bar{d}_{\cdot k} = \frac{1}{n_k} \sum_{i=1}^{n_k} d_{ik}, \quad k = 1, 2. \tag{3.3.4}$$

The difference between sequences (i.e., $\bar{d}_{\cdot 1} - \bar{d}_{\cdot 2}$) is clearly not an unbiased estimator of F unless there are no unequal carryover effects (i.e., $C_R = C_T$) since

$$\begin{aligned} E(\bar{d}_{\cdot 1} - \bar{d}_{\cdot 2}) &= (F_T - F_R) + (C_R - C_T)/2 \\ &= F - C/2, \end{aligned} \tag{3.3.5}$$

where $C = C_T - C_R$.

As a result, if $C_R \neq C_T$, there exists no unbiased estimator for F based on the data from both periods. On the other hand, if $C_R = C_T$, then

$$\begin{aligned} \hat{F} &= \bar{d}_{\cdot 1} - \bar{d}_{\cdot 2} \\ &= \tfrac{1}{2}[(\bar{Y}_{\cdot 21} - \bar{Y}_{\cdot 11}) - (\bar{Y}_{\cdot 22} - \bar{Y}_{\cdot 12})] \\ &= \bar{Y}_T - \bar{Y}_R \end{aligned} \tag{3.3.6}$$

is the MVUE of F, where

$$\bar{Y}_R = \tfrac{1}{2}(\bar{Y}_{\cdot 11} + \bar{Y}_{\cdot 22}) \quad \text{and} \quad \bar{Y}_T = \tfrac{1}{2}(\bar{Y}_{\cdot 21} + \bar{Y}_{\cdot 12}). \tag{3.3.7}$$

Note that $\bar{Y}_R$ and $\bar{Y}_T$ are the so-called least squares (LS) means for the reference and test formulation, respectively. $\hat{F} = \bar{Y}_T - \bar{Y}_R$ is also a linear contrast of the sequence by period means.

In practice, F is often estimated by the difference between the direct sample means for the two formulations. That is,

$$\widehat{F}^* = \overline{Y}_{\mathrm{T}}^* - \overline{Y}_{\mathrm{R}}^*,$$

where

$$\overline{Y}_{\mathrm{R}}^* = \frac{1}{n_1 + n_2}\left\{\sum_{i=1}^{n_1} Y_{i11} + \sum_{i=1}^{n_2} Y_{i22}\right\},$$

and

$$\overline{Y}_{\mathrm{T}}^* = \frac{1}{n_1 + n_2}\left\{\sum_{i=1}^{n_1} Y_{i21} + \sum_{i=1}^{n_2} Y_{i12}\right\}.$$

When $C_{\mathrm{R}} = C_{\mathrm{T}}$, we have

$$E\left(\overline{Y}_{\mathrm{R}}^*\right) = \frac{1}{n_1 + n_2}[(n_1 + n_2)\mu + (n_1 + n_2)F_{\mathrm{R}} + n_1P_1 + n_2P_2]$$

$$E\left(\overline{Y}_{\mathrm{T}}^*\right) = \frac{1}{n_1 + n_2}[(n_1 + n_2)\mu + (n_1 + n_2)F_{\mathrm{T}} + n_1P_2 + n_2P_1].$$

Hence,

$$E\left[\overline{Y}_{\mathrm{T}}^* - \overline{Y}_{\mathrm{R}}^*\right] = (F_{\mathrm{T}} - F_{\mathrm{R}}) + \frac{1}{n_1 + n_2}[(n_2 - n_1)P_1 + (n_1 - n_2)P_2].$$

Therefore, the difference between the direct sample means for the two formulations $\widehat{F}^*$ is not an unbiased estimator for F unless $n_1 = n_2$.

Under assumptions 1–3 as specified in Equation 3.1.4, the difference between the LS means for the two formulations $\widehat{F}$ is normally distributed with mean F and variance

$$V(\widehat{F}) = \sigma_{\mathrm{d}}^2\left(\frac{1}{n_1} + \frac{1}{n_2}\right). \tag{3.3.8}$$

Since $\{d_{i1}\}$, $i = 1, \ldots, n_1$ and $\{d_{i2}\}$, $i = 1, \ldots, n_2$ are two independent samples from normal populations with equal variances when no unequal carryover effects are present, a test for the direct drug effect can be obtained based on an unpaired two-sample t statistic as follows:

$$T_{\mathrm{d}} = \frac{\widehat{F}}{\widehat{\sigma}_{\mathrm{d}}\sqrt{\frac{1}{n_1} + \frac{1}{n_2}}}, \tag{3.3.9}$$

where $\widehat{\sigma}_d^2$ is the pooled sample variance of period differences from both sequences and is an unbiased estimator of σ_d^2. It is given by

$$\widehat{\sigma}_d^2 = \frac{1}{n_1 + n_2 - 2} \sum_{k=1}^{2} \sum_{i=1}^{n_k} (d_{ik} - \bar{d}_{\cdot k})^2. \tag{3.3.10}$$

Since $(n_1 + n_2 - 2)\widehat{\sigma}_d^2$ is distributed as $\sigma_d^2 \chi^2(n_1 + n_2 - 2)$, T_d has a central student t distribution with $(n_1 + n_2 - 2)$ degrees of freedom. A $(1 - \alpha) \times 100\%$ confidence interval for F can then be obtained as follows:

$$\widehat{F} \pm t(\alpha/2,\, n_1 + n_2 - 2)\, \widehat{\sigma}_d \sqrt{\frac{1}{n_1} + \frac{1}{n_2}}. \tag{3.3.11}$$

The presence of the direct drug effect can be examined by testing the hypotheses:

$$\begin{aligned} &\text{H}_0\text{: } F_R = F_T \\ \text{versus } &\text{H}_a\text{: } F_R \neq F_T. \end{aligned} \tag{3.3.12}$$

We reject H_0 if

$$|T_d| > t(\alpha/2,\, n_1 + n_2 - 2). \tag{3.3.13}$$

Note that the above testing procedure is for the equality of the direct drug effects, not for equivalence of direct drug effects, which is discussed in Chapter 4.

As mentioned earlier, $\widehat{F}$ is not an unbiased estimator for F in the presence of unequal carryover effects (i.e., $C_R \neq C_T$). However, an unbiased estimator of F can still be obtained from the data from the first period at the expense of precision. Let $\overline{Y}_{\cdot 11}$ and $\overline{Y}_{\cdot 12}$ be sample means of the two sequences at the first period. Then,

$$\begin{aligned} E(\overline{Y}_{\cdot 12} - \overline{Y}_{\cdot 11}) &= (\mu + P_1 + F_T) - (\mu + P_1 + F_R) \\ &= F_T - F_R \\ &= F. \end{aligned}$$

Denote $\overline{Y}_{\cdot 12} - \overline{Y}_{\cdot 11}$ by $\widehat{F}|C$. Thus, $\widehat{F}|C$ is an unbiased estimator of F in the presence of unequal carryover effects. The variance of $\widehat{F}|C$ is given by

$$V(\widehat{F}|C) = (\sigma_S^2 + \sigma_e^2)\left(\frac{1}{n_1} + \frac{1}{n_2}\right). \tag{3.3.14}$$

Note that

$$V(\widehat{F}|C) - V(\widehat{F}) = \left(\sigma_S^2 + \frac{\sigma_e^2}{2}\right)\left(\frac{1}{n_1} + \frac{1}{n_2}\right). \tag{3.3.15}$$

Hence, in the presence of unequal carryover effects, an unbiased estimator for F can be obtained only by using the data at the first period at the expense of losing the precision by at least 50%, even when $\sigma_S^2 = 0$. Thus, in practice, it is extremely important to have a sufficient length of washout periods between dosing periods to eliminate the residual effects from a previous dosing period before initiating the next dosing period. In the presence of unequal carryover effects, however, a $(1-\alpha)\times 100\%$ confidence interval for F and a test statistic for the hypothesis of no direct drug effect can also be obtained based on an unpaired two-sample t statistic using the data from the first period.

First, an unbiased estimator of $V(\widehat{F}|C)$ is

$$\widehat{V}(\widehat{F}|C) = S_f^2\left(\frac{1}{n_1} + \frac{1}{n_2}\right) \tag{3.3.16}$$

where

$$S_f^2 = \frac{1}{n_1 + n_2 - 2}\sum_{k=1}^{2}\sum_{i=1}^{n_k}(Y_{i1k} - \overline{Y}_{\cdot 1k})^2. \tag{3.3.17}$$

Note that although S_f^2 is an unbiased estimator of $\sigma_e^2 + \sigma_S^2$, individual estimates for σ_e^2 and σ_S^2 are not available based on the data from the first period only. A $(1-\alpha)\times 100\%$ confidence interval for F in the presence of unequal carryover effects is then given by

$$\widehat{F}|C \pm t(\alpha/2,\, n_1 + n_2 - 2)\; S_f\sqrt{\frac{1}{n_1} + \frac{1}{n_2}}. \tag{3.3.18}$$

The null hypothesis of no direct drug effect is rejected if

$$\left|\frac{\widehat{F}|C}{S_f\sqrt{\frac{1}{n_1} + \frac{1}{n_2}}}\right| > t(\alpha/2,\, n_1 + n_2 - 2). \tag{3.3.19}$$

In practice, in the presence of unequal carryover effects, the data in the first period are analyzed to assess the bioequivalence between formulations in bioavailability studies. However, one should be aware of the following consequences:

1. There is little power for detection of a clinically significant difference owing to the increase in variability.

2. The sacrifice of the information in the second period negates the benefit of a crossover design, which removes the inter-subject variability from the comparison of average bioavailability between formulations.

3.4 Period Effect

Define the crossover differences as follows:

$$O_{ik} = \begin{cases} d_{ik} & \text{for subjects in sequence 1} \\ -d_{ik} & \text{for subjects in sequence 2.} \end{cases} \tag{3.4.1}$$

The expected value and variance of the crossover differences are

$$E(O_{ik}) = \begin{cases} \frac{1}{2}[(P_2 - P_1) + (F_T - F_R) + C_R] & \text{for subjects in sequence 1} \\ \frac{1}{2}[(P_1 - P_2) + (F_T - F_R) - C_T] & \text{for subjects in sequence 2} \end{cases} \tag{3.4.2}$$

and $V(O_{ik}) = \sigma_d^2 = \sigma_e^2/2$, respectively.

Let $\overline{O}_{\cdot 1}$ and $\overline{O}_{\cdot 2}$ be the sample means of the crossover differences in sequences 1 and 2. Then,

$$\overline{O}_{ik} = \begin{cases} \overline{d}_{\cdot 1} & \text{for } k = 1 \\ -\overline{d}_{\cdot 2} & \text{for } k = 2. \end{cases} \tag{3.4.3}$$

An unbiased estimator for the period effect P can then be obtained as

$$\begin{aligned} \widehat{P} &= \overline{O}_{\cdot 1} - \overline{O}_{\cdot 2} \\ &= \tfrac{1}{2}[(\overline{Y}_{\cdot 21} - \overline{Y}_{\cdot 11}) - (\overline{Y}_{\cdot 12} - \overline{Y}_{\cdot 22})] \end{aligned} \tag{3.4.4}$$

Because $C_R + C_T = 0$, $\widehat{P}$ is the MVUE for P, regardless of the presence of unequal carryover effects, a $(1 - \alpha) \times 100\%$ confidence interval for P is given as follows:

$$\widehat{P} \pm t(\alpha/2, n_1 + n_2 - 2)\, \widehat{\sigma}_d \sqrt{\frac{1}{n_1} + \frac{1}{n_2}}. \tag{3.4.5}$$

We reject the null hypothesis of no period effect, that is,

$$\begin{aligned} &\text{H}_0\text{: } P_1 = P_2 \\ \text{versus } &\text{H}_a\text{: } P_1 \neq P_2, \end{aligned} \tag{3.4.6}$$

if

$$|T_0| > t(\alpha/2, n_1 + n_2 - 2), \tag{3.4.7}$$

where

$$T_0 = \frac{\widehat{P}}{\widehat{\sigma}_d \sqrt{\frac{1}{n_1} + \frac{1}{n_2}}}. \tag{3.4.8}$$

The statistical inferences for the carryover effects, the direct drug effect, and the period effect for a standard 2×2 crossover design are summarized in Table 3.4.1.

TABLE 3.4.1: Statistical inferences for fixed effects in a standard 2 × 2 crossover design.

Effect	Unequal Carryover Effects	MVUE	$(1-\alpha)\times 100\%$ Confidence Interval	Test Statistic
Carryover	—	$\widehat{C} = \overline{U}_{\cdot 2} - \overline{U}_{\cdot 1}$ $= (\overline{Y}_{\cdot 11} + \overline{Y}_{\cdot 21}) - (\overline{Y}_{\cdot 12} + \overline{Y}_{\cdot 22})$	$\widehat{C} \pm t(\alpha/2, n_1 + n_2 - 2)\, \widehat{\sigma}_{\mathrm{u}} \sqrt{\frac{1}{n_1} + \frac{1}{n_2}}$	$T_{\mathrm{C}} = \frac{\widehat{C}}{\widehat{\sigma}_{\mathrm{u}}\sqrt{\frac{1}{n_1} + \frac{1}{n_2}}}$
Direct drug	No	$\widehat{F} = \overline{d}_{\cdot 1} - \overline{d}_{\cdot 2}$ $= \frac{1}{2}[(\overline{Y}_{\cdot 21} - \overline{Y}_{\cdot 11}) - (\overline{Y}_{\cdot 22} - \overline{Y}_{\cdot 12})]$	$\widehat{F} \pm t(\alpha/2, n_1 + n_2 - 2)\, \widehat{\sigma}_{\mathrm{d}} \sqrt{\frac{1}{n_1} + \frac{1}{n_2}}$	$T_{\mathrm{d}} = \frac{\widehat{F}}{\widehat{\sigma}_{\mathrm{d}}\sqrt{\frac{1}{n_1} + \frac{1}{n_2}}}$
Direct drug	Yes	$\widehat{F}\vert C = \overline{Y}_{\cdot 12} - \overline{Y}_{\cdot 11}$	$\widehat{F}\vert C \pm t(\alpha/2, n_1 + n_2 - 2)\, S_{\mathrm{f}} \sqrt{\frac{1}{n_1} + \frac{1}{n_2}}$	$T_{\mathrm{f}} = \frac{\widehat{F}\vert C}{S_{\mathrm{f}}\sqrt{\frac{1}{n_1} + \frac{1}{n_2}}}$
Period	—	$\widehat{P} = \overline{O}_{\cdot 1} - \overline{O}_{\cdot 2}$ $= \frac{1}{2}[(\overline{Y}_{\cdot 21} - \overline{Y}_{\cdot 11}) - (\overline{Y}_{\cdot 12} - \overline{Y}_{\cdot 22})]$	$\widehat{P} \pm t(\alpha/2, n_1 + n_2 - 2)\, \widehat{\sigma}_{\mathrm{d}} \sqrt{\frac{1}{n_1} + \frac{1}{n_2}}$	$T_{\mathrm{o}} = \frac{\widehat{P}}{\widehat{\sigma}_{\mathrm{d}}\sqrt{\frac{1}{n_1} + \frac{1}{n_2}}}$

Note: MVUE, minimum variance unbiased estimate.

3.5 Analysis of Variance

In previous sections, statistical inferences for the fixed effects in model 3.1.1 for the standard 2×2 crossover design were derived based on unpaired two-sample t statistics. In this section, the method of the analysis of variance that is often considered for a general situation is introduced. The unpaired two-sample t statistic is equivalent to a special case of the method of analysis of variance.

The concept of the analysis of variance is to study the variability in the observed data by partitioning the total sum of squares (SS) of the observations into components of the fixed effects and the random errors. For example, for the standard 2×2 crossover design, we would partition the total SS of the $2(n_1 + n_2)$ observations into components for the carryover effects, the period effect, the direct drug effect, and the error. Let $\overline{Y}_{...}$ be the grand mean of all observations. Then the total corrected SS is given by

$$\begin{aligned} SS_{\text{Total}} &= \sum_{k=1}^{2}\sum_{j=1}^{2}\sum_{i=1}^{n_k}(Y_{ijk} - \overline{Y}_{...})^2 \\ &= \sum_{k=1}^{2}\sum_{j=1}^{2}\sum_{i=1}^{n_k}(Y_{ijk} - \overline{Y}_{i\cdot k} + \overline{Y}_{i\cdot k} - \overline{Y}_{...})^2 \\ &= \sum_{k=1}^{2}\sum_{j=1}^{2}\sum_{i=1}^{n_k}(Y_{ijk} - \overline{Y}_{i\cdot k})^2 + 2\sum_{k=1}^{2}\sum_{i=1}^{n_k}(\overline{Y}_{i\cdot k} - \overline{Y}_{...})^2 \\ &= SS_{\text{within}} + SS_{\text{between}}, \end{aligned} \tag{3.5.1}$$

where

$$\overline{Y}_{i\cdot k} = \frac{1}{2}\sum_{j=1}^{2} Y_{ijk},$$

and SS_{between} is the sum of squares due to subjects (i.e., between subjects) and SS_{within} is the sum of squares for within subjects. As there are $2(n_1 + n_2)$ observations, SS_{total} has $2(n_1 + n_2) - 1$ degrees of freedom. There are $n_1 + n_2$ subjects in both sequences. Thus, SS_{between} and SS_{within} have $(n_1 + n_2 - 1)$ and $n_1 + n_2$ degrees of freedom, respectively. The SS_{between} can be further partitioned into two components, one for the carryover effects and the other for the inter-subject error. That is,

$$SS_{\text{between}} = SS_{\text{carry}} + SS_{\text{inter}}, \tag{3.5.2}$$

where

$$\begin{aligned} SS_{\text{carry}} &= \frac{2n_1 n_2}{n_1 + n_2}\left\{(\overline{Y}_{\cdot 12} + \overline{Y}_{\cdot 22}) - (\overline{Y}_{\cdot 11} + \overline{Y}_{\cdot 21})\right\}^2, \quad \text{and} \\ SS_{\text{inter}} &= \sum_{k=1}^{2}\sum_{i=1}^{n_k}\frac{Y_{i\cdot k}^2}{2} - \sum_{k=1}^{2}\frac{Y_{\cdot\cdot k}^2}{2n_k}, \end{aligned}$$

where $Y_{i\cdot k}$ and $Y_{\cdot\cdot k}$ are the sum of Y_{ijk} over the corresponding indices. SS_{carry} and SS_{inter} have 1 and (n_1+n_2-2) degrees of freedom, respectively. Each SS divided by its degrees of freedom is the corresponding mean squares (MS). The expected value of the mean squares for SS_{carry} and SS_{inter} can be shown to be

$$E(\text{MS}_{\text{carry}}) = \frac{2n_1n_2}{n_1+n_2}(C_{\text{T}}-C_{\text{R}})^2 + 2\sigma_{\text{S}}^2 + \sigma_{\text{e}}^2 \tag{3.5.3}$$

$$E(\text{MS}_{\text{inter}}) = 2\sigma_{\text{S}}^2 + \sigma_{\text{e}}^2. \tag{3.5.4}$$

Therefore, to test the hypotheses in Equation 3.2.4 (i.e., the equality of the carryover effects), we would use the test statistic

$$F_{\text{c}} = \frac{\text{MS}_{\text{carry}}}{\text{MS}_{\text{inter}}}, \tag{3.5.5}$$

which follows an F distribution with degrees of freedom 1 and (n_1+n_2-2) if the null hypothesis in Equation 3.2.4 is true. We reject H_0 if

$$F_{\text{c}} > F(\alpha,\ 1,\ n_1+n_2-2),$$

where $F(\alpha, 1, n_1+n_2-2)$ is the upper α percentile of the F distribution with degrees of freedom 1 and n_1+n_2-2. Note that an F distribution with degrees of freedom 1 and v is equal to the square of a t distribution with degrees of freedom v. Thus, the above test statistic is equivalent to test statistic T_{c} in Equation 3.2.10 since $F_{\text{c}}=T_{\text{c}}^2$.

Similarly, the $\text{SS}_{\text{within}}$ can be further decomposed into three components: SS for the direct drug effect, the period effect, and the intra-subject residuals. That is,

$$\text{SS}_{\text{within}} = \text{SS}_{\text{drug}} + \text{SS}_{\text{period}} + \text{SS}_{\text{intra}}, \tag{3.5.6}$$

where

$$\text{SS}_{\text{drug}} = \frac{2n_1n_2}{n_1+n_2}\left\{\frac{1}{2}[(\overline{Y}_{\cdot 21}-\overline{Y}_{\cdot 11})-(\overline{Y}_{\cdot 22}-\overline{Y}_{\cdot 12})]\right\}^2,$$

$$\text{SS}_{\text{period}} = \frac{2n_1n_2}{n_1+n_2}\left\{\frac{1}{2}[(\overline{Y}_{\cdot 21}-\overline{Y}_{\cdot 11})-(\overline{Y}_{\cdot 12}-\overline{Y}_{\cdot 22})]\right\}^2,$$

$$\text{SS}_{\text{intra}} = \sum_{k=1}^{2}\sum_{j=1}^{2}\sum_{i=1}^{n_k} Y_{ijk}^2 - \sum_{k=1}^{2}\sum_{i=1}^{n_k}\frac{Y_{i\cdot k}^2}{2} - \sum_{k=1}^{2}\sum_{j=1}^{2}\frac{Y_{\cdot jk}^2}{n_k} + \sum_{k=1}^{2}\frac{Y_{\cdot\cdot k}^2}{2n_k}.$$

There is 1 degree of freedom for each of SS_{drug} and $\text{SS}_{\text{period}}$, respectively, and (n_1+n_2-2) degrees of freedom for SS_{intra}. The expected values for their MS follow:

$$E(\text{MS}_{\text{drug}}) = \frac{2n_1n_2}{n_1+n_2}\left[(F_{\text{T}}-F_{\text{R}}) + \frac{C_{\text{R}}-C_{\text{T}}}{2}\right]^2 + \sigma_{\text{e}}^2. \tag{3.5.7}$$

$$E(\mathrm{MS}_{\mathrm{period}}) = \frac{2n_1 n_2}{n_1 + n_2}(P_2 - P_1)^2 + \sigma_e^2, \tag{3.5.8}$$

$$E(\mathrm{MS}_{\mathrm{intra}}) = \sigma_e^2. \tag{3.5.9}$$

Note that $\mathrm{MS}_{\mathrm{intra}} = 2\hat{\sigma}_d^2$, where $\hat{\sigma}_d^2$ is the pooled sample variance of period differences. When $C_R = C_T$, the null hypothesis in Equation 3.3.12 of no direct drug effect can be tested using the following statistic

$$F_d = \frac{\mathrm{MS}_{\mathrm{drug}}}{\mathrm{MS}_{\mathrm{intra}}}, \tag{3.5.10}$$

which is distributed as an F distribution with degrees of freedom 1 and $(n_1 + n_2 - 2)$. We reject the null hypothesis if

$$F_d > F(\alpha, 1, n_1 + n_2 - 2).$$

Test statistic F_d is equivalent to test statistic T_d in Equation 3.3.9, since $F_d = T_d^2$.

For testing the null hypothesis 3.4.6 of no period effect, we may consider the following test statistic

$$F_p = \frac{\mathrm{MS}_{\mathrm{period}}}{\mathrm{MS}_{\mathrm{intra}}}, \tag{3.5.11}$$

which follows an F distribution with degrees of freedom 1 and $(n_1 + n_2 - 2)$. The null hypothesis is then rejected if

$$F_p > F(\alpha, 1, n_1 + n_2 - 2).$$

It can be verified that $F_p = T_0^2$. Thus, test statistic F_p is equivalent to test statistic T_0 in Equation (3.4.8).

For a general crossover design, the method of the analysis of variance is useful in deriving statistical inferences for the fixed effects in model 2.5.1 under some normality assumptions. It can be seen that for the standard 2×2 crossover design, an unpaired two-sample t statistic is equivalent to a special case of the method of the analysis of variance. The analysis of variance table for the standard 2×2 crossover design is summarized in Table 3.5.1.

From Table 3.5.1, in addition, a test for the hypotheses of the presence of the inter-subject variability, that is,

$$\begin{aligned} &\mathrm{H}_0\colon \sigma_S^2 = 0 \\ \text{versus}\quad &\mathrm{H}_a\colon \sigma_S^2 > 0 \end{aligned} \tag{3.5.12}$$

can also be obtained by considering

$$F_v = \frac{\mathrm{MS}_{\mathrm{inter}}}{\mathrm{MS}_{\mathrm{intra}}}, \tag{3.5.13}$$

TABLE 3.5.1: Analysis of variance table for the standard 2 × 2 crossover design.

Source of Variation	Degrees of Freedom (df)	Sum of Squares (SS)	Mean Square (MS) = SS/df	Effect of mean Square (EMS)	*F*
Inter-subjects					
Carryover	1	SS_{carry}	SS_{carry}	$\frac{2n_1n_2}{n_1+n_2}(C_T - C_R)^2 + 2\sigma_S^2 + \sigma_e^2$	$F_C = MS_{carry}/MS_{inter}$
Residuals	n_1+n_2-2	SS_{inter}	$SS_{inter}/(n_1+n_2-2)$	$2\sigma_S^2+\sigma_e^2$	$F_V = MS_{inter}/MS_{intra}$
Intra-subjects					
Direct drug	1	SS_{drug}	SS_{drug}	$\frac{2n_1n_2}{n_1+n_2}\left[(F_T - F_R) + \frac{C_R - C_T}{2}\right]^2 + \sigma_e^2$	$F_d^* = MS_{drug}/MS_{intra}^{a}$
Period	1	SS_{period}	SS_{period}	$\frac{2n_1n_2}{n_1+n_2}(P_2 - P_1)^2 + \sigma_e^2$	$F_P = MS_{period}/MS_{intra}$
Residuals	n_1+n_2-2	SS_{intra}	$SS_{intra}/(n_1+n_2-2)$	σ_e^2	
Total	$2(n_1+n_2)-1$	SS_{total}			

[a] F_d^* is valid only if $C_R = C_T$.

where F_v is distributed as an F distribution with degrees of freedom n_1+n_2-2 and n_1+n_2-2 under H_0. Thus, we reject the null hypothesis of no inter-subject variability if

$$F_v > F(\alpha, n_1+n_2-2, n_1+n_2-2).$$

Statistical inferences for the inter-subject variability (σ_S^2) and the intra-subject variability (σ_e^2) are discussed in Chapter 7.

The standard 2×2 crossover design can provide only estimates and tests for the period effect, the direct drug effect, and the carryover effects. It does not provide any inference on the interactions among these effects and the interactions between fixed and random effects. To draw some statistical inference on the interactions of interest (e.g., the subject-by-formulation, the formulation-by-period, and the sequence-by-period interactions), a higher-order crossover deign is necessary. However, it is important to determine which interaction term is to be examined before an appropriate design is chosen. For example, to test the subject-by-formulation interaction in comparing two formulations, each subject must receive each of the test and reference formulations twice. Consequently, a four-period design will have to be used.

3.6 Example

Example 3.6.1

To illustrate the above statistical inferences for the fixed effects in Equation 3.1.1 for the standard 2×2 crossover design, let us consider the following example concerning the comparison of bioavailability between two formulations of a drug product. This study was conducted with 24 healthy volunteers. During each dosing period, each subject was administered either five 50 mg tablets (test formulation) or 5 mL of an oral suspension (50 mg/mL, reference formulation). Blood samples were obtained at 0 hour before dosing and at various times after dosing. AUC values from 0 to 32 hours, given in Table 3.6.1, were calculated using the trapezoidal method.

For a preliminary examination of the data, the plot of subject profiles for each sequence and sequence-by-period means are useful and presented in Figures 3.6.1 and 3.6.2. Figures 3.6.1 and 3.6.2 indicate that the variability in AUC at the second sequence seems larger than that at the first sequence.

Moreover, some drastic changes in AUC in each sequence were observed. In Figure 3.6.3, 1T and 2T (1R and 2R) are the sample means for test (reference) formulation in sequences 1 and 2, which are given as follows:

Sequence	Period I	Period II	Sequence Mean
1	$1R=\overline{Y}_{\cdot 11}=85.82$	$1T=\overline{Y}_{\cdot 21}=81.80$	$\overline{Y}_{\cdot\cdot 1}=83.81$
2	$2T=\overline{Y}_{\cdot 12}=78.74$	$2R=\overline{Y}_{\cdot 22}=79.30$	$\overline{Y}_{\cdot\cdot 2}=79.02$
Period mean	$\overline{Y}_{\cdot 1\cdot}=82.28$	$\overline{Y}_{\cdot 2\cdot}=80.55$	$\overline{Y}_{\cdot\cdot\cdot}=81.42$

TABLE 3.6.1: AUC(0–32) for test and reference formulations.

Sequence	Subject Number	Period I	Period II	Subject Total	P.D.[a]	C.D.[b]
1						
RT	1	74.675	73.675	148.350	−1.000	−1.000
RT	4	96.400	93.250	189.650	−3.150	−3.150
RT	5	101.950	102.125	204.075	0.175	0.175
RT	6	79.050	69.450	148.500	−9.600	−9.600
RT	11	79.050	69.025	148.075	−10.025	−10.025
RT	12	85.950	68.700	154.650	−17.250	−17.250
RT	15	69.725	59.425	129.150	−10.300	−10.300
RT	16	86.275	76.125	162.400	−10.150	−10.150
RT	19	112.675	114.875	227.550	2.200	2.200
RT	20	99.525	116.250	215.775	16.725	16.725
RT	23	89.425	64.175	153.600	−25.250	−25.250
RT	24	55.175	74.575	129.750	19.400	19.400
2						
TR	2	74.825	37.350	112.175	−37.475	37.475
TR	3	86.875	51.925	138.800	−34.950	34.950
TR	7	81.675	72.175	153.850	−9.500	9.500
TR	8	92.700	77.500	170.200	−15.200	15.200
TR	9	50.450	71.875	122.325	21.425	−21.425
TR	10	66.125	94.025	160.150	27.900	−27.900
TR	13	122.450	124.975	247.425	2.525	−2.525
TR	14	99.075	85.225	184.300	−13.850	13.850
TR	17	86.350	95.925	182.275	9.575	−9.575
TR	18	49.925	67.100	117.025	17.175	−17.175
TR	21	42.700	59.425	102.125	16.725	−16.725
TR	22	91.725	114.050	205.775	22.325	−22.325

[a] P.D. = 2 × (period difference).
[b] C.D. = 2 × (crossover difference).

These results indicate that the mean AUCs for both test and reference formulations in sequence 1 are higher than those in sequence 2. In particular, the mean AUC of the reference formulation in sequence 1 is about 8.2% higher than that in sequence 2. As mentioned earlier, for a 2 × 2 crossover design, the sequence-by-period interaction represents the direct drug effect if there is no carryover effect. Thus, a preliminary test for the presence of carryover effects is necessarily performed before the assessment of average bioequivalence between formulations is made. We now

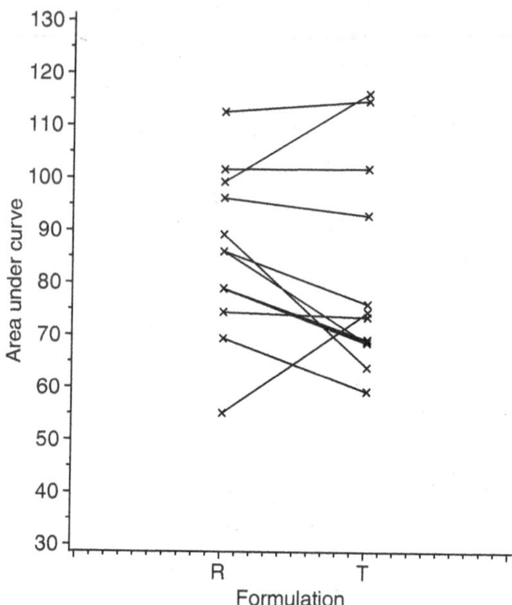

FIGURE 3.6.1: Subject profiles sequence = 1.

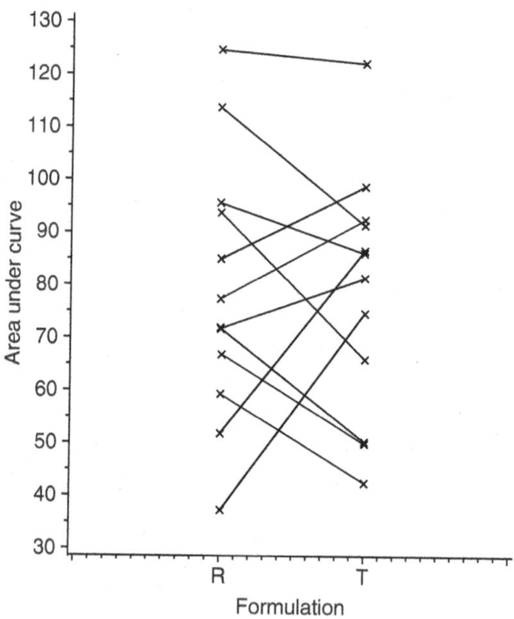

FIGURE 3.6.2: Subject profiles sequence = 2.

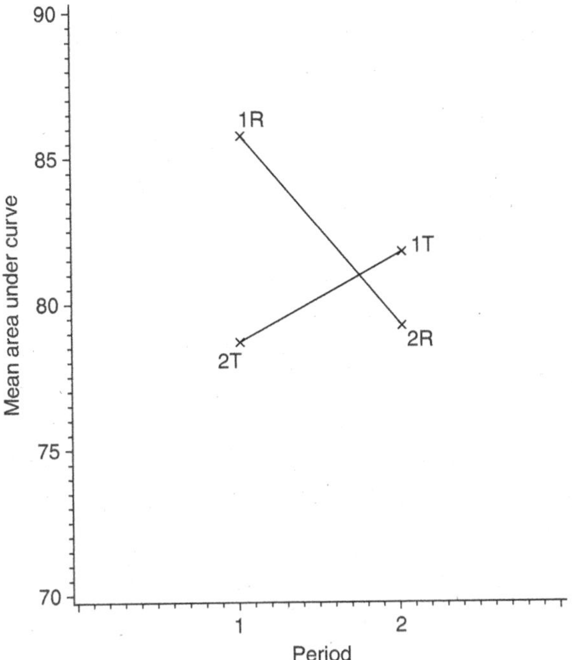

FIGURE 3.6.3: Sequence-by-period means.

carry out the statistical inferences for the fixed effects discussed in previous sections as follows.

3.6.1 Carryover Effects

Since $\overline{U}_{\cdot 1} = 167.63$, $\overline{U}_{\cdot 2} = 158.04$, and $\hat{\sigma}_u^2 = 1473.77$, the test statistic is given by

$$T_c = \frac{158.04 - 167.63}{\sqrt{1473.77\left(\frac{1}{12} + \frac{1}{12}\right)}} = -0.6120.$$

Thus, $|T_c| = 0.612 < t(0.025, 22) = 2.074$. Hence, we fail to reject the hypothesis of no unequal carryover effects. The observed p-value is 0.5468, which also indicates that there is little evidence for the presence of unequal carryover effects. The test result suggests that it may be appropriate to use the data from both periods for inference on the direct drug effect.

3.6.2 Direct Drug Effect

From Table 3.6.1, it can be verified that

$$\overline{d}_{\cdot 1} = -2.0094, \quad \overline{d}_{\cdot 2} = 0.2781, \quad \text{and} \quad \hat{\sigma}_d^2 = 83.623.$$

Thus, the point estimate of F is

$$\widehat{F} = \overline{d}_{\cdot 1} - \overline{d}_{\cdot 2} = -2.29,$$

with a 95% confidence interval

$$\begin{aligned}
&\widehat{F} \pm t(0.025,22)\widehat{\sigma}_{\mathrm{d}}\sqrt{\frac{1}{n_1} + \frac{1}{n_2}} \\
&\quad = -2.29 \pm (2.074)(9.1446)\sqrt{0.1667} \\
&\quad = (-10.03, 5.46).
\end{aligned}$$

As indicated by the 95% confidence interval, no significant direct drug effect was detected. The null hypothesis of the equality in average bioavailability between formulations does not imply the average bioequivalence between formulations. The assessment of average bioequivalence between formulations according to the FDA requirement is discussed extensively in Chapter 4.

3.6.3 Period Effect

From Table 3.6.1, the crossover differences can be obtained as follows:

$$\overline{O}_{\cdot 1} = -2.0094 \quad \text{and} \quad \overline{O}_{\cdot 2} = -0.2781.$$

Thus, the t statistic is given by

$$T_0 = \frac{0.2781 - 2.0094}{\sqrt{(83.623)(0.1667)}} = -0.4637.$$

Hence, we fail to reject the hypothesis of no period effect since $|T_0| = 0.4637 < t(0.025,22) = 2.074$ (p-value = 0.6474).

The results of statistical inferences on the fixed effects obtained from two-sample t statistical are summarized in Table 3.6.2.

TABLE 3.6.2: Statistical interferences for the fixed effects.

Effect	MVUE	Variance Estimate	95% Confidence Interval	T	p-Value
Carryover	−9.59	245.63	(−42.10, 22.91)	−0.612	0.5468
Direct drug	−2.29	13.97	(−10.03, 5.46)	−0.613	0.5463
Period	−1.73	13.97	(−9.47, 6.01)	−0.464	0.6474

TABLE 3.6.3: Analysis of variance table for data in Table 3.6.1.

Source of Variation	Degrees of Freedom (df)	Sum of Squares (SS)	Mean Square (MS)	*F*	*p*-Value
Inter-subject					
Carryover	1	276.00	276.00	0.37	0.5468
Residuals	22	16211.49	736.89	4.41	0.0005
Intra-subject					
Direct drug	1	62.79	62.79	0.38	0.5463
Period	1	35.97	35.97	0.22	0.6474
Residuals	22	3679.43	167.25	—	—
Total	47	20265.68	—	—	—

3.6.4 Analysis of Variance

For the data given in Table 3.6.1, the method of the analysis of variance was also performed. The results are given in Table 3.6.3. It can be easily verified that the results from the method of the analysis of variance are equivalent to the results obtained using unpaired two-sample *t* statistics.

3.6.5 Test for Inter-Subject Variability

It can be seen from the ANOVA table given in Table 3.6.3 that $\mathrm{MS}_{\mathrm{inter}} = 736.885$ and $\mathrm{MS}_{\mathrm{intra}} = 167.246$. Thus, the F statistic for H_0: $\sigma_S^2 = 0$ versus H_a: $\sigma_S^2 > 0$ is

$$F_V = \frac{736.885}{167.246} = 4.41$$

which is greater than $F(0.05, 22, 22) = 2.12$. The observed p-value is 0.0005 which favors the presence of inter-subject variability.

Part II

Average Bioequivalence

Chapter 4

Statistical Methods for Average Bioequivalence

4.1 Introduction

In Chapter 3, statistical tests for the presence of the fixed effects from a crossover design were reviewed. These tests are often used as a preliminary analysis of the data before the assessment of bioequivalence between formulations is made. Failing to reject the null hypothesis of the equality of formulation effects, however, does not imply the bioequivalence between formulations. In this chapter, we introduce several statistical methods based on raw data (or untransformed data), which are derived under a crossover design, for the assessment of average bioequivalence between formulations in average bioavailability.

In practice, it is usually assumed that there are no carryover effects because a washout period of sufficient length can be chosen to completely eliminate the residual effects from one dosing period to the next. In this case, model 2.5.1 for a general crossover design reduces to

$$Y_{ijk} = \mu + S_{ik} + F_{(j,k)} + P_j + e_{ijk}, \tag{4.1.1}$$

where Y_{ijk}, μ, S_{ik}, $F_{(j,k)}$, P_j, and e_{ijk} are defined in Equation 2.5.1. In Equation 4.1.1, the term $F_{(j,k)}$ for formulation is determined when the sequence and period are determined. Occasionally, however, the reduced model is sometimes expressed as follows:

$$Y_{ijk} = \mu + S_{ik} + F_j + P_{(j,k)} + e_{ijk}, \tag{4.1.2}$$

where

Y_{ijk} is the pharmacokinetic (PK) response, possibly log-transformed, of the ith subject in the kth sequence for the jth formulation, in which $i = 1, 2, \ldots, n_k$, $j = 1, 2, \ldots, J$, and $k = 1, 2, \ldots, g$

μ is the overall mean

F_j is the fixed effect for the jth formulation

$P_{(j,k)}$ is the fixed period effect at which the jth formulation in the kth sequence is administered

S_{ik} and e_{ijk} are defined as in model 2.5.1.

It is also assumed that $\{S_{ik}\}$ and $\{e_{ijk}\}$ are mutually independently distributed with mean 0 and variances σ_S^2 and σ_e^2, respectively. The above equations are equivalent, but different representations of the responses. In this chapter, however, unless otherwise stated, all methods for assessing bioequivalence in average bioavailability will be derived under model 4.1.1 for the standard 2×2 crossover design comparing a test formulation with a reference formulation.

To claim bioequivalence in average bioavailability, as indicated in Section 1.6, for the untransformed data, the ± 20 rule requires that the ratio of the two true formulation averages μ_T/μ_R be within (80%, 120%) limits (or the difference $\mu_T - \mu_R$ is within $\pm 20\%$ of μ_R). However, for the logarithmic transformation of PK responses, the 80/125 rule stated in the U.S. FDA guidance (FDA, 2003b) requests that the ratio of two formulation averages of AUC and C_{max} on the original scale be within (80%, 125%) limit in order to claim average bioequivalence. In other words, on the log-scale, the difference $\mu_T - \mu_R$ is within ± 0.2231. The FDA requires that the bioequivalence be concluded with 90% assurance. In this chapter, however, we review the statistical methods using the ± 20 rule based on the original scale instead of the current 80/125 rule based on the log-scale for evaluation of average bioequivalence due to the following two reasons. First, the ± 20 rule was the first original concept and criterion for evaluation of average bioequivalence, which was used to form the interval hypotheses. Second, since the ± 20 rule based on the original scale uses the 20% of the average bioavailability of the reference formulation as the bioequivalence limit, it could be used to illustrate the drawbacks and consequences if one fails to take into consideration the variability associated with the estimate of the bioequivalence limit. The current 80/125 rule based on the log-scale for assessment of the average bioequivalence is discussed in Chapter 6.

Between 1975 and 1995, several methods for assessment of average bioequivalence using the ± 20 rule based on the original scale have been proposed in the literature. These methods include the confidence interval approach, the method of interval hypotheses testing, the Bayesian approach, and nonparametric methods. For the confidence interval approach, for example, relative to the transformed data, we may construct a confidence interval for μ_T/μ_R (Westlake, 1976) and compare the constructed confidence interval with (80%, 120%) limits. If the constructed confidence interval falls within the limits, then the two formulations are considered bioequivalent. Alternatively, we may construct an exact confidence interval for μ_T/μ_R based on Fieller's theorem (Locke, 1984) or construct a confidence region for (μ_R, μ_T) (Chow, 1990; Chow and Shao, 1990), and compare it with the acceptance region R, which is bounded by two straight lines $\mu_T = 0.8\ \mu_R$ and $\mu_T = 1.2\ \mu_R$. For the method of interval hypotheses testing, Schuirmann (1981, 1987) proposed an approach using two one-sided tests. In this approach, two p-values are obtained to evaluate whether the bioavailability of the test formulation is not too low for one side and not too high for the other side. Instead of testing whether or not the true ratio of means is within (80%, 120%), Anderson and Hauck (1983) suggested a test that rejects the null hypothesis of bioinequivalence in favor of bioequivalence for a small p-value. Rodda and Davis (1980) first introduced the idea of Bayesian analysis for assessing bioequivalence. Mandallaz and Mau (1981) proposed a Bayesian method for the ratio, assuming that (1) there are no carryover effects, (2) the subject effects are fixed, and (3) the number of subjects in each sequence is the same. Grieve (1985) considered a Bayesian approach using a prior distribution that takes into account the inter-subject variability. These methods are based mainly on the normality or lognormality assumptions. Other Bayesian methods were also considered in the literature. See, for example, Selwyn et al. (1981), Grieve (1985), Racine-Poon et al. (1986, 1987), and Ghosh and Khattree (2003). Because of the difficulty of testing these assumptions, the search for appropriate nonparametric methods has received tremendous attention (Cornell, 1980; Steinijans and Diletti, 1983, 1985). Several nonparametric methods have been proposed. These methods include the Wilcoxon–Mann–Whitney two one-sided tests procedure (Hauschke et al., 1990; Liu, 1991) and the bootstrap resampling procedure (Chow et al., 1990).

As indicated in Chapter 3, when the numbers of subjects in each sequence are different, the difference in least squares (LS) means is the MVUE of the direct drug effect, but the difference in raw (direct sample) means is not. In practice, the number of randomized subjects in each sequence is often different from the number of subjects who complete the study in each sequence. Thus, to have a correct and valid statistical inference, all statistical methods for the assessment of average bioequivalence discussed in this chapter are based on LS means. Note that if the number of subjects in each sequence is the same, then the LS means are the same as the raw means. For the sake of convenience, the LS means for the test and reference formulations, denoted by $\overline{Y}_{\mathrm{T}}$ and $\overline{Y}_{\mathrm{R}}$, are referred to as the (observed) test and reference means, respectively. It is easily seen that

$$E(\overline{Y}_{\mathrm{R}}) = E[(\overline{Y}_{11} + \overline{Y}_{22})/2] = \mu + F_{\mathrm{R}} \quad \text{and}$$
$$E(\overline{Y}_{\mathrm{T}}) = E[(\overline{Y}_{21} + \overline{Y}_{12})/2] = \mu + F_{\mathrm{T}}.$$

Let $\mu_{\mathrm{R}} = \mu + F_{\mathrm{R}}$ and $\mu_{\mathrm{T}} = \mu + F_{\mathrm{T}}$. Then μ_{R} and μ_{T} are indeed the unknown true reference and test formulation averages. Note that μ_{R} and μ_{T} do not contain any nuisance fixed effects, such as period effects. Therefore, the difference or the ratio of μ_{T} and μ_{R} involves only the direct formulation effects. Thus, in this chapter, various methods using LS means for statistical inferences of either $\mu_{\mathrm{T}} - \mu_{\mathrm{R}}$ or $\mu_{\mathrm{T}}/\mu_{\mathrm{R}}$ are introduced for the assessment of bioequivalence in average bioavailability.

In the following sections, more details on the confidence interval approach, the method of interval hypotheses testing, the Bayesian approach, and some nonparametric methods are given for the untransformed PK responses. All results provided in this chapter, however, can be directly applied to the log-transformed data, which is discussed in details in Chapter 6. The example presented in Section 3.6 is used to illustrate these methods. In Section 4.6, other possible alternatives for the assessment of bioequivalence are discussed. A brief discussion is also included in this section. Some SAS programs for the methods introduced in this chapter are included in Appendix B.

4.2 Confidence Interval Approach

In Chapter 3, a test for the null hypothesis of the equality of the two formulations of a drug product was derived under the standard 2×2 crossover design. Such a test for assessing average bioequivalence, which has been criticized by many researchers (Westlake, 1972; Metzler, 1974; Dunnett and Gent, 1977), is not an appropriate statistical method. Alternatively, Westlake (1976) and Metzler (1974) indicated that the method of confidence interval is an appropriate method for assessing average bioequivalence. On the basis of the confidence interval, Westlake (1981) suggested the following action for decision making.

> If a $(1-2\alpha) \times 100\%$ confidence interval for the difference $(\mu_T - \mu_R)$ or the ratio (μ_T/μ_R) is within the acceptance limits as recommended by the regulatory agency, then conclude that the test formulation (i.e., the test formulation is bioequivalent to the reference formulation); otherwise reject it.

If the ± 20 rule, as indicated in Section 1.6, is adopted, then α is usually chosen to be 0.05 and the acceptance limits (or equivalence limits) are either

1. $\pm 20\%$ of the observed average bioavailability for the reference formulation if the 90% confidence interval for $\mu_T - \mu_R$ is used, or
2. 80% and 120% if the 90% confidence interval for μ_T/μ_R is used.

Thus, we may conclude average bioequivalence if either the 90% confidence interval for the difference in average bioavailability of the two formulations is within $\pm 20\%$ of the observed reference mean or the 90% confidence interval for the ratio of average bioavailability of the two formulations is within 80% and 120% limits. Note that the two decision rules are equivalent when μ_R is known. Although the confidence interval for the difference can be converted to be a confidence interval for the ratio, they may lead to different conclusions of bioequivalence when $\overline{Y}_R$ is assumed to be the true μ_R.

Given the above action of decision making, several methods for constructing a 90% confidence interval for $\mu_T - \mu_R$ or μ_T/μ_R have been proposed under a raw data (or untransformed data) model. These methods include (1) the classic confidence interval, which is also known as the shortest confidence interval; (2) Westlake's symmetric confidence interval; (3) confidence interval for μ_T/μ_R based on Fieller's theorem; and (4) Chow and Shao's joint confidence region for (μ_R, μ_T).

In the following section, these methods are derived under the standard 2×2 crossover design assuming that there are no carryover effects. For a general crossover design with more than two formulations, the methods can be treated similarly.

4.2.1 Classic (Shortest) Confidence Interval

Let $\overline{Y}_T$ and $\overline{Y}_R$ be the respective LS means for the test and reference formulations, which can be obtained from the sequence-by-period means. The classic (or shortest)

$(1-2\alpha)\times 100\%$ confidence interval can then be obtained based on the following t statistic:

$$T=\frac{(\overline{Y}_{\mathrm{T}}-\overline{Y}_{\mathrm{R}})-(\mu_{\mathrm{T}}-\mu_{\mathrm{R}})}{\widehat{\sigma}_{\mathrm{d}}\sqrt{\frac{1}{n_1}+\frac{1}{n_2}}}, \tag{4.2.1}$$

where n_1 and n_2 are the numbers of subjects in sequences 1 and 2, respectively, and $\widehat{\sigma}_{\mathrm{d}}$ is given in Section 3.3. Under normality assumptions, T follows a central Student t distribution with degrees of freedom (n_1+n_2-2). Thus, the classic $(1-2\alpha)\times 100\%$ confidence interval for $\mu_{\mathrm{T}}-\mu_{\mathrm{R}}$ can be obtained as follows:

$$\begin{aligned} L_1&=(\overline{Y}_{\mathrm{T}}-\overline{Y}_{\mathrm{R}})-t(\alpha,\, n_1+n_2-2)\widehat{\sigma}_{\mathrm{d}}\sqrt{\frac{1}{n_1}+\frac{1}{n_2}},\\ U_1&=(\overline{Y}_{\mathrm{T}}-\overline{Y}_{\mathrm{R}})-t(\alpha,\, n_1+n_2-2)\widehat{\sigma}_{\mathrm{d}}\sqrt{\frac{1}{n_1}+\frac{1}{n_2}}. \end{aligned} \tag{4.2.2}$$

The above confidence interval for $\mu_{\mathrm{T}}-\mu_{\mathrm{R}}$ can be converted into a $(1-2\alpha)\times 100\%$ approximate confidence interval for $\mu_{\mathrm{T}}/\mu_{\mathrm{R}}$ by dividing by $\overline{Y}_{\mathrm{R}}$ is the true reference mean (μ_{R}). That is,

$$\begin{aligned} L_2&=(L_1/\overline{Y}_{\mathrm{R}}+1)\times 100\%,\\ U_2&=(U_1/\overline{Y}_{\mathrm{R}}+1)\times 100\%. \end{aligned} \tag{4.2.3}$$

Let θ_{L} and θ_{U} be the respective lower and upper equivalence limits for the difference, Also, let δ_{L} and δ_{U} be the respective lower and upper equivalence limits for the ratio. Then, we conclude average bioequivalence if

$$\begin{aligned} &(L_1,\, U_1)\in(\theta_{\mathrm{L}},\, \theta_{\mathrm{U}}),\\ \text{or}\quad &(L_2,\, U_2)\in(\delta_{\mathrm{L}},\, \delta_{\mathrm{U}}), \end{aligned} \tag{4.2.4}$$

where

$\theta_{\mathrm{L}}=-0.2\ \mu_{\mathrm{R}}$
$\theta_{\mathrm{U}}=0.2\ \mu_{\mathrm{R}}$
$\delta_{\mathrm{L}}=80\%$
$\delta_{\mathrm{U}}=120\%$ for the ± 20 rule.

The use of confidence interval as a tool for assessing average bioequivalence based on Equation 4.2.4 seems intuitively appealing. There is, however, a discrepancy between the concept of the confidence interval and the action of decision making. A $(1-2\alpha)\times 100\%$ confidence interval for $\mu_{\mathrm{T}}-\mu_{\mathrm{R}}$ is a random interval and its associated confidence limits are, in fact, random variables. The fundamental concept of a $(1-2\alpha)\times 100\%$ confidence interval for $\mu_{\mathrm{T}}-\mu_{\mathrm{R}}$ is that if the same study can be repeatedly carried out many times, say B, then $(1-2\alpha)\times 100\%$ times of the B constructed random intervals will cover $\mu_{\mathrm{T}}-\mu_{\mathrm{R}}$ (Bickel and Doksum, 1977). In other words, in the long run, a $(1-2\alpha)\times 100\%$ confidence interval will have at least a $1-2\alpha$ chance to cover the true mean difference (or ratio) because, under the normality assumptions, we have

$$P\{\mu_T - \mu_R \in (L_1, U_1)\} = 1 - 2\alpha.$$

However, the $(1-2\alpha) \times 100\%$ confidence interval does not guarantee that, in the long run, the chance of the $(1-2\alpha) \times 100\%$ confidence interval being within the equivalence limits is at least $1-2\alpha$, that is, the probability

$$P\{(L_1, U_1) \in (\theta_L, \theta_U)\}$$

is not necessarily greater than or equal to $1-2\alpha$. To demonstrate this, as an example, a small simulation study was conducted. A total of 1000 sets of AUC values were generated from the statistical model for the standard 2×2 crossover design under normality assumptions. For simplicity, we assumed there were no period and carry-over effects. The true test and reference formulation means were both chosen to be 100 with $n_1 = n_2 = 9$, 12. Thus, the equivalence limits for the difference are from −20 to 20. The following intra-subject variabilities were considered: $\sigma_e^2 = 400$, 900, and 1600 (or CV = 20%, 30%, and 40%), where CV is defined as $(\sigma_e/\mu_R) \times 100\%$. For each random sample, (L_1, U_1) was calculated. The results are summarized in Table 4.2.1. The results indicate that, for $n_1 = n_2 = 9$, in the long run, 76.8% of confidence intervals (L_1, U_1) will be within the equivalence limits when CV is 20%. However, only 24.7% and 2.1% of confidence intervals will be within the equivalence limits for CV = 30% and 40%, respectively. For $n_1 = n_2 = 12$, a similar pattern was observed. Thus, when there is a large CV (or large variability), the confidence interval approach for assessing bioequivalence in average bioavailability may not have the desired level of assurance required by the FDA. In other words, the probability of correctly concluding bioequivalence may not be of the desired level. In this case, it is suggested that a parametric bootstrap random samples (Efron, 1982) be simulated based on the observed values (i.e., assuming these values are the true population values) to evaluate the performance of (L_1, U_1) in the long run (i.e., to determine the level of assurance of (L_1, U_1)). Note that the probability of correctly concluding bioequivalence for (L_1, U_1) and (L_2, U_2) is the same when μ_R is known.

TABLE 4.2.1: Summary of simulation results.

Sample Size	**Reference Mean**	**Test Mean**	**CV (%)**	**% of CIs Containing 0**	**% of CIs within (−20, 20)**
$n_1 = n_2 = 9$	100	100	20	90.3	76.8
			30	91.3	24.7
			40	90.4	2.1
$n_1 = n_2 = 12$	100	100	20	90.7	91.5
=			30	89.2	43.9
			40	88.6	7.5

Example 4.2.1

To illustrate the use of the classic (shortest) confidence intervals for $\mu_T - \mu_R$ Equation 4.2.2 and μ_T/μ_R Equation 4.2.3, consider the example presented in Section 3.6. On the basis of the AUC values from Table 3.6.1, we have

$$\begin{aligned}\overline{Y}_T &= 80.272;\\ \overline{Y}_R &= 82.559;\\ t(0.05, 22) &= 1.717; \quad \text{and}\\ \widehat{\sigma}_d &= 9.145.\end{aligned}$$

Thus, the equivalence limits for $\mu_T - \mu_R$ are given by -16.51 and 16.51. The confidence interval Equation 4.2.2 for $\mu_T - \mu_R$ can be obtained as follows:

$$(80.272 - 82.559) \pm (1.717)(9.145)\sqrt{0.167}.$$

Thus, $(L_1, U_1) = (-8.698, 4.123)$ and the corresponding approximate 90% confidence interval for μ_T/μ_R, (L_2, U_2), is given by (89.46%, 104.99%). As both (L_1, U_1) and (L_2, U_2) satisfy Equation 4.2.4, we conclude that the test formulation is average bioequivalent to the reference formulation.

The finite samples performance of (L_1, U_1) was also evaluated through a small simulation study. A total of 1000 bootstrap samples were generated from the standard 2×2 crossover model 4.1.1 under normality assumptions with $n_1 = n_2 = 12$, $\mu_R = 82.599$, $\mu_T = 80.272$, and $\sigma_e = 12.933$ (i.e., $\sigma_d = 9.145$). For each bootstrap sample, (L_1, U_1) was calculated. The results indicate that, as expected, 90.6% of the 1000 confidence intervals cover $\mu_T - \mu_R = -2.287$. On the other hand, 98% of these intervals are within the equivalence limits $(-16.51, 16.51)$, where $16.51 = (0.2)\ (82.559)$. The average lower and upper limits for these intervals are -8.68 and 4.00, which are close to $(-8.698, 4.123)$ obtained from the observed data. Thus, there is more than 95% assurance that the observed confidence interval will be within the equivalence limits $(-16.51, 16.51)$ in the long run. This certainly supports the conclusion of average bioequivalence between the two formulations.

Suppose that the observed test and reference means remain the same as 80.272 and 82.559, respectively, but the observed intra-subject variability $\widehat{\sigma}_e$ increases to 27.659 (or $\widehat{\sigma}_d = 19.558$). It can be verified that $(L_1, U_1) = (-15.989, 11.413)$ are totally within the equivalence limits $(-16.51, 16.51)$. Hence, according to Equation 4.2.4, the test formulation is also average bioequivalent to the reference formulation. However, based on simulation study of 1000 bootstrap samples with $\mu_R = 82.559$, $\mu_T = 80.272$, $\sigma_e = 27.659$, and $n_1 = n_2 = 12$, 89.6% of the 1000 90% confidence intervals cover $\mu_T - \mu_R = -2.287$, with the average lower and upper limits being -15.832 and 11.250, but only 26.7% of these 1000 random intervals are within the equivalence limits $(-16.51, 16.51)$. Therefore, the simulation result contradicted the decision made based on the observed 90% confidence interval for $\mu_T - \mu_R$. This example reveals the importance of the intra-subject variability in the assessment of average bioequivalence. Thus, it is suggested that a simulation study be conducted to evaluate the finite sample performance of (L_1, U_1) before a decision on average bioequivalence is made.

4.2.2 Westlake's Symmetric Confidence Interval

It is apparent from Equation 4.2.2 that the classic $(1-2\alpha)\times 100\%$ confidence interval for $\mu_T - \mu_R$ is symmetric about $\overline{Y}_T - \overline{Y}_R$ and not symmetric about 0. Also, it can be seen from Equation 4.2.3 that the confidence interval for μ_T/μ_R is symmetric about $\overline{Y}_T/\overline{Y}_R$, and not about unity. Basically, the classic confidence interval derived from an unpaired two-sample t statistic in Equation 4.2.1 is as follows:

$$|T| < k \quad \text{or} \quad -k < T < k,$$

where k is the upper αth percentile of a central t distribution with degrees of freedom (n_1+n_2-2). In general, a $(1-2\alpha)\times 100\%$ confidence interval for the difference $\mu_T - \mu_R$ can be expressed as

$$k_2 < T < k_1, \tag{4.2.5}$$

where k_1 and k_2 are chosen so that the probability from k_2 to k_1 based on a central t distribution with (n_1+n_2-2) degrees of freedom is $(1-2\alpha)$, that is,

$$\int_{k_2}^{k_1} T\,\mathrm{d}t = 1 - 2\alpha.$$

When $k_2 = -k_1$, Equation 4.2.5 reduces to the classic confidence interval Equation 4.2.2.

As the equivalence limits are usually given in a symmetric form (e.g., -20% to 20%), Westlake (1976) suggested that the confidence interval be adjusted to be symmetric about 0 for the difference (or about unity for the ratio). For the difference, it is desirable to construct a confidence interval as follows:

$$-\Delta < \mu_T - \mu_R < \Delta. \tag{4.2.6}$$

This is, however, equivalent to constructing a confidence interval for the test formulation (μ_T), which is symmetric about the reference mean (μ_R), that is,

$$\mu_R - \Delta < \mu_T < \mu_R + \Delta. \tag{4.2.7}$$

The inequality in Equation 4.2.5 can be rearranged as:

$$\mu_R + k_2\widehat{\sigma}_d\sqrt{\frac{1}{n_1}+\frac{1}{n_2}} - \left(\overline{Y}_R - \overline{Y}_T\right) < \mu_T < \mu_R + k_1\widehat{\sigma}_d\sqrt{\frac{1}{n_1}+\frac{1}{n_2}} - \left(\overline{Y}_R - \overline{Y}_T\right).$$

Hence,

$$\Delta = k_1 \widehat{\sigma}_d \sqrt{\frac{1}{n_1} + \frac{1}{n_2}} - (\overline{Y}_R - \overline{Y}_T)$$
$$= -k_2 \widehat{\sigma}_d \sqrt{\frac{1}{n_1} + \frac{1}{n_2}} + (\overline{Y}_R - \overline{Y}_T).$$

This implies that

$$(k_1 + k_2)\ \widehat{\sigma}_d \sqrt{\frac{1}{n_1} + \frac{1}{n_2}} = 2(\overline{Y}_R - \overline{Y}_T). \tag{4.2.8}$$

The test formulation is concluded to be average bioequivalent with the reference formulation according to the ± 20 rule if $|\Delta| < 0.2\ \mu_R$. To determine the values of k_1 and k_2, an iterative method is needed to solve the equation

$$\int_{k_2}^{k_1} T\,\mathrm{d}t = 1 - 2\alpha$$

for k_1 and k_2 under constraint Equation 4.2.8. This can be done using some statistical software such as SAS. In Appendix B, an SAS program for determination of k_1 and k_2 is given.

Example 4.2.2

For the example in Section 3.6, we can apply the SAS program to determine k_1 and k_2. After several iterations, k_1 and k_2 in Equation 4.2.8 are 2.599 and -1.373, respectively. This gives Δ a value of 7.413. Thus, Westlake's symmetric confidence interval for the true test formulation mean is within 7.413 (or 8.98%) of the true reference mean. Hence, we conclude that the test formulation is average bioequivalent to the reference formulation according to the ± 20 rule.

Let p_w be the coverage probability of Westlake's symmetric confidence interval. It was shown (Westlake, 1976) that

$$\lim_{|\mu_T - \mu_R| \to \infty} p_w = 1 - 2\alpha \leq p_w \leq \lim_{|\mu_T - \mu_R| \to 0} p_w = 1. \tag{4.2.9}$$

Thus, Westlake's symmetric confidence interval approach is somewhat conservative in the determination of average bioequivalence, for it has at least $1 - 2\alpha$ coverage probability.

The concept of using a symmetric confidence interval for assessing average bioequivalence has been discussed and criticized by many researchers since being introduced by Westlake (1976). See, for example, Mantel (1977), Kirkwood (1981), Mandallaz and Mau (1981), Shirley (1976), Steinijans and Diletti (1983), and

Wijnand and Timmer (1983). Among these criticisms, the following are probably the most common:

1. Because Westlake's symmetric confidence interval is symmetric about μ_R, rather than $\overline{Y}_T - \overline{Y}_R$, the interval is, in fact, shifted away from the direction in which the sample difference was observed.

2. The tail probabilities associated with Westlake's symmetric confidence interval is not symmetric. Westlake's symmetric confidence interval moves from a two-sided to a one-sided approach as $\mu_T - \mu_R$ or σ_e^2 increases.

Metzler (1988) argued that Westlake's symmetric confidence interval should be used as a tool for decision making, rather than for estimation or testing. However, it should be recognized that the assessment of bioequivalence depends on the results from valid statistical inference such as estimation or interval hypotheses testing, which should not be separated from the decision making.

4.2.3 Confidence Interval Based on Fieller's Theorem

It can be seen that both the classic confidence interval and Westlake's symmetric confidence interval for the ratio μ_T/μ_R do not take into account the variability of $\overline{Y}_R$ and the correlation between $\overline{Y}_R$ and $\overline{Y}_T - \overline{Y}_R$. To account for the variability of $\overline{Y}_R$, Locke (1984) proposed an approach for constructing a $(1-2\alpha) \times 100\%$ confidence interval for μ_T/μ_R based on Fieller's theorem (Fieller, 1954). This method has become very attractive because (1) it provides an exact $(1-2\alpha) \times 100\%$ confidence interval for μ_T/μ_R, and (2) it does take into account the variability of $\overline{Y}_R$. Recall that in Chapter 2, the responses for the ith subject in sequence 1 at periods I and II, $(Y_{i11}, Y_{i21})'$, had a bivariate normal distribution with mean vector $\boldsymbol{\alpha}_1$ and covariance Σ_1, where

$$\boldsymbol{\alpha}_1 = \begin{bmatrix} \mu + F_R + P_1 \\ \mu + F_T + P_2 \end{bmatrix} \quad \text{and} \quad \boldsymbol{\Sigma}_1 = \begin{bmatrix} \sigma_R^2 + \sigma_S^2 & \sigma_S^2 \\ \sigma_S^2 & \sigma_T^2 + \sigma_S^2 \end{bmatrix}.$$

Similarly, (Y_{i12}, Y_{i22}) are i.i.d. normal with mean vector $\boldsymbol{\alpha}_2$ and covariance $\boldsymbol{\Sigma}_2$, where

$$\boldsymbol{\alpha}_2 = \begin{bmatrix} \mu + F_T + P_1 \\ \mu + F_R + P_2 \end{bmatrix} \quad \text{and} \quad \boldsymbol{\Sigma}_2 = \begin{bmatrix} \sigma_T^2 + \sigma_S^2 & \sigma_S^2 \\ \sigma_S^2 & \sigma_R^2 + \sigma_S^2 \end{bmatrix}.$$

Let $\delta = \mu_T/\mu_R = (\mu + F_T)/(\mu + F_R)$. Define

$$U_{ik}^* = \begin{cases} \frac{1}{2}(Y_{i21} - \delta Y_{i11}), & i = 1, 2, \ldots, n_1, \quad k = 1 \\ \frac{1}{2}(Y_{i12} - \delta Y_{i22}), & i = 1, 2, \ldots, n_2, \quad k = 2. \end{cases} \tag{4.2.10}$$

Then U_{i1}^* are i.i.d. normal with mean $(P_2 - \delta P_1)/2$ and variance $\sigma_\delta^2/4$, where

$$\sigma_\delta^2 = (\sigma_T^2 + \sigma_S^2) - 2\delta\sigma_S^2 + \delta^2(\sigma_R^2 + \sigma_S^2), \quad \text{for} \quad i = 1, 2, \ldots, n_1,$$

and U_{i2}^* are i.i.d. normal with mean $(P_1 - \delta P_2)/2$ and variance $\sigma_\delta^2/4$, for $i = 1, 2, \ldots, n_2$. $\{U_{i1}^*, i=1, 2, \ldots, n_1\}$ and $\{U_{i2}^*, i=1, 2, \ldots, n_2\}$ are two independent samples from normal distributions with equal variances. Thus, a $(1-2\alpha)\times 100\%$ confidence interval for δ can be obtained based on an unpaired two-sample t statistic. First, let $\overline{U}_{\cdot k}^*$ be the sample means of U_{ik}^* for $k=1, 2$ and S_u^2 be the pooled sample variance of U_{ik}^*, that is,

$$\overline{U}_{\cdot k}^* = \frac{1}{n_k}\sum_{i=1}^{n_k} U_{ik}^*, \quad \text{and} \tag{4.2.11}$$

$$S_u^2 = \frac{1}{n_1 + n_2 - 2}\sum_{k=1}^{2}\sum_{i=1}^{n_k}(U_{ik} - \overline{U}_{\cdot k})^2. \tag{4.2.12}$$

Note that $(\overline{U}_{\cdot 1}^* + \overline{U}_{\cdot 2}^*)$ is normally distributed with mean 0 and variance $\omega\sigma_\delta^2$, where

$$\omega = \frac{1}{4}\left(\frac{1}{n_1} + \frac{1}{n_2}\right).$$

Therefore, the statistic

$$T = \frac{\overline{U}_{\cdot 1}^* + \overline{U}_{\cdot 2}^*}{\sqrt{\omega S_u^2}}$$

has a central t distribution with $(n_1 + n_2 - 2)$ degrees of freedom. However, $\overline{U}_1^* + \overline{U}_2^*$ can be expressed in terms of the LS means for the test and reference formulations as follows:

$$\begin{aligned}\overline{U}_{\cdot 1}^* + \overline{U}_{\cdot 2}^* &= \tfrac{1}{2}(\overline{Y}_{\cdot 21} - \delta\overline{Y}_{\cdot 11})\,\tfrac{1}{2}(\overline{Y}_{\cdot 12} - \delta\overline{Y}_{\cdot 22}) \\ &= \tfrac{1}{2}(\overline{Y}_{\cdot 21} - \delta\overline{Y}_{\cdot 12}) - \delta\,\tfrac{1}{2}(\overline{Y}_{\cdot 11} - \delta\overline{Y}_{\cdot 22}) \\ &= \overline{Y}_T - \delta\overline{Y}_R.\end{aligned} \tag{4.2.13}$$

Similarly, it can be verified that

$$S_u^2 = S_{TT}^2 - 2\delta S_{TR} + \delta^2 S_{RR}^2,$$

where

$$S_{RR}^2 = \frac{1}{n_1+n_2-2}\left[\sum_{i=1}^{n_1}(Y_{i11}-\overline{Y}_{\cdot 11})^2 + \sum_{i=1}^{n_2}(Y_{i22}-\overline{Y}_{\cdot 22})^2\right],$$

$$S_{TT}^2 = \frac{1}{n_1+n_2-2}\left[\sum_{i=1}^{n_1}(Y_{i21}-\overline{Y}_{\cdot 21})^2 + \sum_{i=1}^{n_2}(Y_{i12}-\overline{Y}_{\cdot 12})^2\right],$$

$$S_{TR} = \frac{1}{n_1+n_2-2}\left[\sum_{i=1}^{n_2}(Y_{i11}-\overline{Y}_{\cdot 11})(Y_{i21}-\overline{Y}_{\cdot 21}) + \sum_{i=1}^{n_2}(Y_{i12}-\overline{Y}_{\cdot 12})(Y_{i22}-\overline{Y}_{\cdot 22})\right].$$

Thus, T can be rewritten as

$$T = \frac{\overline{Y}_T - \delta\overline{Y}_R}{\left[\omega(S_{TT}^2 - 2\delta S_{TR} + \delta^2 S_{RR}^2\right]^{1/2}}. \tag{4.2.14}$$

Hence, a $(1-2\alpha)\times 100\%$ confidence interval for δ can be obtained as follows:

$$\left\{\delta | T^2 \le t^2(\alpha, n_1+n_2-2)\right\}. \tag{4.2.15}$$

The lower and upper limits of the $(1-2\alpha)\times 100\%$ confidence interval for δ, if they exist, are the two roots of the following quadratic equation

$$(\overline{Y}_T - \delta\overline{Y}_R)^2 - t^2(\alpha, n_1+n_2-2)\,\omega\left(S_{TT}^2 - 2\delta S_{TR} + \delta^2 S_{RR}^2\right), \tag{4.2.16}$$

which are given by

$$\begin{aligned} L_3 &= \frac{1}{1-G}\left[\left\{\frac{\overline{Y}_T}{\overline{Y}_R} - G\frac{S_{TR}}{S_{RR}^2}\right\} - \left\{t(\alpha, n_1+n_2-2)\frac{\sqrt{\omega S_{RR}^2}}{\overline{Y}_R}G^*\right\}\right], \\ U_3 &= \frac{1}{1-G}\left[\left\{\frac{\overline{Y}_T}{\overline{Y}_R} - G\frac{S_{TR}}{S_{RR}^2}\right\} + \left\{t(\alpha, n_1+n_2-2)\frac{\sqrt{\omega S_{RR}^2}}{\overline{Y}_R}G^*\right\}\right], \end{aligned} \tag{4.2.17}$$

where

$$G = \{t(\alpha, n_1+n_2-2)\}^2\left[\frac{\omega S_{RR}^2}{\overline{Y}_R^2}\right],$$

and

$$G_2^* = \left\{\frac{\overline{Y}_T}{\overline{Y}_R}\right\}^2 + \frac{S_{TT}^2}{S_{RR}^2}(1-G) + \frac{S_{TR}}{S_{RR}^2}\left\{G\frac{S_{TR}}{S_{RR}^2} - 2\frac{\overline{Y}_T}{\overline{Y}_R}\right\}.$$

As indicated by Fieller (1954), Kendall and Stuart (1979), and Locke (1984), the solutions to the quadratic Equation 4.2.16 may not result in an actual interval. The conditions for both L_3 and U_3 to be finite positive real numbers are

$$\begin{aligned}&\text{(a)}\ \frac{\overline{Y}_{\mathrm{R}}}{\left[\omega S_{\mathrm{RR}}^2\right]^{1/2}} > t(\alpha, n_1 + n_2 - 2), \quad \text{and} \\ &\text{(b)}\ \frac{\overline{Y}_{\mathrm{T}}}{\left[\omega S_{\mathrm{TT}}^2\right]^{1/2}} > t(\alpha, n_1 + n_2 - 2).\end{aligned} \tag{4.2.18}$$

In other words, it requires that the LS means for both the test and the reference formulations be statistically significantly greater than 0 at the α level of significance. Condition (a) in Equation 4.2.18 implies that if the variability of the reference formulation is large enough for (a) to be false, then there may not exist an interval for δ or the interval may contain imaginary numbers. On the other hand, the interval may contain negative values if the variability of the test formulation is sufficiently large for condition (b) to be false even when the reference formulation satisfies condition (a). Thus, in practice, we conclude average bioequivalence if

1. Both conditions (a) and (b) of Equation 4.2.18 hold;

2. $L_3 > 80\%$ and $U_3 < 120\%$.

Otherwise, we are in favor of average bioinequivalence.

The exact $(1 - 2\alpha) \times 100\%$ confidence interval for $\mu_{\mathrm{T}}/\mu_{\mathrm{R}}$ based on Fieller's theorem takes into account not only the variability of $\overline{Y}_{\mathrm{R}}$ but also the inter-subject variability. In addition, it was derived under a very mild assumption that requires the only normality of the two responses observed on the same subject. Hence, even when $\sigma_{\mathrm{T}}^2 \neq \sigma_{\mathrm{R}}^2$, the exact $(1 - 2\alpha) \times 100\%$ confidence interval for $\mu_{\mathrm{T}}/\mu_{\mathrm{R}}$ by Fieller's theorem is still valid.

Example 4.2.3

For the example in Section 3.6, it can be verified that both conditions (a) and (b) of Equation 4.2.18 are satisfied; that is,

$$\frac{\overline{Y}_{\mathrm{R}}}{\left[\omega S_{\mathrm{RR}}^2\right]^{1/2}} = 19.27 \quad \text{and} \quad \frac{\overline{Y}_{\mathrm{T}}}{\left[\omega S_{\mathrm{TT}}^2\right]^{1/2}} = 18.73,$$

which are both greater than $t(0.05, 22) = 1.717$. Thus, Fieller's theorem will give a positive real interval. It can be found that $G = 0.003$ and $G^* = 0.735$, which leads to a confidence interval for the ratio of (89.78%, 105.19%). Thus, we conclude the two formulations are bioequivalent.

Schuirmann (1989) considered a special case of Equation 4.2.15 by assuming that $\sigma_{\mathrm{R}}^2 = \sigma_{\mathrm{T}}^2$ and $\sigma_{\mathrm{S}}^2 = 0$ (i.e., the subject effects are assumed to be fixed). Schuirmann (1989) refers to such an approach as the fixed Fieller's confidence interval approach. Here, the lower and upper limits of $(1 - 2\alpha) \times 100\%$ confidence interval for δ become

$$L_4 = \frac{1}{1-G_1}\left[\frac{\overline{Y}_T}{\overline{Y}_R} - t(\alpha, n_1+n_2-2)\frac{\sqrt{\omega \text{MS}_{\text{intra}}}}{\overline{Y}_R}\sqrt{\left(\frac{\overline{Y}_T}{\overline{Y}_R}\right)^2 + (1-G_1)}\right],$$

$$U_4 = \frac{1}{1-G_1}\left[\frac{\overline{Y}_T}{\overline{Y}_R} + t(\alpha, n_1+n_2-2)\frac{\sqrt{\omega \text{MS}_{\text{intra}}}}{\overline{Y}_R}\sqrt{\left(\frac{\overline{Y}_T}{\overline{Y}_R}\right)^2 + (1-G_1)}\right], \tag{4.2.19}$$

where

$$G_1 = [t(\alpha, n_1+n_2-2)]^2\left(\frac{\omega \text{MS}_{\text{intra}}}{\overline{Y}_R^2}\right).$$

It can be verified that there exists no interval for the fixed Fieller's confidence interval values $G_1 < 1$.

For the calculation of the lower and upper bound of Fieller's confidence interval, an SAS program has been developed that is given in Appendix B.1. The SAS program also includes the calculation of the above fixed Fieller's confidence interval.

Yee (1986) also attempted to account for the inter-subject variability for construction of a confidence interval for the ratio based on Fieller's theorem through a linear combination of the inter-subject and intra-subject mean-squared errors by a Satterthwaite approximation. His approach, however, is not an exact procedure, but an approximation, since the procedure involves the substitution of an estimate of the intra-subject correlation $\sigma_S^2/(\sigma_S^2 + \sigma_e^2)$ (Schiurmann, 1989).

4.2.4 Chow and Shao's Joint Confidence Region

Instead of constructing $(1-2\alpha) \times 100\%$ confidence intervals for $\mu_T - \mu_R$ and μ_T/μ_R, Chow and Shao (1990) proposed an alternative approach for assessing average bioequivalence by constructing an exact $(1-2\alpha) \times 100\%$ confidence region for (μ_R, μ_T). If the constructed confidence region is within the following bioequivalence region:

$$\{(\mu_R, \mu_T) | \delta_L < \mu_T/\mu_R < \delta_U\},$$

then we conclude that the two formulations are average bioequivalent. In the following, the method will be derived under model 4.1.2. Since S_{ik} consists of the fixed effect of the kth sequence and the random effect of the ith subject in the kth sequence, Equation 4.1.2 can be rewritten as

$$\begin{aligned} Y_{ijk} &= \mu + S_{ik} + F_j + P_{(j,k)} + e_{ijk} \\ &= \mu + G_k + S_{i(k)} + F_j + P_{(j,k)} + e_{ijk}, \end{aligned} \tag{4.2.20}$$

where

Y_{ijk}, μ, F_j, $P_{(j,k)}$, and e_{ijk} are defined as before
G_k is the fixed effect of the kth sequence
$S_{i(k)}$ is the random effect of the ith subject nested in the kth sequence

Thus,

$$\mu_R = \mu + F_R \quad \text{and} \quad \mu_T = \mu + F_T.$$

Under the normality assumptions,

$$\boldsymbol{X}_{ik} = \begin{bmatrix} Y_{i1k} \\ Y_{i2k} \end{bmatrix} \sim N(\boldsymbol{\mu}_k, \boldsymbol{\Sigma}),$$

and $\boldsymbol{X}_{ik}$, $i = 1, 2, \ldots, n_k$, $k = 1, 2$, are mutually independent, where $\Sigma > 0$ is the covariance matrix and

$$\boldsymbol{\mu}_1 = \begin{bmatrix} \mu_R + P_1 + G_1 \\ \mu_T + P_2 + G_1 \end{bmatrix} \quad \text{and} \quad \boldsymbol{\mu}_2 = \begin{bmatrix} \mu_R + P_2 + G_2 \\ \mu_T + P_1 + G_2 \end{bmatrix}. \tag{4.2.21}$$

Chow and Shao (1990) suggested testing the presence of the joint period and sequence effects as the first step for the assessment of bioequivalence. That is, the hypotheses

$$\begin{aligned} &\text{H}_0\text{: } \boldsymbol{\mu}_1 = \boldsymbol{\mu}_2 \\ \text{versus } &\text{H}_a\text{: } \boldsymbol{\mu}_1 \neq \boldsymbol{\mu}_2 \end{aligned} \tag{4.2.22}$$

are tested using the following test statistic

$$T = \frac{n_1 n_2}{2(n_1 + n_2)}(n_1 + n_2 - 3)(\overline{\mathbf{X}}_{\cdot 1} - \overline{\mathbf{X}}_{\cdot 2})'(\mathbf{S}_1 + \mathbf{S}_2)^{-1}(\overline{\mathbf{X}}_{\cdot 1} - \overline{\mathbf{X}}_{\cdot 2}),$$

where

$$\overline{\mathbf{X}}_{\cdot k} = \frac{1}{n_k}\sum_{i=1}^{n_k} \mathbf{X}_{ik},$$

$$\mathbf{S}_k = \sum_{i=1}^{n_k} (\mathbf{X}_{ik} - \overline{\mathbf{X}}_{\cdot k})(\mathbf{X}_{ik} - \overline{\mathbf{X}}_{\cdot k})', \quad k = 1, 2.$$

We reject H_0 in Equation 4.2.22 at the α level of significance if

$$T \geq F(1 - \alpha, 2, n_1 + n_2 - 3),$$

where $F(1 - \alpha, 2, n_1 + n_2 - 3)$ is the $1 - \alpha$ quantile of the F distribution with 2 and $(n_1 + n_2 - 3)$ degrees of freedom.

If we fail to reject H_0 in Equation 4.2.22, then $\mathbf{X}_{ik}$, $i = 1, 2, \ldots, n_k$, $k = 1, 2$ have the same distribution. Let

$$\mathbf{S} = \sum_{k=1}^{2} \sum_{i=1}^{n_k} (\mathbf{X}_{ik} - \overline{\mathbf{X}}_{..})(\mathbf{X}_{ik} - \overline{\mathbf{X}}_{..})',$$

where

$$\overline{\mathbf{X}}_{..} = \frac{1}{\mathbf{n_1} + \mathbf{n_2}} \sum_{k=1}^{2} \sum_{i=1}^{n_k} \mathbf{X}_{ik} = \begin{bmatrix} \overline{\mathbf{Y}}_R^* \\ \overline{\mathbf{Y}}_T^* \end{bmatrix},$$

where $\overline{Y}_R^*$ and $\overline{Y}_T^*$ are the direct sample means for the reference and the test formulation, respectively. Then, $\mathbf{S}$ and $\overline{\mathbf{X}}_{..}$ are independent and

$$T_1 = \frac{(n_1 + n_2)(n_1 + n_2 - 2)}{2} (\overline{\mathbf{X}}_{..} - \boldsymbol{\mu})' \mathbf{S}^{-1} (\overline{\mathbf{X}}_{..} - \boldsymbol{\mu})$$

has an F distribution with degree of freedom 2 and $(n_1 + n_2 - 2)$ and $\boldsymbol{\mu} = (\mu_R, \mu_T)'$. Then, an exact $(1 - 2\alpha) \times 100\%$ confidence region for $\boldsymbol{\mu}$ is

$$\{(\mu_R, \mu_T) | T_1 < F(1 - 2\alpha, 2, n_1 + n_2 - 2)\}. \tag{4.2.23}$$

Note that the confidence region is the interior of an ellipse on a 2×2 plane. Bioequivalence is claimed if, and only if, this ellipse is within the region bounded by two lines $\mu_T = \delta_L \mu_R$ and $\mu_T = \delta_U \mu_R$ (Figure 4.2.1). When average bioequivalence is claimed, we have $(1 - 2\alpha)$ assurance that the true μ_T/μ_R is within (δ_L, δ_U).

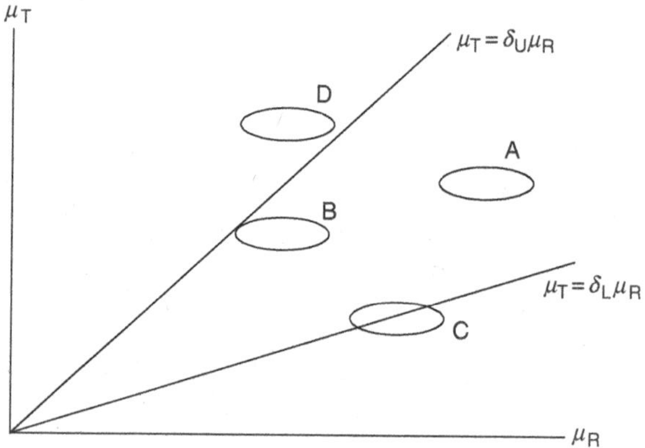

FIGURE 4.2.1: Note that the locations of ellipses A and B indicate that the two formulations are average bioequivalent, whereas locations C and D indicate that the two formulations are not average bioequivalent.

When Y_{ijk} are observed and δ_L and δ_U are given, we can check whether the confidence region Equation 4.2.23 is within $\mu_T = \delta_L/\mu_R$ and $\mu_T = \delta_U\mu_R$ as follows. Let

$$S_{pq} = \sum_{k=1}^{2} \sum_{i=1}^{n_k} (Y_{ipk} - \overline{Y}_{\cdot p \cdot})(Y_{iqk} - \overline{Y}_{\cdot q \cdot}), \quad p, q = 1, 2.$$

Then

$$\mathbf{S} = \begin{bmatrix} S_{11} & S_{12} \\ S_{12} & S_{22} \end{bmatrix} \quad \text{and} \quad \mathbf{S}^{-1} = \frac{1}{S_{11}S_{22} - S_{12}S_{12}} \begin{bmatrix} S_{22} & -S_{12} \\ -S_{12} & S_{11} \end{bmatrix}.$$

Thus, Equation 4.2.23 is equivalent to

$$\begin{aligned} & S_{22}(\overline{Y}_R^* - \mu_R)^2 + S_{11}(\overline{Y}_T^* - \mu_T)^2 - 2S_{12}(\overline{Y}_R^* - \mu_R)(\overline{Y}_T^* - \mu_T) \\ & < \left(\frac{2(S_{11}S_{22} - S_{12}S_{12})}{(n_1 + n_2)(n_1 + n_2 - 2)} \right) F(1 - 2\alpha, 2, n_1 + n_2 - 2) \equiv d. \end{aligned}$$

Therefore, the two formulations are average bioequivalent; that is, the ellipse defined in Equation 4.2.23 is within the region bounded by $\mu_T = \delta_L\mu_R$ and $\mu_T = \delta_U\mu_R$ if, and only if, the following conditions hold simultaneously:

1. $\delta_L < \overline{Y}_T^*/\overline{Y}_R^* < \delta_U$;
2. The following equations have not most one solution:

$$\begin{cases} \mu_T = \delta_U\mu_R \\ S_{22}(\overline{Y}_R^* - \mu_R)^2 + S_{11}(\overline{Y}_T^* - \mu_T)^2 - 2S_{12}(\overline{Y}_R^* - \mu_R)(\overline{Y}_T^* - \mu_T) = d; \end{cases}$$

3. The following equations have at most one solution:

$$\begin{cases} \mu_T = \delta_L\mu_R \\ S_{22}(\overline{Y}_R^* - \mu_R)^2 + S_{11}(\overline{Y}_T^* - \mu_T)^2 - 2S_{12}(\overline{Y}_R^* - \mu_R)(\overline{Y}_T^* - \mu_T) = d. \end{cases}$$

Conditions 1 through 3 are equivalent to following:

(1′) $\delta_L < \overline{Y}_T^*/\overline{Y}_R^* < \delta_U$;

(2′) $$\begin{aligned} & \left(S_{22}\overline{Y}_R^* + \delta_U S_{11}\overline{Y}_T^* - \delta_U S_{12}\overline{Y}_R^* - S_{12}\overline{Y}_T^*\right)^2 \\ & \leq \left(S_{22} + \delta_U^2 S_{11} - 2\delta_U S_{12}\right)\left(S_{22}\overline{Y}_R^{*2} + S_{11}\overline{Y}_T^{*2} - 2S_{12}\overline{Y}_R^*\overline{Y}_T^* - d\right); \end{aligned}$$

(3′) $$\begin{aligned} & \left(S_{22}\overline{Y}_R^* + \delta_L S_{11}\overline{Y}_T^* - \delta_L S_{12}\overline{Y}_R^* - S_{12}\overline{Y}_T^*\right)^2 \\ & \leq \left(S_{22} + \delta_L^2 S_{11} - 2\delta_L S_{12}\right)\left(S_{22}\overline{Y}_R^{*2} + S_{11}\overline{Y}_T^{*2} - 2S_{12}\overline{Y}_R^*\overline{Y}_T^* - d\right). \end{aligned}$$

Thus, we conclude that the two formulations are average bioequivalent if, and only if, conditions 1′ through 3′ hold.

In the case where H_0 in Equation 4.2.22 is rejected, $\overline{\mathbf{X}}_{\cdot\cdot}$ and $\mathbf{S}$ are not independent. However, in this case,

$$E[(\overline{\mathbf{X}}_1 + \overline{\mathbf{X}}_2)/2] = \boldsymbol{\mu},$$

where $(\overline{\mathbf{X}}_1 + \overline{\mathbf{X}}_2)/2 = (\overline{Y}_R, \overline{Y}_T)'$, the vector of the LS means of the reference and test formulations. It can be verified that $(\overline{\mathbf{X}}_{\cdot 1} + \overline{\mathbf{X}}_{\cdot 2})/2$ and $\mathbf{S}_1 + \mathbf{S}_2$ are independent. Therefore,

$$T_2 = \frac{2n_1n_2(n-3)}{n}\{(\overline{\mathbf{X}}_{\cdot 1} + \overline{\mathbf{X}}_{\cdot 2})/2 - \boldsymbol{\mu}\}'(\mathbf{S}_1 + \mathbf{S}_2)^{-1}\{(\overline{\mathbf{X}}_{\cdot 1} + \overline{\mathbf{X}}_{\cdot 2})/2 - \boldsymbol{\mu}\}$$

where $n = n_1 + n_2$ and T_2 has an F distribution with degrees of freedom 2 and $(n_1 + n_2 - 3)$. An exact $(1 - 2\alpha) \times 100\%$ confidence region for $\boldsymbol{\mu}$ is

$$\{(\mu_R, \mu_T) | T_2 < F(1 - 2\alpha, 2, n_1 + n_2 - 3)\}. \tag{4.2.24}$$

Average bioequivalence is claimed if, and only if, the ellipse Equation 4.2.24 is within the region bounded by two lines $\mu_T = \delta_U \mu_R$ and $\mu_T = \delta_L \mu_R$. Thus, we conclude bioequivalence if conditions (1′) through (3′) hold with $\overline{Y}_R^*$, $\overline{Y}_T^*$, S_{pq}, and δ replaced by $\overline{Y}_R$, $\overline{Y}_T$, S'_{pq}, and d', where $\overline{Y}_R$ and $\overline{Y}_T$ are the LS means for the reference and test formulations, respectively, and

$$S'_{pq} = \sum_{k=1}^{2}\sum_{i=1}^{n_k}\left(Y_{ipk} - \overline{Y}'_{\cdot pk}\right)\left(Y_{iqk} - \overline{Y}'_{\cdot qk}\right), \quad p, q = 1, 2,$$

and

$$d' = \frac{n(S_{11'}S_{33'} - S_{12'}S_{12'})}{2n_1n_2(n-3)}F(1 - 2\alpha, 2, n - 3).$$

Note that confidence limits associated with Chow and Shao's 90% joint confidence region approach were derived by Hsu and Lu (1997). They not only provide an easy interpretation of bioequivalence assessment, but also can extend its applicability to both raw-scale and log-transformed data.

Example 4.2.4

To apply the above confidence region approach to the example in Section 3.6, first, the test for the presence of the period and sequence effects is given by

$$T = 3.18 < F(0.95, 2, 21) = 3.47.$$

Therefore, there is no joint presence of period and sequence effects. Furthermore, we have

$$S_{11} = 432.54, \quad S_{12} = 277.65, \quad S_{22} = 445.85, \quad \text{and} \quad d = 1521.40.$$

The observed ratio $\overline{Y}_T^*/\overline{Y}_R^*$ is 97.23%. For $\delta_L = 0.8$ and $\delta_U = 1.2$, it can be verified that the conditions (1′) through (3′) are satisfied. Hence, we conclude that the two formulations are average bioequivalent based on the ±20 rule.

4.3 Methods of Interval Hypotheses Testing

4.3.1 Interval Hypotheses

The assessment of average bioequivalence is based on the comparison of bioavailability profiles between formulations. However, in practice, it is recognized that no two formulations will have exactly the same bioavailability profiles. Therefore, if the profiles of the two formulations differ by less than a (clinically) meaningful limit, the profiles of the two formulations may be considered equivalent. Following this concept, Schuirmann (1981) first introduced the use of interval hypotheses for assessing average bioequivalence.

The interval hypotheses for average bioequivalence can be formulated as

$$\begin{aligned} &\mathrm{H}_0\colon\ \mu_T - \mu_R \leq \theta_L \quad \text{or} \quad \mu_T - \mu_R \geq \theta_U \\ \text{versus} \quad &\mathrm{H}_a\colon\ \theta_L < \mu_T - \mu_R < \theta_U, \end{aligned} \tag{4.3.1}$$

where θ_L and θ_U are some clinically meaningful limits. The concept of interval hypotheses 4.3.1 is to show average bioequivalence by rejecting the null hypothesis of average bioinequivalence. In most bioavailability and bioequivalence studies, θ_L and θ_U are often chosen to be 20% of the reference mean (μ_R). When the natural logarithmic transformation of the data are considered, the hypotheses corresponding to Equation 4.3.1 can be stated as

$$\begin{aligned} &\mathrm{H}_0'\colon\ \mu_T/\mu_R \leq \delta_L \quad \text{or} \quad \mu_T/\mu_R \geq \delta_U \\ \text{versus} \quad &\mathrm{H}_a'\colon\ \delta_L < \mu_T/\mu_R < \delta_U, \end{aligned} \tag{4.3.2}$$

where

$\delta_L = \exp(\theta_L)$
$\delta_U = \exp(\theta_U)$.

Note that the test for hypotheses in Equation 4.3.2 formulated on the log-scale is equivalent to testing for hypotheses 4.3.1 on the raw scale. The interval hypotheses 4.3.1 can be decomposed into two sets of one-sided hypotheses

$$\begin{aligned} &\mathrm{H}_{01}\colon\ \mu_T - \mu_R \leq \theta_L \\ \text{versus} \quad &\mathrm{H}_{a1}\colon\ \mu_T - \mu_R > \theta_L, \end{aligned}$$

and

$$\begin{aligned} &\mathrm{H}_{02}\colon\ \mu_\mathrm{T} - \mu_\mathrm{R} \geq \theta_\mathrm{U} \\ \text{versus}\quad &\mathrm{H}_{a2}\colon\ \mu_\mathrm{T} - \mu_\mathrm{R} < \theta_\mathrm{U}. \end{aligned} \tag{4.3.3}$$

The first set of hypotheses is to verify that the average bioavailability of the test formulation is not too low, whereas the second set of hypotheses is to verify that the average bioavailability of the test formulation is not too high. A relatively low (or high) average bioavailability may refer to the concern of efficacy (or safety) of the test formulation. If one concludes that $\theta_\mathrm{L} < \mu_\mathrm{T} - \mu_\mathrm{R}$ (i.e., reject H_{01}) and $\mu_\mathrm{T} - \mu_\mathrm{R} < \theta_\mathrm{U}$ (i.e., reject H_{02}), then it has been concluded that

$$\theta_\mathrm{L} < \mu_\mathrm{T} - \mu_\mathrm{R} < \theta_\mathrm{U}.$$

μ_T and μ_R, thus, are equivalent. The rejection of H_{01} and H_{02}, which leads to the conclusion of average bioequivalence, is equivalent to rejecting H_0 in Equation 4.3.1.

4.3.2 Schuirmann's Two One-Sided Tests Procedure

Schuirmann (1981, 1987) first introduced the two one-sided tests procedure based on Equation 4.3.3 for assessing average bioequivalence between formulations. The proposed two one-sided tests procedure suggests the conclusion of equivalence of μ_T and μ_R at the α level of significance if, and only if, H_{01} and H_{02} in Equation 4.3.3 are rejected at a predetermined α level of significance. Under the normality assumptions, the two sets of one-sided hypotheses can be tested with ordinary one-sided t tests. We conclude that μ_T and μ_R are average equivalent if

$$T_\mathrm{L} = \frac{(\overline{Y}_\mathrm{T} - \overline{Y}_\mathrm{R}) - \theta_\mathrm{L}}{\hat{\sigma}_\mathrm{d}\sqrt{\frac{1}{n_1} + \frac{1}{n_2}}} > t(\alpha, n_1 + n_2 - 2),$$

and

$$T_\mathrm{U} = \frac{(\overline{Y}_\mathrm{T} - \overline{Y}_\mathrm{R}) - \theta_\mathrm{U}}{\hat{\sigma}_\mathrm{d}\sqrt{\frac{1}{n_1} + \frac{1}{n_2}}} < -t(\alpha, n_1 + n_2 - 2). \tag{4.3.4}$$

The two one-sided t tests procedure is operationally equivalent to the classic (shortest) confidence interval approach; that is, if the classic $(1 - 2\alpha) \times 100\%$ confidence interval for $\mu_\mathrm{T} - \mu_\mathrm{R}$ is within $(\theta_\mathrm{L}, \theta_\mathrm{U})$, then both H_{01} and H_{02} are also rejected at the α level by the two one-sided t tests procedure.

Example 4.3.2

For the example in Section 3.6, we have

$$\overline{Y}_\mathrm{T} = 80.272, \quad \overline{Y}_\mathrm{R} = 82.559, \quad \text{and} \quad \hat{\sigma}_\mathrm{d}^2 = 83.623.$$

Assuming that $\overline{Y}_R$ is the true reference mean, then the lower and upper bioequivalent limits are $-\theta_L = \theta_U = 16.51$. The two sets of one-sided hypotheses corresponding to the interval hypotheses 4.3.1 are

$$\begin{aligned} &H_{01}: \mu_T - \mu_R \leq -16.51 \\ \text{versus } &H_{a1}: \mu_T - \mu_R > -16.51, \end{aligned}$$

and

$$\begin{aligned} &H_{02}: \mu_T - \mu_R \geq 16.51 \\ \text{versus } &H_{a2}: \mu_T - \mu_R < 16.51. \end{aligned}$$

Thus,

$$T_L = \frac{(80.272 - 82.559) + 16.51}{(9.145)\sqrt{0.167}} = 3.810,$$

and

$$T_U = \frac{(80.272 - 82.559) - 16.51}{(9.145)\sqrt{0.167}} = -5.036.$$

As $|T_L|$ and $|T_U|$ are both greater than $t(0.05, 22) = 1.717$, the null hypotheses H_{01} and H_{02} are rejected at the 5% level of significance. Hence, bioequivalence is claimed according to the ± 20 rule.

4.3.3 Anderson and Hauck's Test

For testing the interval hypotheses in Equation 4.3.1, unlike Schuirmann's two one-sided tests procedure, which uses statistics T_L and T_U to evaluate H_{01} and H_{02} rather than testing H_0 directly, Anderson and Hauck (1983) proposed a test statistic that can be used to evaluate H_0 directly. In other words, we would reject the null hypothesis H_0 of bioinequivalence in favor of average bioequivalence for a small p-value. The test statistic is given as

$$T_{AH} = \frac{\overline{Y}_T - \overline{Y}_R - (\theta_L + \theta_U)/2}{\hat{\sigma}_d \sqrt{\frac{1}{n_1} + \frac{1}{n_2}}}. \tag{4.3.5}$$

Under the normality assumptions, T_{AH} follows a noncentral t distribution with noncentrality parameter

$$\delta = \frac{\mu_T - \mu_R - (\theta_L + \theta_U)/2}{\sigma_d \sqrt{\frac{1}{n_1} + \frac{1}{n_2}}}, \tag{4.3.6}$$

where σ_d was defined in Chapter 3.

We reject H_0 in Equation 4.3.1 in favor of average bioequivalence if

$$C_1 < T_{AH} < C_2,$$

where C_1 and C_2 satisfy

$$\begin{aligned} &P[C_1 < T_{AH} < C_2 | \mu_T - \mu_R = \theta_U, \sigma_d] \\ &= P[C_1 < T_{AH} < C_2 | \mu_T - \mu_R = \theta_L, \sigma_d] \\ &= \alpha. \end{aligned} \tag{4.3.7}$$

Because C_1 and C_2 can be chosen to be $C_2 = -C_1 = C$, Equation 4.35 becomes

$$\begin{aligned} &P[|T_{AH}| < C | \mu_T - \mu_R = \theta_U, \sigma_d] \\ &= P[|T_{AH}| < C | \mu_T - \mu_R = \theta_L, \sigma_d] \\ &= \alpha. \end{aligned} \tag{4.3.8}$$

Thus, an α level rejection region can be determined by solving Equation 4.3.8 for C. One of the difficulties of the above test, however, is that δ in Equation 4.3.6 is usually unknown. When δ is known, an empirical significant p-value can be obtained as follows:

$$p = P[|T_{AH}| < |t_{AH}| | \mu_T - \mu_R = \theta_U, \sigma_d], \tag{4.3.9}$$

where t_{AH} is the observed value of T_{AH}.

H_0 is rejected at the α level of significance whenever $p < \alpha$. On the other hand, when δ is unknown, three approximations to Equation 4.3.9, based on noncentral t, central t, and normal distribution, are suggested. Among these approximations as indicated by Anderson and Hauck (1983), the central t approximation appears to be the best in terms of test power. Thus, in the following, the central t approximation to Equation 4.3.9 will be introduced. First, the noncentrality δ can be estimated by

$$\hat{\delta} = \frac{\theta_U - \theta_L}{2\hat{\sigma}_d\sqrt{\frac{1}{n_1} + \frac{1}{n_2}}}. \tag{4.3.10}$$

Then,

$$\begin{aligned} p &= P[|T_{AH}| < |t_{AH}| | \mu_T - \mu_R = \theta_U] \\ &= P[-|t_{AH}| - \hat{\delta} < T_{AH} - \hat{\delta} < |t_{AH}| - \hat{\delta}] \\ &= F_t(|t_{AH}| - \hat{\delta}) - F_t(-|t_{AH}| - \hat{\delta}), \end{aligned} \tag{4.3.11}$$

where

$$T_{AH} - \hat{\delta} = \frac{(\overline{Y}_T - \overline{Y}_R) - \theta_U}{\hat{\delta}_d\sqrt{\frac{1}{n_1} + \frac{1}{n_2}}},$$

and F_t is the central t distribution function with degrees of freedom $(n_1 + n_2 - 2)$.

Note that the approximation in Equation 4.3.11 can also be obtained by using T_L and T_U of Schuirmann's two one-sided t statistics in Equation 4.3.4. Assuming that $t_{AH} > 0$, then

$$|t_{AH}| = \frac{(\overline{Y}_T - \overline{Y}_R) - (\theta_U + \theta_L)/2 - (\theta_U - \theta_L)/2}{\hat{\sigma}_d\sqrt{\frac{1}{n_1} + \frac{1}{n_2}}}$$

$$= \frac{(\overline{Y}_T - \overline{Y}_R) - \theta_U}{\hat{\sigma}_d\sqrt{\frac{1}{n_1} + \frac{1}{n_2}}} = T_U.$$

Similarly, $-|t_{AH}| - \hat{\delta} = -T_L$.

Therefore,

$$\begin{aligned} p &= F_t(|t_{AH}| - \hat{\delta}) - F_t(-|t_{AH}| - \hat{\delta}) \\ &= F_t(T_U) - F_t(-T_L). \end{aligned} \tag{4.3.12}$$

If $t_{AH} < 0$, then $|t_{AH}| - \hat{\delta} = -\ T_L$ and $-\ |t_{AH}| - \hat{\delta} = T_U$ Thus,

$$\begin{aligned} p &= F_t(|t_{AH}| - \hat{\delta}) - F_t(-|t_{AH}| - \hat{\delta}) \\ &= F_t(-T_L) - F_t(T_U). \end{aligned} \tag{4.3.13}$$

From Equations 4.3.12 and 4.3.13, Anderson and Hauck's procedure is always more powerful than Schuirmann's procedure because p may still be smaller than α even if the p-values for T_L and T_U are greater than α. Anderson and Hauck (1983) claim t_{AH} is the most powerful test, but, as a matter of fact, under a normality assumption, there exists no unconditional most powerful, uniformly most powerful, or uniformly powerful unbiased test for the interval hypothesis in Equation 4.3.1 when μ_T, μ_R, and σ_d^2 are unknown (Kendall and Stuart, 1979; Lehmann and Romano, 2005).

In a simulation study, Anderson and Hauck (1983) showed that test procedure Equation 4.3.11 is a more (not the most) powerful test (in the sense of having higher probability of concluding average equivalence), which uniformly dominates both the classic (shortest) confidence interval approach and Westlake's symmetric confidence interval method. In addition, compared to Schuirmann's two one-sided tests procedure, Anderson and Hauck's procedure is always more powerful. This is true when μ_T and μ_R are not equivalent as well as when they are equivalent. The difference in power between the two procedures, however, becomes negligible as the measure of sensitivity

$$\nabla = \frac{\theta_U - \theta_L}{\sigma_d\sqrt{\frac{1}{n_1} + \frac{1}{n_2}}}$$

becomes larger. The drawback of Anderson and Hauck's test is probably that the true level of significance may exceed the nominal level α, particularly for small degrees of freedom associated with the mean-squared error. In addition, Anderson and Hauck's test may still conclude average bioequivalence, even when the intra-subject variability becomes very large because it has an open-ended rejection region, as indicated by Schuirmann (1987). In other words, for a study with low precision, Anderson and Hauck's test may be in favor of average bioequivalence, regardless of the large intra-subject variability.

Example 4.3.3

For the example presented in Section 3.6, since $\overline{Y}_T = 80.272$, $\overline{Y}_R = 82.559$, $\hat{\sigma}_d^2 = 83.623$, and $-\theta_L = \theta_U = 16.51$, the observed t_{AH} can be obtained as

$$t_{AH} = \frac{(80.272 - 82.559) - (-16.51 + 16.51)/2}{(9.145)\sqrt{0.167}} = -0.613.$$

The estimated noncentrality parameter $\hat{\delta}$ is

$$\hat{\delta} = \frac{(16.51 + 16.51)/2}{(9.145)\sqrt{0.167}} = 4.423.$$

Therefore, the empirical p-value is estimated as

$$\begin{aligned} p &= F_t(|-0.613| - 4.423) - F_t(-|-0.613| - 4.423) \\ &= F(-3.810) - F(-5.036) \\ &= 0.000478 - 0.000024 \\ &= 0.000454. \end{aligned}$$

As $p < 0.05$, the interval hypothesis in Equation 4.3.1 is rejected at the 5% level of significance. Thus, we are in favor of average bioequivalence between the two formulations.

4.4 Bayesian Methods

In previous sections, statistical methods for the assessment of bioequivalence were derived based on the sampling distribution of the estimate of the parameter of interest, such as the direct drug effect, which is assumed to be fixed, but unknown. Although statistical inference (e.g., confidence interval and hypothesis testing) on the unknown direct drug effect can be drawn from the sampling distribution of the estimate, there is little information on the probability of the unknown direct drug effect being within the equivalent limits (θ_L, θ_U). As a matter of fact, from sampling theory, the probability that the true direct drug effect is within (θ_L, θ_U) is either 0 or 1, because the true direct drug effect is either within (θ_L, θ_U) or outside (θ_L, θ_U). To have a certain assurance on the probability of the direct drug effect being within (θ_L, θ_U), a Bayesian approach (Box and Tiao, 1973), which assumes that the unknown direct drug effect is a random variable and follows a prior distribution, is useful.

In practice, before a bioavailability and bioequivalence study is conducted, investigators usually have some prior knowledge of the profile of the blood or plasma concentration–time curve. For example, according to past experiments, the investigator may have some information on (1) the inter-subject and the intra-subject variabilities and (2) the ranges of AUC or C_{max} for the test and reference formulations. This information can be used to choose an appropriate prior distribution of the unknown direct drug effect. An appropriate prior distribution can reflect the investigator's belief about the formulations under study. After the study is completed, the observed data can be used to adjust the prior distribution of the direct drug effect, which is called the posterior distribution. Given the posterior distribution, a probability statement on the direct drug effect being within the bioequivalent limits can be made.

A different prior distribution can lead to a different posterior distribution that has an influence on statistical inference on the direct drug effect. Thus, an important issue in a Bayesian approach is how to choose a prior distribution. Box and Tiao (1973) introduced the use of a locally uniform distribution over a possible range of AUC or C_{max} as a noninformative prior distribution. A noninformative prior distribution assumes that there is an equally likely chance for any two points within the possible range being the true state of the location of the direct drug effect. In this case, the resultant posterior distribution can be used to provide the true state of the location of a direct drug effect. In practice, however, it is also desirable to provide an interval showing a range in which most of the distribution of a direct drug effect will fall. We shall refer to such an interval as a highest posterior density (HPD) interval. The HPD interval is also known as a credible interval (Edwards et al., 1963) and a Bayesian confidence interval (Lindley, 1965). An HPD interval possesses the following properties (Box and Tiao, 1973):

1. The density for every point inside the interval is greater than that for every point outside the interval.

2. For a given probability distribution, the interval is the shortest.

It can be verified that the above two properties imply each other. In the following sections, two Bayesian methods with different noninformative priors are discussed under the raw data model.

4.4.1 Rodda and Davis Method

Given the results of a bioavailability and bioequivalence study, Rodda and Davis (1980) proposed a Bayesian evaluation to estimate the probability of a clinically important difference (i.e., the probability that the true direct drug effect will fall within the bioequivalent limits is estimated). As indicated in Chapter 3, under the assumption of normality and equal carryover effects, $\overline{d}_{\cdot 1}$, $\overline{d}_{\cdot 2}$, and $(n_1+n_2-2)\widehat{\sigma}_d{}^2$ are independently distributed as $N(\theta_1, \sigma_d^2/n_1)$, $N(\theta_2, \sigma_d^2/n_2)$, and $\sigma_d^2\chi^2\ (n_1+n_2-2)$,

where

$$\theta_1 = \tfrac{1}{2}[(P_2 - P_1) + (F_T - F_R)], \quad \text{and}$$
$$\theta_2 = \tfrac{1}{2}[(P_2 - P_1) + (F_R - F_T)].$$

Note that $F = \theta_1 - \theta_2 = (\mu + F_T) - (\mu + F_R)$
$= \mu_T - \mu_R.$

Assuming that the noninformative prior distribution for θ_1, θ_2, and log (σ_d) is approximately independent and locally uniformly distributed, then the joint posterior distribution of θ_1, θ_2, and σ_d^2, given data $\mathbf{Y} = \{\mathbf{Y}_{ijk}, i = 1, 2, \ldots, n_k; j, k = 1, 2\}$, is

$$p(\theta_1, \theta_2, \sigma_d^2|\mathbf{Y}) = p(\theta_1|\sigma_d^2, \bar{d}_{\cdot 1})\, p(\theta_2|\sigma_d^2, \bar{d}_{\cdot 2})\, p(\sigma_d^2|\hat{\sigma}_d^2), \tag{4.4.1}$$

where

$$p(\theta_i|\sigma_d^2, \bar{d}_{\cdot i}) = N(\bar{d}_{\cdot i}, \hat{\sigma}_d^2/n_i), \quad i = 1, 2,$$
$$p(\sigma_d^2|\hat{\sigma}_d^2) = (n_1 + n_2)\hat{\sigma}_d^2 \chi^{-2}(n_1 + n_2 - 2),$$

where χ^{-2} $(n_1 + n_2 - 2)$ is the distribution of the inverse of $\chi^2(n_1 + n_2 - 2)$.

Therefore, the joint distribution of $\mu_T - \mu_R$ $(= F)$ and σ_d^2 is given by

$$p(\mu_T - \mu_R, \hat{\sigma}_d^2|\mathbf{Y}) = p(\mu_T - \mu_R|\sigma_d^2, \bar{d}_{\cdot 1} - \bar{d}_{\cdot 2})\, p(\sigma_d^2|\hat{\sigma}_d^2), \tag{4.4.2}$$

where

$$p(\mu_T - \mu_R|\hat{\sigma}_d^2, \bar{d}_{\cdot 1} - \bar{d}_{\cdot 2}) = N\left[\bar{d}_{\cdot 1} - \bar{d}_{\cdot 2}, \hat{\sigma}_d^2\left(\frac{1}{n_1} + \frac{1}{n_2}\right)\right]$$
$$= N\left[\bar{Y}_T - \bar{Y}_R, \hat{\sigma}_d^2\left(\frac{1}{n_1} + \frac{1}{n_2}\right)\right].$$

The marginal posterior distribution of F, given data $\mathbf{Y}$, is

$$p(\mu_T - \mu_R|\mathbf{Y}) = \frac{(\hat{\sigma}_d^2 m)^{-1/2}}{B(1/2, \nu/2)\sqrt{n}} \times \left\{1 + \frac{[(\mu_T - \mu_R) - (\bar{Y}_T - \bar{Y}_R)]^2}{\nu\hat{\sigma}_d^2 m}\right\}^{-(\nu+1)/2} \tag{4.4.3}$$

where
$m = 1/n_1 + 1/n_2$
$\nu = n_1 + n_2 - 2$
$-\infty < \mu_T - \mu_R < \infty$

Equation 4.4.3 indicates that

$$T_{RD} = \frac{(\mu_T - \mu_R) - (\bar{Y}_T - \bar{Y}_R)}{\hat{\sigma}_d\sqrt{\dfrac{1}{n_1} + \dfrac{1}{n_2}}} \tag{4.4.4}$$

has a central Student t distribution with $(n_1 + n_2 - 2)$ degrees of freedom. From Equation 4.4.4, the probability of F being within the bioequivalent limit θ_L and θ_U can be estimated by

$$\begin{aligned} p_{\text{RD}} &= P\{\theta_{\text{L}} < \mu_{\text{T}} - \mu_{\text{R}} < \theta_{\text{U}}\} \\ &= F_t(t_{\text{U}}) - F_t(t_{\text{L}}), \end{aligned} \tag{4.4.5}$$

where F_t is the cumulative distribution function of a central t variable with $(n_1 + n_2 - 2)$ degrees of freedom, and

$$\begin{aligned} t_{\text{U}} &= \frac{\theta_{\text{U}} - (\overline{Y}_{\text{T}} - \overline{Y}_{\text{R}})}{\widehat{\sigma}_{\text{d}}\sqrt{\frac{1}{n_1} + \frac{1}{n_2}}}, \quad \text{and} \\ t_{\text{L}} &= \frac{\theta_{\text{L}} - (\overline{Y}_{\text{T}} - \overline{Y}_{\text{R}})}{\widehat{\sigma}_{\text{d}}\sqrt{\frac{1}{n_1} + \frac{1}{n_2}}}. \end{aligned} \tag{4.4.6}$$

The lower and upper limits of the $(1 - 2\alpha) \times 100\%$ HPD interval are given by

$$\begin{aligned} L_{\text{RD}} &= (\overline{Y}_{\text{T}} - \overline{Y}_{\text{R}}) - t(\alpha, n_1 + n_2 - 2)\widehat{\sigma}_{\text{d}}\sqrt{\frac{1}{n_1} + \frac{1}{n_2}}, \\ U_{\text{RD}} &= (\overline{Y}_{\text{T}} - \overline{Y}_{\text{R}}) + t(\alpha, n_1 + n_2 - 2)\widehat{\sigma}_{\text{d}}\sqrt{\frac{1}{n_1} + \frac{1}{n_2}}. \end{aligned} \tag{4.4.7}$$

Hence, it is verified that the $(1 - 2\alpha) \times 100\%$ HPD interval in Equation 4.4.7 is numerically equivalent to the $(1 - 2\alpha) \times 100\%$ classic confidence interval, given in Equation 4.2.2, obtained from the sampling theory. However, the interpretation of these two intervals is totally different. For example, a 90% classic confidence interval for F indicates that, in the long run, if the study is repeatedly carried out for numerous times, 90% of the times the interval will contain the unknown direct drug effect $\mu_{\text{T}} - \mu_{\text{R}}$. On the other hand, based on the posterior distribution of $\mu_{\text{T}} - \mu_{\text{R}}$, the chance of $\mu_{\text{T}} - \mu_{\text{R}}$ being within the lower and upper limits of a 90% HPD interval is 90%.

From Equations 4.4.5 and 4.4.7, two formulations are average bioequivalent with 90% assurance if either $p_{\text{RD}} > 0.90$ or $(L_{\text{RD}}, U_{\text{RD}})$ is within $(\theta_{\text{L}}, \theta_{\text{U}})$. Furthermore, $p_{\text{RD}} > 0.90$ if and only if $(L_{\text{RD}}, U_{\text{RD}})$ is within $(\theta_{\text{L}}, \theta_{\text{U}})$. Therefore, Equation 4.4.5 is equivalent to Equation 4.4.7 in decision making for average bioequivalence.

Example 4.4.1

To illustrate Rodda and Davis's Bayesian approach, consider the example in Section 3.6. The data give

$$\overline{Y}_{\text{T}} = 80.272, \quad \overline{Y}_{\text{R}} = 82.559, \quad \text{and} \quad \widehat{\sigma}_{\text{d}}^2 = 83.623.$$

From Equation 4.4.4, we have

$$\begin{aligned} t_{\text{U}} &= \frac{16.51 - (80.272 - 82.559)}{(9.145)\sqrt{0.167}} = 5.036, \quad \text{and} \\ t_{\text{L}} &= \frac{-16.51 - (80.272 - 82.559)}{(9.145)\sqrt{0.167}} = -3.810. \end{aligned}$$

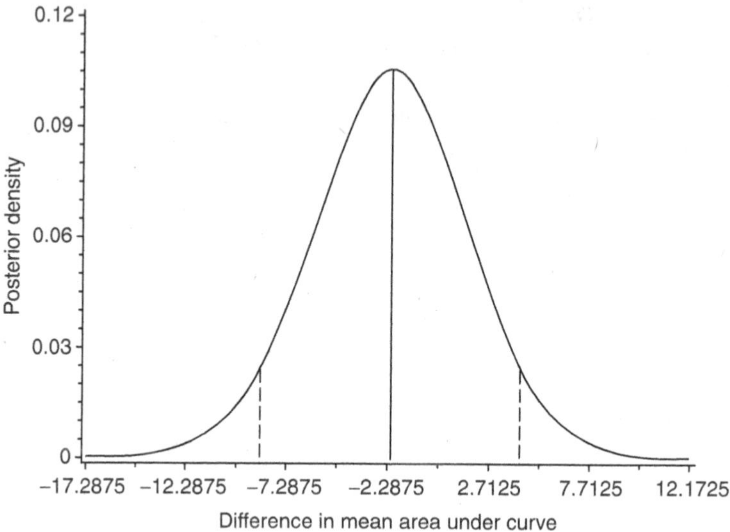

FIGURE 4.4.1: Posterior density of mean area under curve and highest posterior density interval. (From Rodda, B.E. and Davis, R.L., *Clin. Pharmacol. Ther.*, 28, 247, 1980.)

Therefore, $P_{RD} = F_t(5.036) - F_t(-3.810) = 0.9995$ which is greater than 0.9. The 90% HPD-interval is $(-8.698, 4.123)$, and we conclude that the two formulations are average bioequivalent with at least 90% assurance.

The posterior density function for F with a noninformative prior, given data $\mathbf{Y}$, is graphed in Figure 4.4.1.

4.4.2 Mandallaz and Mau's Method

Alternatively, Mandallaz and Mau (1981) proposed a Bayesian method for assessing average bioequivalence for the ratio (μ_T/μ_R) (Fluehler et al., 1981, 1983) under model 4.1.1 with the following assumptions:

1. There are no carryover effects.
2. The effects from subjects are fixed.
3. The numbers of subjects in each sequence are the same (i.e., $n_1 = n_2 = n$).

Under these assumptions, $\overline{Y}_T$ and $\overline{Y}_R$ are independently normally distributed with means μ_T and μ_R and variance σ_d^2/n, where

$$\mu_T = \mu + F_T \quad \text{and} \quad \mu_R = \mu + F_R.$$

Suppose that the prior distribution for μ_T, μ_R, and σ_d has the following improper vague prior distribution of the form:

$$dP = (d\mu_T)(d\mu_R)(d\sigma_d/\sigma_d).$$

The posterior distribution of $\delta = \mu_T/\mu_R$, given data **Y**, can then be approximated by the following statistic

$$T_{MM} = \frac{\hat{\delta} - \delta}{\hat{\sigma}_d\sqrt{(1+\delta^2)/n\overline{Y}_R^2}}, \tag{4.4.8}$$

where $\hat{\delta} = \overline{Y}_T/\overline{Y}_R$ and T_{MM} follows a central t distribution with $2(n-1)$ degrees of freedom.

Therefore, two formulations are considered average bioequivalent with 90% assurance if

$$\begin{aligned} P_{MM} &= P\{\delta_L < \delta < \delta_U\} \\ &= F_t(t_{\delta_L}) - F_t(t_{\delta_U}) > 0.90, \end{aligned} \tag{4.4.9}$$

where

$$\begin{aligned} t_{\delta_U} &= \frac{\hat{\delta} - \delta_U}{\hat{\sigma}_d\sqrt{(1+\delta_U^2)/n\overline{Y}_R^2}}, \\ t_{\delta_L} &= \frac{\hat{\delta} - \delta_L}{\hat{\sigma}_d\sqrt{(1+\delta_L^2)/n\overline{Y}_R^2}}, \quad \text{and} \end{aligned}$$

$F_t(\cdot)$ is the cumulative distribution function of a central t variable with $2(n-1)$ degrees of freedom.

Note that T_{MM} in Equation 4.4.8 can be rewritten as

$$T_{MM} = \frac{\overline{Y}_T - \overline{Y}_R}{\hat{\sigma}_R\sqrt{(1+\delta^2)/n}}, \tag{4.4.10}$$

which is the pivotal quantity used for the construction of a $(1-2\alpha) \times 100\%$ confidence interval of δ in the fixed Fieller's method (Schuirmann, 1989). The Mandallaz and Mau method leads to the same decision for average bioequivalence as that of the fixed Fieller's method when $n_1 = n_2 = n$. To show this, it is sufficient to prove that if δ in Equation 4.4.8 is replaced by L_4 in Equation 4.2.19, then $T_{MM} = t(\alpha, 2(n-1))$. Assuming that $G < 1$, the numerator of Equation 4.4.8 with δ replaced by L_4 is

$$\hat{\delta} - L_4 = \frac{\sqrt{G_1}}{1-G_1}\left[\sqrt{G_1}\hat{\delta} + \sqrt{\hat{\delta}^2 + (1-G_1)}\right].$$

Furthermore, it can be easily verified that

$$1 + L_4^2 = \frac{1}{(1 - G_1)^2}\left[\sqrt{G_1}\hat{\delta} + \sqrt{\hat{\delta}^2 + (1 - G_1)}\right].$$

Thus, the denominator of Equation 4.4.8 can be expressed as

$$\frac{\hat{\delta}_d}{\sqrt{n}\overline{Y}_R(1 - G_1)}\left[\sqrt{G_1}\hat{\delta} + \sqrt{\hat{\delta}^2 + (1 - G_1)}\right].$$

Since $n_1 = n_2$, we have

$$\begin{aligned} G_1 &= [t(\alpha, 2(n-1))]^2\left(\frac{\mathrm{MS_{Intra}}/2n}{\overline{Y}_\mathrm{R}^2}\right) \\ &= [t(\alpha, 2(n-1))]^2\left[\widehat{\sigma}_\mathrm{d}^2\Big/\left(n\overline{Y}_\mathrm{R}^2\right)\right]. \end{aligned}$$

Therefore,

$$\begin{aligned} \frac{\hat{\delta} - L_4}{\widehat{\sigma}_\mathrm{d}\sqrt{\left(1 + L_4^2\right)\Big/\left(n\overline{Y}_\mathrm{R}^2\right)}} &= \frac{\sqrt{G_1}\left[\sqrt{G_1}\hat{\delta} + \sqrt{\hat{\delta}^2 + (1 - G_1)}\right]}{\frac{\widehat{\sigma}_\mathrm{d}}{\sqrt{n}\overline{Y}_\mathrm{R}}\left[\sqrt{G_1}\hat{\delta} + \sqrt{\hat{\delta}^2 + (1 - G_1)}\right]} \\ &= t[\alpha, 2(n-1)]. \end{aligned}$$

When $n_1 = n_2$, since the least squares means $\overline{Y}_\mathrm{T}$ and $\overline{Y}_\mathrm{R}$ are the same as the raw means, denoted by $\overline{Y}_\mathrm{T}^*$ and $\overline{Y}_\mathrm{R}^*$, the above procedure holds with $\overline{Y}_\mathrm{T}$ and $\overline{Y}_\mathrm{R}$ replaced by $\overline{Y}_\mathrm{T}^*$ and $\overline{Y}_\mathrm{R}^*$. However, when $n_1 \neq n_2$, $\overline{Y}_\mathrm{T}$ and $\overline{Y}_\mathrm{R}$ are not the same as $\overline{Y}_\mathrm{T}^*$ and $\overline{Y}_\mathrm{R}^*$. In this case, under the assumptions of no carryover effects and fixed subject effects, we have

$$E\left[\overline{Y}_\mathrm{T}^* - \delta\overline{Y}_\mathrm{R}^*\right] = \frac{1}{n_1 + n_2}[(n_1 - \delta n_2)P_1 + (n_2 - \delta n_1)P_2]. \tag{4.4.11}$$

Hence,

$$T_\mathrm{MM}^* = \frac{\overline{Y}_\mathrm{T}^* - \delta\overline{Y}_\mathrm{R}^*}{\widehat{\sigma}_\mathrm{d}\sqrt{(1 + \delta^2)/n}}$$

is no longer distributed as a central t distribution with $(n_1 + n_2 - 2)$ degrees of freedom. With $n_1 \neq n_2$, T_MM in Equation 4.4.10 still has a central t distribution because $E[\overline{Y}_\mathrm{T} - \delta\overline{Y}_\mathrm{R}] = 0$. In this case, however, whether the posterior distribution of δ can be approximated by T_MM under the same improper vague prior distribution remains unknown.

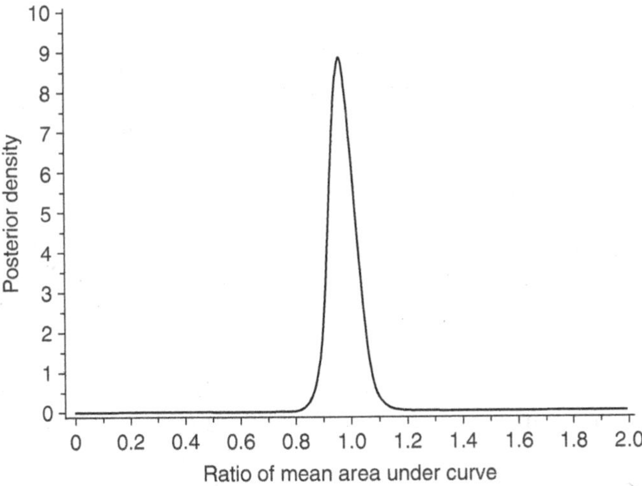

FIGURE 4.4.2: Posterior density of the ratio of mean area under curve. (From Mandallaz, D. and Mau, J., *Biometrics*, 37, 213, 1981.)

Example 4.4.2

For the example in Section 3.6, we have $\overline{Y}_{\mathrm{T}} = 80.272$, $\overline{Y}_{\mathrm{R}} = 82.559$, and $\hat{\delta} = 0.972$. Since $\widehat{\sigma}_{\mathrm{d}}^2 = 83.623$, and $n_1 = n_2 = 12$, we have

$$t_{\delta_{\mathrm{L}}} = \frac{0.972 - 0.8}{\sqrt{(83.623)(1 + 0.64)/(12)(82.559)^2}} = 4.208, \quad \text{and}$$

$$t_{\delta_{\mathrm{U}}} = \frac{0.972 - 1.2}{\sqrt{(83.623)(1 + 1.44)/(12)(82.559)^2}} = -4.559.$$

Therefore,

$$P_{\mathrm{MM}} = F_t(4.208) - F_t(-4.559) = 0.9997,$$

which is greater than 0.90. Thus, we conclude that the formulations are average bioequivalent with at least 90% assurance.

The posterior density function for δ with an improper vague prior distribution, given data $\mathbf{Y}$, is graphed in Figure 4.4.2.

4.5 Nonparametric Methods

In Sections 4.2, 4.3, and 4.4, statistical methods for assessing average bioequivalence between formulations were derived under the assumption that $\{S_{ik}\}$ and $\{e_{ijk}\}$ are mutually independent and normally distributed with mean 0 and variance σ_{S}^2 and σ_{e}^2. Under these normality assumptions, confidence intervals and tests for interval hypotheses were obtained based on either a two-sample t statistic or an F statistic. In practice, however, one of the difficulties commonly encountered in comparing formulations is whether the assumption of normality (for raw or untransformed data) or lognormality (for log-transformed data) is valid. If the normality (or lognormality) is seriously violated, the approach based on a two-sample t statistic or an F statistic is no longer justified. In this situation, a distribution-free (or nonparametric) method is useful. In this section, a nonparametric version of the two one-sided tests procedure for testing interval hypotheses namely, Wilcoxon–Mann–Whitney two one-sided tests procedure, will be derived. The Hodges–Lehmann estimator associated with the Wilcoxon rank sum test will be used to construct a $(1-2\alpha)\times 100\%$ confidence interval for $\mu_T-\mu_R$, the difference in average bioavailability. In addition, the possible use of a bootstrap resampling procedure will be discussed.

For example, t_{max} may be an important pharmacokinetic parameter for evaluation of bioequivalence if there is a clinically relevant claim for rapid onset of action or concerns about adverse events. However, as mentioned before, t_{max} is estimated as the sampling time point at which C_{max} occurs. Its distribution, either on the original scale or on the log-scale, rarely follows a normal distribution. As a result, both the EMEA guidance (2001) and the WHO draft guideline (2005) recommend using the 90% nonparametric confidence interval for assessment of average bioequivalence based on t_{max}.

4.5.1 Wilcoxon–Mann–Whitney Two One-Sided Tests Procedure

Because the standard 2×2 crossover design consist of a pair of dual sequences (i.e., RT and TR), a distribution-free rank sum test can be applied directly to the two one-sided tests procedure (Hauschke et al., 1990; Cornell, 1990; Liu, 1991). We shall refer to this approach as Wilcoxon–Mann–Whitney two one-sided tests procedure. Let $\theta=\mu_T-\mu_R$. The two sets of hypotheses in Equation 4.3.3 can then be rewritten as

$$\begin{aligned} &\mathrm{H_{01}}:\ \theta_L^* \le 0 \\ \text{versus}\quad &\mathrm{H_{a1}}:\ \theta_L^* > 0, \end{aligned}$$

and

$$\begin{aligned} &\mathrm{H_{02}}:\ \theta_U^* \ge 0 \\ \text{versus}\quad &\mathrm{H_{a2}}:\ \theta_U^* < 0, \end{aligned} \tag{4.5.1}$$

where

$$\theta_L^* = \theta - \theta_L$$
$$\theta_U^* = \theta - \theta_U.$$

As discussed in Chapter 3, the estimates of θ_L^* and θ_U^* can be obtained as a linear function of period differences d_{ik}, $i=1, 2, \ldots, n_k$, $k=1, 2$. Let

$$b_{hik} = \begin{cases} d_{ik}-\theta_h & h=L,\ U, \text{ for subjects in sequence 1} \\ d_{ik} & \text{for subjects in sequence 2.} \end{cases} \tag{4.5.2}$$

When there are no carryover effects, the expected value and variance of b_{hik}, where $h = L$, U, $i = 1, 2, \ldots, n_k$, and $k = 1, 2$, are given by

$$E(b_{hik}) = \begin{cases} \frac{1}{2}[(P_2 - P_1) + (\theta - 2\theta_h)] & \text{for} \quad k = 1 \\ \frac{1}{2}[(P_2 - P_1) - \theta] & \text{for} \quad k = 2, \end{cases} \tag{4.5.3}$$

and

$$V(b_{hik}) = V(d_{ik}) = \sigma_{\text{d}}^2 = \sigma_{\text{e}}^2/2.$$

It can be seen that

$$E(b_{hi1}) - E(b_{hi2}) = (\theta - \theta_h) = \theta_h^*.$$

Thus, for a fixed h, $\{b_{hi1}\}$ and $\{b_{hi2}\}$ have the same distribution except for the difference $(=\theta_h^*)$ in location of the true formulation effect. Here, Wilcoxon–Mann–Whitney rank sum test (Wilcoxon, 1945; Mann and Whitney, 1947) for the unpaired two-sample location problem can be directly applied to test each of the two sets of hypotheses given in Equation 4.5.1.

Consider the first set of hypotheses in Equation 4.5.1,

$$\begin{aligned} &\text{H}_{01}\colon\ \theta_{\text{L}}^* \le 0 \\ \text{versus}\quad &\text{H}_{\text{a}1}\colon\ \theta_{\text{L}}^* > 0. \end{aligned}$$

Wilcoxon–Mann–Whitney test statistic can be derived based on $\{b_{Li1}\}$, $i = 1, 2, \ldots, n_1$ and $\{b_{Li2}\}$, $i = 1, 2, \ldots, n_2$. Let $R(b_{Lik})$ be the rank of b_{Lik} in the combined sample $\{b_{Lik}\}$, $i = 1, 2, \ldots, n_k$, $k = 1, 2$. Also, let R_{L} be the sum of the ranks of the responses for subjects in sequence 1; that is

$$R_{\text{L}} = \sum_{i=1}^{n_1} R(b_{\text{L}i1}).$$

Thus, Wilcoxon–Mann–Whitney test statistic for H_{01} is given by

$$W_{\text{L}} = R_{\text{L}} - \frac{n_1(n_1+1)}{2}.$$

We then reject H_{01} if

$$W_{\text{L}} > w(1-\alpha), \tag{4.5.4}$$

where $w(1-\alpha)$ is the $(1-\alpha)$th quantile of the distribution of W_{L} which can be obtained in Table A.5 in Appendix A. Similarly, for the second set of hypotheses in 4.5.1,

$$\text{H}_{02}\colon\ \theta_U^* \geq 0$$
$$\text{versus}\quad \text{H}_{a2}\colon\ \theta_U^* < 0.$$

we reject H_{02} if

$$W_U = R_U - \frac{n_1(n_1+1)}{2} < w(\alpha), \tag{4.5.5}$$

where R_U is the sum of the ranks of $\{b_{Uik}\}$ for subjects in the first sequence. Hence, average bioequivalence is concluded if both H_{01} and H_{02} are rejected; that is,

$$W_L > w(1-\alpha) \quad \text{and} \quad W_U < w(\alpha). \tag{4.5.6}$$

The expected values and variances for W_L and W_U under the null hypotheses H_{01} and H_{02}, when there are no ties, are given by

$$\begin{aligned} E(W_L) &= E(W_U) = \frac{n_1 n_2}{2}, \\ V(W_L) &= V(W_U) = \tfrac{1}{12} n_1 n_2 (n_1 + n_2 + 1). \end{aligned} \tag{4.5.7}$$

When there are ties among observations, average ranks can be assigned to compute W_L and W_U. In this case, however, the expected values and variances of W_L and W_U become

$$\begin{aligned} E(W_L) &= E(W_U) = \frac{n_1 n_2}{2}, \\ V(W_L) &= V(W_U) = \tfrac{1}{12} n_1 n_2 (n_1 + n_2 + 1 - Q), \end{aligned} \tag{4.5.8}$$

where

$$Q = \frac{1}{(n_1+n_2)(n_1+n_2-1)} \sum_{v=1}^{q} (r_v^3 - r_v),$$

where q is the number of tied groups and r_v is the size of the tied group v. Note that if there are no tied observations, $q = n_1 + n_2$, $r_v = 1$ for $v = 1, 2, \ldots, n$, and $Q = 0$, then Equation 4.5.8 reduces to Equation 4.5.7.

Since W_L and W_U are symmetric about their mean $(n_1 n_2)/2$, we have

$$w(1-\alpha) = n_1 n_2 - w(\alpha). \tag{4.5.9}$$

Table A.5 gives the quantiles for $\alpha = 0.001$, 0.005, 0.01, 0.025, 0.05, and 0.1 of the Wilcoxon–Mann–Whitney test statistics. On the basis of Equation 4.5.9, the quantile for $\alpha = 0.90$, 0.95, 0.975, 0.99, 0.995, and 0.999 can be easily obtained. For example, suppose there are 12 subjects in both sequences. From Table A.5, the 5th quantile is 43. Thus, the 95th quantile is given by $w(0.95) = (12)(12) - 43 = 101$.

When $n_1 + n_2$, the total number of subjects, is large (say, $n_1 + n_2 > 40$) and the ratio of n_1 and n_2 is close to 1/2, a large sample approximation using the standard normal distribution can be used to approximate Equation 4.5.6 for average bioequivalence testing; that is, we may conclude bioequivalence if

$$Z_L > z(\alpha) \quad \text{and} \quad Z_U < -z(\alpha),$$

where $z(\alpha)$ is the αth quantile of a standard normal distribution, and

$$Z_L = \frac{W_L - E(W_L)}{\sqrt{V(W_L)}} = \frac{R_L - \left[\dfrac{n_1(n_1+n_2+1)}{2}\right]}{\sqrt{\dfrac{1}{12}n_1n_2(n_1+n_2+1)}},$$
$$Z_U = \frac{W_U - E(W_U)}{\sqrt{V(W_U)}} = \frac{R_U - \left[\dfrac{n_1(n_1+n_2+1)}{2}\right]}{\sqrt{\dfrac{1}{12}n_1n_2(n_1+n_2+1)}}. \tag{4.5.10}$$

Note that the variances in Z_L and Z_U should be replaced with that given in Equation 4.5.8 if these are ties.

Example 4.5.1

To illustrate the above Wilcoxon–Mann–Whitney two one-sided tests procedure, consider the example in Section 3.6. Table 4.5.1 lists the ranks of b_{hik}. The observed reference mean is assumed to be the true mean μ_R. According to the ±20 rule, the average bioequivalence limits are given by

$$-\theta_L = \theta_U = (0.2)(82.559) = 16.51.$$

Thus, the interval hypotheses are

$$\begin{aligned} &\text{H}_0\colon\ \theta < -16.51 \quad \text{or} \quad \theta > 16.51 \\ \text{versus}\quad &\text{H}_a\colon\ -16.51 \le \theta \le 16.51 \end{aligned}$$

which leads to the following two sets of hypotheses

$$\begin{aligned} &\text{H}_{01}\colon\ \theta + 16.51 \le 0 \\ \text{versus}\quad &\text{H}_{a1}\colon\ \theta + 16.51 > 0, \end{aligned}$$

and

$$\begin{aligned} &\text{H}_{02}\colon\ \theta + 16.51 \ge 0 \\ \text{versus}\quad &\text{H}_{a2}\colon\ \theta + 16.51 < 0. \end{aligned}$$

From Table 4.5.1, R_L and R_U can be found to be 207 and 91, respectively. Therefore, W_L and W_U are

$$W_L = 207 - \frac{(12)(12+1)}{2} = 129,$$

TABLE 4.5.1: Ranks of b_{hik} for data in Table 3.6.1.

Sequence	Subject Number	Period I	Period II	Subject Total	P.D.[a]	$2 \times b_{Lik}$[b]	$R(b_{Lik})$	$2 \times b_{Uik}$	$R(b_{Uik})$
1									
RT	1	74.675	73.675	148.350	−1.000	32.024	20	−34.024	10
RT	4	96.400	93.250	189.650	−3.150	29.874	19	−36.174	8
RT	5	101.950	102.125	204.075	0.175	33.199	21	−32.849	11
RT	6	79.050	69.450	148.500	−9.600	23.424	17	−42.624	6
RT	11	79.050	69.025	148.075	−10.025	22.999	16	−43.049	5
RT	12	85.950	68.700	154.650	−17.250	15.774	9	−50.274	2
RT	15	−69.725	59.425	129.150	−10.300	22.724	14	−43.329	3
RT	16	86.275	76.125	162.400	−10.150	22.874	15	−43.174	4
RT	19	112.675	114.875	227.550	2.200	35.224	22	−30.824	12
RT	20	99.525	116.250	215.775	16.725	49.749	23	−16.299	13
RT	23	89.425	65.175	153.600	−25.250	7.774	7	−58.274	1
RT	24	55.175	74.575	129.750	19.400	52.424	24	−13.624	16
2									
TR	2	74.825	37.350	112.175	−37.475	−37.475	1	−37.475	7
TR	3	86.875	51.925	138.800	−34.950	−34.950	2	−34.950	9
TR	3	81.675	72.175	153.850	−9.500	−9.500	5	−9.500	17
TR	8	92.700	77.500	170.200	−15.200	−15.200	3	−15.200	14
TR	9	50.450	71.875	122.325	21.425	21.425	12	21.425	22
TR	10	66.125	94.025	160.150	27.900	27.900	18	27.900	24
TR	13	122.450	124.975	247.425	2.525	2.525	6	2.525	18
TR	14	99.075	85.225	184.300	−13.850	−13.850	4	−13.850	15
TR	17	86.350	95.925	182.275	9.575	9.575	8	9.575	19
TR	18	49.925	67.100	117.025	17.175	17.175	11	17.175	21
TR	21	42.700	59.425	102.125	16.725	16.725	10	12.725	20
TR	22	91.725	114.050	205.775	22.325	22.325	13	22.325	23

[a] P.D., 2 × (period difference).

[b] Assume the observed reference mean is the true mean and $-\theta_L = \theta_U = (0.2)(82.5594) = 16.5119$.

and

$$W_U = 91 - \frac{(12)(12+1)}{2} = 13.$$

From Table A.5 in Appendix A, the 5th quantile of the Wilcoxon–Mann–Whitney statistic for $n_1 = n_2 = 12$ is 43. On the basis of Equation 4.5.8, the 95th quantile of the Wilcoxon–Mann–Whitney statistic can be obtained as

$$w(0.95) = (12)(12) - 43 = 101.$$

As $W_L = 129 > w(0.95) = 101$ and $W_U = 13 < w(0.05) = 43$, both two one-sided null hypotheses (i.e., H_{01} and H_{02}) are rejected at the 5% level of significance. We then conclude average bioequivalence with 90% assurance.

4.5.2 Distribution-Free Confidence Interval Based on the Hodges–Lehmann Estimator

A distribution-free $(1 - 2\alpha) \times 100\%$ confidence interval for θ can be obtained based on the Hodges–Lehmann estimator (Randles and Wolfe, 1979). Let $D_{i,i'}$, $i = 1, 2, \ldots, n_1$; $i' = 1, 2, \ldots, n_2$ be all possible pairwise differences of the period differences between sequence 1 and sequence 2, that is,

$$D_{i,i'} = d_{i1} - d_{i'2}, \quad i = 1, 2, \ldots, n_1; \quad i' = 1, 2, \ldots, n_2.$$

It can be verified that each $D_{i,i'}$ is an unbiased estimate of θ (i.e., $\mu_T - \mu_R$), that is,

$$E(D_{i,i'}) = \theta.$$

Denote the ordered set of $n_1 n_2$ differences $D_{i,i'}$ by

$$D(1) < D(2) < \cdots < D(n_1 n_2).$$

The median of $\{D(i), i = 1, 2, \ldots, n_1 n_2\}$ is then a distribution-free point estimator of $\theta = \mu_T - \mu_R$, which is also known as the Hodges–Lehmann estimator (Hodges and Lehmann, 1963), that is,

$$\tilde{\theta} = \begin{cases} \frac{1}{2}\left[D\left(\frac{n_1 n_2}{2}\right) + D\left(\frac{n_1 n_2}{2} + 1\right)\right] & \text{if } n_1 n_2 \text{ is even,} \\ D\left(\frac{n_1 n_2 - 1}{2} + 1\right) & \text{if } n_1 n_2 \text{ is odd.} \end{cases} \tag{4.5.11}$$

The lower and upper limits for the $(1 - 2\alpha) \times 100\%$ distribution-free confidence interval for $\theta = \mu_T - \mu_R$ are then given by

$$L_w = D[w(\alpha)],$$

and

$$U_w = D[w(1-\alpha)+1], \tag{4.5.12}$$

where $D[w(\alpha)]$ and $D[w(1-\alpha)+1]$ are the $[w(\alpha)]$th and $[w(1-\alpha)+1]$th order statistics of $D(1), D(2), \ldots, D(n_1n_2)$.

For the assessment of average bioequivalence, the distribution-free confidence interval approach is equivalent to the Wilcoxon–Mann–Whitney two one-sided tests procedure. Based on a theorem of Lehmann (1975, p. 87) and Equation 4.5.9, it can be verified that

1. $D[w(\alpha)] > \theta_L$ if and only if $W_L > n_1n_2 - w(\alpha) = w(1-\alpha)$, and
2. $D[w(1-\alpha)+1] < \theta_U$ if and only if $W_U < n_1n_2 - w(1-\alpha) = w(\alpha)$.

Thus, two approaches reach the same decision in determination of average bioequivalence

When the total sample size n_1+n_2 is large, the αth upper percentile $w(\alpha)$ can be approximated by

$$w(\alpha) = \frac{n_1n_2}{2} + z(\alpha)\sqrt{\frac{1}{12}n_1n_2(n_1+n_2+1)}. \tag{4.5.13}$$

Hauschke et al. (1990) examined the true coverage probabilities of (L_w, U_w) for $n_1, n_2 = 4, \ldots, 12$. The results indicate that the distribution-free confidence interval (L_w, U_w) is somewhat conservative, for its coverage probability is always greater than $(1-2\alpha)$ level because the distribution of Wilcoxon–Mann–Whitney statistic is discrete. The true coverage probability of the 90% distribution-free confidence interval for $n_1, n_2 = 4, 5, \ldots, 12$ is given in Hauschke et al. (1990).

Steinijans and Diletti (1983) proposed an alternative distribution-free procedure based on the crossover differences O_{ik} as defined in Chapter 3 using a Wilcoxon signed rank statistic (Wilcoxon, 1945) and a Walsh average (Walsh, 1949). This approach may not be of practical interest because it requires (1) equal period effects and (2) the distribution of the crossover difference to be symmetric, which are not true in general.

Example 4.5.2

For the example described in Section 3.6, from Table 4.5.1, the median of all possible pairwise differences can be found to be −3.263. Since $w(0.05) = 43$ and $w(0.95)+1 = 102$, the lower and upper 90% distribution-free confidence intervals are

$$L_w = D(43) = -10.625 \text{ and } U_w = D(102) = 4.838,$$

respectively. Thus, $(L_w, U_w) = (-10.625, 4.838)$ is within the equivalence limits $(\theta_L, \theta_U) = (-16.51, 16.51)$. Hence, we conclude that the two formulations are average bioequivalent. It can be seen that this conclusion agrees with the confidence interval approaches discussed in Section 4.2. However, $(L_{\text{w}}, U_{\text{w}})$ is wider than the shortest confidence interval, which is given by $(-8.698, 4.123)$. This may be partly explained by the fact that the actual coverage probability for $(L_{\text{w}}, U_{\text{w}})$ is 91.13%, which is higher than the nominal level of 90%.

4.5.3 Bootstrap Confidence Interval

Chow (1990) proposed several alternative approaches for the assessment of average bioequivalence relative to various situations, depending on whether the normally assumptions for $\{S_{ik}\}$ and $\{e_{ijk}\}$ are met. When the distributions of $\{S_{ik}\}$ and $\{e_{ijk}\}$ are both unknown, a nonparametric approach for constructing a $(1-2\alpha)\times 100\%$ confidence interval for the ratio $\delta=\mu_{\text{T}}/\mu_{\text{R}}$ using the bootstrap resampling technique (Efron, 1982) was derived under model 4.2.20. We shall refer to such a confidence interval as a bootstrap confidence interval.

To establish this procedure, the following results are needed. The proofs of these results are straightforward and hence omitted.

THEOREM 4.5.1

Assume that $n_k/n \to \lambda_k$, $k=1,2$, where $n=n_1+n_2$ and $0<\lambda_k$, 1. Then

$$\sqrt{n}\left(\begin{bmatrix}\bar{\mathbf{X}}_{\cdot 1}\\ \bar{\mathbf{X}}_{\cdot 2}\end{bmatrix} - \begin{bmatrix}\boldsymbol{\mu}_1\\ \boldsymbol{\mu}_2\end{bmatrix}\right) \to N(\mathbf{0}, \boldsymbol{\Sigma}),$$

where

$$\boldsymbol{\Sigma} = \begin{pmatrix}\lambda_1\boldsymbol{\Sigma}_1 & 0\\ 0 & \lambda_2\boldsymbol{\Sigma}_2\end{pmatrix},$$

and $\boldsymbol{\mu}_k=E(\mathbf{X}_{ik})$ and $\boldsymbol{\Sigma}_k=\text{Cov}(\mathbf{X}_{ik})$, a 2×2 positive definite matrix.

THEOREM 4.5.2

Let

$$\hat{\delta} = \frac{\bar{Y}_{\cdot 21}+\bar{Y}_{\cdot 12}}{\bar{Y}_{\cdot 11}+\bar{Y}_{\cdot 22}} = \frac{\bar{Y}_{\text{T}}}{\bar{Y}_{\text{R}}}.$$

Then,

$$\sqrt{n}(\hat{\delta}-\delta) \to N(0, \sigma^2),$$

where

$\sigma^2=(C_{22}-2C_{12}\delta+C_{11}\delta^2)/(2\mu_{\text{R}})^2$

C_{uv} is the (u, v)th element of $\lambda_1\boldsymbol{\Sigma}_1+\lambda_2\boldsymbol{\Sigma}_2$.

THEOREM 4.5.3 Almost surely,

$$\frac{n_1}{n}\mathbf{S}_1 + \frac{n_2}{n}\mathbf{S}_2 \rightarrow \lambda_1\mathbf{\Sigma}_1 + \lambda_2\mathbf{\Sigma}_2,$$

where $\mathbf{S}_k$ is given in Section 4.2.4.

THEOREM 4.5.4

Let $\hat{C}_{uv}$ be the (u, v)th element of $(n_1/n)\mathbf{S}_1 + (n_2/n)\mathbf{S}_2$. Then $\hat{\sigma} \rightarrow \sigma^2$ almost surely, where $\widehat{\sigma^2} = (\hat{C}_{22} - 2\hat{C}_{12}\hat{\delta} + \hat{C}_{11}\hat{\delta}^2)/(2\overline{Y}_{\text{R}})^2$.

Combining the above results, we have the following result:

THEOREM 4.5.5

$$\sqrt{n}(\hat{\delta} - \delta)/\widehat{\sigma} \rightarrow N(0, 1).$$

Hence, an approximate $(1 - 2\alpha) \times 100\%$ confidence interval for δ is given by

$$\hat{\delta} \pm z(\alpha)\widehat{\sigma}/\sqrt{n}.$$

The bootstrap procedure can then be applied on this approximate confidence interval as follows:

Step 1. For given $\mathbf{X}_{ik}$, $i = 1, 2, \ldots, n_k$, $k = 1, 2$, draw an i.i.d. bootstrap sample with replacement $\{\mathbf{Z}_{i1}^b, i = 1, 2, \ldots, n_1\}$ from $\{\mathbf{X}_{i1}, i = 1, 2, \ldots, n_1\}$ and an i.i.d. sample $\{\mathbf{Z}_{i2}^b, i = 1, 2, \ldots, n_2\}$ from $\{\mathbf{X}_{i2}, i = 1, 2, \ldots, n_2\}$.

Step 2. On the basis of $\{\mathbf{Z}_i k^b, i = 1, \ldots, n_k; k = 1, 2\}$, calculate $\hat{\delta}_b$, $\widehat{\sigma}_b$, and

$$T_b = \frac{\sqrt{n}(\hat{\delta}_b - \hat{\delta})}{\widehat{\sigma}_b}.$$

Step 3. Repeat step 1 and step 2 many times (say B times) (i.e., $b = 1, 2, \ldots, B$). The bootstrap confidence interval for δ with approximate confidence level of $1 - 2\alpha$ is given by.

$$(\hat{\delta} + \omega(\alpha)\widehat{\sigma}/\sqrt{n}, \hat{\delta} + \omega(1 - \alpha)\widehat{\sigma}/\sqrt{n}),$$

where $\omega(\alpha)$ is the αth quantile of the histogram $\{T_b, b = 1, \ldots, B\}$.

From a simulation study, Chow et al. (1990) showed that the coverage probability for the bootstrap confidence interval is uniformly close to the nominal ones for several combinations of parameters under study and for various distribution assumptions on $\{S_{ik}\}$ and $\{e_{ijk}\}$. However, the drawback of this method is that the bootstrap sampling is based on the asymptotic results (i.e., asymptotic variance), which does not provide the actual variability associated with $\hat{\delta}$.

Example 4.5.3

To illustrate the use of this approach, consider the example given in Section 3.6. The estimates for δ and σ and the critical values $\omega(\alpha)$ and $\omega(1-\alpha)$ obtained from $B = 1000$ bootstrap samples are given as follows:

$$\hat{\delta} = 0.972, \quad \hat{\sigma} = 0.217, \quad \text{and}$$
$$\omega(0.05) = -1.926, \quad \omega(0.95) = 1.543.$$

Thus, the 90% bootstrap confidence interval is given by (92.8%, 104.1%), which is in favor of the conclusion of average bioequivalence.

Note that the above bootstrap procedure can be applied to the confidence interval discussed in Section 4.2 when the normality assumptions of $\{S_{ik}\}$ and $\{e_{ijk}\}$ are seriously violated. In this case, however, the finite sample performance of the bootstrap confidence interval should be examined.

4.6 Discussion and Other Alternatives

4.6.1 Discussion

In this chapter, we have introduced several statistical methods for the assessment of average bioequivalence according to the ± 20 rule. Basically, these methods were derived under the assumption of equal carryover effects and they are summarized in Table 4.6.1. Some of these methods are actually operationally equivalent in the sense that they will reach the same decision on bioequivalence. For example, Schuirmann's two one-sided tests procedure based on a *t*-test is equivalent to the $(1-2\alpha) \times 100\%$ classic (shortest) confidence interval which, in turn, is equivalent to the $(1-2\alpha) \times 100\%$ HPD interval of Bayesian approach proposed by Rodda and Davis. In addition, the *p*-value of Anderson and Hauck's procedure, as shown in Section 4.3.3, can be easily obtained from T_L and T_U, the test statistics for Schuirmann's two one-sided tests procedure. Moreover, the $(1-2\alpha) \times 100\%$ confidence interval for μ_T/μ_R based on the fixed Fieller's theorem is equivalent to the Bayesian method proposed by Mandallaz and Mau. For nonparametric methods, the two one-sided procedure based on the Wilcoxon–Mann–Whitney test is equivalent to the distribution-free $(1-2\alpha) \times 100\%$ confidence interval based on Lehmann–Hodges estimator. Although some of these methods are operationally equivalent in the process of decision making, their interpretations, however, are quite different. For example, the $(1-2\alpha) \times 100\%$ confidence intervals obtained based on sampling theory have a completely different interpretation from the HPD interval obtained from Bayesian methods. Although the $(1-2\alpha) \times 100\%$ confidence internal for $\mu_T - \mu_R$ is statistically equivalent to the hypothesis testing for H_0: $\mu_T = \mu_R$ versus H_a: $\mu_T \neq \mu_R$, the use of a confidence interval as a decision tool for average bioequivalence needs to be carefully examined because the assurance in terms of

TABLE 4.6.1: Summary of methods for assessment of bioequivalence in average bioavailability.

Approach	Method	Parameter	Statistics	Decision on Bioequivalence
Confidence interval	Classical	$\mu_T - \mu_R$	$CI_1 = (\bar{Y}_T - \bar{Y}_R) \pm S$	$CI_1 \in (\theta_L, \theta_U)$
	Westlake	μ_T	$CI_3 = \pm k_i S \pm (\bar{Y}_T - \bar{Y}_R)$	$CI_3 \in (\theta_L, \theta_U)$
	Fieller	μ_T/μ_R	$CI_2 = \frac{1}{1-G}\left[\left(\hat{\delta} - G\frac{S_{TR}}{S_{RR}}G^*\right) \pm \left(t\frac{\sqrt{wS^2_{RR}}}{\bar{Y}_R}\right)\right]$	$CI_2 \in (0.8, 1.2)$
	Fixed Fieller	μ_T/μ_R	$CI_2 = \frac{1}{1-G}\left\{\hat{\delta} \pm t\frac{\sqrt{wMS_{Intra}}}{\bar{Y}_R}[\hat{\delta}^2 + (1-G_1)]^2\right\}$	$CI_2 \in (0.8, 1.2)$
	Chow–Shao	(μ_R, μ_T)	Confidence region (CR) for (μ_R, μ_T)	CR bounded by 0.8 μ_R and 1.2 μ_R
	Nonparametric	$\mu_T - \mu_R$	$CI_1 = (D_{(w(\alpha))}, D_{(w(1-\alpha)+1)})$	$CI_1 \in (\theta_L, \theta_U)$
Hypotheses testing	Schuirmann	$\mu_T - \mu_R$	$T_L = (\overline{Y}_T - \overline{Y}_R - \theta_L)/S$ $T_U = (\overline{Y}_T - \overline{Y}_R - \theta_U)/S$	$T_L > t$ and $T_U > t$
	Anderson–Hauck	$\mu_T - \mu_R$	$p = F_t(T_U) - F_t(-T_L)$ or $p = F_t(-T_L) - F_t(T_U)$	$p < \alpha$
	Nonparametric	$\mu_T - \mu_R$	$W_L = R_L - [n_1(n_1+1)/2]$, $W_U = R_U - [n_1(n_1+1)/2]$	$W_L > w(1-\alpha)$, $W_U < w(\alpha)$
Bayesian	Rodda–Davis	—	$P_{RD} = F_t(t_U) - F_t(t_L)$	$P_{RD} > 0.90$
	Mandallaz–Mau	—	$P_{MM} = F_t(t_{\delta_L}) - F_t(t_{\delta_U})$	$P_{MM} > 0.90$

Note: $t = t(\alpha, n_1 + n_2 - 2)$, $S = \hat{\sigma}_d\sqrt{1/n_1 + 1/n_2}$, $\hat{\delta} = \overline{Y}_T/\overline{Y}_R$, $-\theta_L = \theta_U = 0.2\mu_R$, and others can be found in text.

coverage probability is referred to as $\mu_T - \mu_R$ within the confidence limits, not to the bioequivalence limits stated in the ± 20 rule.

To illustrate the use of these methods, the example described in Section 3.6 was used. The results from each method are summarized in Tables 4.6.2 through 4.6.5. All of the methods led to the conclusion of average bioequivalence. More discussion on the assessment of bioequivalence in terms of average bioavailability as well as the variability of bioavailability is discussed in Chapter 7.

Appendix B.1 gives the SAS program for computation of all procedures discussed in this chapter except the confidence region in Equation 4.6 and bootstrap resampling procedure in Equation 4.53. Note that the SAS programs for Westlake's symmetric confidence interval, Anderson–Hauck's procedure, and Mandallaz–Mau's Bayesian method are modified based on the programs given in Metzler (1988).

As recommended in the FDA guidance on general considerations for bioequivalence studies (FDA, 2003b), the evaluation of bioequivalence consists of three components: (1) a criterion to allow comparison, (2) a confidence interval, and (3) a bioequivalence limit. With respect to the bioequivalence criteria, the U.S. FDA as well as the EMEA and the WHO recommend the continued use of average bioequivalence criterion to compare bioavailability measures for replicate and nonreplicate bioequivalence studies of both immediate- and modified-release products. Therefore, at the 5% significance level, the 90% confidence intervals for the difference (or ratio) of the average bioavailability between the test and reference formulations are constructed. Under the $\pm 20\%$ rule based on the original scale (or 80/125 rule based on the log-scale) for bioequivalence limit, bioequivalence between a test formulation and a reference formulation is claimed at the 5% significance level if the 90% confidence interval for the difference (or ratio) is within $\pm 20\%$ of the reference mean (is within 80% and 125%). Since Schuirmann's two one-sided tests procedure and its nonparametric counterpart are operationally equivalent to their corresponding confidence interval approaches, these two methods are currently recommended by almost all of the regulatory agencies in the world for assessment of average bioequivalence. On the other hand, Fieller's theorem provides the exact confidence interval for the ratio of the average bioavailability on the original scale. It is also recommended that the exact confidence interval constructed by Fieller's theorem be employed to assess bioequivalence for $t_{\max}$.

Since Schuirman's two one-sided tests procedure, which is discussed in Chapter 5, is conservative in the sense that its actual size is smaller than the nominal significance level, Brown et al. (1998) and Munk et al. (2000) proposed an unbiased test for the interval hypothesis which is claimed to be uniformly powerful than the Schuirman's two one-sided tests procedure. However, like the Anderson–Hauck procedure, the unbiased test proposed by Brown et al. (1998) has an open-ended rejection region. Therefore, average bioequivalence can be still concluded if the variability is large. In addition, as demonstrated in Munk et al. (2000), the maximal advantage of the proposed unbiased test and its modified procedures over Schuirman's two one-sided tests procedure occurs when the standard error of $\overline{Y}_T - \overline{Y}_R$ is 4/3 and degrees of freedom is 22 where the power of the proposed unbiased test is only 12%. However, it should be noted that in practice, no one will design a bioequivalence trial with a power less than 80%. But when the power is greater than 70% or standard

TABLE 4.6.2: Summary of results from confidence interval approach for Example 3.6.

Method	Parameter	Decision Making[a]	90% Confidence Interval	Conclusion
Shortest	$\mu_T - \mu_R$	$CI_1 \in (\theta_L, \theta_U)$[b]	$CI_1 = (-8.698, 4.123)$	BE[c]
	μ_T/μ_R	$CI_2 \in (\delta_L, \delta_U)$	$CI_2 = (89.46\%, 104.99\%)$	BE
Westlake	μ_T	$CI_3 \in (-\Delta, \Delta)$	$CI_3 = (-7.413, 7.413)$	BE
Fieller	μ_T/μ_R	$CI_2 \in (\delta_L, \delta_U)$	$CI_2 = (89.78\%, 105.19\%)$	BE
Fixed Fieller	μ_T/μ_R	$CI_2 \in (\delta_L, \delta_U)$	$CI_2 = (89.85\%, 105.20\%)$	BE
Chow and Shao	(μ_R/μ_T)	$T_1 < F(1-2\alpha, 2, n-2)$ and conditions $1'$ through $3'$ in Section 4.2.4 hold	—	BE

[a] CI_1, CI_2, and CI_3 are confidence intervals for $\mu_T - \mu_R$, μ_T/μ_R, and μ_T, respectively.
[b] In most cases, $-\theta_L = \theta_U = 0.2\ \mu_R$; $\delta_L = 80\%$ and $\delta_U = 120\%$; and $\Delta = 20\%$.
[c] BE, bioequivalence.

TABLE 4.6.3: Summary of results from the method of interval hypotheses for Example 3.6.

Method	Hypotheses	Decision Making	p-Value[a]	Conclusion
Schuirmann's two one-sided tests procedure	H_{01}: $\mu_T - \mu_R \leq \theta_L$ H_{02}: $\mu_T - \mu_R \geq \theta_U$	$p_1 < 0.05$ and $p_2 < 0.05$	$p_1 = 0.00002$ $p_2 = 0.00048$	BE
Anderson and Hauck	H_{01}: $\mu_T - \mu_R \leq \theta_L$ or $\mu_T - \mu_R \geq \theta_U$	$p < 0.05$	$p = 0.00045$	BE

[a] p_1 and p_2 are the observed p-values under H_{01} and H_{02}, respectively, whereas p is the observed p-value under H_0.

TABLE 4.6.4: Summary of results from the Bayesian approach for Example 3.6.

Method	Prior	Decision Making	Posterior Probability	Conclusion
Rodda and Davis	Noninformative	$P_{RM} > 0.90$	$P_{RD} = 0.9995$	BE
Mandallaz and Mau	Improper vague prior	$P_{MM} > 0.90$	$P_{MM} = 0.9997$	BE

error of $\overline{Y}_T - \overline{Y}_R$ is smaller than 0.5, the proposed unbiased test and Schuirman's two one-sided tests procedure provide almost identical power. Therefore, we argue that the proposed unbiased test by Brown et al. (1998) is of theoretically sound but of no current practical regulatory applications to evaluation of bioequivalence due to the following reasons:

1. The proposed unbiased test is not uniformly most powerful and the uniformly most powerful unbiased test may not exist (Lehmann and Romano, 2005).
2. It does not provide the corresponding confidence interval.
3. Its real advantage is too negligible to be of any practical use.

Alternatively, other methods have been proposed to evaluate average bioequivalence. For example, Ghosh and Khattree (2003) applied encompassing arithmetic intrinsic Bayes' factor (EIBF) to assess average bioequivalence and Dragilin et al. (2003) suggested the use of Kullback–Leiber divergence as an alternative criterion for average bioequivalence. However, these newly proposed methods do not provide confidence interval as required by the regulatory agencies. The interpretation of their results and performance in terms of size and power require further investigation.

4.6.2 Other Alternatives

As indicated in Section 1.3, the extent and rate of absorption of a drug product are often used to assess bioequivalence between formulations of the drug product. The extent and rate of absorption of the drug product are quantified by the pharmacokinetic measures for systematic exposures such as AUC, C_{max}, and t_{max}, which can be obtained from the blood or plasma concentration–time curve. For the assessment of average bioequivalence, separate univariate analysis of each measure is usually performed based on the methods introduced earlier. However, AUC, C_{max}, and t_{max} are some summarized characteristics of the observed blood or plasma concentration–time curve. Thus, for a single-dose bioavailability and bioequivalent study, instead of studying each measure alone, it may be more appropriate to compare the profiles of the blood or plasma concentration–time curves for the test and reference formulations by use of a repeated measures model (Johnson and Wichern, 1982). In other words, we may consider the blood or plasma concentrations at each sampling time following a dose. For each subject, these concentrations are considered repeated measures. Analysis with a repeated measures model is a

TABLE 4.6.5: Summary of results from nonparametric approaches for Example 3.6.

Method	Parameter or Hypotheses	Decision Making	p-Value or 90% CI	Conclusion
W–M–W two one-sided tests[a]	H_{01}: $\mu_T - \mu_R \leq \theta_L$ H_{02}: $\mu_T - \mu_R \geq \theta_U$	$p_1 < 0.05$ and $p_2 < 0.05$	$p_1 < 0.01$ $p_2 < 0.01$	BE
Hodge–Lehmann	$\mu_T - \mu_R$	$CI_1 \in (\theta_L, \theta_U)$	$(-10.63, 4.84)$	BE
Bootstrap	μ_R/μ_R	$CI_2 \in (\delta_L, \delta_U)$	(92.8%, 104.1%)	BE

[a] W–M–W, Wilcoxon–Mann–Whitney.

comparison of the average concentrations over time. With this model, the difference in the shape of the profile of the blood or plasma concentration–time curve between formulations can be examined by testing the interaction between formulations and sampling times. A significant interaction between formulations and sampling times may indicate that the rates of absorption, distribution, and elimination of the drug are different between formulations. Although a repeated measures model may be appropriate, the following are some difficulties that often occur in practice:

1. This model requires restrictive assumptions about the covariance matrix.
2. It is very difficult to obtain a reliable estimate of the covariance matrix because of the small number of subjects and large number of time points.
3. Unlike AUC, average concentration over time is not a measure of the average amount of drug absorbed in the body.
4. Missing values at some sampling time points often occur which lead to an unbalanced situation and, consequently, complicate the analysis.

Therefore, for the assessment of average bioequivalence using the repeated measures model based on the blood or plasma concentrations, further research is needed to address these concerns.

Several multivariate approaches are also available for the analysis of the blood or plasma concentrations. For example, the method proposed by Grizzle and Allen (1969) can be applied to those blood or plasma concentrations that require no special assumptions on the structure of the covariance matrix. Snee (1972) proposed a method that combines that analysis of variance and principal components for the analysis of continuous curves. This method can be applied to compare the shape of the blood or plasma concentration–time curve between formulations that require less restrictive assumptions about the covariance matrix. Metzler (1974) indicated that other multivariate techniques, such as a multivariate randomization test, could be considered and investigated for their possible application to bioavailability studies.

Given the observed blood or plasma concentrations, another approach, which is often considered as an adjunct to bioavailability studies, is the fitting of a pharmacokinetic model (McQuarrie, 1967; Jacques, 1972). However, the method involves the estimation of parameters from a nonlinear model (one-compartment model or multicompartment model). It is often very difficult to have some desired statistical properties (such as unbiasness and uniformly minimum variance) for estimators of the parameters of interest (e.g., the rate of absorption) owing to the nature of nonlinearity. Besides, as the model may vary from subject to subject, statistical inferences such as estimate and confidence interval of the parameter obtained from a model, which may be able to adequately describe the drug kinetics, may not be meaningful owing to the inter-subject and the intra-subject variabilities. Thus, how to account for the inter-subject and intra-subject variabilities in pharmacokinetic modeling is an important issue. To date, little attention has been paid to this difficulty. Further research in this area would be worthwhile.

Chapter 5

Power and Sample Size Determination

5.1 Introduction

As indicated in Chapter 1, one of the major objectives of a bioavailability and bioequivalence study comparing two formulations (e.g., a test formulation and a reference formulation) of a drug product is to determine whether the two formulations are average bioequivalent. During the planning stage of a bioavailability and bioequivalence study, the following questions concerning the study sample size are of particular interest to the clinicians:

1. How many subjects are needed to have a desired power (e.g., 80%) establishing average bioequivalence between two formulations within clinically important limits (e.g., 20% of the reference mean)?

2. What is the "trade off" if only a small number of subjects are available for the study owing to limited budget or some medical considerations?

To provide answers to these questions, a statistical evaluation for sample size determination is often employed. The most commonly used approach is to perform a prestudy power calculation based on an estimate of the intra-subject from previous studies. In other words, an appropriate sample size is chosen to meet the desired power for assessment of average bioequivalence within clinically important limits, assuming that the estimate of intra-subject variability is the true intra-subject variability.

Determination of a sample size depends on the power function of some test statistics for the hypotheses to be evaluated for assessment of average bioequivalence. A commonly used approach is to choose a sample size based on a power function of the test statistic for the hypothesis of equality between formulation effects (i.e., $\mu_T = \mu_R$). However, as indicated in Chapter 4, the method of hypothesis testing for equality between formulation effects (or point hypotheses) is not an appropriate statistical method for assessment of average bioequivalence. The sample size obtained based on a power function of the test for point hypotheses may not be large enough to provide sufficient power, if other appropriate statistical methods, such as the classic confidence interval approach and Schuirmann's two one-sided tests procedure for interval hypotheses, are used.

For assessment of average bioequivalence, as indicated in Chapter 4, the classic confidence interval approach and Rodda and Davis's Bayesian method are (operationally) equivalent to Schuirmann's two one-sided t tests procedure for interval hypotheses in the sense that they lead to the same conclusion of average bioequivalence. Therefore, in this chapter, without loss of generality, a sample size determination will be evaluated based on the power of Schuirmann's two one-sided t tests procedure for interval hypotheses using the ± 20 rule for assessment of average bioequivalence based on the original scale. This method for sample size determination based on the original scale can be easily extended to the log-scale using the 80/125 rule and is given later in Chapter 9.

In Section 5.2, the concept of type I and type II errors, which occur in interval hypotheses testing, is introduced. In Section 5.3, the powers and sizes of Schuirmann's two one-sided t tests procedure and Anderson and Hauck's procedure is examined. Statistical properties for a commonly used power approach, which are based on the 80/20 rule, for assessment of average bioequivalence are examined. Also included is the comparison of relative efficiencies among methods introduced in Chapter 4. In Section 5.4, a formula for sample size determination is provided based on the power function of Schuirmann's two one-sided t tests procedure. Because the calculation of power for Schuirmann's two one-sided t tests procedure at $\theta = \theta_0 \neq 0$ requires a complicated numerical integration, an empirical power, which can easily be obtained through a simulation study, is introduced to approximate the true power. The power of Schuirmann's two one-sided t tests procedure is also compared with that of Anderson and Hauck's procedure in this section.

5.2 Hypotheses and Type I and Type II Errors

5.2.1 Hypotheses Testing

In bioavailability studies, a hypothesis is a postulation, assumption, or statement that is made about the population relative to a drug product under study, such as a test formulation and a reference formulation of the drug product. The statement that there is a carryover effect (i.e., $C_R \neq C_T$), for example, is a hypothesis for the existence of unequal carryover effects of the drug under study. Another example is the statement that there is a direct formulation effect (i.e., $F \neq 0$). This is a hypothesis for the treatment effect. A random sample is usually drawn through a bioavailability study to evaluate hypotheses about the drug product. To perform a hypothesis testing, the following steps are essential:

1. Choose the hypothesis that is to be tested, denoted by H_0, where H_0 is usually referred to as the null hypothesis.

2. Choose an alternative hypothesis, denoted by H_a, where H_a is usually the hypothesis of particular interest to the investigators.

3. Select a test statistic and define the rejection region (or a rule) for decision making about how and when to reject the null hypothesis and how and when to fail to reject it.

4. Draw a random sample by conducting a bioavailability study.

5. Calculate test statistics.

6. Make conclusions according to the predetermined rule specified in step 3.

5.2.2 Type I and Type II Errors

Basically, two kinds of errors occur when testing hypotheses. If the null hypothesis is rejected when it is true, then a type I error has occurred. If the null hypothesis is not rejected when it is false, then a type II error has been made. The probabilities of making type I and type II errors are given as

$$\begin{aligned} \alpha &= P(\text{type I error}) \\ &= P(\text{reject H}_0 \text{ when H}_0 \text{ is true}). \end{aligned}$$

$$\begin{aligned} \beta &= P(\text{type II error}) \\ &= P(\text{fail to reject H}_0 \text{ when H}_0 \text{ is false}). \end{aligned}$$

The probability of making a type I error, α, is called the level of significance. In practice, α is also known as the consumer's risk, while β is sometimes referred to as the producer's risk. Table 5.2.1 summarizes the relation between type I and type II errors when testing hypotheses.

Power of the rest is defined as the probability of correctly rejecting H_0 when H_0 is false; that is,

$$\begin{aligned} \text{Power} &= 1 - \beta \\ &= P(\text{reject H}_0 \text{ when H}_0 \text{ is false}). \end{aligned}$$

TABLE 5.2.1: Relationship between type I and type II errors.

I. General Case

		If H_0 is	
		True	**False**
When	Fail to reject H_0	No error	Type II error
	Reject H_0	Type I error	No error

II. Bioequivalence Trial

	True State H_0	
Decision	**Bioinequivalent**	**Bioequivalent**
Bioinequivalent (fail to reject H_0)	Right decision	Type II error
Bioequivalent (reject H_0)	Type I error	Right decision

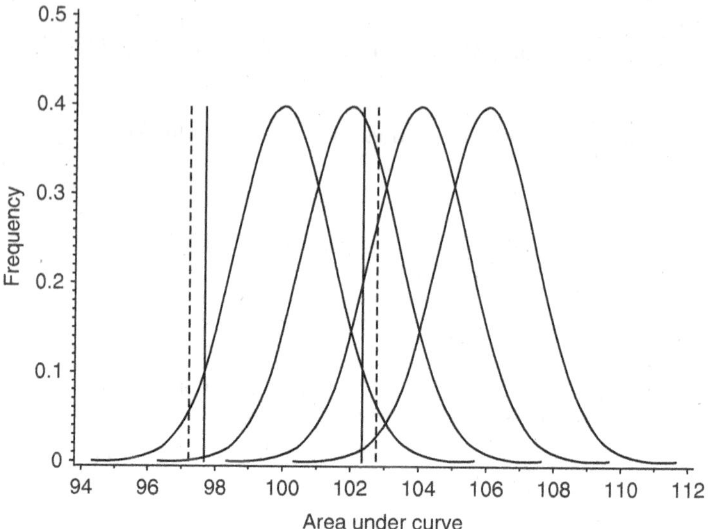

FIGURE 5.2.1: Relationship between probabilities of type I and II errors: Hypothesis of equality. The null hypothesis is mean AUC = 100. Solid line corresponds to the test at the 10% nominal level. Dashed line corresponds to the test at the 5% nominal level.

To illustrate the relationship between α and β (or power), a plot based on the hypothesis of equality is presented in Figure 5.2.1, which shows various β's under H_0 (i.e., AUC = 100) for various alternatives (i.e., AUC = 102, 104, and 106) at $\alpha = 5\%$ and 10%. It can be seen that α decreases as β increases and α increases as β decreases. The only way of decreasing both α and β is to increase the sample size. In practice, because a type I error is usually considered to be a more important or serious error, which one would like to avoid, a typical approach in hypothesis testing is to control α at an acceptable level and try to minimize β by choosing an appropriate sample size. In other words, the null hypothesis can be tested at a predetermined level (or nominal level) of significance with a desired power. From Figure 5.2.1, it can be seen that for a fixed α, β increases when H_a moves toward H_0. This means that we will not have sufficient power to detect a small difference between H_0 and H_a. On the other hand, β decreases when H_a moves away from H_0.

5.2.3 Hypotheses Setting

In practice, the null hypothesis H_0 and the alternative hypothesis H_a are sometimes reversed and evaluated for different interests. However, a test for H_0 versus H_a is not equivalent to a test for $H_0' = H_a$ versus $H_a' = H_0$. Two tests under different null hypotheses may lead to a totally different conclusion. For example, a test for

H_0 versus H_a may lead to the rejection of H_0 in favor of H_a. However, a test for $H_0' = H_a$ versus $H'_a = H_0$ may reject the alternative hypothesis. Thus, the choice of the null hypothesis and the alternative hypothesis may have some influence on the parameter to be tested. The following criteria are commonly used as rule of thumb for choosing the null hypothesis.

Rule 1. Choose H_0 based on the importance of a type I error. Under this rule, we believe that a type I error is more important and serious than that of a type II error. We would like to control the chance of making a type I error at a tolerable limit (i.e., α). Thus, H_0 is chosen so that the maximum probability of making a type I error [i.e., P (reject H_0 when H_0 is true)] will not exceed the α level.

Rule 2. Choose the hypothesis we wish to reject as H_0 (Colton, 1974; Ott, 1984; Ware et al., 1986). The purpose of this rule is to establish H_a by rejecting H_0. Note that we will never be able to prove that H_0 is true even though the data fail to reject it.

Occasionally, for a given set of hypotheses, it may be easy to determine whether a type I error is more important or serious than a type II error. If a type II error appears to be more important or serious than a type I error, *Rule 1* suggests that the null hypothesis and the alternative hypothesis be reversed. Frequently, however, the relative importance of the type I error and the type II error is usually very subjective. In this case, *Rule 2* is useful in choosing H_0 and H_a. To illustrate the use of these two criteria, consider the following three examples.

Example 5.2.1 Example of Patient–Doctor

Suppose that there is a very sick patient who is about to die and his/her life depends on a life-support equipment. The situation that exists here is that when no sign of life (e.g., no pulse or heart beat) is detectable on the equipment, the physician will have to make a decision whether the patient is still alive. The consequence of this decision is that if the patient is pronounced dead, the life-support equipment will be removed; otherwise, the life-support equipment will remain and a rescue action will be taken. When a decision is made of whether the patient is dead or still alive, the following errors may occur:

1. The doctor declares the patient is dead when, in fact, the patient is still alive. As a consequence of this wrong decision, the life-support equipment will be removed, and the patient will then be dead. The cost of this error is a human life.

2. The doctor concludes that the patient is still alive when, in fact, the patient is dead. Here, the life-support equipment will remain. The consequence of this wrong decision is that the life-support equipment will not be available for other patients who are in critical condition and need the support of this equipment.

A wrong decision on the death of a patient when he or she is still alive is clearly more serious than the mistake made by concluding that the patient is alive when, in fact, he or she is dead. A doctor will want to avoid, or at least minimize, the chance of making this error of wrongly concluding the death of a patient. In this case, *Rule 1* may be used to choose H_0 as follows:

$$\begin{aligned} &H_0\text{: the patient is alive} \\ \text{versus } &H_a\text{: the patient is dead.} \end{aligned}$$

Therefore, the probability of making a type I error will not exceed a tolerable limit (e.g., 1%). In this case, to reject the null hypothesis that the patient is alive in favor of the alternative hypothesis that the patient is dead, strong evidence or more information (e.g., brain death) is needed before a decision can be made.

However, we cannot prove that the patient is still alive even if we fail to reject H_0. On the basis of *Rule 2*, we are, in fact, more interested in proving that the patient is dead. On the other hand, if we are interested in proving that the patient is alive, we may want to consider the following hypotheses based on *Rule 2*:

$$\begin{aligned} &H_0\text{: the patient is dead} \\ \text{versus } &H_a\text{: the patient is alive.} \end{aligned}$$

Example 5.5.2 Example of Criminal–Jury

Suppose that there is a suspect who is charged with first degree murder and is currently on trial. The situation that exists here is that if the suspect is found guilty, he or she will then be sentenced to death (or a life sentence). On the other hand, if he or she is found innocent, he or she will then be released. The jury will have to determine whether he or she is guilty. Again, there are two kinds of mistakes that the jury can make:

1. The jury can conclude that the suspect is guilty when, in fact, he or she is innocent. The consequence of this mistake is that the person may lose his or her life or spend the rest of his or her life in jail. Human rights would be seriously violated.

2. The suspect is set free when, in fact, he or she is guilty of first degree murder. The consequence of this mistake is that the suspect may again kill or threaten other people's lives. In this situation, the safety of the society is of great concern.

Unlike the patient–doctor example, it is not clear which mistake is more important and serious. Different persons may have different viewpoint(s) on this issue. However, if you believe that human rights are more important than anything else, you probably want to minimize the chance of making the first kind of error. In other words, based on *Rule 1*, one would be interested in testing the following hypotheses:

$$\begin{aligned} &H_0\text{: the suspect is innocent} \\ \text{versus } &H_a\text{: the suspect is guilty.} \end{aligned}$$

To prove the suspect is guilty by rejecting H_0, more evidence will be needed so that the chance of making a type I error is controlled at a tolerable limit (e.g., 1%). On the basis of the above hypotheses, we will not be able to prove that the suspect is innocent, even when we fail to reject H_0. However, in the current judicial system, a suspect is assumed innocent until he or she is proved guilty. Note that, based on *Rule 2*, the purpose of the above hypotheses is to prove that the suspect is guilty.

On the other hand, if the safety of the community is of greatest concern, we may want to minimize the probability of making the second kind of mistake. Therefore, the hypotheses are set up as follows:

$$\begin{aligned} &H_0\text{: the suspect is guilty} \\ \text{versus}\quad &H_a\text{: the suspect is innocent.} \end{aligned}$$

To avoid making the mistake of wrongly concluding the suspect is innocent when, in fact, he or she is guilty, a careful evaluation is necessary before the suspect is concluded to be innocent. The purpose of the above hypotheses is, therefore, to prove that the suspect is innocent.

Example 5.2.3 Example of Bioinequivalence–Bioequivalence

Similarly, the following two errors occur in the assessment of bioequivalence when comparing two formulations in average bioavailabilities:

1. We conclude bioequivalence when, in fact, the test formulation is not bioequivalent with the reference formulation.
2. We conclude bioinequivalence when, in fact, the test formulation is bioequivalent with the reference formulation.

In the interest of controlling the chance of making a type I error, the FDA may consider hypothesis 1 is more important than hypothesis 2 and, consequently, prefer the following hypothesis:

$$\begin{aligned} &H_0\text{: bioinequivalence} \\ \text{versus}\quad &H_a\text{: bioequivalence.} \end{aligned} \tag{5.2.1}$$

On the other hand, pharmaceutical companies may want to eliminate the probability of wrongly rejecting the null hypothesis of bioequivalence. Thus, the following hypotheses are used:

$$\begin{aligned} &H_0\text{: bioinequivalence} \\ \text{versus}\quad &H_a\text{: bioinequivalence.} \end{aligned} \tag{5.2.2}$$

It is very subjective whether hypothesis 1 is more important than hypothesis 2 or hypothesis 2 is more important than hypothesis 1 when comparing two formulations of the same drug product.

In bioavailability studies, *Rule 2* is usually applied to choose H_0. For example, when a new formulation is developed by the innovator, the innovator will want to show bioequivalence between the new formulation and the reference formulation by disproving the hypothesis of bioinequivalence. In this case, hypothesis 5.2.1 may be considered. On the other hand, if the formulation is prepared by generic companies, the innovator will be in favor of the hypothesis of bioinequivalence. In this latter case, hypothesis in 5.2.2 is preferred.

5.3 Power and Relative Efficiency

5.3.1 Power and Size of Tests

Because, based on *Rule 2* for hypothesis setting, the purpose of a bioavailability study is to establish average bioequivalence between formulations, the hypotheses in Equation 5.2.1 is considered, which can be stated in terms of interval hypotheses in Equation 4.3.1.

Without loss of generality, the equivalence limits (θ_L, θ_U) can be chosen such that $-\theta_L = \theta_U = \Delta > 0$. Thus, the hypotheses in 5.2.1 become:

$$\begin{aligned} &H_0: \theta \leq -\Delta \quad \text{or} \quad \theta \geq \Delta \text{ (i.e., average bioinequivalence)} \\ \text{versus} \quad &H_a: -\Delta < \theta < \Delta \text{ (i.e., average bioequivalence)} \end{aligned} \qquad (5.3.1)$$

where $\theta = \mu_T - \mu_R$.

From hypotheses 5.3.1, it can be seen that the true difference in formulation means θ could be any real number between $-\infty$ and ∞. Under H_0, θ is either in $(-\infty, -\Delta]$ or $[\Delta, \infty)$, while θ could be any number between $-\Delta$ and Δ under H_a. Let

$$\Omega_0 = \{(-\infty, \ -\Delta]U[\Delta, \infty)\} \quad \text{and} \quad \Omega_a = \{(-\Delta, \Delta)\}, \qquad (5.3.2)$$

where Ω_0 and Ω_a are usually referred to as the parameter space corresponding to H_0 and H_a, respectively.

The hypotheses in 5.3.1 are then equivalent to

$$\begin{aligned} &H_0: \ \theta \in \Omega_0 \\ \text{versus} \quad &H_a: \ \theta \in \Omega_a. \end{aligned} \qquad (5.3.3)$$

A test is said to have a significance level of α if the probability of committing a type I error is less than or equal to α, $0 < \alpha < 1$, for $\theta \in \Omega_0$, that is,

$$\begin{aligned} &P\{\text{reject } H_0 \text{ given average bioinequivalence}\} \\ &\quad = P\{\text{reject } H_0 \text{ given } \theta \in \Omega_0\} \\ &\quad \leq \alpha. \end{aligned}$$

A test is said to have a size of α if

$$\max_{\theta \in \Omega_0} P\{\text{reject H}_0 \text{ given } \theta \in \Omega_0\} = \alpha.$$

Similarly, the probability of correctly concluding average bioequivalence or power of the test of hypotheses in 5.3.1 or 5.3.3 is given by

$$\begin{aligned}\phi(\theta) &= 1 - \beta \\ &= P\{\text{reject H}_0 \text{ given } \theta \in \Omega_a\} \\ &= P\{\text{reject H}_0 \text{ given average bioequivalence}\},\end{aligned}$$

where β is the probability of wrongly concluding average bioequivalence; that is,

$$\begin{aligned}\beta &= P\{\text{fail to reject H}_0 \text{ given } \theta \in \Omega_a\} \\ &= P\{\text{fail to reject H}_0 \text{ given average bioequivalence}\}.\end{aligned}$$

5.3.2 Power of Schuirmann's Two One-Sided *t* Tests Procedure

Let

$$Y = \overline{Y}_T - \overline{Y}_R, \quad m = \sqrt{\frac{1}{n_1} + \frac{1}{n_2}},$$
$$t = t(\alpha, n_1 + n_2 - 2), \quad \text{and} \quad s = \widehat{\sigma}_d.$$

Schuirmann's two one-sided t tests procedure for hypothesis in Equations 5.3.1 or 5.3.3 then leads to the rejection of H_0 at the α level of significance if

$$t_1 = \frac{Y + \Delta}{ms} > t \quad \text{and} \quad t_2 = \frac{Y - \Delta}{ms} < -t.$$

In other words, the null hypothesis, H_0, of average bioinequivalence is rejected at the α level of significance if the observed value of Y is within the following rejection region:

$$P = \{(Y, s) | -\Delta + tms < Y < \Delta - tms\}. \tag{5.3.4}$$

Note that the acceptance region (i.e., the region that leads to the conclusion of average bioinequivalence) is the complement of $\mathcal{R}$; that is,

$$P^c = \{(Y, s) | Y <-\Delta + tms \quad \text{or} \quad Y \geq \Delta - tms\}.$$

Schuirmann (1987) examined the rejection region $\mathcal{R}$ in terms of the relationship between Y (observed difference is least square (LS) means between formulations) and ms (standard error). For example, Figure 5.3.1 gives the rejection region (the triangular area) at the α level of significance for the case where $\Delta = 20$ and $n_1 = n_2 = 6$. The results indicate that we will never reject H_0 (or conclude bioequivalence) if the

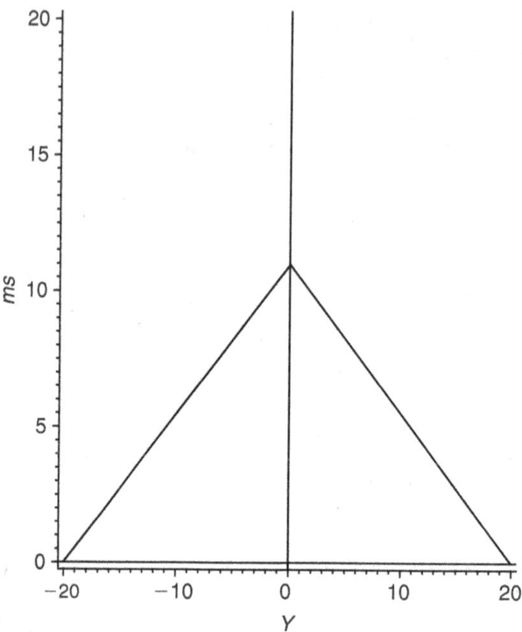

FIGURE 5.3.1: Rejection region of Schuirmann's two one-sided tests procedure for $\Delta = 20$, $n_1 = n_2 = 6$, and the 0.05 nominal level. (From Schuirmann, D.J., *J. Pharmacokinet. Biopharm.*, 15, 657, 1987.)

standard error of Y (i.e., ms) is greater than Δ/t, even when $Y = 0$. On the other hand, if the standard error of Y is small, a large value of Y would possibly lead to the rejection of H_0 as long as Y is within $(-\Delta, \Delta)$.

On the basis of hypotheses given in Equations 5.3.1 or 5.3.3, the power for Schuirmann's two one-sided tests procedure (or the probability of correctly concluding average bioequivalence) is given as

$$\begin{aligned} \phi_s(\theta) &= P\{\text{reject } H_0 \text{ given average bioequivalence}\} \\ &= P\{(Y, s), P \text{ given } \theta \in \Omega_a\}. \end{aligned} \tag{5.3.5}$$

The power can be evaluated at $\theta = \theta_0$ as follows:

$$\begin{aligned} \phi_s(\theta_0) &= P\left\{\frac{-\theta_0}{m\sigma_d} + \frac{-\Delta + tms}{m\sigma_d} < \frac{Y - \theta_0}{m\sigma_d} < \frac{-\theta_0}{m\sigma_d} + \frac{\Delta - tms}{m\sigma_d}\right\} \\ &= E\left[P\left\{\frac{-\theta_0}{m\sigma_d} - \frac{(\Delta - tms)}{m\sigma_d} < \frac{Y - \theta_0}{m\sigma_d} < \frac{-\theta_0}{m\sigma_d} + \frac{\Delta - tms}{m\sigma_d}\middle| s\right\}\right], \end{aligned} \tag{5.3.6}$$

where the expectation is taken over the distribution of s^2/σ_d^2 which is a $\chi^2\,(n_1 + n_2 - 2)/(n_1 + n_2 - 2)$.

Denote

$$a = \frac{\theta_0}{m\sigma_d}, \quad b = \frac{\Delta - tms}{m\sigma_d}, \quad \text{and} \quad Z = \frac{Y - \theta_0}{m\sigma_d}.$$

Then, Equation 5.3.6 becomes

$$\begin{aligned}\phi_s(\theta_0) &= E[P\{-a - b < Z < -a + b|s\}] \\ &= E[\Phi(-a+b) - \Phi(-a-b)],\end{aligned} \qquad (5.3.7)$$

where Φ is the cumulative distribution function of the standard normal distribution.

If $\theta = -\theta_0$, the power is given by

$$\phi_s(-\theta_0) = E[\Phi(a+b) - \Phi(a-b)].$$

Since $\Phi(a+b) - \Phi(a-b) = \Phi(-a+b) - \Phi(-a-b)$, the power function $\phi_s(\theta)$ is symmetric about $(\theta_L + \theta_U)/2$. In particular, $\phi_s(\theta)$ is symmetric about 0 when $-\theta_L = \theta_U > 0$. The maximum power occurs at $\theta = 0$. It can be seen that the power decreases as θ moves away from 0; that is, $\phi_s(\theta') < \phi_s(\theta'')$ if either $\theta' > \theta'' > 0$ or $\theta' < \theta'' < 0$. Therefore, the size of Schuirmann's two one-sided t tests procedure can be evaluated at $\theta = \Delta$ or $\theta = -\Delta$; that is,

$$\max_{\theta \in \Omega_0} \phi_s(\theta) = \phi_s(\Delta) = \phi_s(-\Delta).$$

Note that

$$\begin{aligned}\phi_s(\Delta) &= P\left\{\frac{-2\Delta}{ms} + t < \frac{Y - \Delta}{ms} < -t\right\} \\ &\leq P\left\{\frac{Y - \Delta}{ms} < -t\right\} \\ &= \alpha.\end{aligned} \qquad (5.3.8)$$

As a result, Schuirmann's two one-sided t tests procedure is a test of significance level α. However, in general, it does not provide a size of α because

$$\max_{\theta \in \Omega_0} \phi_s(\theta) = \phi_s(\Delta) \leq \alpha.$$

Schuirmann (1987) also examined $\phi_s(\theta)$ in terms of the so-called index of sensitivity, which is defined as the ratio of width of the average bioequivalence interval (2Δ) to standard error of the difference in LS means, that is,

$$\nabla = \frac{2\Delta}{\sigma_d\sqrt{\frac{1}{n_1} + \frac{1}{n_2}}}. \qquad (5.3.9)$$

TABLE 5.3.1: Values of the index of sensitivity.

	Coefficient of Variation						
Sample Size	**10%**	**15%**	**20%**	**25%**	**30%**	**35%**	**40%**
8	8.00	5.33	4.00	3.20	2.67	2.29	2.00
10	8.94	5.96	4.47	3.58	2.98	2.56	2.34
12	9.80	6.53	4.90	3.92	3.27	2.80	2.45
14	10.58	7.06	5.29	4.23	3.53	3.02	2.65
16	11.31	7.54	5.66	4.53	3.77	3.23	2.83
18	12.00	8.00	6.00	4.80	4.00	3.43	3.00
20	12.65	8.43	6.32	5.06	4.22	3.61	3.16
22	13.27	8.84	6.63	5.31	4.42	3.79	3.32
24	13.86	9.24	6.93	5.54	4.62	3.96	3.46

According to the ±20 rule, $\Delta/\mu_R = 20\%$. Therefore, ∇ can be expressed in terms of $CV = \sigma_e/\mu_R$ as follows:

$$\nabla = \frac{2\Delta/\mu_R}{(\sigma_e/\mu_R)\sqrt{\frac{1}{2}\left(\frac{1}{n_1}+\frac{1}{n_2}\right)}} = \frac{40}{CV\sqrt{\frac{1}{2}\left(\frac{1}{n_1}+\frac{1}{n_2}\right)}}. \tag{5.3.10}$$

Table 5.3.1 gives value of ∇ for different combinations of CVs, n_1, and n_2 which are encountered in most bioequivalence studies. The results indicate that ∇ increases as sample size increases and as CV decreases. Schuirmann (1987) examined the size of two one-sided test at $\theta = \Delta$ as a function of ∇. For example, Figure 5.3.2 plots $\phi_s(\Delta)$ against ∇ for $n_1 = n_2 = 22$. It appears that the size is close to the nominal level α when ∇ approaches 5 or 6. In view of Table 5.3.1, 38% of ∇'s (24 out of 63) are less than 5. In other words, the size of Schuirmann's two one-sided t tests procedure for about 38% of the combinations is lower than the nominal level α. Furthermore, Figure 5.3.3 presents the power curve $\phi_s(\theta)$ for the case $\nabla = 4$ and $n_1 = n_2 = 22$. It can be seen that the maximum power which occurs at $\theta = 0$ is about 25%. This is due to a tremendous intra-subject variability (about 47%). When the intra-subject variability is large, the size of Schuirmann's two one-sided t tests procedure is less than the nominal level and the procedure may lose power for correctly concluding average bioequivalence.

Note that for evaluation of $\phi_s(\theta)$ at $\theta = \theta_0$, Equation 5.3.6 is rather complicated, requiring a numerical integration from s^2/σ_d^2 to $(\Delta/m\sigma_d)^2/t^2$ as indicated by Schuirmann (1987) and Müller-Cohrs (1990). Phillips (1990) suggested a method using a bivariate noncentral t distribution, in which the correlation between the two variables is 1, to calculate the power of Schuirmann's two one-sided t tests procedure. The idea is to show that T_L and T_U of Equation 4.3.4 follow a bivariate noncentral t distribution with $(n_1 + n_2 - 2)$ degrees of freedom and noncentrality parameters

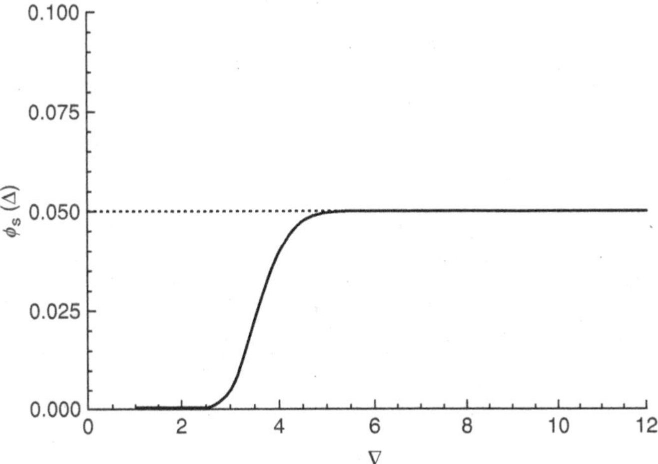

FIGURE 5.3.2: $\phi_s(\Delta)$ versus ∇ for Schuirmann's two one-sided tests procedure for $n_1 = n_2 = 22$, and the nominal level $= 0.05$. (From Schuirmann, D.J., *J. Pharmacokinet. Biopharm.*, 15, 657, 1987.)

$$\mathrm{NC_L} = \frac{\theta + \Delta}{m\sigma_d}, \quad \text{and} \qquad \mathrm{NC_U} = \frac{\theta - \Delta}{m\sigma_d}. \tag{5.3.11}$$

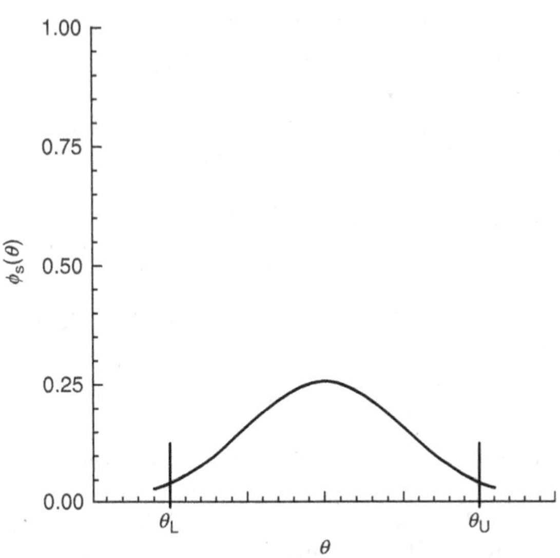

FIGURE 5.3.3: Power function $\phi_s(\theta)$ of Schuirmann's two one-sided tests procedure for $\nabla = 4$, $\Delta = 20$, $n_1 = n_2 = 22$, and the nominal level $= 0.05$. (From Schuirmann, D.J., *J. Pharmacokinet. Biopharm.*, 15, 657, 1987.)

Let X be a normal random variable with mean 0 and variance σ_d^2. $Y+\Delta$ and $Y-\Delta$ can then be expressed in terms of X as follows:

$$\begin{aligned} Y+\Delta &= X+\theta+\Delta \sim N(\theta+\Delta,\, m\sigma_d^2), \quad \text{and} \\ Y-\Delta &= X+\theta-\Delta \sim N(\theta-\Delta,\, m\sigma_d^2). \end{aligned} \tag{5.3.12}$$

It can be seen that the correlation between $Y+\Delta$ and $Y-\Delta$ is equal to 1. Now, $(n_1+n_2-2)s^2/\sigma_d^2$ is distributed as $\chi^2(n_1+n_2-2)$ and is independent of Y. Therefore, the joint distribution of $T_L=(Y+\Delta)/ms$ and $T_U=(Y-\Delta)/ms$ follows a bivariate noncentral t distribution with (n_1+n_2-2) degrees of freedom, correlation $=1$, and noncentrality parameters NC_L and NC_U. Thus, the power $\phi_s(\theta)$ at $\theta=\theta_0$ and $\sigma_d^2=\sigma_0^2$ can be evaluated by

$$P\{T_L > t \text{ and } T_U < -t|\theta_0,\, \sigma_0^2\}. \tag{5.3.13}$$

Owen (1965) showed that the integral of a bivariate noncentral t distribution can be expressed as the difference of the integrals between two univariate noncentral distributions when the correlation is 1. Although Owen's formulae are rather complicated and involve a define integral, these formulae can be programmed using statistical software such as SAS (Phillips, 1990).

From the above discussion, the computation of power for Schuirmann's two one-sided t tests procedure requires special programs for numerical integration based on either Equation 5.3.6 or Equation 5.3.13. To examine the performance of power, instead we may consider an empirical power, which can easily be obtained by conducting a simulation study with fixed θ, σ_d, and sample size, to estimate the true power. This simulation study can be carried out using any standard statistical package such as SAS. The procedure for obtaining an empirical power is outlined as follows:

Step 1. Generate a random sample of size n_1+n_2 according to Equation 4.1.1 with prespecified μ_T, μ_R, σ_d^2, and σ_S^2.

Step 2. For a given equivalence limit Δ (or θ_L and θ_U), calculate T_L and T_U.

Step 3. Repeat steps 1 and 2 many times, say B times.

Step 4. The empirical power is the proportion of B random samples such that $T_L > t$ and $T_U < -t$.

5.3.3 Power of Anderson and Hauck's Test Procedure

Let $p_1=P(T_L>t)$ and $p_2=P(T_U<-t)$. Anderson–Hauck's test produce for interval hypotheses 5.3.1 rejects H_0 and concludes average bioequivalence at the α level of significance if

$$|p_1-p_2| < \alpha. \tag{5.3.14}$$

TABLE 5.3.2: The actual size of Anderson–Hauck's procedure at the nominal levels of $\alpha = 0.05$ and $\alpha = 0.01$.

Degrees of Freedom	$\alpha = 0.05$	$\alpha = 0.01$
10	0.0613	0.0140
20	0.0560	0.0121
50	0.0525	0.0109
100	0.0513	0.0105

Source: From Frick, H., *Communications in Statistics—Theory Methods*, 16, 2771, 1987 and Müller-Cohrs, J., *Biometric. J.*, 32, 259, 1990.

Anderson–Hauck's test procedure is always more powerful than Schuirmann's two one-sided tests procedure at the same nominal level α because Schuirmann's procedure rejects H_0 if

$$p_1 < \alpha \quad \text{and} \quad p_2 < \alpha. \tag{5.3.15}$$

However, Anderson–Hauck's procedure has two major drawbacks that are criticized by the FDA (see Attachment No. 5 of the Report by the Bioequivalence Task Force, January 1988), which are described in the following.

Frick (1987) pointed out that the real size of Anderson–Hauck's procedure does not depend on the prespecified equivalence limit Δ, but only on the sample size (or degrees of freedom) and the nominal level α. Table 5.3.2 lists the actual sizes of Anderson–Hauck's procedure at nominal levels $\alpha = 0.05$ and $\alpha = 0.01$ for various degrees of freedom. The results indicate that the actual size of Anderson–Hauck's procedure is always larger than the nominal level (also see Müller-Cohrs, 1990). Therefore, Anderson–Hauck's procedure can lead to a high probability of committing a type I error (wrongly concluding average bioequivalence).

Furthermore, Figure 5.3.4 gives the rejection of Anderson–Hauck's procedure at $\alpha = 0.05$ nominal level with $\Delta = 20$, $n_1 = n_2 = 6$. The nonconvex shape of the rejection region indicates that any observed LS means difference $\overline{Y}_Y - \overline{Y}_R$ might reject the hypothesis of bioinequivalence and conclude bioequivalence if the observed standard error of $\overline{Y}_T - \overline{Y}_R$ is sufficiently large (also see Rocke, 1984; Schuirmann, 1987; Müller-Cohrs, 1990).

Similar to Schuirmann's two one-sided t tests procedure, calculation of the power of Anderson–Hauck's procedure also requires a complicated numerical integration. Müller-Cohrs (1990) compared the power of Schuirmann's two one-sided tests procedure with that of Anderson–Hauck's procedure at the same real size. The results indicate that Schuirmann's procedure is slightly more powerful than Anderson–Hauck's procedure if the index of sensitivity is greater than 6 (or CV is less than 20%) and the sample size is moderate (e.g., 18–24). This suggests that Schuirmann's procedure is preferred over Anderson–Hauck's procedure for assessment of bioequivalence in average bioavailability in the case where the sample size is between 18 and 24 and a prior CV is less than 20%.

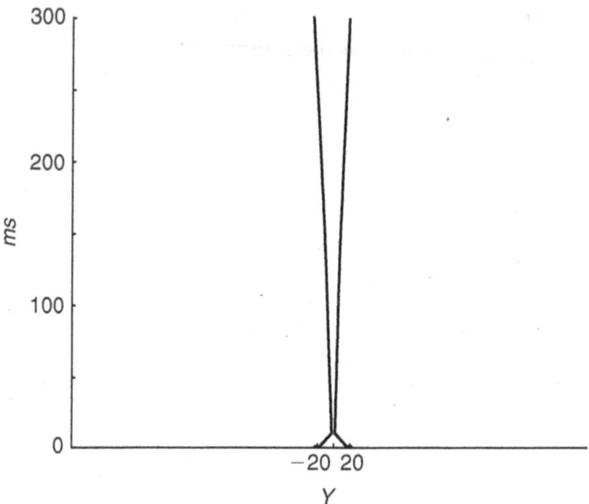

FIGURE 5.3.4: Rejection region of Anderson–Hauck's procedure for $\Delta = 20$, $n_1 = n_2 = 6$, and the 0.05 nominal level. (From Schuirmann, D.J., *J. Pharmacokinet. Biopharm.*, 15, 657, 1987.)

5.3.4 Power Approach for Assessing Average Bioequivalence

The power approach, according to the 80/20 rule, consists of two steps. The first step is to test the hypothesis of equality between two formulations at the α level, that is,

$$\begin{aligned} & \mathrm{H}_0': \theta = 0 \\ \text{versus} \quad & \mathrm{H}_a': \theta \neq 0, \end{aligned} \tag{5.3.16}$$

where $\theta = \mu_T - \mu_R$.

If H_0' is rejected at the α level of significance, we then cannot conclude that the two formulations are bioequivalent in average bioavailability. However if H_0' is not rejected, we proceed to examine whether the power for detection of a difference of $\Delta = 0.2\mu_R$ is greater than 80%. We conclude average bioequivalence if the power is greater than 80%. Let

$$T_P = \frac{Y}{ms} = \frac{\overline{Y}_T - \overline{Y}_R}{\widehat{\sigma}_d \sqrt{\frac{1}{n_1} + \frac{1}{n_2}}}. \tag{5.3.17}$$

Also, let $t(\alpha/2)$ be the upper $\alpha/2$ quantile of a central t distribution with $(n_1 + n_2 - 2)$ degrees of freedom. Then, the power approach concludes that two formulations are bioequivalent in average bioavailability if

$$\begin{aligned} &1.\ |T_p| < t(\alpha/2), \text{ and} \\ &2.\ P\{|T_p| > t(\alpha/2) \text{ given } |\theta| = \Delta\} > 0.80. \end{aligned} \tag{5.3.18}$$

Note that the power in (2) of Equation 5.3.18 can be approximated by a central t distribution, i.e.,

$$P\{|T_p| > t(\alpha/2) \text{ given } |\theta| = \Delta\}$$
$$\cong P\{T > t(\alpha/2) - (\Delta/ms)\},$$

where T has a central t distribution with $(n_1 + n_2 - 2)$ degrees of freedom.

Therefore, the power approach leads to the rejection of average bioinequivalence between the two formulations if

$$t(\alpha/2) - \frac{\Delta}{ms} < -t(0.2).$$

As a result, no value of Y (or $\overline{Y}_T - \overline{Y}_R$) will lead to the conclusion of average bioequivalence if

$$ms \geq \frac{\Delta}{t(\alpha/2) + t(0.2)}. \tag{5.3.19}$$

Note that (1) of Equation 5.3.18 is the acceptance region of the null hypothesis of equality which is bounded by $Y = mst(\alpha/2)$ and $Y = -mst(\alpha/2)$. Hence, the region for conclusion of average bioequivalence using the power approach based upon the 80/20 rule is the intersection of

$$\{(Y, s)| - mst(\alpha/2) < Y < mst(\alpha/2)\} \quad \text{and} \quad \left\{s|s < \frac{\Delta/m}{t(\alpha/2) + t(0.2)}\right\}.$$

Figure 5.3.5 provides the rejection region of the power approach for $\Delta = 20$, $\alpha = 0.05$, and $n_1 + n_2 = 12$. The shape of the rejection region is an upside down triangle, which indicates a major drawback of the power approach. As ms (or the standard error of $\overline{Y}_T - \overline{Y}_R$) decreases, the rejection region of the power approach becomes smaller and smaller. When $ms = 0$, Y has to be 0 to conclude average bioequivalence. This suggests that if the same LS mean difference is observed in two bioequivalence studies, the probability of correctly concluding average bioequivalence is smaller for the study with smaller intra-subject variability than the study with larger intra-subject variability. This undesirable property is a direct consequence of the incorrect use of T_p for testing the hypothesis of equality for the assessment of average bioequivalence. The test statistic T_p is the uniformly most powerful unbiased test for the hypothesis of equality. It has the maximum power for detection of a difference among all unbiased tests when there is difference between two formulations. The power of T_p for detecting a difference increases as ms decreases. This implies that the rejection region for the hypothesis of equality

$$\{(Y, s)|Y > mst(\alpha/2) \quad \text{and} \quad Y < -mst(\alpha/2)\}.$$

increases as ms decreases. However, hypothesis (1) of Equation 5.3.18 is just the complement of the rejection for the hypothesis of equality which becomes smaller as ms decreases.

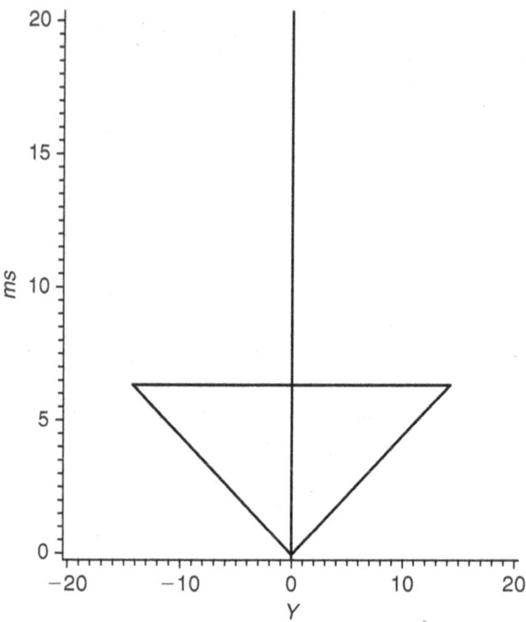

FIGURE 5.3.5: Rejection region of the power approach for $\Delta = 20$, $n_1 = n_2 = 6$, and the nominal level $= 0.05$. (From Schuirmann, D.J., *J. Pharmacokinet. Biopharm.*, 15, 657, 1987).

Schuirmann (1987) pointed out that the power approach for assessment of average bioequivalence cannot control the size at the nominal level. The size of the power approach is an increasing function of degrees of freedom. As an example, Table 5.3.3 lists the size of the power approach at $\theta = \Delta$ for various degrees of freedom.

TABLE 5.3.3: The size of power approach for the interval hypotheses at $\theta = \Delta$.

Degrees of Freedom	Size
10	0.0605
16	0.0722
20	0.0779
26	0.0847
30	0.0884
40	0.0958
50	0.1016
100	0.1188

Source: From Schuirmann, D.J., *J. Pharmacokinet. Biopharm.*, 15, 657, 1987.

The results indicate that it requires a large sample size (degrees of freedom = 50) to reach a size of 0.1016. The size of the power approach converges to 0.2 when sample size approaches infinity.

5.3.5 Relative Efficiency

In previous sections, test powers for Schuirmann's two one-sided *t* tests procedure, Anderson–Hauck's test procedure, and the power approach were discussed. Schuirmann's two one-sided *t* tests procedure and Anderson–Hauck's test procedure are based on interval hypotheses, whereas the power approach is based on the hypothesis of equality. One of the major drawbacks of Anderson–Hauck's test procedure is that it has an open-ended rejection region as *ms* increases. For the power approach, the region for conclusion of average bioequivalence becomes smaller as *ms* decreases. Among these test procedures, Schuirmann's two one-sided *t* tests procedure appears to be a reasonable approach to the interval hypotheses; despite that it is somewhat conservative when the index of sensitivity is small. Schuirmann's two one-sided *t* tests procedure is equivalent to the classic confidence approach as well as Rodda and Davis's Bayesian method in the same that they all reach the same conclusion on average bioequivalence. In other words, the probability of correctly concluding average bioequivalence is the same for these methods.

For interval hypothesis testing, little has been done in the comparison of Schuirmann's two one-sided tests procedure based upon a *t* test with that based on a Wilcoxon–Mann–Whitney rank sum test. For the hypothesis of equality, Wilcoxon–Mann–Whitney rank sum test is a locally most powerful test for detection of a location shift under logistic distribution (Randles and Wolfe, 1979). Its asymptotic Pitman's relative efficiency against at two-sample *t* test is $3/\pi = 95.5\%$ under normal distribution. However, it is not known whether the same property remains for the nonparametric two one-sided procedure for interval hypotheses discussed in Section 4.5.1. To compare the performance of a nonparametric two one-sided tests procedure based on the Wilcoxon–Mann–Whitney rank sum test with parametric two one-sided tests procedure based upon a *t* test, a small simulation study was conducted to examine the size and power of the two procedures at the $\alpha = 0.05$ nominal level. The sizes were evaluated at either $\mu_T = 80$ and $\mu_R = 100$ or $\mu_T = 120$ and $\mu_R = 100$ (i.e., $\theta = \Delta = \pm 20$). The powers were obtained at $\theta = 0$ or $\mu_T = \mu_R = 100$. A total of 1000 normal random samples were generated for each combinations of μ_T, μ_R, CV (10%, 20%, 30%, and 40%), and sample size $n_1 = n_2 = 9$, 12. We computed the proportion of 1000 random samples, which leads to a conclusion of average bioequivalence for each combination. Table 5.3.4 summarizes the results of the simulation study. From Table 5.3.4, it seems that the size of the nonparametric procedure is larger than the parametric, whereas the power of the parametric procedure is greater than that of the nonparametric procedure. However, the differences in size and power between the two procedures are very small (less than 2%) for all combinations considered. Therefore, even for the normal distribution, the Wilcoxon–Mann–Whitney two one-sided tests procedure is very competitive. Comparison of the size and power between the parametric and nonparametric two one-sided tests procedures for other distributions can be found in Liu and Weng (1994).

TABLE 5.3.4: The empirical size and power of parametric and nonparametric two one-sided procedures under normal distribution.

			$n_1 = n_2 = 9$		$n_1 = n_2 = 12$	
CV (%)	μ_T	μ_R	**Parametric**[a]	**Nonparametric**[b]	**Parametric**	**Nonparametric**
10	80	100	6.2%	6.4%	3.8%	4.8%
	120	100	5.2%	5.6%	4.2%	4.6%
	100	100	100.0%	100.0%	100.0%	100.0%
15	80	100	5.8%	6.3%	4.6%	5.1%
	120	100	5.9%	6.3%	4.4%	4.7%
	100	100	98.0%	96.8%	99.1%	98.6%
20	80	100	4.4%	4.8%	5.7%	4.9%
	120	100	4.9%	5.3%	5.3%	5.7%
	100	100	77.1%	75.9%	89.9%	88.5%
30	80	100	4.0%	4.5%	3.8%	4.3%
	120	100	3.4%	4.1%	4.6%	4.3%
	100	100	25.9%	27.2%	43.2%	42.0%
40	80	100	0.6%	1.5%	1.5%	2.1%
	120	100	1.2%	1.7%	1.9%	2.0%
	100	100	3.0%	4.8%	10.7%	9.2%

Note: Size and power are evaluated at $\mu_T - \mu_R = \pm 20$ and $\mu_T = \mu_R = 100$, respectively. Calculation was done based on 1000 normal random samples.

[a] Calculated based upon 90% classic confidence interval.

[b] Calculated based upon 90% nonparametric confidence interval.

Schuirmann (1989) compared the methods of confidence approach for three intervals (L_2, U_2), (L_3, U_3), and (L_4, U_4), given in Section 4.2, which are for the interval hypotheses in Equation 4.3.2 expressed by a ratio, in terms of their actual sizes and powers. He referred to (L_2, U_2), (L_3, U_3), and (L_4, U_4) as the approximate method, the exact method, and the fixed Fieller's method, respectively. Note that the fixed Fieller's method is equivalent to the Bayesian method proposed by Mandallaz and Mau (1981) as shown in the previous chapter. Some of these results are summarized in Figures 5.3.6 through 5.3.10, which are discussed separately in the following.

Figure 5.3.6 plots the actual size of these three intervals against Δ for $r=1$ and $\rho=0.9$, where $\Delta = \overline{Y}_R/\sqrt{w\sigma_R^{*2}}$, r is the ratio of the standard deviation of $\overline{Y}_Y$ to Y_R, ρ is the correlation between $\overline{Y}_T$ and $\overline{Y}_R$, and σ_R^{*2} is the variance of $\overline{Y}_R$. The results indicate that these three intervals are very conservative when Δ is small. However, the exact method can always control the actual size under the nominal level of $\alpha=0.05$. The approximate method produces a larger actual size compared with $\alpha=0.05$ when $\delta_U=1.2$ ($f=0.2$ in the figures), while it controls the actual size under the nominal level of 0.05 when $\delta_L=0.8$ ($f=-0.2$ in the figures). The fixed Fieller's method has an actual size greater than $\alpha=0.05$ as Δ increases.

Figure 5.3.7 plots the actual size of the three methods against Δ for $\rho=0.9$ and $r=0.5$ which is the case where the intra-subject variability of the test formulation is smaller than that of the reference formulation. It appears that the exact method controls actual size under the nominal level, whereas the approximate and fixed Fieller's methods are somewhat conservative (size <0.05) when $\delta_L=0.8$ and slightly liberal (size >0.05) when $\delta_U=1.2$. Schuirmann (1989) also showed that when $\rho=0.9$ and $r=2$, which holds when the intra-subject variability of the test formulation is greater than that of reference formulation, both the approximate and fixed Fieller's methods are liberal (size >0.05) when $\delta_L=0.8$ and conservative (size <0.05) when $\delta_U=1.2$.

Figure 5.3.8 plots the actual size of the three procedures against $\rho=$ for $r=1$, $\Delta=40$, $\delta_L=0.8$, and $\delta_U=1.2$. The actual size of the exact Fieller's method under these conditions is independent of ρ and exactly at the nominal level of 0.05. As ρ approaches 1, the actual size of the approximate method and the fixed Fieller's method converges to 0.5.

Figure 5.3.9 gives the same graphs as those in Figure 5.3.6 except that it provides the actual size for the case of unknown variance for fixed Fieller's method and the approximate method when $n_1=n_2=6$. The results from Figure 5.3.9 are similar to those from Figure 5.3.6 discussed earlier.

Finally, Figure 5.3.10 presents the power curves of the three methods over the range from $\delta_L=0.8$ to $\delta_U=1.2$ for $r=1$, $\rho=0.9$, $\Delta=10$, 20, and 40. It is deceptive to conclude that the power curves of the three methods are symmetric about 0 because they are not, owing to the results from Figures 5.3.6 and 5.3.9. In addition, these power curves are those compared at the same nominal level of 0.05, not at the same actual size. Therefore, it is not fair to say that these three methods have the same power as those shown in Figures 5.3.6, 5.3.8, and 5.3.9. The actual size of the approximate method and the fixed Fieller's method is such larger than 0.05 when $\rho=0.9$.

Given the above arguments, among these three methods, the exact Fieller's method is the recommended method for interval hypotheses expressed by a ratio in the assessment of bioequivalence for average bioavailability under a raw data model.

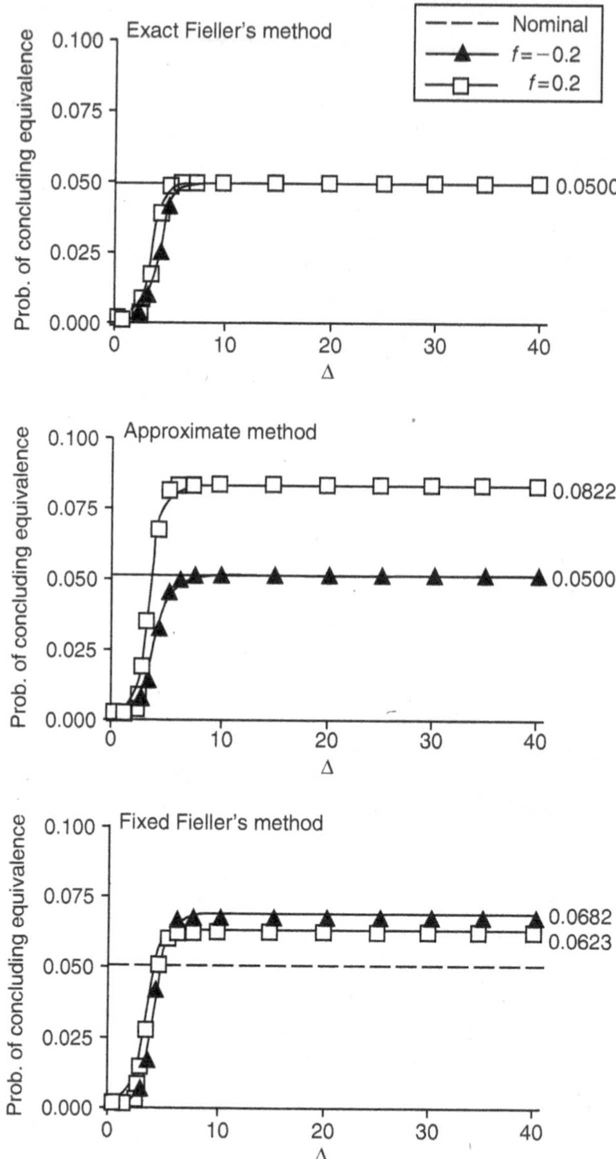

FIGURE 5.3.6: Actual size of exact Fieller's, approximate, and fixed Fieller's methods as a function of Δ, for $\rho = 0.9$, $r = 1$. (From Schuirmann, D.J. Confidence intervals for the ratio of two means from a cross-over study. *Proceedings of the Biopharmaceutical Section of the American Statistical Association*, Washington, DC, pp. 121–126, 1989.)

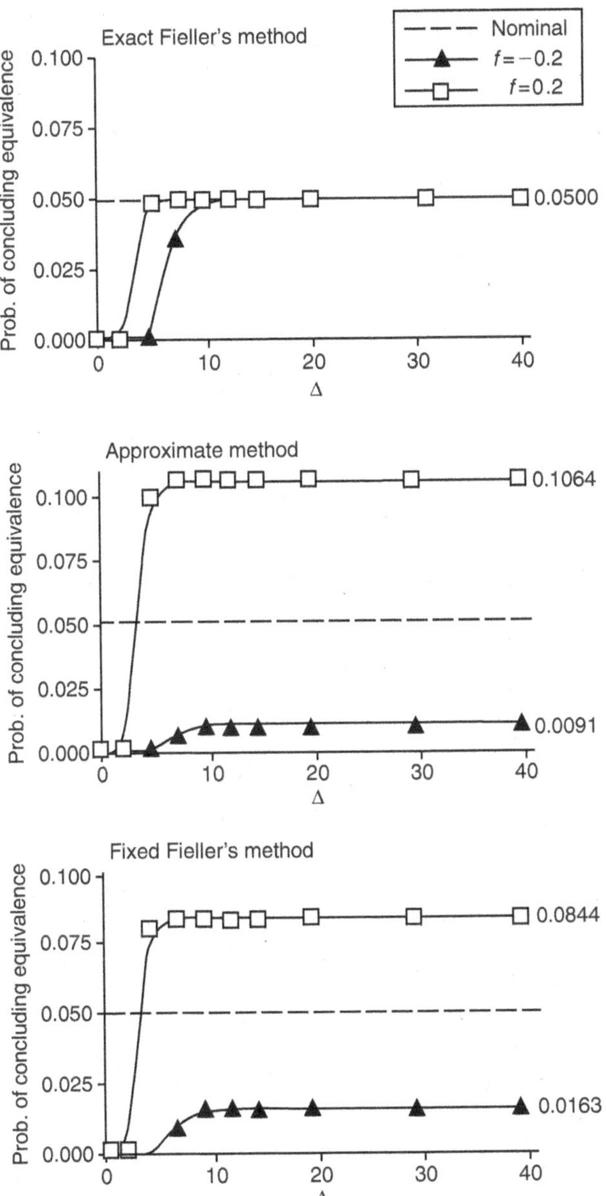

FIGURE 5.3.7: Actual size of exact Fieller's, approximate, and fixed Fieller's methods as a function of Δ, for $\rho = 0.9$, $r = 0.5$. (From Schuirmann, D.J. Confidence intervals for the ratio of two means from a cross-over study. *Proceedings of the Biopharmaceutical Section of the American Statistical Association*, Washington, DC, pp. 121–126, 1989.)

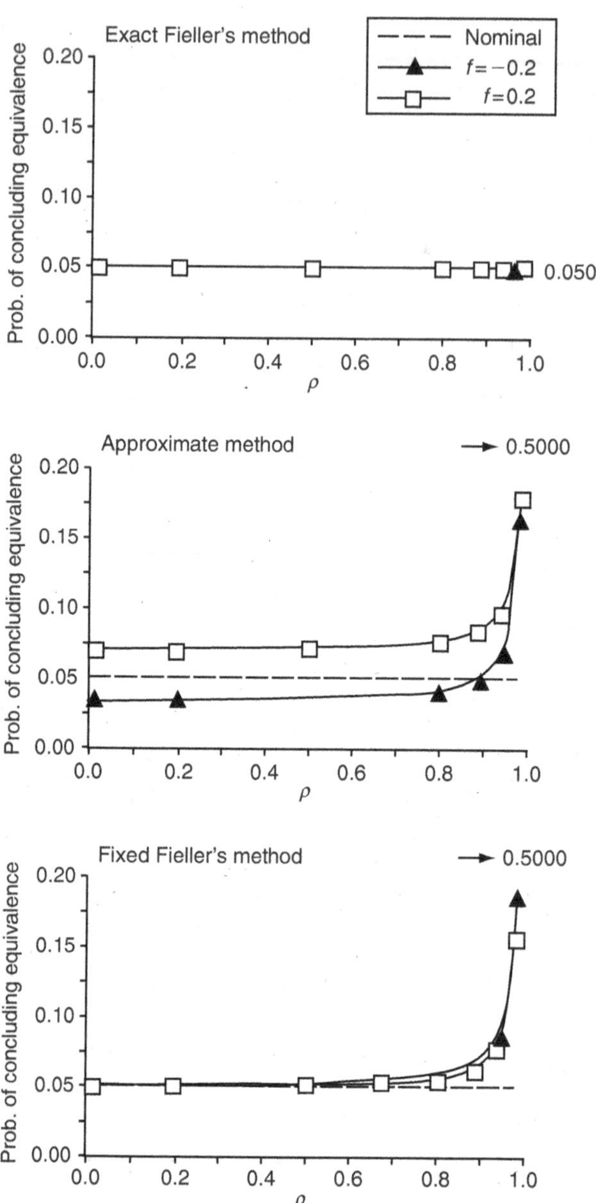

FIGURE 5.3.8: Actual size of exact Fieller's, approximate, and fixed Fieller's methods as a function of ρ for $\Delta = 40$, $r = 1$. (From Schuirmann, D.J. Confidence intervals for the ratio of two means from a cross-over study. *Proceedings of the Biopharmaceutical Section of the American Statistical Association*, Washington, DC, pp. 121–126, 1989.)

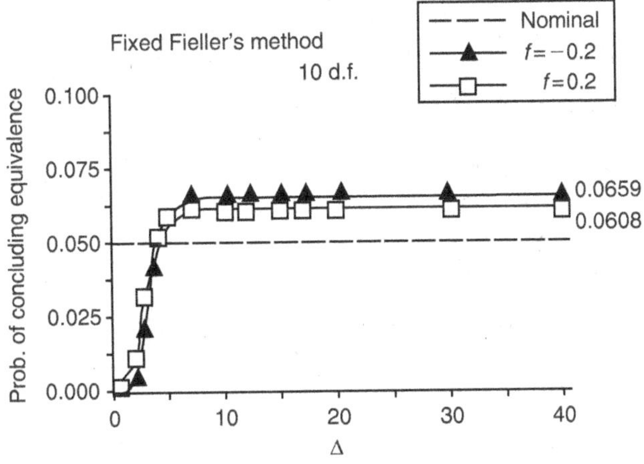

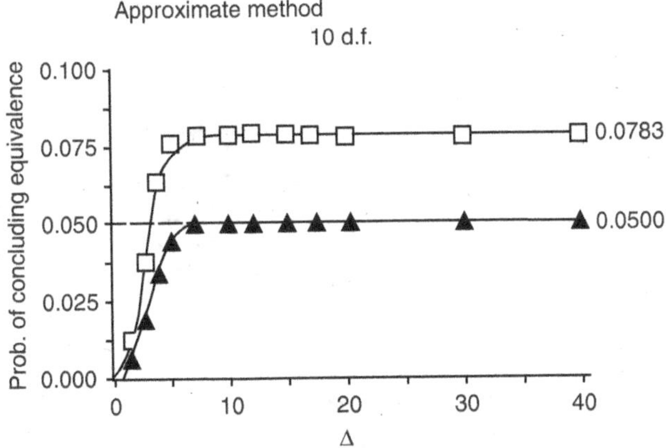

FIGURE 5.3.9: Actual size of fixed Fieller's and approximate methods as a function of Δ, for $\rho = 0.9$, $r = 1$ and $n_1 = n_2 = 6$. (From Schuirmann, D.J. Confidence intervals for the ratio of two means from a cross-over study. *Proceedings of the Biopharmaceutical Section of the American Statistical Association*, Washington, DC, pp. 121–126, 1989.)

5.4 Sample Size Determination

In bioavailability studies, how large a sample size is required to have a desired power to establish average bioequivalence within meaningful limits is a question of particular interest to the investigator. To provide an answer to this question, we will first discuss the calculation of sample size for the hypothesis of equality under the standard 2×2 crossover model 4.1.1.

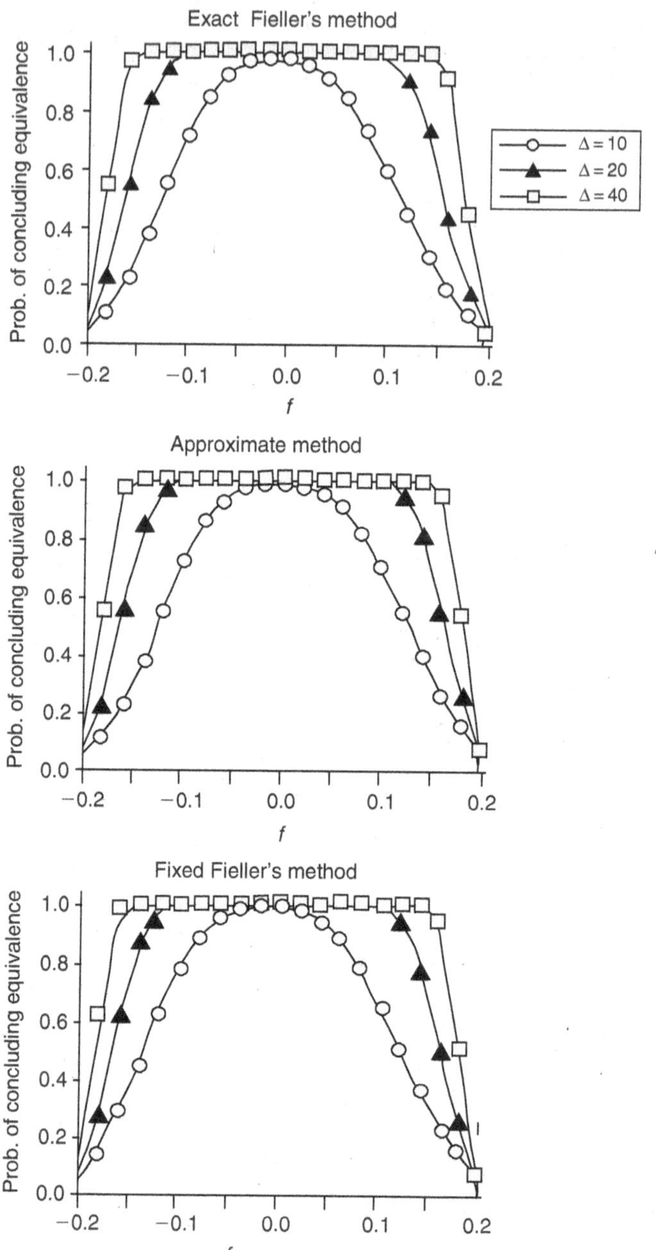

FIGURE 5.3.10: Full power curves of exact Fieller's, approximate, and fixed Fieller's methods as a function of f, for $\rho = 0.9$, $r = 1$. (From Schuirmann, D.J. Confidence intervals for the ratio of two means from a cross-over study. *Proceedings of the Biopharmaceutical Section of the American Statistical Association*, Washington, DC, pp. 121–126, 1989.)

5.4.1 Sample Size for Point Hypotheses

Let α be the nominal level of significance (i.e., the probability of committing a type I error that one is willing to tolerate); and $\phi = 1 - \beta$, the power one wishes to have to detect a difference of at least Δ magnitude, where β is the probability of making a type II error. In the interest of balance, we assume $n_1 = n_2 = n_e$. In other words, each sequence will be allocated the same number of subjects at random. The sample size per sequence n_e for the hypotheses of equality Equation 5.3.1 can be determined by the formulation given in the following:

$$n_e \geq 2[t(\alpha/2,\, 2n-2) + t(\beta,\, 2n-2)]^2[\widehat{\sigma}_d/\Delta]^2, \tag{5.4.1}$$

where $\widehat{\sigma}_d$ can usually be obtained from previous studies. According to the power approach used on the 80/20 rule, the sample size should be large enough to provide a power of 80% for detection of a difference of the magnitude at least 20% of the unknown reference mean. Thus, Equation 5.4.1 can be simplified as

$$n_e \geq [t(\alpha/2,\, 2n-2) + t(\beta,\, 2n-2)]^2[\mathrm{CV}/20]^2, \tag{5.4.2}$$

where

$$\mathrm{CV} = 100 \times \frac{\sqrt{2\widehat{\sigma}_d^2}}{\mu_R} = 100 \times \frac{\sqrt{\mathrm{MSE}}}{\mu_R}.$$

The total number of subjects required for the standard 2×2 crossover design is $N = 2n_e$. Since the degrees of freedom $(2n-2)$ in both Equations 5.4.1 and 5.4.2 are unknown, a numerical iterative procedure is required to solve for n_e. To illustrate this, let us consider the following example.

Example 5.4.1

Suppose we would like to conduct a bioequivalence study to compare average bioavailability of a new formulation with a reference formulation as discussed in Example 3.6.1. The design was chosen to be the standard 2×2 crossover design and the 80/20 rule will be used to determine bioequivalence in average bioavailability between two formulations. The next question then is how many subjects are needed to have 80% power to detect a 20% difference. From the data from Example 3.6.1, we have

$$\mathrm{CV} = 100 \times \frac{\sqrt{167.246}}{82.559} = 15.66.$$

Let us first guess $n_e = 9$. This gives degrees of freedom $2n - 2 = 18 - 2 = 16$, $t(0.025,\, 16) = 2.12$ and $t(0.2,\, 16) = 0.865$. By Equation 5.4.2,

$$n_e = (2.12 + 0.865)^2(15.66/20)^2 = 5.5 \cong 6.$$

We then start with $n_e = 6$ and repeat the same calculation, which gives degrees of freedom $= 12 - 2 = 10$,

$$t(0.025,\ 10) = 2.228,$$
$$t(0.2,\ 10) = 0.879.$$

Again, by Equation 5.4.2, we have

$$n_e = (2.228 + 0.879)^2(15.66/20)^2 = 5.9 \cong 6,$$

which is very close to the previous solution.

Therefore, a total of $N = (2)(6) = 12$ subjects are needed based on the 80/20 rule.

As we have pointed out earlier, the power approach based on the 80/20 rule is an ad hoc method for assessment of average bioequivalence that may not be statistically valid. The sample size determined by Equation 5.4.1 or Equation 5.4.2 may not be large enough to provide sufficient power if other methods for interval hypotheses such as Schuirmann's two one-sided tests procedure are used.

5.4.2 Sample Size for Interval Hypotheses

As discussed in Chapter 4, the classic (or shortest) confidence interval, Schuirmann's two one-sided tests procedure, as well as Rodda and Davis's Bayesian method can lead to the same conclusion for determination of bioequivalence in average bioavailability. Therefore, in this section, we will focus on sample size determination based upon Schuirmann's two one-sided tests procedure for interval hypotheses.

As indicated in Section 5.3, the power function $\phi_s(\theta)$ for Schuirmann's two one-sided t tests procedure is symmetric about 0 when the ± 20 rule is used for the assessment of average bioequivalence. Furthermore, the intra-subject variability has an influence on the power function. To illustrate this, Phillips (1990) provided several graphs for the power of Schuirmann's two one-sided t tests procedure for various sample sizes and CVs. Some graphs are presented in Figure 5.4.1. Because calculation for the exact power for Schuirmann's two one-sided t tests procedure requires complicated numerical integration as discussed in Section 5.3, the sample size determination based on the power function is complicated and difficult to obtain. However, an approximate sample size based on the power function can be obtained using some familiar traditional methods (Liu and Chow, 1992a).

We first consider the case where $\theta = \mu_T - \mu_R = 0$ and $n_1 = n_2 = n$. Here,

$$\frac{Y}{\sqrt{\frac{2}{n}\hat{\sigma}_d^2}}$$

has a central t distribution with $2n - 2$ degrees of freedom. The power at $\theta = 0$ is then given by

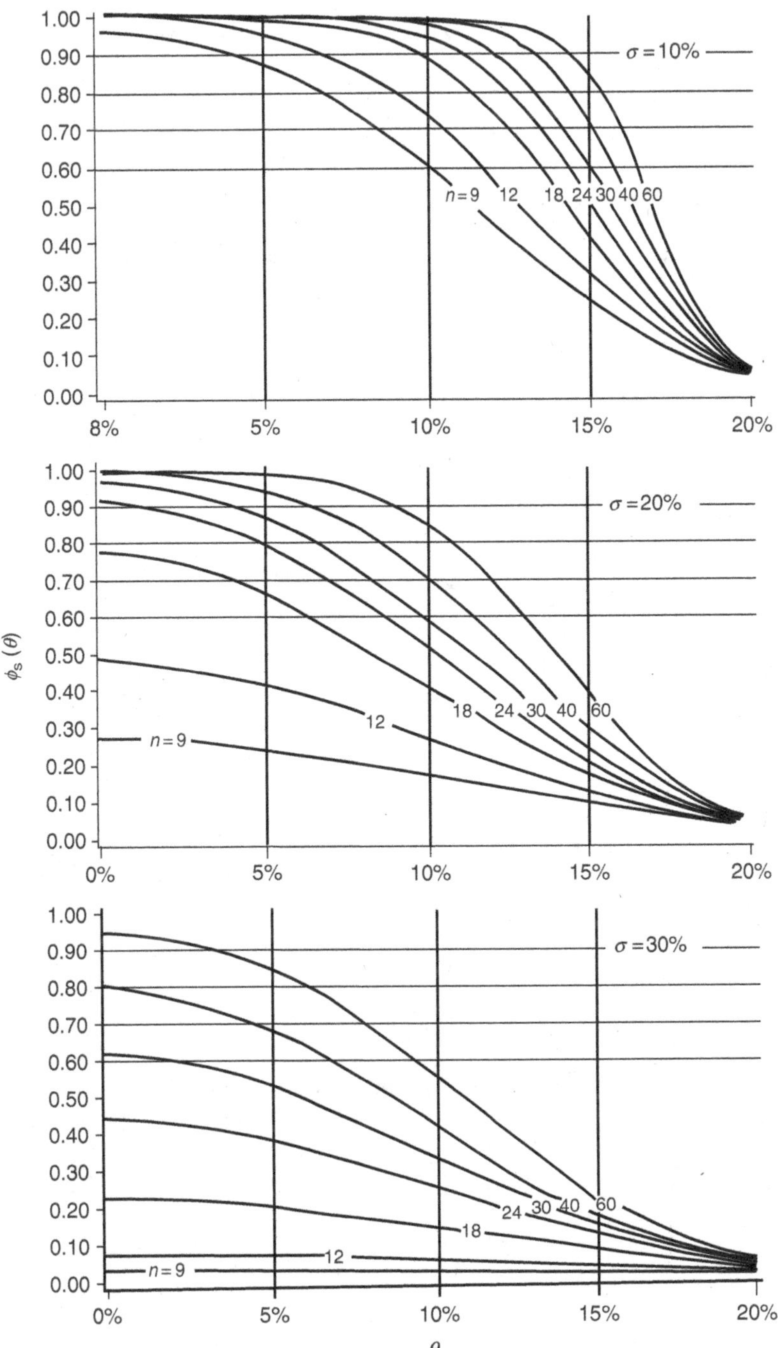

FIGURE 5.4.1: Power curves of Shuirmann's two one-sided tests procedure for total sample size of 9, 12, 18, 24, 30, 40, and 60 at the 0.05 nominal level and $\Delta = 0.2\mu_R$. (From Phillips, K.F., *J. Pharmacokinet. Biopharm.*, 18, 137, 1990.)

$$\phi_s(0) = P\left\{-\Delta + t(\alpha, 2n-2)\sqrt{\frac{2}{n}\widehat{\sigma}_d^2} < Y < \Delta - t(\alpha, 2n-2)\sqrt{\frac{2}{n}\widehat{\sigma}_d^2}\right\}$$

$$= P\left\{\frac{-\Delta}{\sqrt{\frac{2}{n}\widehat{\sigma}_d^2}} + t(\alpha, 2n-2) < \frac{Y}{\sqrt{\frac{2}{n}\widehat{\sigma}_d^2}} < \frac{\Delta}{\sqrt{\frac{2}{n}\widehat{\sigma}_d^2}} - t(\alpha, 2n-2)\right\}. \qquad (5.4.3)$$

As a central t distribution is symmetric about 0, the lower and upper endpoints of Equation 5.4.3 are also symmetric about 0, that is,

$$\frac{\Delta}{\sqrt{\frac{2}{n}\widehat{\sigma}_d^2}} - t(\alpha, 2n-2) = -\left\{\frac{-\Delta}{\sqrt{\frac{2}{n}\widehat{\sigma}_d^2}} + t(\alpha, 2n-2)\right\}.$$

Therefore, $\phi_s(0) \geq 1 - \beta$ implies that

$$\left|\frac{\Delta}{\sqrt{\frac{2}{n}\widehat{\sigma}_d^2}} - t(\alpha, 2n-2)\right| \geq t(\beta/2, 2n-2) \qquad (5.4.4)$$

or

$$n_I \geq 2[t(\alpha, 2n-2) + t(\beta/2, 2n-2)]^2\left(\frac{\widehat{\sigma}_d}{\Delta}\right)^2. \qquad (5.4.5)$$

where n_I is the sample size required to achieve $1-\beta$ power at the α level of significance for interval hypotheses in 4.3.1. If the ± 20 rule is used with $D = 0.2\mu_R$, Equation 5.4.5 becomes

$$n_I \geq [t(\alpha, 2n-2) + t(\beta/2, 2n-2)]^2\left(\frac{CV}{20}\right)^2. \qquad (5.4.6)$$

The sample size is exact for $\theta = 0$ either by Equation 5.4.5 or 5.4.6. Note that Westlake (1986) also derived Equation 5.4.5 using the $(1-2\alpha) \times 100\%$ classic confidence interval.

We will now consider the case where $\theta \neq 0$. Because the power of Schuirmann's two one-sided t tests procedure is symmetric about 0, without loss of generality, we will consider a sample size determination for the case where $\theta > 0$ only. When $0 < \theta = \theta_0 > \Delta$,

$$\frac{Y - \theta_0}{\sqrt{\frac{2}{n}\widehat{\sigma}_d^2}}$$

has a central distribution with $2n-2$ degrees of freedom. The power for Schuirmann's two one-sided t tests procedure at θ_0 is

$$\phi_s(\theta_0) = P\left\{\frac{-\Delta - \theta_0}{\sqrt{\frac{2}{n}\widehat{\sigma}_d^2}} + t(\alpha, 2n-2) < \frac{Y - \theta_0}{\sqrt{\frac{2}{2}\widehat{\sigma}_d^2}} < \frac{\Delta - \theta_0}{\sqrt{\frac{2}{n}\widehat{\sigma}_d^2}} - t(\alpha, 2n-2)\right\}. \tag{5.4.7}$$

Note that, unlike the case where $\theta = 0$, the lower and upper endpoints of Equation 5.4.7 are not symmetric about 0 because

$$-\left[\frac{\Delta - \theta_0}{\sqrt{\frac{2}{n}\widehat{\sigma}_d^2}} - t(\alpha, 2n-2)\right] = \frac{-\Delta + \theta_0}{\sqrt{\frac{2}{n}\widehat{\sigma}_d^2}} + t(\alpha, 2n-2)$$

$$> \frac{-\Delta - \theta_0}{\sqrt{\frac{2}{n}\widehat{\sigma}_d^2}} + t(\alpha, 2n-2).$$

Therefore, if we choose

$$\frac{\Delta - \theta_0}{\sqrt{\frac{2}{n}\widehat{\sigma}_d^2}} - t(\alpha, 2n-2) = t(\beta/2, 2n-2),$$

then the resultant sample size might be too large to be of practical interest. The power may be more than we require. A compromise method, which is less conservative, for sample size determination can be obtained using the following inequality:

$$\phi_s(\theta_0) \leq P\left\{\frac{Y - \theta_0}{\sqrt{\frac{2}{n}\widehat{\sigma}_d^2}} < \frac{\Delta - \theta_0}{\sqrt{\frac{2}{n}\widehat{\sigma}_d^2}} - t(\alpha, 2n-2)\right\}. \tag{5.4.8}$$

As a result, $\phi_s(\theta_0) \geq 1 - \beta$ gives

$$\frac{\Delta - \theta_0}{\sqrt{\frac{2}{n}\widehat{\sigma}_d^2}} - t(\alpha, 2n-2) = t(\beta, 2n-2),$$

or

$$n_1(\theta_0) \geq 2[t(\alpha, 2n-2) + t(\beta, 2n-2)]^2 \left(\frac{\widehat{\sigma}_d}{\Delta - \theta_0}\right)^2. \tag{5.4.9}$$

If the ±20 rule is used with $\Delta = 0.2\mu_R$, then Equation 5.4.9 becomes

$$n_1(\theta_0) \geq [t(\alpha, 2n-2) + t(\beta, 2n-2)]^2 \left(\frac{CV}{20 - \theta_0'}\right), \tag{5.4.10}$$

where $\theta_0' = 100 \times \theta_0/\mu_R$.

On the basis of Equation 5.4.10, Table 5.4.1 gives the total sample sizes needed to achieve a desired power for the standard 2×2 crossover design for various combinations of θ and CVs. The values in Table 5.4.1 agree with those numbers given in

TABLE 5.4.1: Sample sizes for Schuirmann's two one-sided t tests procedure at $\Delta = 0.2\mu_R$ and $\alpha = 0.05$ nominal level.

		$100 \times (\mu_T - \mu_R)/\mu_R$			
Power	**CV (%)[a]**	**0%**	**5%**	**10%**	**15%**
80%	10	8	8	16	52
	12	8	10	20	74
	14	10	14	26	100
	16	14	16	34	126
	18	16	20	42	162
	20	20	24	52	200
	22	24	28	62	242
	24	28	34	74	288
	26	32	40	86	336
	28	36	46	100	390
	30	40	52	114	448
	32	46	58	128	508
	34	52	66	146	574
	36	58	74	162	644
	38	64	82	180	716
	40	70	90	200	794
90%	10	10	10	20	70
	12	10	14	28	100
	14	14	18	36	136
	16	16	22	46	178
	18	20	28	58	224
	20	24	32	70	276
	22	28	40	86	334
	24	34	46	100	396
	26	40	54	118	466
	28	44	62	136	540
	30	52	70	156	618
	32	58	80	178	704
	34	66	90	200	794
	36	72	100	224	890
	38	80	112	250	992
	40	90	124	276	1098

Source: From Liu, J.P. and Chow, S.C., *J. Pharmacokinet. Biopharm.*, 20, 101, 1992a.

[a] $CV = 100 \times \left(\sqrt{MSE}/\mu_R\right)$.

Phillips (1990). An approximate formula for sample size calculations can be found in Liu and Chow (1992a). The results indicate that more subjects are needed to achieve the same power, if intra-subject variability and θ increase. In the following, the data presented in Section 3.6 will be used to illustrate the calculations for sample sizes to achieve 80% power for $\theta = 0$ and 5% of μ_R.

Example 5.4.2

First, let us consider the case where $\theta = 0$. We start with an initial guess of 9, i.e., $n_R(0) = 9$. This gives a degree of freedom of $2n - 2 = 16$ and

$$t(0.05, 16) = 1.746 \quad \text{and} \quad t(0.1, 16) = 1.337.$$

By Equation 5.4.6, we have

$$n_I(0) = (1.746 + 1.337)^2(15.66/20)^2 = 5.8 \cong 6.$$

We then use $n_I(0) = 6$ as a starting value for the next iteration. This gives degrees of freedom $= 10$;

$$t(0.05, 10) = 1.812,$$
$$t(0.1, 10) = 1.372.$$

Therefore, by Equation 5.4.6,

$$n_I(0) = (1.812 + 1.372)^2(15.66/20)^2 = 6.2 \cong 6.$$

Because these two iterations give a similar result of 6 subjects per sequence, a total of 12 subjects would be needed to have an 80% power to detect a 20% difference for the case $\theta = 0$.

On the other hand, when $\theta = 0.05\mu_R$, we may apply a similar iterative procedure. Let us start with $n_I(5\%) = 6$. As $t(0.2, 10) = 0.879$, by Equation 5.4.10, we have

$$n_I(5\%) \geq (1.8.12 + 0.879)^2[15.66/(20 - 5)]^2 = 7.9 \cong 8.$$

We then use $n_I(5\%) = 8$ as an initial value for the next iteration. With $n = 8$, the degrees of freedom is equal to 14. Thus, $t(0.05, 14) = 1.761$ and $t(0.2, 14) = 0.868$. By Equation 5.4.10,

$$n_I(5\%) \geq (1.761 + 0.868)^2[15.66/(20 - 5)]^2 = 7.5 \cong 8.$$

Therefore, a total of 16 subjects would be needed to achieve an 80% power, if θ is 5% of the reference mean.

TABLE 5.4.2: Empirical power by simulation for Example 5.5 at $\alpha = 0.05$ nominal level.

Procedure	$n_I(0) = 6$ (%)	$n_I(5\%) = 8$
Schuirmann's two one-sided	81.8	82.0
Nonparametric two one-sided	82.9	80.2
Anderson–Hauck	93.1	91.4

Sample sizes $n_I(0)$ and $n_I(5\%)$ were also verified by means of empirical powers at $\alpha = 0.05$ level through a simulation study with 1000 random samples using the procedure described in Section 5.3. The results are summarized in Table 5.4.2. The results indicate that both sample sizes calculated using Equation 5.4.4 for $\theta = 0$ and Equation 5.4.10 for $\theta = 5\%$ are large enough to provide at least 80% power. This result is also true for Wilcoxon–Mann–Whitney two one-sided tests procedure and Anderson–Hauck's procedure. As expected, Anderson–Hauck's procedure has a better power because its actual size is greater than the nominal level.

Chapter 6

Transformation and Analysis of Individual Subject Ratios

6.1 Introduction

In Chapter 4, based on the ± 20 rule, we introduced several statistical methods for assessment of average bioequivalence. Most of these methods were derived under a raw data model [i.e., model 4.1.1 or 4.1.2] for the standard 2×2 crossover design, with normality assumptions on the between-subject and within-subject random variables. The intra-subject variability is assumed to be the same from subject to subject and from formulation to formulation. As a result, the responses (e.g., AUC or C_{max}) are assumed to be normally distributed. One of the difficulties commonly encountered in bioavailability studies, however, is whether the assumption of normality is valid. Often, distributions of the responses are positively skewed and exhibit a lack of homogeneity of variances (e.g., variance being dependent on the mean). In this situation, a log-transformation on the responses is often considered to reduce the skewness and to achieve an additive model with relatively homogeneous variances. In addition, the FDA guidances on *Statistical Approaches to Establishing Bioequivalence*, issued in 2001, and *Bioavailability and Bioequivalence Studies for Orally Administrated Drug Products–General Considerations*, issued in 2003, suggest the routine use of logarithmic transformation for $AUC_{0-\infty}$ and C_{max} for assessment of average bioequivalence. A justification of multiplicative (or a log-transformed) model is provided by the guidance. From the transformed data, the methods introduced in Chapter 4 can then be applied directly and followed by an antilog-transformation to assess average bioequivalence.

Under a multiplicative model, the ratio of means, which is usually considered as a measure of average bioequivalence, may be confounded with the period effect or intra-subject variabilities. Therefore, in this chapter, we consider several estimators for the ratio of average bioavailabilities that reflect the effect caused by only differences in the formulations. These estimators include the maximum likelihood estimator and the minimum variance unbiased estimator (Liu and Weng, 1992). These estimators are derived under the multiplicative model with normality assumptions on the transformed data. Based on these estimators, a $(1 - 2\alpha) \times 100\%$

confidence interval for the ratio of average bioavailabilities can be obtained to assess bioequivalence.

If the normality assumptions are seriously violated and there is no period effect, Peace (1986) suggested studying individual subject ratios to remove the heterogeneity of intra-subject variability from the comparison between formulations. Under his model, however, distribution of the ratios is unknown; therefore, the statistical procedures are not exact. Under the assumption of no period effects, Tse (1990) examined several approaches, which are derived assuming that the ratios follow a lognormal distribution, for constructing the confidence interval for mean and median of individual subject ratios. Anderson and Hauck (1990) also examined individual bioequivalence using individual subject ratios. Peace (1990) recommended the use of individual subject ratios as a preliminary test for assessment of bioequivalence. In this chapter, the ratio of least squares means (RM) and the least squares mean of individual subject ratios (MIR), which are often considered as alternative estimators for the average bioavailabilities ratio, are examined.

This chapter is organized as follows: In Section 6.2, a brief description of a multiplicative model for the standard 2×2 crossover design is given. Various bioequivalence measures are discussed in Section 6.3. The maximum likelihood estimator, the minimum variance unbiased estimator, the mean of individual subject ratios, and the ratio of least square (LS) means for estimation of the ratio of average bioavailabilities are described from Sections 6.4 through 6.7. Section 6.8 provides statistical evaluation for the performances of these methods using a simulation study. An example concerning the comparison of two erythromycin formulations is presented in Section 6.9. Finally, a brief discussion is given in Section 6.10.

6.2 Multiplicative (or Log-Transformed) Model

As indicated earlier, the distributions of responses, such as AUC and $C_{\max}$, are often positively skewed and exhibit a lack of homogeneity of variances. Therefore, the normality assumption on AUC and $C_{\max}$ may not be appropriate. In this situation, the assessment of average bioequivalence based upon a raw data model and normality assumptions may not be appropriate. Therefore, to reduce the skewness and achieve an additive model with relatively homogeneous variances, a log-transformation on AUC or $C_{\max}$ is usually considered. This leads to the following multiplicative model (or log-transformed model):

$$X_{ijk} = \tilde{\mu}\tilde{S}_{ik}\tilde{P}_j\tilde{F}_{(j,k)}\tilde{C}_{(j-1,k)}\,\tilde{e}_{ijk}, \tag{6.2.1}$$

or equivalently

$$Y_{ijk} = \log(X_{ijk}) = \mu + S_{ik} + P_j + F_{(j,k)} + C_{(j-1,k)} + e_{ijk},$$

where $i = 1, 2, \ldots, n_k$ and j, $k = 1, 2$ for the standard 2×2 crossover design and μ, S_{ik}, P_j, $F_{(j,k)}$, $C_{(j-1,k)}$, and e_{ijk} are as defined in Equation 2.5.1. From the above multiplicative model, it can be seen that $\widetilde{\mu} = \exp(\mu)$, $\widetilde{S}_{ik} = \exp(S_{ik})$, $\widetilde{P}_j = \exp(P_j)$, $\widetilde{F}_{(j,k)} = \exp(F_{(j,k)})$, $\widetilde{C}_{(j-1,k)} = \exp(C_{(j-1,k)})$, and $\widetilde{e}_{ijk} = \exp(e_{ijk})$. If $\{S_{ik}\}$ and e_{ijk} are independent and normally distributed with covariance structure, as specified in Equation 2.5.5, then X_{ijk} is said to follow a lognormal linear model (Bradu and Mundlak, 1970; Shimizu, 1988). Equation 6.2.1 can also be expressed as

$$X_{ijk} = \exp\{\mu + S_{ik} + P_j + F_{(j,k)} + C_{(j-1,k)} + e_{ijk}\}. \tag{6.2.2}$$

Note that, under the normality assumptions of $\{S_{ik}\}$ and $\{e_{ijk}\}$, the vector, $(X_{i1k}, X_{i2k})'$, of pair responses observed on the ith subject in the kth sequence follows a bivariate lognormal distribution (Crow and Shimizu, 1988).

6.3 Bioequivalence Measures

In practice, the ratio of means of X_{ijk} between the test and reference formulations is usually considered as a measure of average bioequivalence. Because the distribution of X_{ijk} is often positively skewed, some researchers suggest that the ratio of medians, instead of the ratio of means, be used as an alternative measure of average bioequivalence because the median is a better representative of the central location of the corresponding distribution (Metzler and Huang, 1983; Chinchilli and Durham, 1989). However, the ratio of means and the ratio of medians may be confounded with the period effect or the intra-subject variabilities under Equation 6.2.1. Table 6.3.1 gives the means and medians of X_{ijk} by sequence and period assuming that there are no carryover effects. The results indicate that means of X_{ijk} involve the inter-subject variability σ_S^2, and the intra-subject variabilities σ_T^2 and σ_R^2 of the log-transformed data Y_{ijk}, whereas medians of X_{ijk} consist of only the fixed effects $\widetilde{\mu}$, $\widetilde{P}_j$, and $\widetilde{F}_{(j,k)}$.

Therefore, for assessment of average bioequivalence, we may consider the following ratio of average bioavailabilities on the original scale, which reflects only the effect caused by the difference in average between the two formulations:

TABLE 6.3.1: Sequence-by-period means and medians for model 6.2.1.

Sequence		Period I	Period II
1	Mean	$\exp[(\mu + P_1 + F_R) + \frac{1}{2}(\sigma_R^2 + \sigma_S^2)]$	$\exp[(\mu + P_2 + F_T) + \frac{1}{2}(\sigma_T^2 + \sigma_S^2)]$
	Median	$\exp(\mu + P_1 + F_R)$	$\exp(\mu + P_2 + F_T)$
2	Mean	$\exp[(\mu + P_1 + F_T) + \frac{1}{2}(\sigma_T^2 + \sigma_S^2)]$	$\exp[(\mu + P_2 + F_R) + \frac{1}{2}(\sigma_R^2 + \sigma_S^2)]$
	Median	$\exp(\mu + P_1 + F_T)$	$\exp(\mu + P_2 + F_R)$

$$\begin{aligned}\delta &= \widetilde{F} \\ &= \exp(F) \\ &= \exp(F_{\mathrm{T}} - F_{\mathrm{R}}) \\ &= \frac{\widetilde{F}_{\mathrm{T}}}{\widetilde{F}_{\mathrm{R}}} \\ &= \frac{\exp(\mu + F_{\mathrm{T}})}{\exp(\mu + F_{\mathrm{R}})} \\ &= \frac{\widetilde{\mu}\widetilde{F}_{\mathrm{T}}}{\widetilde{\mu}\widetilde{F}_{\mathrm{R}}} \\ &= \frac{\widetilde{\mu}_{\mathrm{T}}}{\widetilde{\mu}_{\mathrm{R}}}.\end{aligned} \tag{6.3.1}$$

where

$\widetilde{\mu}_{\mathrm{T}} = \widetilde{\mu}\widetilde{F}_{\mathrm{T}}$
$\widetilde{\mu}_{\mathrm{R}} = \widetilde{\mu}\widetilde{F}_{\mathrm{R}}$

Note that there are several measures of relative average bioavailability, for example, the ratio of the marginal test formulation mean to the reference mean, which is given by

$$\delta_{\mathrm{M}} = \begin{cases} \exp\left[P + F + \frac{1}{2}\left(\sigma_{\mathrm{T}}^2 - \sigma_{\mathrm{R}}^2\right)\right], & k = 1, \\ \exp\left[-P + F + \frac{1}{2}\left(\sigma_{\mathrm{T}}^2 - \sigma_{\mathrm{R}}^2\right)\right], & k = 2. \end{cases}$$

Under the assumption of no period effect, δ_{M} reduces to

$$\delta_{\mathrm{M}} = \exp\left[F + \frac{1}{2}\left(\sigma_{\mathrm{T}}^2 - \sigma_{\mathrm{R}}^2\right)\right].$$

It can be seen that δ_{M} is a measure of average bioavailability that assesses bioequivalence by combining the information of the fixed direct formulation effect and difference in intra-subject variabilities on the logarithmic scale. When $\sigma_{\mathrm{T}}^2 = \sigma_{\mathrm{R}}^2$, δ_{M} is the ratio of the marginal median of the test formulation to the reference formulation. Another appealing measure of relative bioavailability is the mean of individual subject ratios, which is given as

$$\delta_{\mathrm{I}} = \begin{cases} \exp\left[P + F + 2\sigma_{\mathrm{d}}^2\right], & k = 1, \\ \exp\left[-P + F + 2\sigma_{\mathrm{d}}^2\right], & k = 2, \end{cases}$$

where $\sigma_{\mathrm{d}}^2 = \left(\frac{1}{4}\right)\left(\sigma_{\mathrm{T}}^2 + \sigma_{\mathrm{R}}^2\right)$.

If there is no period effect, δ_I reduces to

$$\delta_I = \exp\left(F + 2\sigma_d^2\right).$$

Hence, assessment of average bioequivalence using δ_I involves not only the fixed direct formulation effect, but also the average of intra-subject variabilities. Consequently, even if the direct fixed formulation effect on the logarithmic scale is zero, two formulations may still be concluded bioinequivalent because of intra-subject variabilities. On the other hand, the median of individual subject ratio reduces to δ in the absence of period effect. Since δ involves only the fixed direct formulation effect on the logarithmic scale, we focus on point estimation of δ in this section. The concept of individual subject ratio is suggested to assess individual bioequivalence, which are discussed in detail in Chapters 11 and 12 (Anderson and Hauck, 1990; Liu and Chow, 1997a,b). In the following sections, we consider several estimators for estimation of δ. These estimators include the maximum likelihood (ML) estimator, the minimum variance unbiased estimator (MVUE), mean of individual subject ratios (MIR), and ratio of least squares means (RM). On the basis of these estimators, a corresponding $(1 - 2\alpha) \times 100\%$ confidence interval for δ may be obtained to assess average bioequivalence.

6.4 Maximum Likelihood Estimator

If the skewness of X_{ijk} can be removed by means of a log-transformation and the log-transformed data are approximately normally distributed, then average bioequivalence can be assessed using statistical methods described in Chapters 3 and 4. In other words, a point estimate and a $(1 - 2\alpha) \times 100\%$ confidence interval for the mean formulation difference on the logarithmic scale (i.e., $\mu_T - \mu_R$) can be obtained based on the log-transformed data, which are given by $\hat{F} = \overline{Y}_T - \overline{Y}_R$ and (L_1, U_1), respectively, where L_1 and U_1 are defined as in Equation 4.2.2. Thus, a point estimate and a $(1 - 2\alpha) \times 100\%$ confidence interval for $\delta = \tilde{\mu}_T/\tilde{\mu}_R$ on the original scale can be obtained by inverse (or back) transformation (i.e., antilog) of the corresponding estimate and interval on the logarithmic scale.

From Equation 3.3.6, we have

$$\begin{aligned}
\hat{F} = \overline{Y}_T - \overline{Y}_R &= \frac{1}{2}\left[\left(\overline{Y}_{\cdot 21} + \overline{Y}_{\cdot 12}\right) - \left(\overline{Y}_{\cdot 11} + \overline{Y}_{\cdot 22}\right)\right] \\
&= \frac{1}{2}\left[\left(\overline{Y}_{\cdot 21} - \overline{Y}_{\cdot 11}\right) - \left(\overline{Y}_{\cdot 22} - \overline{Y}_{\cdot 12}\right)\right] \\
&= \overline{d}_{\cdot 1} - \overline{d}_{\cdot 2},
\end{aligned}$$

where $\bar{d}_{\cdot k}$ are the sample means of period differences d_{ik} defined in Equation 3.3.1 for the transformed data. Note that

$$\begin{aligned} d_{ik} &= \tfrac{1}{2}(Y_{i2k} - Y_{i1k}) \\ &= \tfrac{1}{2}(\log X_{i2k} - \log X_{i1k}) \\ &= \tfrac{1}{2}\log\left(\frac{X_{i2k}}{X_{i1k}}\right) \\ &= \tfrac{1}{2}\log(r_{ik}), \end{aligned} \tag{6.4.1}$$

where $r_{ik} = X_{i2k}/X_{i1k}$ are the period ratios, $i = 1, 2, \ldots, n_k$, $k = 1, 2$. Under the assumption of no carryover effects, r_{ik} can be expressed as

$$r_{ik} = \frac{X_{i2k}}{X_{i1k}} = \begin{cases} \dfrac{\widetilde{P}_2\widetilde{F}_{\mathrm{T}}\widetilde{e}_{i2k}}{\widetilde{P}_1\widetilde{F}_{\mathrm{R}}\widetilde{e}_{i1k}} & \text{if } k = 1, \\[2ex] \dfrac{\widetilde{P}_2\widetilde{F}_{\mathrm{R}}\widetilde{e}_{i2k}}{\widetilde{P}_1\widetilde{F}_{\mathrm{T}}\widetilde{e}_{i1k}} & \text{if } k = 2. \end{cases} \tag{6.4.2}$$

As indicated in Chapter 4, for the standard 2×2 crossover design, the inter-subject variability can be eliminated with the use of the period differences under an additive model 4.1.1. Similarly, the period ratios r_{ik} can remove the inter-subject variability from the comparison of average bioavailability between formulations when a multiplicative model is used.

Since $\widehat{F}$ is the ML estimator of $\mu_{\mathrm{T}} - \mu_{\mathrm{R}}$, the estimator obtained from the inverse transformation (i.e., exponential) is also the ML estimator for $\delta = \widetilde{\mu}_{\mathrm{T}}/\widetilde{\mu}_{\mathrm{R}}$, which is given as

$$\widehat{\delta}_{\mathrm{ML}} = \exp(\widehat{F}) = \exp(\overline{Y}_{\mathrm{T}} - \overline{Y}_{\mathrm{R}}). \tag{6.4.3}$$

Note that the relation between the difference of least squares means on the logarithmic scale and the period ratios on the original scale can be examined as follows

Let R_k be the geometric mean of period ratios r_{ik} obtained from sequence k, which is given by

$$R_k = \left(\prod_{i=1}^{n_k} r_{ik}\right)^{1/n_k}, \quad k = 1, 2.$$

It can be verified that

$$\widehat{\delta}_{\mathrm{ML}} = \left(\frac{R_1}{R_2}\right)^{1/2}.$$

Therefore, the best linear unbiased estimator (BLUE) of $\widehat{F}$ on the logarithmic scale is the log transformation of the square root of the ratio of geometric means of the period ratios of sequence 1 to sequence 2 [i.e., $\widehat{F} = \log(\delta_{\mathrm{ML}})$]. As a result, $\widehat{\delta}_{\mathrm{ML}}$ follows a univariate lognormal distribution with mean $\delta \exp(m\sigma_{\mathrm{d}}^2/2)$, which indicates that $\widehat{\delta}_{\mathrm{ML}}$ is not an unbiased estimator of $\delta = \widetilde{\mu}_{\mathrm{T}}/\widetilde{\mu}_{\mathrm{R}}$.

The corresponding $(1 - 2\alpha) \times 100\%$ confidence interval for δ can be obtained as follows:

$$[\exp(L_1),\ \exp(U_1)]. \tag{6.4.4}$$

As, under the normality assumption, the exact $(1 - 2\alpha) \times 100\%$ confidence interval (L_1, U_1) is the shortest confidence interval for $\mu_{\mathrm{T}} - \mu_{\mathrm{R}}$, the exact $(1 - 2\alpha) \times 100\%$ confidence interval $\exp(L_1)$, $\exp(U_1)$ is also the shortest confidence interval for $\widetilde{\mu}_{\mathrm{T}}/\widetilde{\mu}_{\mathrm{R}}$ (Land, 1988). According to the 80/125 rule specified in the guidances by most regulatory agencies in the world (see, e.g., EMEA, 2001; FDA, 2003b; WHO, 2005), we conclude that two formulations are average bioequivalent if

$$\exp(L_1) > 80\% \text{ and } \exp(U_1) < 125\%,$$

or

$$L_1 > -0.2231 = \log 0.8 \text{ and } U_1 < 0.2231 = \log 1.25.$$

The reasons that most guidances select the range of 80%–125% for the ratio of average bioavailabilities as the criterion for average bioequivalence over the ± 20 rule (80%–120%) are given as:

1. The equivalence limits are symmetric about 0 on the log-scale.
2. The maximum power of concluding average bioequivalence is reached if the ratio of the averages is 1 on the original scale (i.e., is 0 on the log-scale).
3. The power for ± 20 rule to conclude average bioequivalence is at a maximum when the ratio of the averages is 0.98.

Extending the results in Chapter 5, the sample size n required to achieve a $1 - \beta$ power at the α nominal level for the standard 2×2 crossover design after the logarithmic transformation is determined by the following equations:

$$\begin{aligned} &n \geq [t(\alpha, 2n-2) + t(\beta/2, 2n-2)]^2[\mathrm{CV}/\log 1.25]^2, \text{ if } \delta = 1, \\ &n \geq [t(\alpha, 2n-2) + t(\beta, 2n-2)]^2[\mathrm{CV}/(\log 1.25 - \log\delta)]^2, \text{ if } 1 < \delta < 1.25, \end{aligned} \tag{6.4.5}$$

and

$$n \geq [t(\alpha,\ 2n-2) + t(\beta,\ 2n-2)]^2\ [\mathrm{CV}/(\log 0.8 - \log\delta)]^2, \quad \text{if } 0.8 < \delta < 1,$$

where $CV = \sqrt{\exp(\sigma^2) - 1}$ and σ^2 is the variance of the intra-subject residuals obtained from the ANOVA table in Table 3.5.1 based on the log-transformed pharmacokinetic measures.

6.5 Minimum Variance Unbiased Estimator

As it can be seen from Section 6.4, the maximum likelihood estimator $\widehat{\delta}_{\mathrm{ML}}$ overestimates δ when the intra-subject variability is large and the sample size is small. The bias could be substantial. Consequently, the mean-squared error of the estimate could be too large to draw a meaningful statistical inference on δ. In the interest of unbiasedness, we may consider MVUE of $\delta = \widetilde{\mu}_{\mathrm{T}}/\widetilde{\mu}_{\mathrm{R}}$, which is given by

$$\widehat{\delta}_{\mathrm{MVUE}} = \widehat{\delta}_{\mathrm{ML}}\Phi_f(-m\mathrm{SSD}), \tag{6.5.1}$$

where $m = 1/n_1 + 1/n_2$, SSD is the pooled sum of squares of the period differences of the transformed data $\left(\text{i.e., SSD} = (n_1 + n_2 - 2)\widehat{\sigma}_{\mathrm{d}}^2\right)$, f is the degrees of freedom $[n_1 + n_2 - 2]$), and

$$\Phi_f(-m\mathrm{SSD}) = \sum_{j=0}^{\infty} \frac{\Gamma(f/2)}{\Gamma[(f/2)+j]j!}[(-m/4)\,\mathrm{SSD}]^j, \tag{6.5.2}$$

where $\Gamma(\cdot)$ is the gamma function.

From Equation 6.5.2, although $\Phi_f(-m\mathrm{SSD})$ involves an infinite series, it, in fact, converges at a much faster rate than $\exp(-m\mathrm{SSD})$ because $\Gamma(f/2)/\Gamma[(f/2)+j!] < 1$. To obtain $\widehat{\delta}_{\mathrm{MVUE}}$ for δ as given in Equation 6.5.1, the calculation of $\Phi_f(-m\mathrm{SSD})$ is necessary. Our experience indicates that, in most cases, the first five terms of $\Phi_f(-m\mathrm{SSD})$ are sufficient to provide a reasonable approximation at accuracy up to 10^{-8} for a small size (e.g., ≤ 24). An SAS program for the calculation of $\widehat{\delta}_{\mathrm{MVUE}}$ is included in Appendix B.3.

The function of Φ_f was first introduced by Neyman and Scott (1960). The properties of Φ_f, which have been examined by several researchers (Hoyle, 1968; Mehran, 1973; Smith, 1988), are summarized as follows

LEMMA 6.5.1

If SSD is distributed as $\sigma_{\mathrm{d}}^2\chi^2(f)$, then for any number $c \neq 0$, we have

$$\begin{aligned} &1.\ E[\Phi_f(c\mathrm{SSD})] = \exp\left[(c/2)\sigma_{\mathrm{d}}^2\right]; \\ &2.\ E\left\{\left[\Phi_f(c\mathrm{SSD})\right]^2\right\} = \exp\left(c\sigma_{\mathrm{d}}^2\right)\Phi_f\left(c\sigma_{\mathrm{d}}^4\right). \end{aligned} \tag{6.5.3}$$

PROOF A proof can be found in Neyman and Scott (1960) and Mehran (1973).

Let σ_d^2 be the variance of period differences in log scale [i.e., $\sigma_d^2 = \left(\sigma_T^2 + \sigma_R^2\right)/4$]. When $\sigma_T^2 = \sigma_R^2 = \sigma_e^2$, $\sigma_d^2 = \sigma_e^2/2$. The following results can be obtained using the above lemma.

THEOREM 6.5.1

Under model 6.2.1 with the assumption of no carryover effects, the bias, mean-squared error (MSE) of $\widehat{\delta}_{ML}$, the variance of $\widehat{\delta}_{MVUE}$, the relative efficiency of MVUE to MLE, and an unbiased estimator of the variance of MVUE are given as

1. $\text{Bias}(\widehat{\delta}_{ML}) = \delta\{\exp\left[(m/2)\sigma_d^2\right] - 1\};$ (6.5.4)

2. $\text{MSE}(\widehat{\delta}_{ML}) = \delta^2\left\{\left[\exp\left(m\sigma_d^2\right) - 1\right]^2 + 2\exp\left(m\sigma_d^2/2\right)\left[\exp\left(m\sigma_d^2/2\right) - 1\right]\right\};$ (6.5.5)

3. $\text{Var}(\widehat{\delta}_{MVUE}) = \delta^2\left\{\exp\left(m\sigma_d^2\right)\Phi_f\left[\left(m\sigma_d^2\right)^2\right] - 1\right\};$ (6.5.6)

4. The relative efficiency of MVUE to MLE is

$$\text{eff}(\widehat{\delta}_{MVUE}, \widehat{\delta}_{ML}) = \text{MSE}(\widehat{\delta}_{ML})/\text{Var}(\widehat{\delta}_{MVUE}); \tag{6.5.7}$$

5. An unbiased estimator of $\text{Var}(\widehat{\delta}_{MVUE})$ is given by

$$\text{Var}(\widehat{\delta}_{MVUE}) = \exp\left[2(\overline{Y}_T - \overline{Y}_R)\right]\left\{\left[\Phi_f(-m\text{SSD})\right]^2 - \Phi_f(-4m\text{SSD})\right\}. \tag{6.5.8}$$

PROOF

1. The result follows from the fact that

$$E(\widehat{\delta}_{ML}) = \delta\exp\left(m\sigma_d^2/2\right).$$

2. Since

$$\text{Var}(\widehat{\delta}_{ML}) = \delta^2\exp\left(m\sigma_d^2\right)\left[\exp\left(m\sigma_d^2\right) - 1\right],$$

the result follows from

$$\text{MSE}(\widehat{\delta}_{ML}) = \text{Var}(\widehat{\delta}_{ML}) + \left[\text{Bias}\left(\widehat{\delta}_{ML}\right)\right]^2.$$

3. $$\begin{aligned}\mathrm{Var}(\widehat{\delta}_{\mathrm{MVUE}}) &= E(\widehat{\delta}_{\mathrm{MVUE}}) - \delta^2 \\ &= E\{\exp[2(\overline{Y}_{\mathrm{T}} - \overline{Y}_{\mathrm{R}})]\}E\{[\Phi_f(-m\mathrm{SSD})]^2\} - \delta^2 \\ &= \{\delta^2 \exp(2m\sigma_{\mathrm{d}}^2)\}\{\exp(-m\sigma_{\mathrm{d}}^2)\Phi_f(m^2\sigma_{\mathrm{d}}^4)\} - \delta^2 \\ &= \delta^2\left\{\exp(m\sigma_{\mathrm{d}}^2)\Phi_f\left[(m_{\mathrm{d}}^2)^2\right] - 1\right\}.\end{aligned}$$

4 and 5 can be easily verified.

Because $\exp\left[(m/2)\sigma_{\mathrm{d}}^2\right]$ is greater than 1, $\widehat{\delta}_{\mathrm{ML}}$ always overestimates δ, $\widehat{\delta}_{\mathrm{ML}}$ is asymptotically unbiased for a large sample size (i.e., n_1 and n_2 are large). In most bioequivalence studies, however, the sample size ranges from small (e.g., 6) to moderate (e.g., 24). Therefore, if the intra-subject variability σ_{d}^2 in log-scale is rather large, then the bias of $\widehat{\delta}_{\mathrm{ML}}$ could be substantial if the ± 20 rule is used for assessment of average bioequivalence.

6.6 Mean of Individual Subject Ratios

When there are no period effects, Peace (1986) and Anderson and Hauck (1990) suggested use of individual subject ratios for assessment of bioequivalence. Peace (1990) proposed a method using the Tchebycheff inequality that is based on individual subject ratios as a preliminary test for assessment of average bioequivalence. The individual subject ratios for the standard 2×2 crossover design are defined as follows:

$$\widetilde{r}_{ik} = \begin{cases} r_{ik} & \text{if } k = 1, \\ 1/r_{ik} & \text{if } k = 2, \end{cases} \tag{6.6.1}$$

where r_{ik} are defined in Equation (6.4.2).

As indicated earlier, the individual subject ratios can remove inter-subject variability. However, it cannot remove the period effect. Therefore, if we use the mean of individual subject ratios to estimate δ, the bias could be substantial. Note that $\widetilde{r}_{ik}$ is independently lognormally distributed; that is, $\log(\widetilde{r}_{ik})$ is independently normally distributed with mean $\mu + (F_{\mathrm{T}} - F_{\mathrm{R}}) + (P_2 - P_1)$ for $k = 1$ and $\mu + (F_{\mathrm{T}} - F_{\mathrm{R}}) + (P_1 - P_2)$ for $k = 2$ and variance $\sigma_{\mathrm{T}}^2 + \sigma_{\mathrm{R}}^2$. Tse (1990) compared several methods for constructing a confidence interval for δ based on mean of individual subject ratios $(\widetilde{r}_{ik})$ under a lognormal distribution assumption. The results indicate that the resultant confidence intervals for δ lead to a poor coverage probability.

For estimation of δ, the least squares mean of individual subject ratios, denoted by $\widehat{\delta}_{\mathrm{MIR}}$, is usually considered; that is,

$$\widehat{\delta}_{\mathrm{MIR}} = \frac{1}{2}\sum_{k=1}^{2}\frac{1}{n_k}\sum_{i=1}^{n_k}\widetilde{r}_{ik}. \tag{6.6.2}$$

Under Equation 6.2.1, with assumption of no carryover effects, the expected value and variance of $\widehat{\delta}_{\mathrm{MIR}}$ are given by

$$E(\widehat{\delta}_{\text{MIR}}) = \frac{1}{2}\delta \exp\left(\frac{\sigma_{\text{T}}^2 + \sigma_{\text{R}}^2}{2}\right)\{\exp(P_1 - P_2) + \exp(P_2 - P_1)\}, \tag{6.6.3}$$

$$\text{Var}(\widehat{\delta}_{\text{MIR}}) = \frac{1}{4}V_{\text{MIR}}^*\left\{\frac{1}{n_1}\exp[2(P_2 - P_1)] + \frac{1}{n_2}\exp[2(P_1 - P_2)]\right\}, \tag{6.6.4}$$

where

$$V_{\text{MIR}}^* = \exp\left[2(F_{\text{T}} - F_{\text{R}}) + \left(\sigma_{\text{T}}^2 + \sigma_{\text{R}}^2\right)\right]\left\{\exp\left(\sigma_{\text{T}}^2 + \sigma_{\text{R}}^2\right) - 1\right\}.$$

Therefore, the bias of $\widehat{\delta}_{\text{MIR}}$ is given by

$$\text{Bias}(\widehat{\delta}_{\text{MIR}}) = \frac{1}{2}\delta\left\{\left[\exp\left(\frac{\sigma_{\text{T}}^2 + \sigma_{\text{R}}^2}{2}\right)\right][\exp(P_1 - P_2) + \exp(P_2 - P_1)] - 2\right\}. \tag{6.6.5}$$

It can be seen from Equation 6.6.5 that (1) the bias of $\widehat{\delta}_{\text{MIR}}$ is independent of the sample size and (2) the bias involves intra-subject variabilities as well as the period effect. Hence, unlike $\widehat{\delta}_{\text{ML}}$, we cannot reduce the bias by increasing the sample size. In addition, $\widehat{\delta}_{\text{MIR}}$ is not an unbiased estimator of δ, even when there is no period effect. These undesirable statistical properties certainly argue against its use in the assessment of average bioequivalence.

To compare the relative performances in terms of bias between $\widehat{\delta}_{\text{ML}}$ and $\widehat{\delta}_{\text{MIR}}$, Figures 6.6.1 and 6.6.2 plot their relative biases against $\sigma_{\text{T}}^2 + \sigma_{\text{R}}^2$ for $n_1 = n_2 = 10{,}15$ under the assumption of no period and carryover effects. The

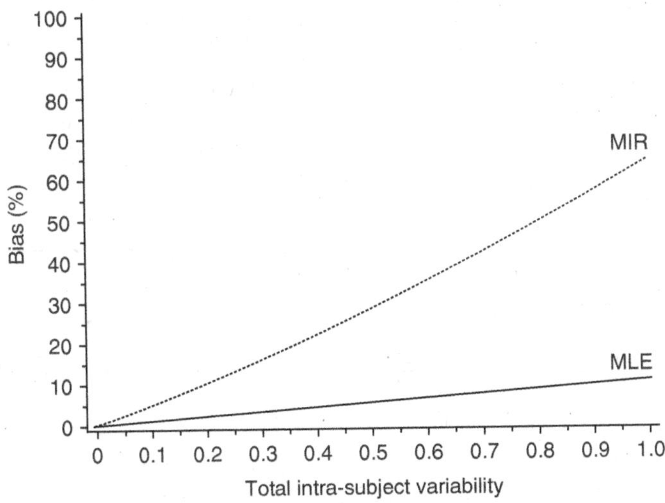

FIGURE 6.6.1: Bias of MLE and LS mean of individual subject ratios: sample size per sequence = 10; direct formulation effect in log scale = 0.

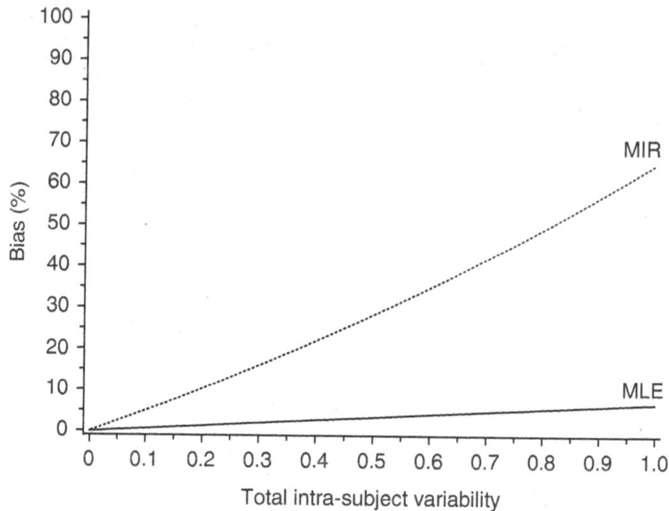

FIGURE 6.6.2: Bias of MLE and LS mean of individual subject ratios: sample size per sequence = 15; direct formulation effect in log scale = 0.

results indicate that the biases of $\widehat{\delta}_{\text{ML}}$ and $\widehat{\delta}_{\text{MIR}}$ are an increasing function of the intra-subject variability. Therefore, one way to reduce the bias is to reduce the intra-subject variability. In addition, the bias of $\widehat{\delta}_{\text{MIR}}$ is always larger than that of $\widehat{\delta}_{\text{ML}}$. For example, when the total intra-subject variability (in log scale) is 1.0 and $n_1 = n_2 = 10$, the bias of $\widehat{\delta}_{\text{MIR}}$ is about 60%, whereas the bias of $\widehat{\delta}_{\text{ML}}$ is about 8%. The bias of $\widehat{\delta}_{\text{ML}}$ reduces to about 3% as the sample size increases to $n_1 = n_2 = 15$, whereas the bias of $\widehat{\delta}_{\text{MIR}}$ remains the same as the sample size increases because the bias is not a function of sample size. As a result, the bias of $\widehat{\delta}_{\text{ML}}$ can be reduced either by increasing the sample size, or by decreasing the intra-subject variability, and the bias of $\widehat{\delta}_{\text{MIR}}$ can be reduced only by decreasing the intra-subject variability.

6.7 Ratio of Formulation Means

From model 6.2.1, the least squares means for test and reference formulations are

$$\overline{X}_{\text{T}} = \frac{1}{2}\,(\overline{X}_{\cdot 21} + \overline{X}_{\cdot 12}),$$

$$\overline{X}_{\text{R}} = \frac{1}{2}\,(\overline{X}_{\cdot 11} + \overline{X}_{\cdot 22}).$$

Therefore, the ratio of least squares means is given by

$$\widehat{\delta}_{\mathrm{RM}} = \frac{\overline{X}_{\mathrm{T}}}{\overline{Y}_{\mathrm{R}}},$$

which is usually considered for assessment of average bioequivalence. For example, in Section 4.5.3, we introduced a bootstrap method for constructing a confidence interval for δ based on $\widehat{\delta}_{\mathrm{RM}}$. It, however, should be noted that the exact distribution of $\overline{X}_{\mathrm{T}}/\overline{X}_{\mathrm{R}}$ is rather complicated and is, thus, not trackable. In this section, the results in Section 4.5.3 are used to examine the asymptotic bias of $\widehat{\delta}_{\mathrm{RM}}$ under Equation 6.2.1.

Let $\overline{\boldsymbol{X}} = (\overline{X}_{\cdot 11}, \overline{X}_{\cdot 21}, \overline{X}_{\cdot 12}, \overline{X}_{\cdot 22})'$ and $\lambda_k = n_k/n$, where $n = n_1 + n_2$; $k = 1, 2$. Under model 6.2.1 and by Theorem 4.5.1, we then have

$$\overline{\boldsymbol{X}} \xrightarrow{d} (\boldsymbol{\mu}, \boldsymbol{\Sigma}/n),$$

where

$$\boldsymbol{\mu} = (\mu_{11}, \mu_{21}, \mu_{12}, \mu_{22})',$$

and

$$\boldsymbol{\Sigma} = \begin{bmatrix} \lambda_2\boldsymbol{\Sigma}_1 & 0 \\ 0 & \lambda_2\boldsymbol{\Sigma}_2 \end{bmatrix} = \begin{bmatrix} V_{11} & V_{12} & & \\ V_{12} & V_{22} & & 0 \\ & 0 & V_{33} & V_{34} \\ & & V_{34} & V_{34} \end{bmatrix},$$

where

$$\begin{aligned}
\mu_{11} &= \exp\left[(\mu + P_1 + F_{\mathrm{R}}) + \left(\sigma_{\mathrm{R}}^2 + \sigma_{\mathrm{S}}^2\right)/2\right]; \\
\mu_{21} &= \exp\left[(\mu + P_2 + F_{\mathrm{T}}) + \left(\sigma_{\mathrm{T}}^2 + \sigma_{\mathrm{S}}^2\right)/2\right]; \\
\mu_{12} &= \exp\left[(\mu + P_1 + F_{\mathrm{T}}) + \left(\sigma_{\mathrm{T}}^2 + \sigma_{\mathrm{S}}^2\right)/2\right]; \\
\mu_{22} &= \exp\left[(\mu + P_2 + F_{\mathrm{R}}) + \left(\sigma_{\mathrm{R}}^2 + \sigma_{\mathrm{S}}^2\right)/2\right]; \\
V_{11} &= \exp\left[2(\mu + P_1 + F_{\mathrm{R}}) + \left(\sigma_{\mathrm{R}}^2 + \sigma_{\mathrm{S}}^2\right)\right]\left[\exp\left(\sigma_{\mathrm{R}}^2 + \sigma_{\mathrm{S}}^2\right) - 1\right]; \\
V_{22} &= \exp\left[2(\mu + P_2 + F_{\mathrm{T}}) + \left(\sigma_{\mathrm{T}}^2 + \sigma_{\mathrm{S}}^2\right)\right]\left[\exp\left(\sigma_{\mathrm{T}}^2 + \sigma_{\mathrm{S}}^2\right) - 1\right]; \\
V_{33} &= \exp\left[2(\mu + P_1 + F_{\mathrm{T}}) + \left(\sigma_{\mathrm{T}}^2 + \sigma_{\mathrm{S}}^2\right)\right]\left[\exp\left(\sigma_{\mathrm{T}}^2 + \sigma_{\mathrm{S}}^2\right) - 1\right]; \\
V_{44} &= \exp\left[2(\mu + P_2 + F_{\mathrm{R}}) + \left(\sigma_{\mathrm{R}}^2 + \sigma_{\mathrm{S}}^2\right)\right]\left[\exp\left(\sigma_{\mathrm{R}}^2 + \sigma_{\mathrm{S}}^2\right) - 1\right]; \\
V_{12} &= V_{34} = \exp\left[2\mu + \left(\sigma_{\mathrm{R}}^2 + \sigma_{\mathrm{T}}^2 + 2\sigma_{\mathrm{S}}^2\right)/2\right]\left[\exp\left(\sigma_{\mathrm{S}}^2\right) - 1\right].
\end{aligned} \tag{6.7.1}$$

Thus, the random vector $(\overline{X}_{\mathrm{T}}, \overline{X}_{\mathrm{R}})'$ is also asymptotically normal with mean vector $\boldsymbol{\mu}^* = (\mu_{\mathrm{T}}^*, \mu_{\mathrm{R}}^*)'$ and covariance matrix

$$\frac{1}{4n}\boldsymbol{\Sigma}^* = \begin{bmatrix} V_{\mathrm{TT}} & V_{\mathrm{TR}} \\ V_{\mathrm{TR}} & V_{\mathrm{RR}} \end{bmatrix},$$

where

$$\begin{aligned}
\mu_T^* &= \frac{1}{2}\{\exp[(\mu + F_T) + (\sigma_T^2 + \sigma_S^2)/2]\}\{\exp(P_1) + \exp(P_2)\};\\
\mu_R^* &= \frac{1}{2}\{\exp[(\mu + F_R) + (\sigma_R^2 + \sigma_S^2)/2]\}\{\exp(P_1) + \exp(P_2)\};\\
V_{TT} &= \exp\left[2(\mu + F_T) + (\sigma_T^2 + \sigma_S^2)\right]\left[\exp(\sigma_T^2 + \sigma_S^2) - 1\right]\\
&\quad [\lambda_1 \exp(2P_2) + \lambda_2 \exp(2P_1)];\\
V_{RR} &= \exp\left[2(\mu + F_R) + (\sigma_R^2 + \sigma_S^2)\right]\left[\exp(\sigma_R^2 + \sigma_S^2) - 1\right]\\
&\quad [\lambda_1 \exp(2P_1) + \lambda_2 \exp(2P_2)];\\
V_{TR} &= \exp\left[2\mu + (\sigma_T^2 + \sigma_R^2 + 2\sigma_S^2)/2\right]\left[\exp(\sigma_S^2) - 1\right].
\end{aligned} \tag{6.7.2}$$

The asymptotic bias $\widehat{\delta}_{RM}$ is given in the following theorem.

THEOREM 6.7.1

Suppose that there are no carryover effects. Under model 6.2.1, the asymptotic bias of $\widehat{\delta}_{RM}$, denoted by ABias ($\widehat{\delta}_{RM}$), is then given by

$$\begin{aligned}
\text{ABias}(\widehat{\delta}_{RM}) &= E(\widehat{\delta}_{RM}) - \delta\\
&= \delta\left\{\exp\left[\frac{\sigma_T^2 - \sigma_R^2}{2}\right]\left[1 + \frac{1}{n\pi_1}\left\{\pi_2\left[\exp(\sigma_R^2 + \sigma_S^2) - 1\right]\right.\right.\right.\\
&\quad \left.\left.\left. - \left[\exp(\sigma_S^2) - 1\right]\right\}\right]\right\} - \delta,
\end{aligned} \tag{6.7.3}$$

where

$$\pi_1 = [\exp(P_1) + \exp(P_2)]^2,$$

and

$$\pi_2 = [\lambda_1 \exp(2P_1) + \lambda_2 \exp(2P_2)].$$

PROOF Consider Taylor expansion of $\widehat{\delta}_{RM}$ around μ_T^*/μ_R^* up to the second order term. We then have

$$\begin{aligned}
\widehat{\delta}_{RM} &= \frac{\overline{X}_T}{\overline{X}_R}\\
&= \frac{\mu_T^*}{\mu_R^*} + \frac{1}{\mu_R^*}(\overline{X}_T - \mu_T^*) - \frac{\mu_T^*}{\mu_R^{*2}}(\overline{X}_R - \mu_R^*) + \frac{2 \cdot \mu_T^*}{\mu_R^{*3}}(\overline{X} - \mu_R^*)^2\\
&\quad - \frac{1}{\mu_R^{*2}}(\overline{X}_T - \mu_T^*)(\overline{Y}_R - \mu_R^*) + O(n^{-2}).
\end{aligned}$$

Therefore, the asymptotic bias is

$$\begin{aligned}\text{Bias}(\widehat{\delta}_{\text{RM}}) &= E(\widehat{\delta}_{\text{RM}}) - \delta \\ &= \frac{\mu_{\text{T}}^*}{\mu_{\text{R}}^*} + \frac{\mu_{\text{T}}^*}{\mu_{\text{R}}^{*3}} V_{\text{RR}} - \frac{V_{\text{TR}}}{\mu_{\text{R}}^{*2}} + E[O(n^{-2})] - \delta.\end{aligned}$$

As $E[O(n^{-2})]$ is negligible as n tends to infinity, the result follows.

COROLLARY 6.7.1

When there is no period effect and $\lambda_1 = \lambda_2 = 1/2$, then the asymptotic bias becomes

$$\text{ABias}(\widehat{\delta}_{\text{RM}}) = \delta\left\{\exp\left[\frac{\sigma_{\text{T}}^2 - \sigma_{\text{R}}^2}{2}\right]\left[1 + \frac{1}{4n}\exp(\sigma_{\text{S}}^2)\left[\exp(\sigma_{\text{R}}^2) - 1\right]\right] - 1\right\}. \quad (6.7.4)$$

Note that the asymptotic bias of $\widehat{\delta}_{\text{RM}}$ contains inter-subject variability.

6.8 Comparison of MLE, MVUE, MIR, and RM

Thus far, we have introduced four estimators for δ. They are the maximum likelihood estimator ($\widehat{\delta}_{\text{RM}}$), minimum variance unbiased estimator ($\widehat{\delta}_{\text{MVUE}}$), mean of individual subject ratios ($\widehat{\delta}_{\text{MIR}}$), and ratio of formulation means ($\widehat{\delta}_{\text{RM}}$). Under model 6.2.1, the results for biases, variances, and mean-squared errors for $\widehat{\delta}_{\text{ML}}$, $\widehat{\delta}_{\text{MVUE}}$, and $\widehat{\delta}_{\text{MIR}}$ are exact. For the ratio of means $\widehat{\delta}_{\text{RM}}$, however, only asymptotic results are obtained. To evaluate their relative performances in small samples, a simulation study (Liu and Weng, 1992) was conducted to compare these estimators in terms of relative bias [i.e., $100 \times (\text{bias}/\delta)$], variance and mean-squared error under model 6.2.1. In this simulation study, we consider combinations of three sample sizes ($n_1 = n_2 = 7, 10$, and 15), six covariance structures (in log scale), two formulation effects ($F_{\text{T}} - F_{\text{R}} = 0$ and 0.5), and two period effects ($P_1 - P_2 = 0$ and 2). For each combination, a total of 1000 random samples were generated to compute average relative bias and average variance/mean-squared error for the four estimators. The random samples were obtained by generating normal random samples according to model 4.1.1 and following an inverse transformation. The results are summarized in Table 6.8.1 (relative bias) and Table 6.8.2 (variance and mean-squared error), respectively.

From Table 6.8.1, the results indicate that the biases of $\widehat{\delta}_{\text{ML}}$ and $\widehat{\delta}_{\text{RM}}$ decrease as either sample size increases or the intra-subject variability decreases when $\sigma_{\text{T}}^2 = \sigma_{\text{R}}^2 = \sigma_{\text{e}}^2$. In addition, as expected, the biases of $\widehat{\delta}_{\text{ML}}$ are not affected by period effects. However, the biases of $\widehat{\delta}_{\text{RM}}$ and $\widehat{\delta}_{\text{MIR}}$ increase substantially when there is a

TABLE 6.8.1: Relative average bias (%) of estimators.

Covariance Structure		Estimator	$F_T - F_R = 0$, $P_1 - P_2 = 0$			$F_T - F_R = 0$, $P_1 - P_2 = 0$		
			7	**10**	**15**	**7**	**10**	**15**
0.5	0.25	MVUE	0.41	0.11	0.39	−1.0	<0.1	0.37
	0.5	MLE	1.4	1.2	1.2	0.79	1.2	0.45
		RM	1.7	1.3	1.8	6.2	5.1	2.2
		MIR	27.8	28.9	29.0	375.9	382.4	380.0
1	0.5	MVUE	0.85	−0.98	−0.25	0.12	0.84	0.29
	1	MLE	4.6	1.5	1.4	3.8	3.8	2.0
		RM	7.7	3.9	2.4	17.0	15.0	8.9
		MIR	66.5	64.6	63.2	510.6	535.7	533.9
2	1	MVUE	1.1	−1.1	−0.41	−0.83	−0.29	0.36
	2	MLE	8.8	4.0	3.0	6.6	4.8	3.7
		RM	23.1	12.5	9.7	45.6	29.2	20.1
		MIR	173.5	186.6	171.0	942.2	886.3	911.9
0.5	$\sqrt{0.125}$	MVUE	0.69	0.39	−0.31	0.77	−0.69	<0.1
	1	MLE	3.5	2.4	1.0	3.6	1.3	1.3
		RM	−14.5	−18.0	−19.4	−9.7	−12.9	−16.0
		MIR	48.2	48.3	48.4	469.0	452.7	455.6
0.5	0.5	MVUE	0.39	−0.18	0.18	0.56	0.44	1.3
	2	MLE	5.7	3.7	2.7	6.1	4.3	3.9
		RM	−39.1	−43.7	−46.1	−32.9	−38.4	−41.6
		MIR	104.5	112.0	110.6	723.1	717.2	712.0
0.5	$\sqrt{0.5}$	MVUE	−0.58	0.94	−0.79	−0.42	0.22	−0.48
	4	MLE	11.3	9.1	4.5	11.3	8.1	4.7
		RM	−66.2	−69.8	−74.0	−58.8	−64.2	−70.5
		MIR	361.2	380.5	367.6	1674.8	1643.3	1611.1

0.5	0.25	MVUE	0.13	0.72	0.40	0.33	−0.24	−0.12
	0.5	MLE	1.9	2.0	1.2	2.1	1.0	0.72
		RM	3.0	2.3	1.7	6.1	3.9	3.5
		MIR	28.5	29.3	29.0	381.1	381.5	384.0
1	0.5	MVUE	0.20	0.93	−0.18	0.61	1.23	0.53
	1	MLE	3.9	3.5	1.5	4.2	3.7	1.1
		RM	6.0	5.98	3.0	14.5	13.0	7.2
		MIR	66.3	68.1	63.1	515.1	524.8	507.9
2	1	MVUE	<0.1	−1.8	−1.1	−0.88	0.55	0.22
	2	MLE	7.4	3.3	2.3	6.3	5.7	3.6
		RM	17.4	12.6	9.0	33.7	26.5	16.3
		MIR	173.7	171.7	168.7	862.8	895.8	930.1
0.5	$\sqrt{0.125}$	MVUE	−0.42	−0.47	0.49	−0.39	0.20	<0.1
	1	MLE	2.4	1.6	1.8	2.5	2.2	1.4
		RM	−16.6	−18.6	−18.6	−10.4	−12.2	−16.2
		MIR	47.6	49.1	49.5	457.7	453.9	457.6
0.5	0.5	MVUE	−0.21	−0.35	0.12	−0.40	1.3	<0.1
	2	MLE	5.3	3.5	2.4	5.1	5.1	2.4
		RM	−41.2	−44.1	−46.6	−32.3	−38.2	−42.2
		MIR	109.0	113.3	112.8	679.1	720.4	692.4
0.5	$\sqrt{0.5}$	MVUE	−0.87	2.4	−0.48	<0.1	1.1	−0.15
	4	MLE	10.7	10.6	4.7	11.6	9.2	5.1
		RM	−65.4	−69.8	−73.2	−57.5	−64.5	−70.5
		MIR	376.8	380.2	364.5	1619.6	1698.7	1612.3

Source: From Liu, J.P. and Weng, C.S., *Stat. Med.*, 11, 881, 1992.

Note: Relative average bias (%) = 100 [average bias/(exp($F_T - F_R$))]; MVUE, minimum variance unbiased estimator; MLE, maximum likelihood estimator; RM, ratio of means; MIR, mean of individual ratios.

TABLE 6.8.2: Average mean-square error and variance of estimators.

Covariance Structure		Estimator	$F_T - F_R = 0$, $P_1 - P_2 = 0$			$F_T - F_R = 0$, $P_1 - P_2 = 0$		
			7	**10**	**15**	**7**	**10**	**15**
0.5	0.25	MVUE	0.036	0.027	0.018	0.033	0.024	0.016
	0.5	MLE	0.037	0.028	0.018	0.034	0.025	0.016
		RM	0.050	0.036	0.026	0.141	0.095	0.057
		MIR	0.151	0.140	0.122	15.878	16.082	15.380
1	0.5	MVUE	0.068	0.045	0.034	0.066	0.054	0.034
	1	MLE	0.076	0.048	0.035	0.072	0.57	0.036
		RM	0.146	0.098	0.069	0.511	0.344	0.180
		MIR	0.756	0.649	0.540	33.440	35.580	33.420
2	1	MVUE	0.153	0.098	0.066	0.171	0.104	0.075
	2	MLE	0.182	0.110	0.071	0.200	0.117	0.082
		RM	0.706	0.434	0.269	6.771	1.325	0.840
		MIR	5.633	4.839	4.409	204.709	122.727	119.150
0.5	$\sqrt{0.125}$	MVUE	0.060	0.045	0.026	0.054	0.036	0.026
	1	MLE	0.065	0.043	0.027	0.058	0.038	0.027
		RM	0.088	0.075	0.067	0.156	0.129	0.096
		MIR	0.418	0.361	0.320	26.504	23.840	23.280
0.5	0.5	MVUE	0.107	0.083	0.051	0.115	0.177	0.061
	2	MLE	0.121	0.091	0.054	0.132	0.084	0.065
		RM	0.230	0.245	0.246	0.279	0.252	0.244
		MIR	1.911	2.000	1.691	97.100	90.890	64.377
0.5	$\sqrt{0.5}$	MVUE	0.250	0.158	0.113	0.261	0.186	0.103
	4	MLE	0.323	0.193	0.127	0.336	0.223	0.116
		RM	0.506	0.526	0.570	0.477	0.486	0.537
		MIR	32.762	32.940	25.590	1200.760	698.380	529.244

0.5	0.25	MVUE	0.101	0.072	0.044	0.097	0.071	0.041
	0.5	MLE	0.105	0.074	0.045	0.101	0.073	0.045
		RM	0.151	0.111	0.070	0.424	0.269	0.177
		MIR	0.433	0.383	0.324	44.840	43.940	42.761
1	0.5	MVUE	0.217	0.144	0.091	0.196	0.134	0.082
	1	MLE	0.236	0.155	0.094	0.214	0.144	0.085
		RM	0.475	0.350	0.184	1.021	0.789	0.498
		MIR	2.169	1.951	1.466	96.199	91.890	79.790
2	1	MVUE	0.444	0.293	0.175	0.394	0.281	0.197
	2	MLE	0.517	0.325	0.188	0.458	0.317	0.213
		RM	2.442	1.290	0.743	5.362	2.600	2.235
		MIR	17.171	15.319	12.184	371.444	346.882	340.516
0.5	$\sqrt{0.125}$	MVUE	0.155	0.102	0.078	0.159	0.108	0.078
	1	MLE	0.164	0.106	0.081	0.171	0.114	0.080
		RM	0.249	0.213	0.177	0.434	0.353	0.279
		MIR	1.096	1.003	0.921	71.582	65.301	63.510
0.5	0.5	MVUE	0.303	0.227	0.140	0.302	0.213	0.147
	2	MLE	0.343	0.247	0.148	0.344	0.236	0.156
		RM	0.662	0.668	0.684	0.738	0.687	0.675
		MIR	5.650	6.309	4.845	203.713	207.342	171.998
0.5	$\sqrt{0.5}$	MVUE	0.612	0.500	0.303	0.650	0.480	0.284
	4	MLE	0.795	0.604	0.338	0.831	0.576	0.320
		RM	1.325	1.455	1.525	1.281	1.304	1.467
		MIR	111.466	139.567	81.574	3285.000	2790.540	1428.850

Source: From Liu, J.P. and Weng, C.S., *Stat. Med.* 11, 881, 1992.

Note: MVUE, minimum variance unbiased estimator; MLE, maximum likelihood estimator; RM, ratio of means; MIR, mean of individual ratios.

period effect. For the case where $\sigma_T^2 < \sigma_R^2$, the bias of $\widehat{\delta}_{ML}$ does not change much. This is because it depends on only the total intra-subject variabilities $\sigma_T^2 + \sigma_R^2$. On the other hand, the bias of $\widehat{\delta}_{RM}$ becomes negative and does not change much regardless of the presence of a period effect. This is because the leading term of the asymptotic bias of $\widehat{\delta}_{RM}$ is $\exp(\sigma_T^2 - \sigma_R^2)$ and is not a function of sample size, whereas the first-order term, which contains the period effect, is a decreasing function of sample size. In general, the absolute magnitude of the bias of $\widehat{\delta}_{MIR}$ is much larger than that of $\widehat{\delta}_{RM}$ for the combinations considered.

The empirical relative bias of $\widehat{\delta}_{MVUE}$ is always less than 2%, except for one combination. The absolute magnitudes of the maximum relative biases for $\widehat{\delta}_{ML}$, $\widehat{\delta}_{RM}$, and $\widehat{\delta}_{MIR}$ are 11.6%, −74%, and 1700%, respectively.

From Table 6.8.2, the results indicate that the empirical variances and mean-squared errors of the four estimators decrease as the sample size increases and increase in the presence of formulation effect. As shown in Table 6.8.2, as expected, empirical variances and mean-squared errors for $\widehat{\delta}_{MVUE}$ and $\widehat{\delta}_{ML}$ do not change much regardless of the presence of period effect. However, the mean-squared errors of $\widehat{\delta}_{MIR}$ and $\widehat{\delta}_{RM}$ increase dramatically when there is period effect. In general, $\widehat{\delta}_{MIR}$ has the largest mean-squared error among the four estimators. The mean-squared errors for $\widehat{\delta}_{ML}$ are quite close to the variance of $\widehat{\delta}_{MVUE}$.

In summary, for estimation of δ (or for assessment of bioequivalence), the minimum variance unbiased estimator should be used, whereas the maximum likelihood estimator is competitive when the total intra-subject variabilities (on log-scale) is small (e.g., < 0.5) and sample size is moderate (e.g., $n_1 = n_2 > 10$). However, bias of the maximum likelihood estimator involves the intra-subject variability, which may have some influence on the assessment of bioequivalence in average bioavailability when the ± 20 rule is applied.

6.9 Example

To illustrate the use of estimators of δ discussed is the previous sections, we consider the AUC data from two erythromycin formulations in a bioavailability study published by Clayton and Leslie (1981). In this study, a standard 2×2 crossover experiment was conducted with 18 subjects to compare a new erythromycin formulation (i.e., erythromycin stearate) with a reference formulation (i.e., erythromycin base). The new formulation and the reference formulation are denoted by formulations C and D, respectively. As no sequence identification of each subject was provided in Clayton and Leslie (1981), for the purpose of this illustration, we adapt the order of periods given in Weiner (1989) and assign subjects 1 through 9 to sequence 1 and the remaining subjects to sequence 2. Table 6.9.1 gives the original AUCs and log-transformed AUCs as well as the individual subject ratios and their log transformation.

Note that this data set has been analyzed by many researchers because of its possible violation of the normality assumption in raw data and the existence of

TABLE 6.9.1: AUCs for two erythromycin formulations.

		C (Stearate)		D (Base)		Ratio C/D	
Subject	**Sequence**	**Raw**	**Log(Raw)**	**Raw**	**Log(Raw)**	**Raw**	**Log(Raw)**
1	CD	2.52	0.9243	5.47	1.6993	0.4607	−0.7750
2	CD	8.87	2.1827	4.84	1.5769	1.8326	0.6058
3	CD	0.79	−0.2357	2.25	0.8109	0.3511	−1.0467
4	CD	1.68	0.5188	1.82	0.5988	0.9231	−0.0800
5	CD	6.95	1.9387	7.87	2.0631	0.8831	−0.1243
6	CD	1.05	0.0488	3.25	1.1787	0.3231	−1.1299
7	CD	0.99	−0.0101	12.39	2.5169	0.0800	−2.5269
8	CD	5.60	1.7228	4.77	1.5624	1.1740	0.1604
9	CD	3.16	1.1506	1.88	0.6313	1.6809	0.5193
10	DC	3.19	1.1600	4.98	1.6054	0.6406	−0.4454
11	DC	9.83	2.2854	7.14	1.9657	1.3768	0.3197
12	DC	2.91	1.0682	1.81	0.5933	1.6077	0.4748
13	DC	4.58	1.5217	7.34	1.9933	0.6240	−0.4716
14	DC	7.05	1.9530	4.25	1.4469	1.6588	0.5061
15	DC	3.41	1.2267	6.66	1.8961	0.5120	−0.6694
16	DC	2.49	0.9123	4.76	1.5603	0.5231	−0.6480
17	DC	6.18	1.82313	7.16	1.9685	0.8631	−0.1472
18	DC	2.85	1.0473	5.52	1.7084	0.5163	−0.6611

Source: From Clayton, D. and Leslie, A., *J. Int. Med. Res.*, 9, 470, 1981.

potential outliers (Metzler and Huang, 1983; Hauck and Anderson, 1984; Anderson and Hauck, 1990). Furthermore, the conclusion drawn by these authors does not support Clayton and Leslie's claim on average bioequivalence between the two formulations. This data set, however, is also used for checking the normality assumption and for detection of outliers in later chapters.

Table 6.9.2 presents a table of analysis of variance for the log-transformed data. The results show no evidence of unequal carryover effects (p-value > 0.10) and

TABLE 6.9.2: Analysis of variance for log-transformed data in Table 6.9.1.

Source of Variation	Degrees of Freedom (df)	SS	MS	F	p-Value
Inter-subject					
Carryover	1	1.3053	1.3053	2.50	0.1332
Residuals	16	8.3434	0.5215	1.69	
Intra-subject					
Formulation	1	1.0470	1.0470	3.39	0.0843
Period	1	0.1959	0.1959	0.63	0.4376
Residuals	16	4.9440	0.3090		

period effect (p-value > 0.4). However, the test for inter-subject variability by F_v in Equation 3.5.13 is not significant at the 10% level. This indicates that the intra-subject variability might be larger than the inter-subject variability. A close examination of the data reveals that possible outlying observations may occur in subject 7, because the AUCs for the two formulations are quite different (0.99 vs. 12.39 in the original scale or −0.01 vs. 2.52 in log scale). The estimated CV is about 36.55% which is high, but not unusual in bioavailability and bioequivalence studies. The index of sensitivity defined in Equation 5.3.10 is estimated to be about 3.28. Therefore, as discussed in Section 5.3.2, this study has little power to conclude bioequivalence if Schuirmann's two one-sided procedure and the ±20 rule are applied.

In the following, for estimation of δ, the estimators and their corresponding biases, variances, and mean-squared errors are obtained based upon the AUC data in Table 6.9.1.

6.9.1 Maximum Likelihood Estimator $\widehat{\delta}_{ML}$

From Table 6.9.1, the LS means, $\widehat{F}$, SSD, $\widehat{\sigma}_d^2$, and the classical 90% confidence interval for $\widehat{F}$, based on log-transformed data, can be obtained as follows:

$$\overline{Y}_T = 1.1798,\ \overline{Y}_R = 1.5209,\ \widehat{F} = -0.3411,\ \text{SD} = 2.4720,\ \widehat{\sigma}_d^2 = 0.1545,$$

and

$$(L_1, U_1) = (-0.6646,\ -0.0176).$$

Therefore, the maximum likelihood estimate of δ is given by

$$\widehat{\delta}_{ML} = \exp(-0.3411) = 0.7110.$$

The 90% confidence interval for δ according to Equation 6.4.4 is then given by

$$[\exp(-0.6646),\ \exp(-0.0176)] = (0.5145,\ 0.9826).$$

Because the confidence interval for δ is not within the bioequivalence limits (80%, 125%), we conclude that the two erythromycin formulations are not average bioequivalent according to the 80/125 rule.

From Theorem 6.5.1, the estimates for bias and variance of $\widehat{\delta}_{ML}$ can be obtained as follows:

$$\begin{aligned}\widehat{\text{Bias}}(\widehat{\delta}_{ML}) &= \widehat{\delta}_{ML}\left[\exp\left(m\widehat{\sigma}_d^2/2\right) - 1\right] \\ &= (0.7110)\ [\exp(0.1545/9) - 1] \\ &= 0.0123, \\ \widehat{\text{Var}}(\widehat{\delta}_{ML}) &= \widehat{\delta}_{ML}^2 \exp\left(m\widehat{\sigma}_d^2\right)\left[\exp\left(m\widehat{\sigma}_d^2\right) - 1\right] \\ &= 0.0183.\end{aligned}$$

Hence, the estimate of mean-squared error of $\widehat{\delta}_{\text{ML}}$ is given by

$$\begin{aligned}\widehat{\text{MSE}}(\widehat{\delta}_{\text{ML}}) &= 0.0183 + (0.0123)^2 \\ &= 0.0184.\end{aligned}$$

6.9.2 Minimum Variance Unbiased Estimator $\widehat{\delta}_{\text{MVUE}}$

For the minimum variance unbiased estimate of δ, as $\Phi_f(-m\text{SSD}) = 0.9831$, we have

$$\begin{aligned}\widehat{\delta}_{\text{MVUE}} &= \widehat{\delta}_{\text{ML}}\Phi_f(-m\text{SSD}) \\ &= (0.7110)(0.9831) \\ &= 0.6990.\end{aligned}$$

From Equation 6.5.6, the estimate for the variance of $\widehat{\delta}_{\text{MVUE}}$ can be obtained as follows:

$$\begin{aligned}\widehat{\text{Var}}(\widehat{\delta}_{\text{MVUE}}) &= \widehat{\text{MSE}}(\widehat{\delta}_{\text{MVUE}}) \\ &= \widehat{\delta}^2_{\text{ML}}\left\{\left[\Phi_f(-m\text{SSD})\right]^2 - \Phi_f(-4m\text{SSD})\right\} \\ &= (0.7110)^2[(0.9831)^2 - 0.9354] \\ &= 0.0157.\end{aligned}$$

As a result, the relative efficiency of $\widehat{\delta}_{\text{MVUE}}$ to $\widehat{\delta}_{\text{ML}}$ is estimated as

$$\begin{aligned}\text{eff}(\widehat{\delta}_{\text{MVUE}}, \widehat{\delta}_{\text{ML}}) &= \frac{0.0184}{0.0157} \\ &= 117.39\%.\end{aligned}$$

Therefore, for this data set, for the estimation of δ, the minimum variance unbiased estimator is not only an unbiased estimator, but also is about 17% more efficient than the maximum likelihood estimator.

6.9.3 Mean of Individual Subject Ratios $\widehat{\delta}_{\text{MIR}}$

The mean of individual subject ratios based on the raw data is given by $\widehat{\delta}_{\text{MIR}} = 0.8906$, which is much higher than $\widehat{\delta}_{\text{ML}}$ and $\widehat{\delta}_{\text{MVUE}}$. Since $\widehat{P} = P_2 - P_1 = 0.1475$, the bias of $\widehat{\delta}_{\text{MIR}}$ can be estimated using Equation 6.6.5, which is given as

$$\begin{aligned}\widehat{\text{Bias}}(\widehat{\delta}_{\text{MIR}}) &= \frac{1}{2}\,\widehat{\delta}_{\text{ML}}\left\{\left[\exp\left(2\widehat{\sigma}^2_{\text{d}}\right)\right]\left[\exp\left(-\widehat{P}\right) + \exp\left(\widehat{P}\right)\right] - 2\right\} \\ &= 0.2680.\end{aligned}$$

Similarly, an estimate of the variance of $\widehat{\delta}_{\text{MIR}}$ can be obtained using Equation 6.6.4 which is given by 0.0465. Hence, the mean-squared error for $\widehat{\delta}_{\text{MIR}}$ can be estimated by 0.1183.

6.9.4 Ratio of Formulation Means $\widehat{\delta}_{\text{RM}}$

Because the least squares means based upon the raw data are

$$\overline{X}_{\text{T}} = 4.1167 \quad \text{and} \quad \overline{X}_{\text{R}} = 5.2311,$$

then, the ratio of least squares means is given by

$$\widehat{\delta}_{\text{RM}} = \overline{X}_{\text{T}}/\overline{X}_{\text{R}} = 4.1167/5.2311 = 0.7870.$$

Under the assumption of no carryover and period effects, the sample covariance matrix, based on 17 degrees of freedom, can be obtained as follows:

$$\begin{bmatrix} 0.3093 & 0.1326 \\ 0.1326 & 0.5607 \end{bmatrix}.$$

Consequently, the estimates for $\sigma_{\text{T}}^2 - \sigma_{\text{R}}^2$, σ_{R}^2, and σ_{S}^2, by the method of moments, are 0.2514, 0.1767, and 0.1326, respectively. Therefore, by Equation 6.7.4 in Corollary 6.7.1, the asymptotic bias is estimated by

$$\begin{aligned}\widehat{\text{Bias}}(\widehat{\delta}_{\text{RM}}) = \widehat{\delta}_{\text{ML}} \Bigg\{ &[\exp(0.2514/2)] \\ &\times \left\{ 1 + \frac{1}{72}[\exp(0.1326)][\exp(0.1767) - 1] \right\} - 1 \Bigg\} = 0.0977.\end{aligned}$$

Table 6.9.3 summarizes the results of estimates of the biases, variances, and mean-squared errors for Clayton and Leslie's data. Although the estimated bias of the maximum likelihood estimator is very small, the estimated variance is about 17% larger than that of the minimum variance unbiased estimator. The estimated biases

TABLE 6.9.3: Estimates for biases, variances, and mean-squared errors of MLE, MVUE, MIR, and RM.

Estimator	Estimate	Estimated Bias	Estimated Variance/MSE
MVUE ($\widehat{\delta}_{\text{MVUE}}$)	0.6990	—	0.01570
MLE ($\widehat{\delta}_{\text{ML}}$)	0.7110	0.0123	0.01840
MIR ($\widehat{\delta}_{\text{MIR}}$)	0.8906	0.2680	0.11830
RM ($\widehat{\delta}_{\text{RM}}$)	0.7870	0.0977[a]	—

Source: From Lin, J.P. and Weng, C.S., *Stat. Med.*, 11, 881, 1992.

[a] Asymptotic bias when there is no period effect.

for the least squares mean of individual subject ratios and the ratio of the least squares means are both greater than 10%. The estimated mean-squared error of the least squares mean of individual subject ratios is about seven times as large as those of the maximum likelihood estimator and the minimum variance unbiased estimator. These results strongly suggest that, under model 6.2.1, the least squares mean of individual subject ratios and the ratio of the least squares means should not be used for estimation of δ.

6.10 Discussion

In this chapter, we considered several estimators for estimation of δ, the ratio of average bioavailabilities which is used as a bioequivalence measure under model 6.2.1. Based on these estimators, a $(1 - 2\alpha) \times 100\%$ confidence intervals for δ can be obtained to assess average bioequivalence. For example, from the maximum likelihood estimator $\widehat{\delta}_{ML}$, an exact $(1 - 2\alpha) \times 100\%$ confidence interval for δ is given in Equation 6.4.4. Currently, the U.S. FDA, the EMEA, and the WHO recommend the use of the confidence interval approach based on the maximum likelihood approach to evaluate average bioequivalence using 80/125 rule for the log-transformed AUC and C_{max}. The sample size determination is also provided in this chapter for the evaluation of average bioequivalence using 80/125 rule under the multiplicative model 6.2.1. However, it should be noted again that the point estimator of δ by the maximum likelihood is always upward biased. For other estimators, although no exact confidence intervals for δ are available, approximate confidence intervals may be obtained using a nonparametric bootstrap resampling procedure. These confidence intervals can then be used to determine average bioequivalence. In other words, we conclude average bioequivalence if the confidence interval is within bioequivalent limits (e.g., 80% and 125%) according to the 80/125 rule.

For the analysis of individual subject ratios, although the least squares mean of individual subject ratios is commonly used for assessment of average bioequivalence, the expected value of individual subject ratios is not equal to 1 [i.e., $E(r_{ik}) \neq 1$] even when X_{i1k} and X_{i2k} have exactly the same distribution. Because the distribution of individual subject ratios is often positively skewed, it may be more appropriate to use the median of individual subject ratios as an alternative bioequivalence measure. Tse (1990) examined the relative performances of confidence intervals for the true mean and median of individual subject ratios, which were obtained under the assumption that the ratios follow a log-normal distribution, in terms of their coverage probabilities. The results indicate that the confidence interval for the median of individual subject ratios provides a better coverage probability. As a result, it may suggest that the ratio of medians of X_{ijk} under model 6.2.1 or the true median of individual subject ratios be used as alternative measures of average bioequivalence. However, statistical inference on the ratio of medians or the median of individual subject ratios is more complicated to obtain.

In practice, although a log-transformation may be able to reduce skewness and achieve an additive model with relatively homogeneous variances, the log-transformed data may not follow a normal distribution owing to unknown distributions of the transformed random subject effects. Distribution of the transformed data for a different formulation may be of a different type owing to different distributions of transformed random subject effects. To remove the unknown random subject effects, assuming that there are no period effects, Chow et al. (1991) proposed a method using log-transformed individual subject ratios followed by an inverse transformed under a semiparametric multiplicative model. However, the method proposed by Chow et al. is similar to a method proposed by Steinijans and Diletti (1985), which is derived to construct a confidence interval for a bioavailability ratio using a Wilcoxon signed rank test.

Chapter 7

Assessment of Inter- and Intra-Subject Variabilities

7.1 Introduction

In previous chapters, we only considered the assessment of equivalence in average bioavailabilities between formulations. However, as indicated in Section 1.5, bioequivalence between formulations, in fact, depends on whether the marginal distributions of the pharmacokinetic parameters of interest, such as AUC and C_{max}, for the two formulations are equivalent. This equivalence is usually referred to as population bioequivalence (Anderson and Hauck, 1990). Under normality assumptions, the equivalence between distributions can be determined by the equivalence between their first moment (average) and second moment (variability). For assessment of bioequivalence, however, the U.S. FDA, the EMEA, and the WHO only require that evidence of equivalence in average bioavailabilities between formulations be provided (EMEA, 2001; FDA, 2003b; WHO, 2005). The conclusion of bioequivalence based on only average bioavailability may be somewhat misleading because the safety and exchangeability of the test formulations are questionable (Hauck and Anderson, 1992; Chow and Liu, 1995a).

In practice, because individual subjects may differ widely in their response to the drug, in addition to equivalence in average bioavailability, it is important to compare the variability of bioavailability. If the variability of the test formulation is much larger than that of the reference formulation, then the safety of the test formulation may be of concern, and the exchangeability between two formulations is questionable, even when the two formulations are equivalent in average bioavailability. This is because the equivalence of average bioavailability does not take into account the difference in variabilities (Liu, 1991). Suppose a patient switches from the reference formulation (with a smaller intra-subject variability) to a test formulation (with a much larger intra-subject variability). It is very likely that the AUC of the patient will be outside the therapeutic range. If the AUC is below the therapeutic range, the test formulation may not be effective. On the other hand, if the AUC is above the therapeutic range, the safety of the test formulation is of great concern because it may cause severe adverse experiences. As a result, equivalence in average bioavailability does not guarantee that the two formulations are therapeutically equivalent and exchangeable (Anderson, 1993; Liu and Chow, 1995). For example, for comparison of an intranasal formulation with an intravenous formulation of a drug product (e.g., insulin for diabetes or butorphanol for migraine headaches), bioequivalence in average bioavailability may be concluded. However, they may not be therapeutically equivalent because the intra-subject variability of the intranasal formulation is usually much larger than that of the intravenous formulation.

The objective of this chapter, then, is to investigate the assessment of equivalence in variabilities of bioavailability between formulations. In Section 7.2, possible decision rules for assessing equivalence in intra-subject variabilities between formulations are discussed. Point and interval estimates for the inter-subject and intra-subject variabilities are provided in Section 7.3. The commonly used Pitman–Morgan's adjusted F test for equality of variabilities is outlined in Section 7.4. A distribution-free test procedure based on Spearman's rank correlation coefficient is also included in this section. In Section 7.5, two test procedures for interval hypotheses of equivalence in variability of bioavailability are presented. In Section 7.6, a conditional random effects model is considered to assess the intra-subject variability in terms of the common coefficient of variation (CV) when the intra-subject variabilities vary subject to subject. A brief discussion is presented in Section 7.7.

7.2 Variability and Decision Making

As indicated earlier, for assessment of bioequivalence, it is important to compare variability (the inter- and intra-subject variability) of bioavailability between formulations because individual subjects may differ widely in their responses to the drug. Levy (1986) pointed out that knowledge of inter- and intra-subject variabilities may provide valuable information in the assessment of bioequivalence. In Chapter 4, several methods were introduced for assessment of equivalence in average bioavailability. One of the primary assumptions of variability is that the intra-subject variabilities between formulations are assumed to be the same (i.e., $\sigma_T^2 = \sigma_R^2$). It is then of interest to examine whether these methods are still valid when there is a significant difference in intra-subject variabilities. As these methods are operationally equivalent, as indicated in Chapter 4, in what follows without loss of generality, we will examine only whether the two one-sided tests procedure is valid when there is a difference in intra-subject variabilities.

For a bioavailability and bioequivalence study with the standard 2×2 crossover design, as indicated in Section 4.2, the two one-sided tests procedure (parametric or nonparametric) is based on the period differences d_{ik}, as defined in Equation 3.3.1. If there is no unequal carryover effect, under model 4.1.2 and assumptions given in 3.1.4, the expected value and variance are given by

$$E(d_{ik}) = \begin{cases} \frac{1}{2}[(P_2 - P_1) + (F_T - F_R)] & \text{for } k = 1, \\ \frac{1}{2}[(P_2 - P_1) + (F_R - F_T)] & \text{for } k = 2, \end{cases}$$

and

$$\text{Var}(d_{ik}) = \sigma_d^2 = \tfrac{1}{4}\left(\sigma_R^2 + \sigma_T^2\right).$$

Therefore $\{d_{i1}, i = 1, 2, \ldots, n_1\}$ and $\{d_{i2}, i = 1, 2, \ldots, n_2\}$ are two independent samples with equal variance σ_d^2. Note that σ_d^2 is half of the average of the intra-subejct variability of the test and reference formulations. As a result, the two one-sided tests procedure for assessing equivalence in average bioavailability is still valid, even when the intra-subject variabilities between formulations are different $\left(\text{i.e., } \sigma_T^2 \neq \sigma_R^2\right)$. In other words, for assessment of equivalence in average bioavailability, the methods introduced in Chapter 4, which depend on the period differences, completely ignore difference of intra-subject variabilities between formulations. The difference in intra-subject variabilities, however, may have an important influence on the safety and exchangeability of the test formulation. Therefore, in addition to equivalence in average bioavailability, it is imperative to demonstrate equivalence in variability of bioavailability.

Similar to the ± 20 rule, we may conclude the two formulations are equivalent in variability of bioavailability if σ_T^2 is within $\pm\Delta\%$ of σ_R^2 where Δ is a clinically important difference. On the basis of this decision rule, we may test the following interval hypotheses to establish equivalence in variability of bioavailability:

$$\begin{aligned} &\text{H}_0\text{: } \sigma_T^2 - \sigma_R^2 \leq -\Delta\sigma_R^2 \quad \text{or} \quad \sigma_T^2 - \sigma_R^2 \geq \Delta\sigma_R^2, \\ \text{versus} \quad &\text{H}_a\text{: } -\Delta\sigma_R^2 < \sigma_T^2 - \sigma_R^2 < \Delta\sigma_R^2. \end{aligned} \tag{7.2.1}$$

The selection of Δ depends on the characteristics of the drug routes of administration. A discussion for selection of Δ based on the collected data is given in Section 7.7. Similar to testing for average bioequivalence, we may consider interval hypotheses for the difference in variances or the ratio of variances as follows:

$$\begin{aligned} &\text{H}_0\text{: } \sigma_T^2 - \sigma_R^2 \leq -\theta_1 \quad \text{or} \quad \sigma_T^2 - \sigma_R^2 \geq \theta_2, \\ \text{versus} \quad &\text{H}_a\text{: } \theta_1 < \sigma_T^2 - \sigma_R^2 < \theta_2. \end{aligned} \tag{7.2.2}$$

and

$$\begin{aligned} &\text{H}_0\text{: } \sigma_T^2/\sigma_R^2 \leq \delta_1 \quad \text{or} \quad \sigma_T^2/\sigma_R^2 \geq \delta_2, \\ \text{versus} \quad &\text{H}_a\text{: } \delta_1 < \sigma_T^2/\sigma_R^2 < \delta_2. \end{aligned} \tag{7.2.3}$$

where θ_1 and θ_2 are equivalent limits for the difference in variances and δ_1 and δ_2 are equivalent limits for the ratio of variances. The choices of θ_1, θ_2 and δ_1, δ_2 are rather subjective. Note that hypotheses 7.2.2 reduce to hypotheses 7.2.1 if $\theta_2 = -\theta_1 = \Delta\sigma_R^2$, which depend on the unknown parameter σ_R^2.

7.3 Point and Interval Estimates

7.3.1 Point Estimates

The assumptions of model 3.1.1 in Chapter 3 for the standard 2×2 crossover design, as stated in 3.1.4, are

1. $\{S_{jk}\}$ are i.i.d. normal with mean 0 and variance σ_S^2;
2. $\{e_{ijk}\}$ are i.i.d. normal with mean 0 and variance σ_e^2;
3. $\{S_{jk}\}$ and $\{e_{ijk}\}$ are mutually independent.

Under model 3.1.1, σ_S^2 and σ_e^2 are indicative of the inter- and intra-subject variability, respectively. The information of σ_S^2 and σ_e^2 is useful in bioavailability studies. For example, prior information of σ_S^2 and σ_e^2 can be used for sample size determination in the planning stage of a bioavailability study. On the other hand, estimates of σ_S^2 and σ_e^2, which can be obtained from the data, are usually used to interpret the inter- and intra-subject variabilities. Note that the sum of inter- and intra-subject variabilities $(\text{i.e., } \sigma_S^2 + \sigma_e^2)$ is the variance of the marginal distribution of Y_{ijk}. As discussed in previous chapters, under a crossover design, the comparison of average bioavailabilities between formulations can be made using period differences based only on the intra-subject variability. Therefore, the gain in precision for using the intra-subject variability alone can be expressed by

$$\rho_I = \frac{\sigma_S^2}{\sigma_S^2 + \sigma_e^2},$$

which is known as the intraclass correlation between responses of the two formulations. Although σ_S^2, σ_e^2, and ρ_I are indicative of the inter-subject variability, the intra-subject variability, and the intraclass correlation, respectively, in practice, they are unknown population parameters and must be estimated from the data. Therefore, in this section, we investigate point and interval estimates for σ_S^2, σ_e^2, and ρ_I.

Under model 3.1.1, the structure of the crossover design with random components $\{S_{ik}\}$ and $\{e_{ijk}\}$ is, in fact, a balanced two-stage nested design. Therefore, standard estimation procedures for a balanced two-stage nested design can be used to obtain point and interval estimates for σ_S^2, σ_e^2, and ρ_I. Recall that from the analysis of variance table (Table 3.5.1), under the assumptions of 3.1.4, distributions of sum of squares of inter- and intra-subject residuals are

$$\begin{aligned} SS_{\text{inter}} &\sim (\sigma_e^2 + 2\sigma_S^2)\chi^2(n_1 + n_2 - 2) \quad \text{and} \\ SS_{\text{intra}} &\sim \sigma_e^2\chi^2(n_1 + n_2 - 2), \end{aligned} \tag{7.3.1}$$

where SS_{inter} and SS_{intra} were defined in Section. 3.5. The expected values of the mean squares for the inter- and intra-subject variabilities are then given by

$$E(\text{MS}_{\text{inter}}) = E\left(\frac{\text{SS}_{\text{inter}}}{n_1+n_2-2}\right) = \sigma_e^2 + 2\sigma_S^2,$$
$$E(\text{MS}_{\text{intra}}) = E\left(\frac{\text{SS}_{\text{intra}}}{n_1+n_2-2}\right) = \sigma_e^2. \qquad (7.3.2)$$

Therefore, the analysis of variance estimates of σ_e^2 and σ_S^2 can be obtained by equating the observed mean squares and their expected values as follows:

$$\widehat{\sigma}_e^2 = \text{MS}_{\text{intra}} \quad \text{and} \quad \widehat{\sigma}_S^2 = \frac{\text{MS}_{\text{inter}} - \text{MS}_{\text{intra}}}{2}. \qquad (7.3.3)$$

Note that, under model 3.1.1 with assumptions of Equation 3.1.4, the estimators $\widehat{\sigma}_e^2$ and $\widehat{\sigma}_S^2$ are minimum variance unbiased quadratic estimators for σ_e^2 and σ_S^2, respectively (Searle, 1971). Furthermore, it can be verified that the distribution of $\widehat{\sigma}_e^2$ is

$$\frac{\sigma_e^2}{n_1+n_2-2}\chi^2(n_1+n_2-2),$$

and $\widehat{\sigma}_S^2$ is distributed as

$$\widehat{\sigma}_S^2 \sim \frac{\sigma_e^2+2\sigma_S^2}{2(n_1+n_2-2)}\chi^2(n_1+n_2-2) - \frac{\sigma_e^2}{2(n_1+n_2-2)}\chi^2(n_1+n_2-2). \qquad (7.3.4)$$

From Equation 7.3.4, it can be seen that there is no closed form for the distribution of $\widehat{\sigma}_S^2$ because the equation's coefficients involve unknown parameters σ_e^2 and σ_S^2, and the coefficient of its second term is negative (Searle, 1971). However, because SS_{inter} and SS_{intra} are independent, the variance of $\widehat{\sigma}_S^2$ and $\widehat{\sigma}_e^2$ can easily be obtained as follows:

$$\text{Var}(\widehat{\sigma}_e^2) = \frac{2\sigma_e^4}{n_1+n_2-2} \quad \text{and}$$
$$\text{Var}(\widehat{\sigma}_S^2) = \frac{1}{2(n_1+n_2-2)}\left[\left(\sigma_e^2+2\sigma_S^2\right)^2 + \sigma_e^4\right]. \qquad (7.3.5)$$

As $\widehat{\sigma}_S^2$ is based on the difference in mean squares between inter- and intra-subject residuals, it is possible to obtain a negative estimate if $\text{MS}_{\text{inter}} < \text{MS}_{\text{intra}}$. Searle (1971) provided a formula for calculation of the probability for obtaining a negative estimate of σ_S^2, which is given by

$$P\{\widehat{\sigma}_S^2 < 0\} = P\left\{F(n_1+n_2-2,\, n_1+n_2-2) < \frac{\sigma_e^2}{\sigma_e^2+2\sigma_S^2}\right\}, \qquad (7.3.6)$$

where $F(n_1+n_2-2,\, n_1+n_2-2)$ is a central F distribution with (n_1+n_2-2) and (n_1+n_2-2) degrees of freedom. Since σ_e^2 and σ_S^2 in Equation 7.3.6 are unknown, an estimate for $\sigma_e^2/(\sigma_e^2+2\sigma_S^2)$ is necessary to evaluate the probability. $\sigma_e^2/(\sigma_e^2+2\sigma_S^2)$ can be estimated by $1/F_v$, where

$$F_v = \frac{\text{MS}_{\text{inter}}}{\text{MS}_{\text{intra}}}.$$

Note that the probability given in 7.3.6 could be substantial when σ_S^2/σ_e^2 is small. A negative estimate may indicate that model 3.1.1 is incorrect or sample size is too small. More details on negative estimates in analysis of variance components can be found in Hocking (1985).

To avoid negative estimates, a typical approach is to consider the following estimator:

$$\begin{aligned}\widehat{\sigma}_S^2 &= \max\{0, \widehat{\sigma}_S^2\}\\ &= \begin{cases}\widehat{\sigma}_S^2 & \text{if MS}_{\text{inter}} \geq \text{MS}_{\text{intra}},\\ 0 & \text{if MS}_{\text{inter}} < \text{MS}_{\text{intra}},\end{cases}\end{aligned} \tag{7.3.7}$$

and

$$\widehat{\sigma}_e^2 = \begin{cases}\widehat{\sigma}_e^2 & \text{if MS}_{\text{inter}} \geq \text{MS}_{\text{intra}},\\ \widehat{\sigma}^2 & \text{if MS}_{\text{inter}} < \text{MS}_{\text{intra}},\end{cases}$$

where

$$\widehat{\sigma}^2 = \frac{\text{SS}_{\text{inter}} + \text{SS}_{\text{intra}}}{2(n_1+n_2)}.$$

The above estimators are known as the restricted maximum likelihood (REML) estimators. (Hocking, 1985; Searle et al., 1992).

For estimation of the intraclass correlation ρ_I, Snedecor and Cochran (1980) suggested the following estimator:

$$\widehat{\rho}_I = \frac{\text{MS}_{\text{inter}} - \text{MS}_{\text{intra}}}{\text{MS}_{\text{inter}} + \text{MS}_{\text{intra}}}. \tag{7.3.8}$$

It can be seen that ρ_I, again, could be negative because its numerator is the difference of mean squares between inter- and intra-subject variabilities. A negative estimate of ρ_I indicates that two responses on the same subjects are negatively correlated.

7.3.2 Confidence Intervals

To obtain interval estimates for σ_e^2, σ_S^2, and ρ_I, it is helpful to define the following quantiles for a chi-square and an F distribution. Let

$$\chi_L^2 = \chi^2(\alpha/2,\, n_1+n_2-2);$$
$$\chi_U^2 = \chi^2(1-\alpha/2,\, n_1+n_2-2);$$
$$F_L = F(\alpha/2,\, n_1+n_2-2,\, n_1+n_2-2);$$
$$F_U = F(1-\alpha/2,\, n_1+n_2-2,\, n_1+n_2-2).$$

$(1-\alpha)\times 100\%$ confidence intervals for σ_e^2 and ρ_I are then given by (L_e, U_e) and (L_ρ, U_ρ), respectively, where

$$L_e = \frac{SS_{intra}}{\chi_U^2} \quad \text{and} \quad U_e = \frac{SS_{intra}}{\chi_L^2}, \tag{7.3.9}$$

and

$$L_\rho = \frac{F_v/F_U - 1}{F_v/F_U + 1} \quad \text{and} \quad U_\rho = \frac{F_v/F_L - 1}{F_v/F_L + 1}. \tag{7.3.10}$$

The $(1-\alpha)\times 100\%$ confidence interval for ρ_I in Equation 7.3.10 was derived by Graybill (1961). Confidence intervals Equations 7.3.9 and 7.3.10, however, are not the shortest confidence intervals because we assign equal probability of $\alpha/2$ to the upper and lower tails of χ^2 or F distributions. These confidence intervals can provide at least $(1-\alpha)\times 100\%$ coverage probability for the respective parameters.

For interval estimates of σ_S^2, there exists no exact $(1-\alpha)\times 100\%$ confidence interval (Graybill, 1976). Turkey (1951) and Williams (1962), however, derived a confidence interval that has a confidence level between $(1-2\alpha)\times 100\%$ and $(1-\alpha)\times 100\%$. We will refer to this confidence interval as William–Turkey's confidence interval. William–Turkey's confidence interval, denoted by (L_S, U_S), is given as

$$L_S = \frac{(SS_{inter})(1 - F_U/F_v)}{2\chi_U^2} \quad \text{and} \quad U_S = \frac{(SS_{inter})(1 - F_L/F_v)}{2\chi_L^2}. \tag{7.3.11}$$

In a simulation study comparing Equation 7.3.11 with eight other approximate confidence intervals, Boardman (1974) recommended that William–Turkey's confidence interval be used for obtaining a $(1-\alpha)\times 100\%$ confidence interval for σ_S^2 because it yields approximately $(1-\alpha)\times 100\%$ coverage probability. Wang (1990), further, showed that the lower bound of the confidence interval of the William–Turkey intervals is indeed $1-\alpha$.

Example 7.3.1

To illustrate the use of these point and interval estimates for σ_e^2, σ_S^2 and ρ_I, we, once again, use AUC data given in Table 3.6.1. From the analysis of variance table (Table 3.6.3), we have

$$SS_{inter} = 16211.49 \quad \text{and} \quad SS_{intra} = 3679.43.$$

As $n_1 + n_2 - 2 = 22$, $\hat{\sigma}_e^2$, $\hat{\sigma}_S^2$, and $\hat{\rho}_I$ are given by

$$\hat{\sigma}_e^2 = \text{MS}_{\text{intra}} = \frac{\text{SS}_{\text{intra}}}{n_1 + n_2 - 2} = \frac{3679.43}{22} = 167.25,$$

$$\hat{\sigma}_S^2 = \frac{\text{MS}_{\text{inter}} - \text{MS}_{\text{intra}}}{2} = \frac{736.886 - 167.25}{2} = 284.82\,,$$

$$\hat{\rho}_I = \frac{\text{MS}_{\text{inter}} - \text{MS}_{\text{intra}}}{\text{MS}_{\text{inter}} + \text{MS}_{\text{intra}}} = \frac{736.886 - 167.25}{736.886 + 167.25} = 0.63.$$

For interval estimation, as

$$\chi^2(0.025, 22) = 10.982, \quad \chi^2(0.975, 22) = 36.781,$$
$$F(0.025, 22, 22) = 0.424, \quad F(0.975, 22, 22) = 2.358, \quad \text{and}$$
$$F_v = \text{MS}_{\text{inter}}/\text{MS}_{\text{intra}} = 4.406,$$

the 95% confidence intervals for σ_e^2 and ρ_I are

$$L_e = \frac{3679.43}{36.781} = 100.037, \quad U_e = \frac{3679.43}{10.982} = 335.032, \quad \text{and}$$
$$L_\rho = \frac{(4.406/2.358) - 1}{(4.406/2.358) + 1} = 0.303, \quad U_\rho = \frac{(4.406/0.424) - 1}{(4.406/0.424) + 1} = 0.824,$$

respectively. In addition, the 95% confidence interval for σ_S^2 based on William–Turkey's confidence interval is given by

$$L_S = \frac{(16211.49)[1 - (2.358/4.406)]}{2(36.781)} = 102.443,$$

$$U_S = \frac{(16211.49)[1 - (0.424/4.406)]}{2(10.982)} = 667.027.$$

The probability of obtaining a negative estimate of σ_S^2 is also evaluated using Equation 7.3.6. Since $F_v = 4.406$, which is an estimate of $\left\{\sigma_e^2/\left(\sigma_e^2 + 2\sigma_S^2\right)\right\}^{-1}$, the probability can be obtained as follows:

$$P\{\hat{\sigma}_S^2 < 0\} = P\{F(22, 22) < 1/4.406\} = 0.00048.$$

Therefore, the chance of obtaining a negative estimate for σ_S^2 based on the AUC data in Table 3.6.1 is negligible. The above results are summarized in Table 7.3.1.

Example 7.3.2

For another example, point and interval estimates for σ_e^2, σ_S^2, and ρ_I for Clayton–Leslie's example given in Table 6.9.1 were also obtained based on log-transformed data. The results are also summarized in Table 7.3.1.

TABLE 7.3.1: Summary of point and interval estimation of inter- and intra-subject variability for data sets in Examples 3.6.1 and 6.9.1.

Data Set	Parameter	Point Estimate	95% Confidence Interval
Example 3.6.1	σ_e^2	167.25	(100.04, 335.03)
	σ_S^2	284.82	(102.44, 667.03)
	ρ_I	0.63	(0.30, 0.82)
	$P\{\hat{\sigma}_S^2 < 0\}$	0.00048	—
Example 6.9.1	σ_e^2	0.31	(0.17, 0.72)
	σ_S^2	0.11	(−0.09, 0.47)
	ρ_I	0.26	(−0.24, 0.65)
	$P\{\hat{\sigma}_S^2 < 0\}$	0.15	—

Note: Based on log-transformed AUC data.

In Clayton–Leslie's example, although we obtained positive estimates for σ_e^2, σ_S^2, and ρ_I, the probability for obtaining a negative estimate for σ_S^2 is about 15% which is non-negligible. This may be partly due to the two completely opposite responses observed on subject 7 for test and reference formulations. A high probability of obtaining a negative estimate may lead to a confidence interval with a negative lower confidence limit. It is clear that the negative portion of the interval is meaningless, for σ_S^2 is always positive. Although one may ignore the negative portion and simply use the positive portion as the confidence interval for σ_S^2, whether the truncated confidence interval is still of the same confidence level is questionable. More discussion on this issue is given in Section 7.7.

7.4 Tests for Equality of Variabilities

In Chapter 4, we introduced several methods for assessment of equivalence in average bioavailabilities between formulations. These methods were derived under model 4.1.1 [or equivalently model 4.1.2] for the standard 2×2 crossover design with assumptions described in 3.1.4. Under these assumptions, one assumes that the intra-subject variabilities for the test and reference formulations are the same $\left(\text{i.e., } \sigma_T^2 = \sigma_R^2 = \sigma_e^2\right)$. As indicated in previous sections, if the intra-subject variabilities between formulations are different, then equivalence in average bioavailabilities between formulations does not imply that the two formulations are therapeutically equivalent and are, thus, interchangeable. In this situation, the effectiveness and safety of the test formulation may be of great concern. Therefore, it is important to examine whether the intra-subject variability of the test formulation is the same as that of the reference formulation.

In the following section, we introduce both parametric and nonparametric test procedures for testing equality of intra-subject variabilities between formulations under the assumption of no period effects. In the presence of period effects, these test procedures can still be applied with some modifications.

7.4.1 Pitman–Morgan's Adjusted *F* Test

In bioavailability studies, the most commonly used test procedure for equality of variabilities is probably the so-called Pitman–Morgan's adjusted *F* test, which is derived in the following:

Under model 4.1.2, let $\mathbf{X}_{ik}$ be a bivariate random vector of the two responses observed on subject i of sequence k, that is,

$$\mathbf{X}_{ik} = \begin{bmatrix} Y_{i\mathrm{R}k} \\ Y_{i\mathrm{T}k} \end{bmatrix}, \quad i = 1, 2 \ldots, n_k; \quad k = 1, 2. \tag{7.4.1}$$

If the intra-subject variabilities for the test and reference formulations are different $\left(\text{i.e., } \sigma_{\mathrm{T}}^2 \neq \sigma_{\mathrm{R}}^2\right)$, then, according to Equation 2.5.5, the covariance matrix of $\mathbf{X}_{ik}$ is

$$\mathbf{\Sigma} = \begin{bmatrix} \sigma_{\mathrm{R}}^2 + \sigma_{\mathrm{S}}^2 & \sigma_{\mathrm{S}}^2 \\ \sigma_{\mathrm{S}}^2 & \sigma_{\mathrm{T}}^2 + \sigma_{\mathrm{S}}^2 \end{bmatrix}. \tag{7.4.2}$$

Note that

$$\begin{aligned} \mathrm{Var}(Y_{i\mathrm{T}k}) - \mathrm{Var}(Y_{i\mathrm{R}k}) &= \left(\sigma_{\mathrm{T}}^2 + \sigma_{\mathrm{S}}^2\right) - \left(\sigma_{\mathrm{R}}^2 + \sigma_{\mathrm{S}}^2\right) \\ &= \sigma_{\mathrm{T}}^2 - \sigma_{\mathrm{R}}^2. \end{aligned} \tag{7.4.3}$$

Therefore, under Equation 7.4.2, the difference in variances between the marginal distributions of the two formulations is, in fact, the difference in intra-subject variabilities between the two formulations. Haynes (1981) first introduced Pitman–Morgan's test for equality of the variances of the marginal distributions of two correlated variables in bioavailability and bioequivalence studies. Under Equations 7.4.2 and 7.4.3, the hypotheses for testing equality of variance of marginal distributions between the test and reference formulations become

$$\begin{aligned} &\mathrm{H_0}\colon \sigma_{\mathrm{T}}^2 = \sigma_{\mathrm{R}}^2 \\ \text{versus} \quad &\mathrm{H_a}\colon \sigma_{\mathrm{T}}^2 \neq \sigma_{\mathrm{R}}^2. \end{aligned} \tag{7.4.4}$$

By applying the idea proposed by Pitman (1939) and Morgan (1939), a test statistic can be obtained based on the correlation between the crossover differences defined in Equation 3.4.1 and subject totals defined in Equation 3.2.1.

Under the assumption of no carryover effects, we first consider the situation where there are no period effects. It can be seen that $\mathbf{X}_{ik}$ are i.i.d. bivariate random vectors with mean

$$\mu = \begin{bmatrix} \mu + F_{\mathrm{R}} \\ \mu + F_{\mathrm{T}} \end{bmatrix},$$

and covariance matrix as defined in Equation 7.4.2.

Let V_{ik} be twice of the crossover differences O_{ik} defined in Equation 3.4.1, that is,

$$V_{ik} = 2(O_{ik}) = Y_{iTk} - Y_{iRk},\ i = 1, 2, \ldots, n_k, \text{ and } k = 1, 2\,.$$

Also, let U_{ik} be subject totals as defined in Equation 3.2.1, that is,

$$U_{ik} = Y_{iTk} + Y_{iRk}.$$

The bivariate random vectors $\mathbf{B}_{ik} = (V_{ik}, U_{ik})$ are the i.i.d. with mean vector

$$\boldsymbol{\mu}_B = \begin{bmatrix} F_T - F_R \\ 2\mu \end{bmatrix}, \tag{7.4.5}$$

and covariance matrix

$$\Sigma_B = \begin{bmatrix} \sigma_T^2 + \sigma_R^2 & \sigma_T^2 - \sigma_R^2 \\ \sigma_T^2 - \sigma_R^2 & 4\sigma_S^2 + \sigma_T^2 + \sigma_R^2 \end{bmatrix}. \tag{7.4.6}$$

From Equation 7.4.6, it can be seen that the covariance between V_{ik} and U_{ik} is just the difference in intra-subject variabilities between the test and reference formulations. Therefore, the hypotheses, in Equation 7.4.4, are equivalent to the hypotheses for testing the presence of correlation between the crossover differences V_{ik} and subject totals U_{ik}, that is,

$$\begin{aligned} &\text{H}_0\colon\ \rho_{VU} = 0 \\ \text{versus}\quad &\text{H}_a\colon\ \rho_{VU} \neq 0. \end{aligned} \tag{7.4.7}$$

Hence, the following standard F test for correlation between two random variables can be applied to test hypotheses Equation 7.4.4.

Under model 4.1.2 with assumptions of Equation 3.1.4, the Pearson correlation coefficient between V_{ik} and U_{ik} is given by

$$r_{VU} = \frac{S_{VU}}{\sqrt{S_{VV}^2 S_{UU}^2}}, \tag{7.4.8}$$

where

$$S_{VV}^2 = \frac{1}{n_1 + n_2 - 1} \sum_{k=1}^{2} \sum_{i=k}^{n_k} (V_{ik} - \overline{V})^2,$$

$$S_{UU}^2 = \frac{1}{n_1 + n_2 - 1} \sum_{k=1}^{2} \sum_{i=1}^{n_k} (U_{ik} - \overline{U})^2,$$

$$S_{VU}^2 = \frac{1}{n_1 + n_2 - 1} \sum_{k=1}^{2} \sum_{i=1}^{n_k} (V_{ik} - \overline{V})(U_{ik} - \overline{U}),$$

$$\overline{V} = \frac{1}{n_1 + n_2} \sum_{k=1}^{2} \sum_{i=1}^{n_k} V_{ik},$$

$$\overline{U} = \frac{1}{n_1 + n_2} \sum_{k=1}^{2} \sum_{i=k}^{n_k} U_{ik}.$$

We then reject H_0 at the α level, if

$$F_{\mathrm{VU}} = \frac{(n-2)r_{\mathrm{VU}}^2}{1 - r_{\mathrm{VU}}^2} > F(\alpha, 1, n_1 + n_2 - 2), \tag{7.4.9}$$

where $F(\alpha, 1, n_1 + n_2 - 2)$ is the upper αth quantile $(0 < \alpha < 1)$ of an F distribution with degrees of freedom 1 and $(n_1 + n_2 - 2)$.

From Equation 7.4.9, it can be seen that test statistic F_{VU} is obtained based on the transformed data V_{ik} and U_{ik}. To relate Equation 7.4.9 to Y_{ijk}, let S_{tt}^2, S_{rr}^2, and S_{tr} be the sample variances and covariances of $Y_{i\mathrm{T}k}$ and $Y_{i\mathrm{R}k}$, that is,

$$S_{\mathrm{tt}}^2 = \frac{1}{n_1 + n_2 - 1} \sum_{k=1}^{2} \sum_{i=1}^{n_k} (Y_{i\mathrm{T}k} - \overline{Y}_{\mathrm{T}})^2,$$

$$S_{\mathrm{rr}}^2 = \frac{1}{n_1 + n_2 - 1} \sum_{k=1}^{2} \sum_{i=1}^{n_k} (Y_{i\mathrm{R}k} - \overline{Y}_{\mathrm{R}})^2,$$

$$S_{\mathrm{tr}} = \frac{1}{n_1 + n_2 - 1} \sum_{k=1}^{2} \sum_{i=1}^{n_k} (Y_{i\mathrm{T}k} - \overline{Y}_{\mathrm{T}})(Y_{i\mathrm{R}k} - \overline{Y}_{\mathrm{R}}),$$

$$\overline{Y}_{\mathrm{T}} = \frac{1}{n_1 + n_2} \sum_{k=1}^{2} \sum_{i=1}^{n_k} Y_{i\mathrm{T}k},$$

$$\overline{Y}_{\mathrm{R}} = \frac{1}{n_1 + n_2} \sum_{k=1}^{2} \sum_{i=1}^{n_k} Y_{i\mathrm{R}k}.$$

It can then be easily verified that

$$\begin{aligned} S_{\mathrm{VV}}^2 &= S_{\mathrm{tt}}^2 + S_{\mathrm{rr}}^2 - 2S_{\mathrm{tr}}, \\ S_{\mathrm{UU}}^2 &= S_{\mathrm{tt}}^2 + S_{\mathrm{rr}}^2 - 2S_{\mathrm{tr}}, \\ S_{\mathrm{VU}} &= S_{\mathrm{tt}}^2 + S_{\mathrm{rr}}^2. \end{aligned} \tag{7.4.10}$$

Therefore,

$$r_{\mathrm{VU}}^2 = \frac{(S_{\mathrm{tt}} - S_{\mathrm{rr}})^2}{\left(S_{\mathrm{tt}}^2 + S_{\mathrm{rr}}^2\right)^2 - 4S_{\mathrm{tr}}^2},$$

and

$$1 - r_{\mathrm{VU}}^2 = \frac{4\left(S_{\mathrm{tt}}^2 S_{\mathrm{rr}}^2 - S_{\mathrm{tr}}^2\right)}{\left(S_{\mathrm{tt}}^2 + S_{\mathrm{rr}}^2\right)^2 - 4S_{\mathrm{tr}}^2}.$$

It follows that

$$
\begin{aligned}
F_{\mathrm{VU}} &= \frac{(n_1+n_2-2)r_{\mathrm{VU}}^2}{1-r_{\mathrm{VU}}^2} \\
&= \frac{(n_1+n_2-2)\left(S_{\mathrm{tt}}^2-S_{\mathrm{rr}}^2\right)^2}{4\left(S_{\mathrm{tt}}^2S_{\mathrm{rr}}^2-S_{\mathrm{tr}}^2\right)} \\
&= \frac{(n_1+n_2-2)\left[\dfrac{S_{\mathrm{tt}}^2}{S_{\mathrm{rr}}^2}-1\right]^2}{4\left[\dfrac{S_{\mathrm{tt}}^2}{S_{\mathrm{rr}}^2}\right]\left[1-\dfrac{S_{\mathrm{tr}}^2}{S_{\mathrm{tt}}^2S_{\mathrm{rr}}^2}\right]}.
\end{aligned}
$$

If we let $F_{\mathrm{tr}} = S_{\mathrm{tt}}^2/S_{\mathrm{rr}}^2$ and $r_{\mathrm{tr}} = S_{\mathrm{tr}}/(S_{\mathrm{tt}}S_{\mathrm{rr}})$, then F_{VU} becomes the familiar Pitman–Morgan's adjusted F test, as introduced by Haynes (1981):

$$
F_{\mathrm{PM}} = \frac{(n_1+n_2-2)[F_{\mathrm{tr}}-1]^2}{4F_{\mathrm{tr}}\left(1-r_{\mathrm{tr}}^2\right)}. \tag{7.4.11}
$$

Note that Pitman–Morgan's adjusted F test is the uniformly most powerful test for hypotheses Equation 7.4.4. We then reject H_0 in Equation 7.4.4 if

$$
F_{\mathrm{PM}} > F(\alpha, 1, n_1+n_2-2).
$$

Example 7.4.1

For AUC data given in Table 3.6.1, assuming that there are no period effects, we have

$$
\begin{aligned}
S_{\mathrm{VV}}^2 &= 323.08, \quad S_{\mathrm{UU}}^2 = 1433.69, \quad S_{\mathrm{VU}} = 13.32, \\
S_{\mathrm{tt}}^2 &= 445.85, \quad S_{\mathrm{rr}}^2 = 432.53, \quad S_{\mathrm{tr}} = 277.65.
\end{aligned}
$$

The Pearson correlation coefficient between crossover differences and subject totals is then given by

$$
r_{\mathrm{VU}} = \frac{13.32}{\sqrt{(323.03)(1433.69)}} = 0.0196.
$$

This gives

$$
F_{\mathrm{VU}} = \frac{(22)(0.0196)^2}{1-(0.0196)^2} = 0.00843.
$$

with a p-value of 0.93. Therefore, we fail to reject H_0: $\alpha_{\mathrm{T}}^2 = \sigma_{\mathrm{R}}^2$ at the 5% level of significance. On the other hand, as

$$F_{tr} = \frac{445.85}{432.53} = 1.0308 \quad \text{and}$$

$$r_{tr} = \frac{277.65}{\sqrt{(445.85)(432.53)}} = 0.6323.$$

Pitman–Morgan's test statistic Equation 7.4.11 is then given by

$$F_{PM} = \frac{(22)(1.0308 - 1)^2}{(4)(1.0308)[1 - (0.6323)^2]} = 0.00843,$$

which agrees with the value obtained based on F_{VU}.

Similarly, the above tests can also be applied to Clayton and Leslie's example (Table 6.9.1). It can be verified that, based on the log-transformed data, $r_{VU} = 0.3035$ and $F_{PM} = 1.6231$, which yields a p-value of 0.22. Therefore, we fail to reject the null hypothesis of equality in intra-subject variabilities between the two erythromycin formulations.

7.4.2 Distribution-Free Test Based on Spearman's Rank Correlation Coefficient

In the previous section, if normality assumptions on $\{S_{ik}\}$ and $\{e_{ijk}\}$ are seriously violated, neither test statistic Equation 7.4.9 nor Equation 7.4.11 follows an F distribution. In other words, Pitman–Morgan's adjusted F test for the hypothesis of equality in intra-subject variabilities between formulations is not valid. In this situation, alternatively, the following distribution-free test based upon Spearman's rank correlation coefficient is useful.

Let $R(V_{jk})$ and $R(U_{ik})$ be the rank of V_{ik} and U_{ik} in the combined sequence of $\{V_{ik}\}$ and $\{U_{ik}\}, k = 1, 2;\ i = 1, 2, \ldots, n_k$, respectively. Spearman's rank correlation coefficient r_S can be obtained by replacing V_{ik} and U_{ik} in Equation 7.4.8 with their corresponding ranks $R(V_{ik})$ and $R(U_{ik}), k = 1, 2;\ i = 1, 2, \ldots, n_k$. If there are no ties, then r_S is given by

$$r_S = \frac{12 \sum_{k=1}^{2} \sum_{i=1}^{n_k} \left[R(V_{ik}) - \frac{n_1 + n_2 - 1}{2}\right]\left[R(U_{ik}) - \frac{n_1 + n_2 + 1}{2}\right]}{(n_1 + n_2)[(n_1 + n_2)^2 - 1]}. \tag{7.4.12}$$

If there are ties, then r_S should be calculated as follows:

$$r_S = \frac{\sum_{k=1}^{2} \sum_{i=1}^{n_k} R(V_{ik})R(U_{ik}) - K_S}{\left\{\left[\sum_{k=1}^{2} \sum_{i=1}^{n_k} R^2(V_{ik}) - K_S\right]\left[\sum_{k=1}^{2} \sum_{i=1}^{n_k} R^2(U_{ik}) - K_S\right]\right\}^{1/2}}, \tag{7.4.13}$$

where $K_S = (n_1 + n_2)[(n_1 + n_2)/2]^2$.

We then reject H_0 in Equation 7.4.4 at the α level if

$$|r_S| > r_S(\alpha/2, n_1 + n_2),$$

where $r_S(\alpha/2, n_1 + n_2)$ is the αth quantile of the distribution of Spearman's rank correlation coefficient based on the $n_1 + n_2$ observations. When $n_1 + n_2 > 30$, the αth upper quantile of r_S can be approximated by

$$r_S(\alpha, n_1 + n_2) \approx \frac{Z_\alpha}{\sqrt{n_1 + n_2 - 1}}, \tag{7.4.14}$$

where Z_α is the αth upper quantile of a standard normal variable.

As can be seen, Pitman–Morgan's adjusted F test is derived based on Pearson's correlation coefficient, r_{VU}, under normality assumptions. In most bioavailability and bioequivalence studies, however, the normality assumption is not easy to verify. Therefore, the above distribution-free test based on Spearman's rank correlation coefficient is usually considered as an alternative to Pitman–Morgan's adjusted F test for testing the equality of intra-subject variabilities if the normality assumption is in doubt. When the normality assumption is violated, McCulloch (1987) showed that the asymptotic variance of Pearson's correlation coefficient r_{VU} depends on the common kurtosis between the crossover differences and subject totals. The actual size of the test Equation 7.4.8 is larger (smaller) than the nominal level if the common kurtosis is larger (smaller) than 0. From a simulation study, McCulloch (1987) pointed out that Spearman's test is the only test among five tests under study, including test Equation 7.4.8, that controls the actual size at the nominal level with a very competitive power for a variety of different distributions. Hence, Spearman's test (Equation 7.4.12 or Equation 7.4.13) is recommended for testing the equality between intra-subject variabilities.

Example 7.4.2

To illustrate the use of Spearman's test for equality of variabilities, similarly, we consider the two examples given in Sections 3.6 and 6.9.

For AUC data in Table 3.6.1, it can be verified that Spearman's rank correlation coefficient between crossover differences and subject totals based on the raw data is 0.1165 with a p-value of 0.59. Similar to the Pearson correlation coefficient and Pitman–Morgan's test, we fail to reject H_0 at the 5% level of significance. However, the p-value of r_S is much smaller than that of the Pearson correlation coefficient.

For Clayton and Leslie's example, based on log-transformed AUC, we have $r_S = 0.3684$, which yields a p-value of 0.13. Thus, we fail to reject H_0 at the 5% level of significance. This result agrees with that from the Pitman–Morgan test.

7.4.3 Tests in the Presence of Period Effects

In previous sections, in addition to the assumption of no carryover effects, we assume that there are no period effects to derive Pitman–Morgan's adjusted F test.

This result does not generally hold because Pitman–Morgan's adjusted F test depends on S_{tt}^2, S_{rr}^2, and S_{tr}, the expected values of which include the period effects (Ho and Patel, 1988). In this situation, Pitman–Morgan's adjusted F test can be modified as follows.

Assuming that there are no unequal carryover effects, under model 4.1.2 with normality assumptions, we have

$$\mathbf{X}_{ik} \sim \mathrm{N}(\boldsymbol{\mu}_k, \boldsymbol{\Sigma}), \quad i = 1, 2, \ldots, n_k; \quad k = 1, 2,$$

where $\boldsymbol{\Sigma}$ is the covariance matrix as defined in Equation 7.4.2 and

$$\boldsymbol{\mu}_1 = \begin{bmatrix} \mu + F_\mathrm{R} + P_1 \\ \mu + F_\mathrm{T} + P_2 \end{bmatrix} \quad \text{and} \quad \boldsymbol{\mu}_2 = \begin{bmatrix} \mu + F_\mathrm{R} + P_2 \\ \mu + F_\mathrm{T} + P_1 \end{bmatrix}.$$

The pooled sample covariance matrix $\widehat{\boldsymbol{\Sigma}}$ is an unbiased estimator of $\boldsymbol{\Sigma}$, which is given as

$$\begin{aligned} \widehat{\boldsymbol{\Sigma}} &= \frac{1}{n_1 + n_2 - 2}(\mathbf{S}_1 + \mathbf{S}_2) \\ &= \begin{bmatrix} S_\mathrm{RR}^2 & S_\mathrm{TR} \\ S_\mathrm{TR} & S_\mathrm{TT}^2 \end{bmatrix}, \end{aligned}$$

where $\mathbf{S}_1$ and $\mathbf{S}_2$ are defined in Section 4.2.4 and S_RR^2, S_TT^2, and S_TR are defined in Section 4.2.3, which were used to construct a $(1 - 2\alpha) \times 100\%$ confidence interval for $\mu_\mathrm{T}/\mu_\mathrm{R}$ based on Fieller's theorem. As there are $(n_1 + n_2 - 2)$ degrees of freedom for $\widehat{\boldsymbol{\Sigma}}$, the adjusted F statistic for the Pitman–Morgan's test becomes

$$\widetilde{F}_\mathrm{PM} = \frac{(n_1 + n_2 - 3)(F_\mathrm{TR} - 1)^2}{4F_\mathrm{TR}(1 - r_\mathrm{TR}^2)}, \tag{7.4.15}$$

where $F_\mathrm{TR} = S_\mathrm{TT}^2/S_\mathrm{RR}^2$ and $r_\mathrm{TR}^2 = S_\mathrm{TR}^2/\left(S_\mathrm{TT}^2 S_\mathrm{RR}^2\right)$.

We then reject H_0 at the α level if

$$\widetilde{F}_\mathrm{PM} > F(\alpha, 1, n_1 + n_2 - 3). \tag{7.4.16}$$

Note that the above test is equivalent to Pearson's correlation coefficient between the crossover differences and subject totals based on the residuals from the sequence-by-period means, that is,

$$\mathbf{R}_{ik} = \mathbf{X}_{ik} - \overline{\mathbf{X}}_k = \begin{bmatrix} X_{i\mathrm{R}k} - \overline{X}_{\cdot\mathrm{R}k} \\ X_{i\mathrm{T}k} - \overline{X}_{\cdot\mathrm{T}k} \end{bmatrix}, \quad i = 1, 2, \ldots, n_k; \quad k = 1, 2,$$

where

$$\overline{\mathbf{X}}_k = \frac{1}{n_k}\mathbf{X}_{ik} = \begin{bmatrix} \frac{1}{n_k}\sum_{i=1}^{n_k} X_{iRk} \\ \frac{1}{n_k}\sum_{i=1}^{n_k} X_{iTk} \end{bmatrix}, \quad k = 1, 2.$$

Similarly, Spearman's test can also be computed based on the ranks of the residuals from sequence-by-period means using either Equation 7.4.12 or 7.4.13. We will denote this test statistic by $\widetilde{r}_S$ and reject H_0 at the α level if

$$|\widetilde{r}_S| > r_S(\alpha/2, n_1 + n_2 - 2). \tag{7.4.17}$$

Example 7.4.3

To illustrate use of Pitman–Morgan's test and Spearman's test in the presence of period effects, again, we consider AUC data in Table 3.6.1 and log-transformed AUC data given in Table 6.9.1.

When they are period effects, the Pitman–Morgan test should be applied to the residuals from the sequence-by-period means. From Table 3.6.1, it can be found that

$$S^2_{TT} = 463.557, \quad S^2_{RR} = 440.576, \quad \text{and} \quad S_{TR} = 284.82.$$

This leads to

$$F_{TR} = \frac{463.557}{440.576} = 1.0522,$$

and

$$r_{TR} = \frac{284.82}{\sqrt{(463.557)(440.576)}} = 0.6302.$$

The Pitman–Morgan adjusted test statistic is then given by

$$\widetilde{F}_{PM} = \frac{(21)(1.0522 - 1)^2}{(4)(1.0522)[1 - (0.6302)^2]} = 0.0225,$$

which gives a p-value of 0.8821.

Hence, we also fail to reject the hypothesis of no difference in intra-subject variabilities between formulations.

One can also easily verify that Spearman's rank correlation coefficient based on the residuals from the sequence-by-period is given by 0.1017 with a p-value of 0.65.

TABLE 7.4.1: Test results for equality of variabilities.

Example	Method	Test[a] (p-Value)	Test[b] (p-Value)
3.6.1	Pearson	0.0196 (0.93)	0.0327 (0.88)
	Pitman–Morgan	0.0084 (0.93)	0.0225 (0.88)
	Spearman	0.1165 (0.59)	0.1017 (0.65)
6.9.1[c]	Pearson	0.3035 (0.22)	0.2540 (0.33)
	Pitman–Morgan	1.6231 (0.22)	1.0345 (0.33)
	Spearman	0.3684 (0.13)	0.3560 (0.15)

[a] Based on raw data.
[b] Based on residuals from sequence-by-period means.
[c] Based on log-transformed AUC data.

For log-transformed AUC in Clayton and Leslie's example, it can be verified that $\widetilde{F}_{\mathrm{PM}} = 1.0345$ (p-value $= 0.33$) and $\widetilde{r}_{\mathrm{S}} = 0.3560$ (p-value $= 0.15$). Both tests fail to reject the null hypothesis of no difference in intra-subject variabilities between the two erythromycin formulations.

Test results for the two examples (one from Section 3.6 and the other from Section 6.9) with and without period effects are summarized in Table 7.4.1.

7.5 Equivalence in Variability of Bioavailability

Under normality assumptions, Pitman–Morgan's adjusted F test is the uniformly most powerful test for the hypotheses of equality of variances between the marginal distributions of the test and reference formulations. However, it is not an appropriate test for equivalence in variability between formulations. Similar to the interval hypotheses given in 4.3.1, for the difference in means, and hypotheses given in 4.3.2, for the ratio of means, for assessment of average bioavailability, equivalence in variability of bioavailability can be assessed by testing interval hypotheses 7.2.2 or 7.2.3. Hypotheses 7.2.3 for the ratio of variances can be decomposed into two one-sided hypotheses as follows:

$$\begin{aligned} &\mathrm{H}_{01}\colon\ \sigma_{\mathrm{T}}^2/\sigma_{\mathrm{R}}^2 \leq \delta_1 \\ \text{versus}\quad &\mathrm{H}_{\mathrm{a}1}\colon\ \sigma_{\mathrm{T}}^2/\sigma_{\mathrm{R}}^2 > \delta_1, \end{aligned}$$

and

$$\begin{aligned} &\mathrm{H}_{02}\colon\ \sigma_{\mathrm{T}}^2/\sigma_{\mathrm{R}}^2 \geq \delta_2 \\ \text{versus}\quad &\mathrm{H}_{\mathrm{a}2}\colon\ \sigma_{\mathrm{T}}^2/\sigma_{\mathrm{R}}^2 > \delta_2. \end{aligned} \tag{7.5.1}$$

On the other hand, hypotheses 7.2.2 for the difference in variances can be decomposed into the following two one-sided hypotheses:

$$\begin{aligned} &H_{01}\colon \sigma_T^2 - \sigma_R^2 \le \theta_1 \\ \text{versus}\quad &H_{a1}\colon \sigma_T^2 - \sigma_R^2 > \theta_1, \end{aligned}$$

and

$$\begin{aligned} &H_{02}\colon \sigma_T^2 - \sigma_R^2 \ge \theta_2 \\ \text{versus}\quad &H_{a2}\colon \sigma_T^2 - \sigma_R^2 < \theta_2. \end{aligned} \tag{7.5.2}$$

For testing hypotheses 7.5.1, the idea in Section 7.4.1 can be extended to derive a test (Liu and Chow, 1992b). Define

$$\begin{aligned} V_{ik} &= Y_{iTk} - Y_{iRk}, \quad \text{and} \\ U_{ik} &= Y_{iTk} + \delta Y_{iRk}, \end{aligned}$$

where $\delta > 0$. It can be easily verified that, in the absence of period effects,

$$E(V_{ik}) = F_T - F_R, \quad E(U_{ik}) = (1+\delta)\mu + (\delta - 1)F_T,$$

and

$$\text{Var}(V_{ik}) = \sigma_T^2 + \sigma_R^2, \quad \text{Var}(U_{ik}) = \sigma_T^2 + \delta^2\sigma_R^2 + (1+\delta)^2\delta_S^2.$$

The covariance between V_{ik} and U_{ik} is then given by

$$\begin{aligned} \text{Cov}(V_{ik}, U_{ik}) &= \text{Cov}(Y_{iTk} - Y_{iRk}, Y_{iTk} + \delta Y_{iRk}) \\ &= \text{Var}(Y_{iTk}) + (\delta - 1)\,\text{Cov}(Y_{iTk}, Y_{iRk}) - \delta\,\text{Var}(Y_{iRk}) \\ &= \sigma_T^2 - \delta\sigma_R^2. \end{aligned}$$

Therefore, $\text{Cov}(V_{ik}, U_{ik})$ is the difference between σ_T^2 and $\delta\sigma_R^2$. Hypotheses Equation 7.5.1 are equivalent to the following two one-sided hypotheses:

$$\begin{aligned} &H_{01}\colon \sigma_T^2 - \delta_1\sigma_R^2 \le 0 \\ \text{versus}\quad &H_{a1}\colon \sigma_T^2 - \delta_1\sigma_R^2 > 0, \end{aligned} \tag{7.5.3}$$

and

$$\begin{aligned} &H_{02}\colon \sigma_T^2 - \delta_2\sigma_R^2 \ge 0 \\ \text{versus}\quad &H_{a2}\colon \sigma_T^2 - \delta_2\sigma_R^2 < 0, \end{aligned}$$

which are equivalent to the hypotheses for testing the presence of a positive correlation between V_{ik} and U_{Lik} and the presence of a negative correlation between V_{ik} and U_{Uik}, respectively, where

$$\begin{aligned} U_{Lik} &= Y_{iTk} + \delta_1 Y_{iRk} \quad \text{and} \\ U_{Uik} &= Y_{iTk} + \delta_2 Y_{iRk}. \end{aligned}$$

In other words, hypotheses 7.5.3 are equivalent to the following two one-sided hypotheses:

$$\begin{aligned} &\text{H}_{01}\colon\ \rho_{\text{L}} \leq 0 \\ \text{versus}\quad &\text{H}_{\text{a}1}\colon\ \rho_{\text{L}} > 0, \end{aligned} \tag{7.5.4}$$

and

$$\begin{aligned} &\text{H}_{02}\colon\ \rho_{\text{U}} \geq 0 \\ \text{versus}\quad &\text{H}_{\text{a}2}\colon\ \rho_{\text{U}} < 0, \end{aligned}$$

where ρ_{L} and ρ_{U} are correlation coefficients between $V_{ik}, U_{\text{L}ik}$, and $V_{ik}, U_{\text{U}ik}$, respectively.

Let r_{L} and r_{U} be the sample Pearson correlation coefficients between V_{ik} and $U_{\text{L}ik}$, and between V_{ik} and $U_{\text{U}ik}$, respectively. H_{01} is then rejected at the α level of significance if

$$t_{\text{L}} = \frac{r_{\text{L}}}{\left[\dfrac{1 - r_{\text{L}}^2}{n_1 + n_2 - 2}\right]^{1/2}} > t(\alpha, n_1 + n_2 - 2), \tag{7.5.5}$$

and H_{02} is rejected at the α level of significance if

$$t_{\text{U}} = \frac{r_{\text{U}}}{\left[\dfrac{1 - r_{\text{U}}^2}{n_1 + n_2 - 2}\right]^{1/2}} < -t(\alpha, n_1 + n_2 - 2). \tag{7.5.6}$$

We conclude that σ_{T}^2 and σ_{R}^2 are equivalent if both H_{01} and H_{02} are rejected.

Note that tests given in 7.5.5 and 7.5.6 can be directly applied to obtain a distribution-free test by simply replacing r_{L} and r_{U} with their corresponding Spearman's rank correlation coefficient when normality assumptions are in doubt.

In the presence of period effects, the above procedure can be carried out using residuals from sequence-by-period means as raw data with degrees of freedom $(n_1 + n_2 - 3)$. In other words, test statistics t_{L} and t_{U} can be expressed in terms of $S_{\text{TT}}^2, S_{\text{RR}}^2$, and S_{TR} as follows:

$$t_{\text{L}} = (F_{\text{L}})^{1/2} \quad \text{and} \quad t_{\text{U}} = (F_{\text{U}})^{1/2},$$

where

$$F_{\text{U}} = \frac{(n_1 + n_2 - 3)\left[S_{\text{TT}}^2 - \delta_1 S_{\text{RR}}^2 + (\delta_1 - 1)S_{\text{TR}}\right]^2}{(1 + \delta_1)^2 (S_{\text{TT}}^2 S_{\text{RR}}^2 - S_{\text{TR}}^2)},$$

and

$$F_{\mathrm{U}} = \frac{(n_1 + n_2 - 3)\left[S_{\mathrm{TT}}^2 - \delta_2 S_{\mathrm{RR}}^2 + (\delta_2 - 1)S_{\mathrm{TR}}\right]^2}{(1+\delta_2)^2(S_{\mathrm{TT}}^2 S_{\mathrm{RR}}^2 - S_{\mathrm{TR}}^2)}.$$

We then reject H_{01} at the α level if $S_{\mathrm{TT}}^2 - \delta_1 S_{\mathrm{RR}}^2 + (\delta_1 - 1)S_{\mathrm{TR}} > 0$, and

$$|t_{\mathrm{L}}| > t(\alpha, n_1 + n_2 - 3), \tag{7.5.7}$$

and reject H_{02} at the α level if $S_{\mathrm{TT}}^2 - \delta_2 S_{\mathrm{RR}}^2 + (\delta_2 - 1)S_{\mathrm{TR}} < 0$, and

$$|t_{\mathrm{U}}| > t(\alpha, n_1 + n_2 - 3). \tag{7.5.8}$$

Appendix B.4 provides SAS programs for testing hypotheses 7.4.4 and 7.5.1 based on the residuals from sequence-by-period means.

For testing hypotheses 7.5.2, Liu (1991) proposed a two one-sided tests procedure based upon the idea of orthogonal transformations introduced by Cornell (1980). An orthogonal transformation is used to transform the $n_1 + n_2$ independent bivariate random vectors $\mathbf{Y}_{ik}$ into $n_1 + n_2 - 2$ independent bivariate random vectors $\mathbf{Z}_{gk}$ with mean 0 and covariance matrix $\mathbf{\Sigma}_k$, where $i = 1, 2, \ldots, n_k$; $g = 1, 2, \ldots, n_k - 1$; $k = 1, 2$. The difference of the squares of the two components of each $\mathbf{Z}_{gk}$ is then unbiased estimates of the difference of intra-subject variabilities between the two formulations. Consequently, the nonparametric two one-sided tests procedure for average bioavailability described in Chapter 4 can be directly applied to hypotheses 7.5.2 based on the differences of the squares of two components of $\mathbf{Z}_{gk}$.

Let $\mathbf{Y}_{jk} = (Y_{1jk}, \ldots, Y_{n_k jk})'$, be the vector of n_k responses observed on subjects during period j in sequence k. Also let c_{gk} be an $n_k \times 1$ vector of coefficients of normalized linear orthogonal contrasts of degree n_k such that $\mathbf{I}'\ \mathbf{c}_{gk} = 0, \mathbf{c}'_{gk}\mathbf{c}_{gk} = 1$, and $\mathbf{c}'_{gk}\mathbf{c}_{g'k} = 0$, for $g \neq g'$, where $g = 1, 2, \ldots, n_k - 1$; $j = 1, 2$; $k = 1, 2$. If we define

$$\begin{aligned} Z_{gjk} &= \mathbf{c}'_{gk}\mathbf{Y}_{jk}, \quad \text{and} \\ \mathbf{Z}_{gk} &= (Z_{g1k}, Z_{g2k})', \end{aligned} \tag{7.5.9}$$

where
$g = 1, 2, \ldots, n_k - 1$; $j = 1, 2$; $k = 1, 2$, then, $\mathbf{Z}_{gk}$, $g = 1, 2, \ldots, n_k$; $k = 1, 2$, are independent bivariate normal vectors with mean vector $\mathbf{0}$ and covariance matrix $\mathbf{\Sigma}_k$, where $\mathbf{\Sigma}_k$ is defined in Equation 2.5.5. Because orthogonal transformations are linear, the units of the original data are maintained in the transformed data. In addition, orthogonal transformation preserves the covariance structure of the original data. Define the period difference of the squares of Z_{gjk} as follows:

$$Q_{gk} = \frac{1}{2}\left(Z_{g2k}^2 - Z_{g1k}^2\right), \quad g = 1, 2, \ldots, n_k - 1, \quad k = 1, 2. \tag{7.5.10}$$

Q_{gk} then follow a distribution as a half of the difference of two correlated χ^2 random variables (each with 1 degree of freedom). Under the normality assumptions of $\{S_{ik}\}$

and $\{e_{ijk}\}$ as described in hypotheses 2.5.5, Q_{gk} are independently distributed with mean

$$E(Q_{gk}) = \begin{cases} \frac{1}{2}\left(\sigma_T^2 - \sigma_R^2\right) & \text{for } k = 1, \\ \frac{1}{2}\left(\sigma_R^2 - \sigma_T^2\right) & \text{for } k = 2, \end{cases}$$

and common variance

$$\text{Var}(Q_{gk}) = \tfrac{1}{4}\left[\left(\sigma_T^4 + \sigma_R^4\right) + 2\sigma_S^2\left(\sigma_T^2 + \sigma_R^2\right)\right].$$

As $\{Q_{g1}, g = 1, 2, \ldots, n_1 - 1\}$ and $\{Q_{g2}, g = 1, 2, \ldots, n_2 - 1\}$ are two independent samples from the distributions with a common variance and a location difference of $\sigma_T^2 - \sigma_R^2$, Wilcoxon–Mann–Whitney's two one-sided procedure and the distribution-free confidence interval based on Hodges–Lehmann's estimator, discussed in Chapter 4, can be directly applied to $\{Q_{gk}, g = 1, 2, \ldots, n_k - 1, k = 1, 2\}$ to test interval hypotheses of equivalence in intra-subejct variabilities. Similar to the nonparametric procedures for average bioavailability as discussed in Sections 4.5.1 and 4.5.2, the resultant nonparametric two one-sided tests procedure for hypotheses 7.5.2 is also operationally equivalent to the corresponding distribution-free confidence interval.

Note that, in computation of W_L and W_U, the $n_1 + n_2 - 2Q_{gk}$ values should be treated as raw data and quantiles $w(\alpha)$ and $w(1-\alpha)$ are based on sample sizes $n_1 - 1$ and $n_2 - 1$. The orthogonal transformations based on Equation 7.5.9 can be easily obtained using statistical software such as the ORPOL function of SAS IML.

Compared with tests for hypotheses 7.5.1, one disadvantage of Liu's test procedure is that the equivalent limits θ_1 and θ_2 depend on the estimate of σ_R^2, which can certainly introduce bias to the procedure.

Sometimes, as pointed out by Anderson and Hauck (1990), to maintain a comparable safety profile, it is desirable to test whether variability of the test formulation does not exceed that of the reference formulation by at least some specific amount. In this situation, one needs to test only the second set of hypotheses in Equation 7.5.1 or 7.5.2 (i.e., H_{02} vs. H_{a2}), which has the same form as the hypotheses for evaluation of equivalence of efficacy in clinical trials considered by others (e.g., Blackwelder, 1982). Note that the hypotheses H_{02} versus H_{a2} can be tested using test statistics, either t_U for hypotheses 7.5.1 or w_U for hypotheses 7.5.2.

For testing hypotheses Equation 7.5.2, Esinhart and Chinchilli (1990) also proposed several test procedures based upon Wald's test, Rao's score test, and the likelihood ratio test. Esinhart and Chinchilli (1991) also proposed the use of generalized estimating equations (GEEs; Liang and Zeger, 1986) for analysis of average and variability of bioavailability. However, these test procedures are based on asymptotic results. The GEES procedure was originally developed for analysis of epidemiology studies that involve a large number of patients (sometimes in the thousands). In practice, because the number of subjects involved in a bioavailability/bioequivalence study is usually small (e.g., 12–24), the application of these procedures needs further investigation.

Although the asymptotic GEEs procedure requires only that distributions be expressed in an exponential form with the first two moments, unlike the nonparametric two one-sided procedure for average bioavailability, it is not general enough to include some distributions, such as Cauchy, which do not have any moments greater than or equal to 1. In addition, the asymptotic $(1 - 2\alpha) \times 100\%$ confidence intervals, based on these tests, may not provide sufficient $(1 - 2\alpha) \times 100\%$ coverage probability in small samples. Furthermore, it is doubtful that these confidence intervals are operationally equivalent to their corresponding test procedures.

Example 7.5.1

We first use AUC data from Example 3.6.1 to illustrate the two one-sided tests procedure given in 7.5.5 and 7.5.6 for testing hypotheses 7.5.1 of equivalence in variability of bioavailability. For the purpose of illustration, we choose $\delta_1 = 0.8$ and $\delta_2 = 1.2$. Pearson's correlation coefficients between V_{ik} and $U_{\mathrm{L}ik}$ and between V_{ik} and $U_{\mathrm{U}ik}$, based on the residuals from the sequence-by-period means, are given by 0.0854 and −0.0106, respectively. This gives

$$t_{\mathrm{L}} = \frac{0.0854}{\left[\dfrac{1 - (0.0854)^2}{21}\right]^{1/2}} = 0.3928 \quad \text{and}$$

$$t_{\mathrm{U}} = \frac{-0.0106}{\left[\dfrac{1 - (-0.0106)^2}{21}\right]^{1/2}} = -0.0485.$$

Therefore, we fail to reject H_{01} (p-value = 0.3492) and H_{02} (p-value = 0.4809) at the 5% level of significance. We then conclude that the two formulations are not bioequivalent in variability.

Similarly, it can be verified that Spearman's rank correlation coefficients between V_{ik} and $U_{\mathrm{L}ik}$ and between V_{ik} and $U_{\mathrm{U}ik}$ are 0.1635 and 0.0217. This leads to the same conclusion that the two formulations are not equivalent in variability (p-values > 0.1). Note that t_{L} and t_{U} can also be obtained from the squared root of F_{L} and F_{U} with values of S^2_{TT}, S^2_{RR}, and S_{TR} given in Example 7.4.3.

The above results are summarized in Table 7.5.1, which also gives test results of Clayton and Leslie's example that were obtained based on log-transformed AUC. The results indicate that the two erythromycin formulations are not equivalent in variability.

For the nonparametric two one-sided tests procedure for hypotheses 7.5.2, for the purpose of illustration, we choose $\theta_2 = -\theta_1 = 168$, which is an estimate of the intra-subject variability obtained from the analysis of variance table (Table 3.6.3). Therefore, we will conclude equivalence in intra-subject variabilities if the 90% confidence interval for $\sigma^2_{\mathrm{T}} - \sigma^2_{\mathrm{R}}$ is within ±168.

Table 7.5.2 gives Z_{gjk} and Q_{gk}, which are obtained after orthogonal transformations. On the basis of these values, Hodges–Lehmann's estimator yields an estimate of 9.66 and a distribution-free 90% confidence interval of (−216.76, 263.28). Since

TABLE 7.5.1: Summary of test results for equivalence in variability based on the ratio of variances.

Example	Method	Test[a] (p-Value)
3.1	Pearson	$r_L = 0.0854$ (0.3492)
		$r_U = -0.0106$ (0.4809)
	Spearman	$r_L = 0.1635$ (>0.1)
		$r_U = 0.0217$ (>0.5)
6.1[b]	Pearson	$r_L = 0.3312$ (0.0970)
		$r_U = 0.1869$ (0.7637)
	Spearman	$r_L = 0.3829$ ($0.05 < p < .1$)
		$r_U = 0.2632$ (>0.5)

[a] Based on the residuals from the sequence-by-period means.
[b] Based on the log-transformed AUC data.

TABLE 7.5.2: Results of orthogonal transformation for data in Table 3.6.1.

Sequence	Z_{g1k}	Z_{g2k}	Q_{gk}
1	43.4344	−11.0164	−1765.19
	−35.7584	−13.2207	−1103.88
	23.4740	2.7537	−543.45
	35.2714	26.8370	−523.85
	31.3209	54.0996	1945.77
	4.9200	8.4439	47.09
	−7.0244	−25.3875	595.18
	15.1894	0.3349	−230.61
	2.1556	23.7542	559.61
	−22.0535	−23.3809	60.31
	−15.7381	−12.1105	−101.03
2	3.6063	−5.0457	12.45
	4.3842	−13.8096	171.48
	−19.3074	−20.0137	27.77
	−40.5814	−39.4527	−90.33
	22.4712	6.1321	−467.35
	26.5541	3.3575	−693.85
	22.6315	5.7194	−479.43
	16.6862	1.0559	−277.32
	−14.8249	−20.4558	198.66
	1.2681	−2.8886	6.94
	0.2745	5.0672	25.60

TABLE 7.5.3: Summary of test results for equivalence in variability based on the difference in variances.

Example	Point Estimate	Distribution-Free 90% Confidence Intervals
3.1	9.660	(−216.76, 263.28)
6.1[a]	0.035	(−0.26, 0.32)

[a] Based on log-transformed AUC data.

the 90% confidence interval is not within (−168, 168), we conclude that there is not enough evidence to support the equivalence in intra-subject variabilities between the two formulations. It can be verified that this result agrees with that obtained using nonparametric two one-sided tests procedure based upon Q_{gk}.

Test results for Clayton and Leslie's example based on log-transformed AUC data are also obtained and summarized in Table 7.5.3. However, in Clayton and Leslie's example, $\theta_2 = -\theta_1$ was chosen to be 0.30, which is the mean squared error obtained from the analysis of variance table given in Table 6.9.2. From Table 7.5.3, it can be seen that the two formulations from Example 3.6.1 are equivalent in average bioavailability, but not in variability of bioavailability. On the other hand, the two erythromycin formulations are not equivalent in both average and variability of bioavailability.

Recently, in addition to average bioavailability, more attention has been paid to the issue of equivalence or noninferiority of intra-subject variability of the test formulation with respect to the reference formulation. Lee et al. (2002) and Chow et al. (2003b) have proposed some procedures for determination of sample size on evaluation of equivalence in intra-subject variability. Although sometimes closed-form formulas may not be available, sample size required for assessment of equivalence in intra-subject variability can always be empirically obtained through the simulation by the following steps:

1. With respect to model 4.1.2 and the assumptions given in 3.1.4, specify the parameters of fixed-effects, inter-subject variance, and intra-subject variances for both test and reference formulations.

2. Choose the appropriate test statistics with equivalence limits, sample size, and the significance level (say 5%), and the desired power (say 80%).

3. Generate a large number of random samples of the data (say 2000), according to the specifications of parameters and intra-subject variances in (1) and sample size in (2).

4. For each sample generated, perform the test for evaluation of equivalence in intra-subject variability according to the statistics chosen in (2).

5. Compute the proportion of random samples that reject the null hypothesis and conclude the equivalence in intra-subject variability at the 5% significance level. This proportion is referred to as the empirical power.

6. If the empirical power is too low or too high, go to step (2) to either increase or decrease the sample size.

7. Repeat (2) to (5) until the empirical power is within the prespecified margin of the desired power (say $\pm 2\%$).

8. The corresponding sample size is the sample size for the study on evaluation of equivalence in intra-subject variability.

However, in most bioavailability studies, sample sizes are chosen such that there is sufficient power for detection of significant difference in average bioavailability between formulations, which may not be large enough for assessment of equivalence in variability of bioavailability. Therefore, a nonsignificant test result for interval hypotheses of variability may imply that the sample size is too small to declare equivalence in variability if the two formulations are indeed equivalent. However, sample size required for assessment of equivalence in variability as compared to those for equivalence in average requires further investigation.

7.6 CV Assessment

As indicated in previous sections, it is important to compare the inter- and intra-subject variabilities between formulations in addition to average bioavailability. Therefore, it is helpful to estimate the inter- and intra-subject variabilities for each formulation. In practice, if the drug has a short half-life, it is possible that each subject has replicates for each formulation (i.e., each subject receives several administrations of the sequence of formulations). On the basis of these replicates, the inter- and intra-subject variabilities can then be estimated using the methods introduced in Section 7.3. However, frequently, each subject may have a different intra-subject mean and intra-subject variability for the parameter under study. In this case, assessment of the inter-subject variability and the intra-subject variability is not possible because standard statistical methods assume that intra-subject variability is the same from subject to subject. However, if we assume that the CV for each subject is the same from subject to subject, then intra-subject variability can be assessed in terms of the common CV. Assuming that there are no period effects, Chow and Tse (1988, 1990b) provided several estimators for the common CV under a conditional one-way random effects model. The conditional one-way random effects are described in the next section.

7.6.1 Conditional One-Way Random Effects Model

Let Y_{ij} be the response of a bioavailability parameter, say AUC, of the jth replicate of the ith subject for a given formulation of a drug. To estimate the inter- and intra-subject variabilities, the following one-way random effects model is usually considered:

$$Y_{ij} = \mu + S_i + e_{ij}, \quad i = 1, 2, \ldots, k, \quad j = 1, 2, \ldots, n, \tag{7.6.1}$$

where

μ is the overall mean

S_i's and e_{ij}'s are independently distributed as $N(0, \sigma_S^2)$ and $N(0, \sigma_e^2)$, respectively.

Under model 7.6.1 the inter- and the intra-subject variability of the AUC are described by σ_S^2 and σ_e^2, respectively.

However, this model is based on the assumption that the intra-subject variability is the same from subject to subject. To account for the different intra-subject means and variances, Chow and Tse (1988, 1990b) considered the following conditional one-way random effects model:

$$Y_{ij} = \mu + S_i + e_{ij}, \quad i = 1, 2, \ldots, k; \quad j = 1, 2, \ldots, n, \tag{7.6.2}$$

where

μ is the overall mean

S_i's are independently distributed as $N(0, \sigma_S^2)$ and given $S_i = a_i$, the e_{ij}'s are independently distributed as $N(0, \sigma_i^2)$; that is,

$$e_{ij} | S_i = a_i \sim N(0, \sigma_i^2).$$

The difference between models 7.6.1 and 7.6.2 is that the variance of the e_{ij}'s in the latter model differs from subject to subject.

Suppose μ_i and σ_i^2 are the mean and variance for the ith subject. The CV of the ith subject is then given by

$$\lambda_i = \sigma_i / \mu_i.$$

Under the assumption that the CV is the same from subject to subject, we have

$$\lambda = \lambda_i, \quad i = 1, \ldots, k.$$

Therefore, the expected value and variance of Y_{ij} given $S_i = a_i$ are given as

$$E(Y_{ij} | S_i = a_i) = \mu_i = \mu + a_i \quad \text{and}$$
$$\mathrm{Var}(Y_{ij} | S_i = a_i) = \sigma_i^2 = \lambda^2 \mu_i^2 = \lambda^2 (\mu + a_i)^2.$$

It appears that model 7.6.2 is useful because it can account for the different intra-subject means and variances. Note that, instead, one could suggest using a log-transformed model to stabilize the intra-subject variabilities. However, this method may not be effective in a typical bioavailability/bioequivalence study, which often involves the comparison of bioavailability among several formulations. In this case, the attempt to stabilize the variabilities fails if the CVs are different from formulation to formulation. However, model 7.6.2 can be extended to the case where there are several formulations.

7.6.2 Estimators for the Common CV

Let $\overline{Y}_i$ and $\widehat{\sigma}_i$ be the sample mean and sample standard deviation of the ith subject. Under model 7.6.2, the following estimators of the common CV are considered by Chow and Tse (1990b):

$$1.\ \widehat{\lambda}_1 = \frac{1}{k}\sum_{i=1}^{k}(\widehat{\sigma}_i/\overline{Y}_i),$$

$$2.\ \widehat{\lambda}_2 = \left[\frac{1}{k}\sum_{i=1}^{k}(\widehat{\sigma}_i/\overline{Y}_i)^2\right]^{1/2},$$

$$3.\ \widehat{\lambda}_3 = \left[\sum_{i=1}^{k}\widehat{\sigma}_i\overline{Y}_i\right]\bigg/\left[\sum_{i=k}^{k}\overline{Y}_i^2\right],$$

$$4.\ \widehat{\lambda}_4 = \left\{\left[\sum_{i=1}^{k}\widehat{\sigma}_i^2\overline{Y}_i^2\right]\bigg/\left[\sum_{i=1}^{k}\overline{Y}_i^4\right]\right\}^{1/2},$$

$$5.\ \widehat{\lambda}_5 = \left[\frac{M_2}{\overline{Y}^2 + \sigma_S^2}\right]^{1/2},$$

where

$$\sigma_S^2 = (M_1 - M_2)/n,$$

and

$$M_1 = \frac{n}{k-1}\sum_{i=1}^{k}(\overline{Y}_i - \overline{Y})^2,$$

$$M_2 = \frac{1}{k(n-1)}\sum_{i=j}^{k}\sum_{j=1}^{n}(Y_{ij} - \overline{Y}_i)^2.$$

The first two estimators are derived by taking the average of the estimates of λ_i and λ_i^2 (i.e., $\widehat{\sigma}_i/\overline{Y}_i$ and $\widehat{\sigma}_i^2/\overline{Y}_i^2$), respectively. The third and fourth estimators are obtained by fitting a least regression function (through the origin) of $\widehat{\sigma}_i$ and $\widehat{\sigma}_i^2$ on $\overline{Y}$ and $\overline{Y}_i^2$, respectively, based on the fact that $\sigma_i = \lambda\mu_i$ and $\sigma_i^2 = \lambda^2\mu_i^2$. The fifth estimator is the analysis of variance estimator, which is obtained by equating M_1 and M_2 to their expectations and solving for λ', that is,

$$M_1 = E(M_1) = n\sigma_S^2 + \mu^2\lambda^2 + \sigma_S^2,$$

and

$$M_2 = E(M_2) = \mu^2\lambda^2 + \sigma_S^2\lambda^2.$$

Chow and Tse (1990b) compared the above estimators in terms of the asymptotic order terms for their biases and mean squared errors. The results indicate that, for large n and k, the biases can be approximated by

$$\text{Bias}(\widehat{\lambda}_1) \approx -5\lambda c^4/2,$$
$$\text{Bias}(\widehat{\lambda}_2) \approx 13\lambda c^4/8,$$
$$\text{Bias}(\widehat{\lambda}_3) \approx -5\lambda c^4/8,$$
$$\text{Bias}(\widehat{\lambda}_4) \approx -19\lambda c^4/8,$$
$$\text{Bias}(\widehat{\lambda}_5) \approx [\lambda c^2(1 + c^2)^{-1}]/2k,$$

where $c = \sigma_S/\mu$.

The results show that these estimators, except for $\widehat{\lambda}_2$, underestimate λ. In addition, $\widehat{\lambda}_5$ is asymptotically unbiased. All the other four estimators are with biases of order O(1). On the basis of a simulation study, Chow and Tse (1990b) indicated that $\widehat{\lambda}_5$ usually gives the best performance. When λ is small, $\widehat{\lambda}_2$, λ_3, and $\widehat{\lambda}_4$ may be possible contenders; however, they perform miserably for large λ.

Example 7.6.2

Chow and Tse (1990b) considered an example concerning the comparison of bioavailability between two intranasal formulations and one intravenous formulation of a drug product. To assess the intra-subject variability in terms of the common CV, each subject was administered the same formulation three times. For the purpose of illustration, let us consider the intravenous formulation. Table 7.6.1 gives AUCs of 14 subjects for the intravenous formulation. The results indicate that the subjects have different intra-subject means and intra-subject variances. Therefore, the usual one-way random effects model is not an appropriate model due to the heterogeneity of intra-subject variability among subjects. As the CVs are similar from subject to subject, we then consider model 7.6.2 to assess the intra-subject variability in terms of the common CV. Estimates of the common CV for the intravenous formulation using $\widehat{\lambda}_1$ through $\widehat{\lambda}_5$ are

$$\widehat{\lambda}_1 = 18.36\%, \quad \widehat{\lambda}_2 = 18.69\%, \quad \widehat{\lambda}_3 = 18.56\%,$$
$$\widehat{\lambda}_4 = 19.05\%, \quad \text{and} \quad \widehat{\lambda}_5 = 18.94\%.$$

These results indicate that intra-subject variability for the AUC of the formulation is less than 20%.

TABLE 7.6.1: AUCs for an intravenous formulation.

Subject	AUC (mμ × min/mL)			Mean	SD	CV
1	7462.7	6212.8	5782.5	6486.0	872.78	0.1346
2	7533.9	5337.7	7371.4	6747.7	1223.76	0.1814
3	6509.3	10084.6	6665.4	7753.1	2020.67	0.2606
4	6184.8	6042.9	8026.9	6751.5	1106.76	0.1639
5	5693.1	7139.3	8597.7	7263.4	1635.81	0.2252
6	9551.9	6550.8	8987.1	8363.3	1594.82	0.1907
7	8643.5	6153.3	8800.0	7865.6	1484.93	0.1888
8	9167.8	6756.3	6192.9	7372.3	1580.22	0.2143
9	7900.5	6767.8	9123.3	7930.5	1178.01	0.1485
10	6522.4	8040.5	6236.0	6932.9	969.77	0.1399
11	8178.9	6329.5	9211.0	7906.5	1459.93	0.1847
12	6835.5	7002.1	8906.8	7581.4	1150.78	0.1518
13	6533.7	6948.9	9669.3	7717.3	1703.26	0.2207
14	5876.9	8066.4	6511.7	6818.3	1126.46	0.1652

Source: From Chow, S.C. and Tse, S.K., *Biometric. J.*, 32, 597, 1990b.

7.7 Discussion

In Section 7.2, we briefly discussed the decision rule for assessing equivalence in variability of bioavailability. In most of the current guidances by the U.S. FDA, the EMEA, and the WHO, there is no discussion as to how much difference in variability would be considered of clinically meaningful significance. On the other hand, some suggestions for evaluation of equivalence in intra-subject variability have been proposed for individual bioequivalence as described in the *Guidance on Statistical Approaches to Establishing Bioequivalence* by the U.S. FDA (FDA, 2001). On the basis of the logarithmic scale, the U.S. FDA guidance recommends an allowance of 0.02 for the difference in intra-subject variability between the test and the reference formulations. However, for the standard 2 × 2 crossover design, under model 4.1.2 and assumptions given in 3.1.4, the difference in total variability between test and reference formulations is the difference in intra-subject variability between the two references. Therefore, for individual bioequivalence, the FDA guidance implies that, on the logarithmic scale, an increase larger than 0.02 for intra-subject variability of test formulation over the reference will be of clinical significance.

Furthermore, the formulation for assessment of equivalence in variability in the FDA guidance is in the form of difference. As a result, the second set of hypotheses given in 7.5.1 with equivalence limit of 0.02

$$\begin{aligned} &\mathrm{H}_{02}\colon\ \sigma_T^2 - \sigma_R^2 \geq 0.02 \\ \text{versus}\quad &\mathrm{H}_{a2}\colon\ \sigma_T^2 - \sigma_R^2 < 0.02 \end{aligned} \tag{7.7.1}$$

should be employed to assess equivalence in variability under the standard 2×2 crossover design and logarithmic scale. Consequently, the procedures based on orthogonal transformation proposed by Liu (1991) can be directly applied to test the hypothesis in Equation 7.7.1. The null hypothesis given in 7.7.1 is rejected at the α significance level if the upper $(1 - \alpha)$ 100% confidence limit constructed based on Hodges–Lehmann's estimator is greater than the allowable equivalence limit of 0.02.

For a hypothesis formulated in terms of the ratio of $\theta = \sigma_T^2/\sigma_R^2$, Guilbaud (1993) and Wang (1997) proposed some exact or unbiased tests. Guilbaud considered the following function of σ_T^2/σ_R^2,

$$\gamma = \frac{(\sigma_T^2 - \sigma_R^2)}{(\sigma_T^2 + \sigma_R^2)}. \tag{7.7.2}$$

Note that γ is an increasing function of $\sigma_T^2/\sigma_R^2 > 0$ and $-1 < \gamma < 1$. Because

$$\gamma = \frac{(\theta - 1)}{(\theta + 1)}, \tag{7.7.3}$$

therefore, the hypothesis given in 7.2.3 can be reformulated in terms of γ as

$$\begin{aligned} &H_0\colon\ \gamma \le \gamma_U \quad \text{or} \quad \gamma \ge \gamma_L \\ \text{versus}\quad &H_a\colon\ \gamma_L < \gamma < \gamma_U, \end{aligned} \tag{7.7.4}$$

where γ_U and γ_L are obtained by replacing θ in Equation 7.7.3 by θ_U and θ_L, respectively. An estimator of γ is given as

$$\widehat{\gamma} = \frac{S_{VU}}{S_{VV}^2}, \tag{7.7.5}$$

and the $(1 - 2\alpha)$ 100% confidence interval is given by (L_γ, U_γ), where

$$L_\gamma(U_\gamma) = \widehat{\gamma} + t(\alpha,\, n_1 + n_2 - 3)S_\gamma,$$

$$S_\gamma^2 = \frac{\left[S_{UU}^2/(S_{VV}^2 - \widehat{\gamma}^2)\right]}{(n_1 + n_2 - 3)},$$

and $t(\alpha, n_1 + n_2 - 3)$ is αth upper quantile of a central t distribution.

The null hypothesis in Equation 7.7.4 is rejected at the α significance level if (L_γ, U_γ) is completed contained (γ_L and γ_U). However, a serious drawback for this approach is that it does not guarantee that the point estimator γ and the confidence interval for γ will be in the interval of $(-1, 1)$. As a matter of fact, the example in Guilbaud (1993) using the data set given in Liu (1991) gave an estimate of 1.870 and an interval of (1.58, 2.16) for γ.

Both Schuirmann's two one-sided tests procedure in Equation 4.3.4 and Pitman–Morgan's two one-sided tests procedure given in 7.5.7 and 7.5.8 are based on t-tests. Brown et al. (1998) proposed an unbiased test for evaluation of average bioequivalence in terms of interval hypothesis 4.3.1. Therefore, Wang (1997) extended the results to an unbiased test for hypothesis of equivalence in intra-subject variability. The improvement of power for their methods over the Schuirmann or Pitman–Morgan two one-sided tests procedure is the addition of an open-end rejection region. The width of this open-end addition is an increasing function of variability of the corresponding response. Furthermore, the width of the open-end rejection region will be even larger than the length of equivalence interval. In other words, a sloppily conducted bioequivalence study with a large variability will be more likely than a carefully executed study with better precision of the estimators to conclude equivalence not only in average but also in variability. On the other hand, as mentioned earlier, relative to the FDA guidance, the assessment of equivalence in variability will be based on the second one-sided hypothesis given in 7.5.1. As a result, the test procedure based on t statistics given in 7.5.6 will be the uniformly most powerful unbiased test.

In Section 7.3, several estimators for σ_S^2 are considered to assess the inter-subject variability. The restricted maximum likelihood estimator and maximum likelihood estimator are commonly used to avoid negative estimates by truncating the estimates at 0. However, these estimators are likely to yield a zero estimate when σ_S^2 is small. This is because there is a high probability of obtaining a negative estimate for small σ_S^2. To avoid negative and zero estimates in variance components models, Chow and Shao (1988) proposed an estimation procedure for variance components and their ratios that has lower mean squared error than the customary estimators over a large range of parameters space. In the interest of obtaining a positive estimate for σ_S^2, this estimation procedure can be applied, with some modification under model 3.1.1. For interval estimate of σ_S^2, the lower confidence limit for σ_S^2 could be less than 0, especially for small σ_S^2. The portion $(L_S, 0)$ would not be meaningful because σ_S^2 is always positive. Here, a modification by truncating at zero is usually considered [i.e., L_S is set to be $\max(0, L_S)$]. However, with this modification, the confidence level may no longer be $1 - \alpha$. In addition, the expected width of (L_S, U_S) may be too wide to be useful. As an alternative approach, Chow (1985) considered a nonparametric procedure using the jackknife technique in conjunction with the ideas of grouping, truncation, and shifting to construct an approximate $(1 - \alpha) \times 100\%$ confidence interval for σ_S^2. On the basis of a simulation study, the resultant confidence interval has approximately $(1 - \alpha) \times 100\%$ coverage probability, with a much narrower confidence interval. This procedure is useful, yet complicated, and hence is not included.

The two one-sided tests procedure for average bioavailability, such as Schuirmann's procedure, together with the two one-sided tests procedure for variability of bioavailability can be used to assess population bioequivalence between test and reference formulations if the responses (or logarithmic transformation) are approximately normally distributed. However, when data are not normal, we still can establish equivalence in only average and variability, and hence population equivalence, using nonparametric methods described in Chapter 4 and this chapter. For more discussion of population bioequivalence using nonparametric procedures, see Cornell (1990) and Liu and Chow (1992b).

From Chapter 4, it can be seen that both the parametric and nonparametric two one-sided tests procedure for assessing equivalence in average bioavailability are based on the mean period differences, which are linear combinations of the sequence-by-period means. For hypotheses 7.5.3, it is suggested that the test statistics be calculated based on the residuals from the sequence-by-period means because the resultant statistics does not involve fixed period effects and they are independent of the sequence-by-period means. Furthermore, the test statistics, proposed by Liu (1991), for hypotheses 7.5.2 are based on the orthogonal transformation, which are also independent of the sequence-by-period means. Therefore, the two one-sided tests procedure for variability of bioavailability are independent of the two one-sided tests procedure for average bioavailability. For assessment of bioequivalence between formulations, some researchers (Metzler and Huang, 1983) suggested that the equivalence in variability of bioavailability be tested before the assessment of equivalence in average bioavailability is performed. However, testing for equivalence between variances generally requires much larger sample sizes than does testing for difference in averages. In addition, testing for equivalence in variability of bioavailability and testing for equivalence in average bioavailability are done either separately or simultaneously, an appropriate justification on the α level should be considered to have a predetermined overall type I error rate.

Instead of testing for equivalence in both average bioavailability and variability of bioavailability, testing for equivalence in CV may be useful if the CV is the same from subject to subject. Let μ_T and μ_R be the means for test and reference formulation, respectively. Also, let λ_T and λ_R be the corresponding CV (i.e., $\lambda_T = \sigma_T/\mu_T$ and $\lambda_R = \sigma_R/\mu_R$). Bioequivalence between formulations may then be determined by testing the following hypotheses:

$$\begin{aligned} &\mathrm{H_0}\colon \lambda_T - \lambda_R \leq \lambda_L \quad \text{or} \quad \lambda_T - \lambda_R \geq \lambda_U \\ \text{versus} \quad &\mathrm{H_a}\colon \lambda_L < \lambda_T - \lambda_R < \lambda_U, \end{aligned} \tag{7.7.6}$$

where λ_L and λ_U are equivalence limits. It can be seen that if $\sigma_T^2 = \sigma_R^2$, then hypotheses 7.7.1 reduces to hypotheses 4.3.1 for average bioavailability. On the other hand, if $\mu_T = \mu_R$, then testing for hypotheses 7.7.1 is equivalent to testing for hypotheses 7.5.2.

Chapter 8

Assumptions of Outlier Detection for Average Bioequivalence

8.1 Introduction

For the standard 2×2 crossover design, as indicated in Chapter 2, the following model is usually considered for assessing bioequivalence between formulations

$$Y_{ijk} = \mu + S_{ik} + F_{(j,k)} + C_{(j-1,k)} + P_j + e_{ijk}, \tag{8.1.1}$$

where

$i = 1, 2, \ldots, n_k$
$j = 1, 2$
$k = 1, 2.$

Several statistical methods for assessment of bioequivalence in average bioavailability between formulations were discussed under model 8.1.1 with the following normality assumptions:

$$\begin{aligned} &1.\ \{S_{ik}\} \text{ are i.i.d. normal with mean 0 and variance } \sigma_S^2. \\ &2.\ \{e_{ijk}\} \text{ are i.i.d. normal with mean 0 and variance } \sigma_e^2. \\ &3.\ \{S_{ik}\} \text{ and } \{e_{ijk}\} \text{ are mutually independent.} \end{aligned} \tag{8.1.2}$$

In most bioavailability studies, the above assumptions may not hold. The validation of assumptions 8.1.2 has an influence on the assessment of bioequivalence in average bioavailability in the following ways.

8.1.1 Model Selection

In a bioavailability study, because the methods introduced in Chapter 4 can be applied to either raw data or log-transformed data, it is important to check the assumptions before an appropriate statistical model is chosen. A different model may result in a different conclusion for bioequivalence (Chow, 1990).

8.1.2 Drug Safety and Exchangeability

As indicated in Chapter 7, a significant difference in intra-subject variability between formulations may raise a great concern in drug safety and exchangeability of the test formulations (Liu, 1991; Liu and Chow, 1992b). Assumptions 8.1.2 basically require that the intra-subject variabilities be the same from subject to subject and from formulation to formulation. In practice, this is often not true, for individual subjects may differ widely in their responses to a drug (Wagner, 1971; Chow and Tse, 1988, 1990b). Therefore, assumptions 8.1.2 should be examined before assessment of bioequivalence. More discussion about drug safety and exchangeability is provided in Chapters 11 and 12.

8.1.3 Outlying Data

One of the problems commonly encountered in bioavailability and bioequivalence studies is that the data set sometimes contains either some extremely large or small observations. We refer to these extreme values as outlying data. These outlying data may have dramatic effects on the bioequivalence test. Results with inclusion of the outlying observations could be totally different from those without inclusion of the outlying observations in a marginal case (Chow and Tse, 1990a). Therefore, it is important to examine the outlying data under model 8.1.1 carefully.

The objectives of this chapter are then to (1) provide some tests for assumptions that can be used for model selection between the raw data model and the log-transformation model, and (2) introduce several statistical test procedures for detection of outlying data under model 8.1.1.

In Section 8.2, several tests for assumptions using the inter-subject and intra-subject residuals are discussed. We then describe three different types of outlying observations that often occur in bioavailability and bioequivalence studies in Section 8.3. In Sections 8.4 and 8.5, statistical tests for detection of outlying subjects and outlying observations are presented. A brief discussion is given in Section 8.6.

8.2 Tests for Assumptions

For the standard 2×2 crossover design, under model 8.1.1 with assumptions 8.1.2, as indicated in Chapter 3, the total sum of squares can be partitioned into the between-subject sum of squares ($SS_{between}$) and the within-subject sum of squares (SS_{within}). $SS_{between}$ can be further partitioned into the sum of squares of carryover effects and the sum of squares of inter-subject error (SS_{inter}). The within-subject sum of squares can be further decomposed into sum of squares of formulation effects (SS_{drug}), sum of squares of period effects (SS_{period}), and sum of squares of intra-subject residuals (SS_{intra}). For testing assumptions 8.1.2, Jones and Kenward (2003) suggested the use of the inter-subject and intra-subject residuals. In the following, tests for assumptions using the intra-subject and inter-subject residuals are outlined. We first consider the use of intra-subject residuals.

8.2.1 Intra-Subject Residuals

The intra-subject residual for subject i within sequence k during period j, denoted by $\widehat{e}_{ijk}$, is defined as the difference between the observed response Y_{ijk} and its predicted value $\widehat{Y}_{ijk}$ which can be obtained under model 8.1.1, that is,

$$\begin{aligned}\widehat{e}_{ijk} &= Y_{ijk} - \widehat{Y}_{ijk} \\ &= Y_{ijk} - \overline{Y}_{i\cdot k} + \overline{Y}_{\cdot jk} - \overline{Y}_{\cdot\cdot k},\end{aligned} \tag{8.2.1}$$

where

$$\widehat{Y}_{ijk} = \overline{Y}_{i\cdot k} - \overline{Y}_{\cdot jk} + \overline{Y}_{\cdot\cdot k},$$

and

$$\begin{aligned}\overline{Y}_{i\cdot k} &= \frac{1}{2}\sum_{j=1}^{2} Y_{ijk} = \frac{Y_{i\cdot k}}{2}, \\ \overline{Y}_{\cdot jk} &= \frac{1}{n_k}\sum_{i=1}^{n_k} Y_{ijk} = \frac{Y_{\cdot jk}}{n_k}, \\ \overline{Y}_{\cdot\cdot k} &= \frac{1}{2n_k}\sum_{j=1}^{2}\sum_{i=1}^{n_k} Y_{ijk} = \frac{Y_{\cdot\cdot k}}{2n_k} = \frac{1}{2}\sum_{j=1}^{2}\overline{Y}_{\cdot jk},\end{aligned} \tag{8.2.2}$$

where
$i = 1, 2, \ldots, n_k$
$j, k = 1, 2.$

From Equation 8.2.2, it can be verified that

$$Y_{i\cdot k} = 2\overline{Y}_{i\cdot k},$$

and

$$2\overline{Y}_{\cdot\cdot k} = \overline{Y}_{\cdot 1k} + \overline{Y}_{\cdot 2k}.$$

It follows that

$$\widehat{e}_{i1k} + \widehat{e}_{i2k} = 0, \tag{8.2.3}$$

or equivalently,

$$\widehat{e}_{i1k} = -\widehat{e}_{i2k} \quad \text{for} \quad i = 1, 2, \ldots, n_k \quad \text{and} \quad k = 1, 2.$$

Also, for $k = 1, 2$

$$\begin{aligned}\sum_{i=1}^{n_k}\widehat{e}_{ijk} &= \sum_{i=1}^{n_k}(Y_{ijk} - \overline{Y}_{i\cdot k} - \overline{Y}_{\cdot jk} + \overline{Y}_{\cdot\cdot k}) \\ &= n_k(\overline{Y}_{\cdot jk} - \overline{Y}_{\cdot\cdot k} - \overline{Y}_{\cdot jk} + \overline{Y}_{\cdot\cdot k}) = 0.\end{aligned} \tag{8.2.4}$$

Because there are $n_1 + n_2$ constraints in Equation 8.2.3 and two constraints in Equation 8.2.4, the degrees of freedom for the sum of squares of the intra-subject residuals (SS_{intra}) is $2(n_1 + n_2) - (n_1 + n_2) - 2 = n_1 + n_2 - 2$.

The variances and covariances of $\widehat{e}_{ijk}$ under the second assumption of assumptions 8.2.1 are given by

$$\mathrm{Var}(\widehat{e}_{ijk}) = \frac{(n_k - 1)}{2n_k}\sigma_e^2, \tag{8.2.5}$$

and

$$\mathrm{Cov}(\widehat{e}_{ijk}, \widehat{e}_{i'j'k'}) = \begin{cases} -\dfrac{n_k - 1}{2n_k}\sigma_e^2 & \text{if } i = i', j \neq j', k = k', \\ -\sigma_e^2/2n_k & \text{if } i \neq i', j = j', k = k', \\ \sigma_e^2/2n_k & \text{if } i \neq i', j \neq j', k = k', \\ 0 & \text{if } k \neq k'. \end{cases} \tag{8.2.6}$$

From Equations 8.2.3 and 8.2.6, it can be seen that there is a perfect negative correlation (i.e., $\rho = -1$) between the two intra-subject residuals within the same subject. Thus, it is sufficient to examine intra-subject residuals at the first period; that is,

$$\widehat{e}_{i1k}, i = 1, 2, \ldots, n_k, \quad k = 1, 2.$$

If σ_e^2 is known, we may consider the following standardized intra-subject residuals

$$e_{i1k}^* = \frac{\widehat{e}_{i1k}}{\left[\dfrac{n_k - 1}{2n_k}\sigma_e^2\right]^{1/2}} \quad i = 1, 2, \ldots, n_k \quad k = 1, 2. \tag{8.2.7}$$

The marginal distribution of e_{i1k}^* is the standard normal distribution with mean 0 and variance 1. Owing to the constraints of Equation 8.2.4, the joint distribution of $\{e_{i1k}^*\}$ is an $n_1 + n_2$ dimensional singular multivariate distribution with mean vector $\mathbf{0}$ and covariance matrix

$$\mathrm{Cov}(e_{i1k}^*, e_{i1k'}^*) = \begin{cases} 1 & \text{if } i = i', k = k' \\ -\dfrac{1}{n_k} & \text{if } i \neq i', k = k' \\ 0 & \text{if } k \neq k'. \end{cases} \tag{8.2.8}$$

In practice, however, σ_e^2 is usually unknown, but can be estimated unbiasedly by MS_{intra}. Substituting σ_e^2 in Equation 8.2.7 with MS_{intra} yields the following studentized intra-subject residuals:

$$\widetilde{e}_{i1k} = \frac{\widetilde{e}_{i1k}}{\left[\frac{n_k - 1}{2n_k} \text{MS}_{\text{intra}}\right]^{1/2}}, \quad i = 1, 2, \ldots, n_k, \quad k = 1, 2. \tag{8.2.9}$$

Although $\widetilde{e}_{i1k}$ also has mean 0 and variance 1, the joint distribution of the studentized intra-subject residuals is quite complicated. In practice, we can treat $\widetilde{e}_{i1k}$ as standard normal random variables to evaluate assumptions 8.1.2.

Based on $\{\widetilde{e}_{i1k}\}$ and $\{\widehat{Y}_{i1k}\}$ where $i = 1, 2, \ldots, n_k$ and $k = 1, 2$, assumptions 8.1.1 and the adequacy of model 8.1.1 can be examined in terms of the normal probability plot of $\{\widetilde{e}_{i1k}\}$ or the residual plot between $\{\widetilde{e}_{i1k}\}$ and $\{\widehat{Y}_{i1k}\}$. The normal probability plot of $\{\widetilde{e}_{i1k}\}$ is used to examine the normality assumption on the intra-subject variability of e_{ijk}, whereas the residual plot between $\{\widetilde{e}_{i1k}\}$ and $\{\widehat{Y}_{i1k}\}$ is used to examine whether model 8.1.1 is adequate. Note that the residual plot and normal probability plot can also provide preliminary information of potential outlying data.

The normal probability plot is obtained by plotting $\widetilde{e}_{i1k}$ against the expected normal order statistics (or normal scores), which can be easily computed using some statistical software programs such as PROC RANK in SAS. If e_{ijk} is, indeed, normally distributed, then the normal probability plot should be a straight line. Therefore, any marked deviation from a straight line may indicate that the normality assumption of e_{ijk} does not hold for the data set under study. Alternatively, the normality of e_{ijk} can also be examined using the test of Shapiro and Wilk (1965) on $\widetilde{e}_{i1k}$. This can be accomplished using PROC UNIVARIATE in SAS. It, however, should be noted that Shapiro and Wilk's test requires that the observations be independent. Therefore, the p-value for the normality test of Shapiro and Wilk based upon the studentized intra-subject residuals should be used with caution, especially with a small sample size, because they are not independent.

For the residual plot, if model 8.1.1 is an appropriate model, then $\widetilde{e}_{i1k}$ should be randomly scattered between -2 and 2 on the plot. Any distinct pattern observed in the plot may indicate that the model is not adequate to describe the data. In this case, additional terms or covariates may be added to the model. In addition, if there are some extremely large or small unusual values [i.e., outside interval $(-2, 2)$] observed on the plot, the corresponding subjects may possibly be outlying subjects. These subjects should be carefully examined in terms of their demographic information, plasma concentration, and other important factors.

8.2.2 Inter-Subject Residuals

Similarly, the inter-subject residuals can be used to evaluate the normality assumption imposed on the inter-subject variability of S_{ik}. The inter-subject residuals, denoted by $\widehat{S}_{ik}$, are given as

$$\widehat{S}_{ik} = Y_{i \cdot k} - \overline{Y}_{\cdot \cdot k}, \quad i = 1, 2, \ldots, n_k, \quad k = 1, 2. \tag{8.2.10}$$

Under the first assumption of assumptions 8.1.2, the variances and covariances of $\widehat{S}_{ik}$ are given by

$$\mathrm{Var}(\widehat{S}_{ik}) = \frac{2(n_k - 1)}{n_k}\left(2\sigma_S^2 + \sigma_e^2\right), \tag{8.2.11}$$

and

$$\mathrm{Cov}(\widehat{S}_{ik}, \widehat{S}_{i'k'}) = \begin{cases} -\dfrac{2\left(2\sigma_S^2 + \sigma_e^2\right)}{n_k} & \text{if } i \neq i', k = k', \\ 0 & \text{if } k \neq k'. \end{cases} \tag{8.2.12}$$

The studentized inter-subject residuals are then given by

$$\widetilde{S}_{ik} = \frac{\widehat{S}_{ik}}{\left[\frac{2(n_k-1)}{n_k}\mathrm{MS_{inter}}\right]^{1/2}}, \quad i = 1, 2, \ldots, n_k, \quad k = 1, 2. \tag{8.2.13}$$

Therefore, the normality assumption of S_{ik} can be checked by either examining the normal probability plot of $\{\widetilde{S}_{ik}\}$ or performing Shapiro–Wilk's test on $\{\widetilde{S}_{ik}\}$.

Note that the assumption 3 of independence between $\{S_{ik}\}$ and $\{e_{ijk}\}$ in Equation 8.1.2 can also be checked by examining either Pearson's correlation coefficient or Spearman's rank correlation coefficient between $\{\widehat{e}_{i1k}\}$ and $\{\widetilde{S}_{ik}\}$.

Example 8.2.1

We use AUC data (both raw data and log-transformed data) of the two erythromycin formulations in Clayton and Leslie's study to illustrate procedures for examination of assumptions 8.1.2 through the inter-subject and intra-subject residuals.

Raw Data

Table 8.2.1 provides studentized intra-subject and inter-subject residuals of the raw AUC data, which were obtained by plugging the values of $\mathrm{MS_{intra}}(=5.992)$ and $\mathrm{MS_{inter}}(=8.911)$ into Equations 8.2.9 and 8.2.13, respectively. Note that only studentized intra-subject residuals at the first period are given in Table 8.2.1. The residual plot of predicted values versus studentized intra-subject residuals is given in Figure 8.2.1. Figure 8.2.1 exhibits a slightly downward pattern of distribution of the studentized intra-subject residuals. It can be seen that studentized intra-subject residuals corresponding to approximately the same value of $\widehat{Y}_{i1k}$ for three subjects are quite different. These three subjects are subject 2 (6.137 vs. 1.675), subject 7 (5.972 vs. −3.053), and subject 14 (6.046 vs. −1.101). As a matter of fact, these three subjects yield the largest three studentized intra-subject residuals in absolute magnitude, although they are in the opposite direction. In addition, subject 7 of sequence 1 has a very large studentized intra-subject residual (−3.053). Therefore, the first normality assumption of 8.1.2 on the intra-subject variability is questionable. From Table 6.9.1, which gives the raw AUC data, it can be seen that the AUC of

TABLE 8.2.1: Intra-subject and inter-subject residuals of raw AUC for Clayton and Leslie's study at the first period.

Subject	Y_{i1k}	$\widehat{Y}_{i1k}$	$\widehat{e}_{i1k}$	$\widetilde{e}_{i1k}$	$Y_{i\cdot k}$	$\overline{Y}_{\cdot k}$	$\widehat{S}_{ik}$	$\widehat{S}_{ik}$
1	2.52	3.277	−0.757	−0.464	7.99	8.461	−0.471	−0.118
2	8.87	6.137	2.733	1.675	13.71	8.461	5.249	1.319
3	0.79	0.802	−0.012	−0.007	3.04	8.461	−5.421	−1.362
4	1.68	1.032	0.648	0.397	3.50	8.461	−4.961	−1.247
5	6.95	6.692	0.258	0.158	14.82	8.461	6.359	1.598
6	1.05	1.432	−0.382	−0.234	4.30	8.461	−4.161	−1.046
7	0.99	5.972	−4.982	−3.053	13.38	8.461	4.919	1.236
8	5.60	4.467	1.133	0.695	10.37	8.461	1.909	0.480
9	3.16	1.802	1.358	0.832	5.04	8.461	−3.421	−0.860
10	4.98	4.481	0.499	0.306	8.17	10.234	−2.064	−0.519
11	7.14	8.881	−1.741	−1.069	16.97	10.234	6.736	1.692
12	1.81	2.756	−0.946	−0.580	4.72	10.234	−5.514	−1.386
13	7.34	6.356	0.984	0.603	11.92	10.234	1.686	0.424
14	4.25	6.046	−1.796	−1.101	11.30	10.234	1.066	0.268
15	6.66	5.431	1.229	0.753	10.07	10.234	−0.164	−0.041
16	4.76	4.021	0.739	0.453	7.25	10.234	−2.984	−0.750
17	7.16	7.066	0.094	0.058	13.34	10.234	3.106	0.780
18	5.52	4.851	0.939	0.575	8.37	10.234	−1.864	−0.469

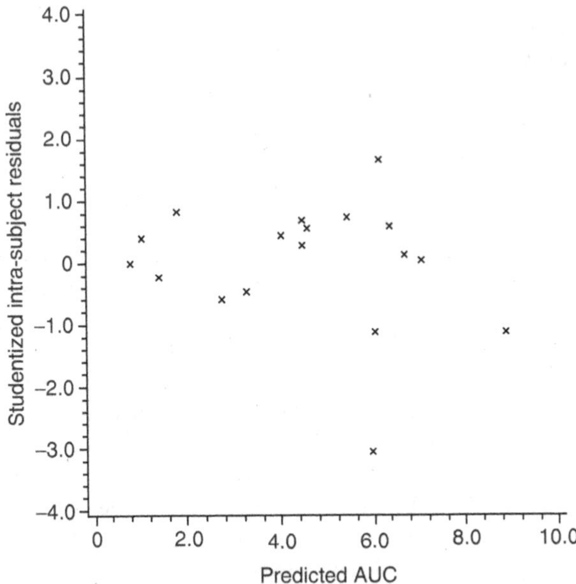

FIGURE 8.2.1: Predicted AUC versus studentized intra-subject residuals.

TABLE 8.2.2: Hourly plasma erythromycin concentrations (μg/mL) for subject 7 in Clayton and Leslie's study.

	Erythromycin	
H	**Stearate**	**Base**
0.0	0.00	0.00
0.5	0.09	0.07
1.0	0.10	0.07
1.5	0.13	0.07
2.0	0.18	0.07
3.0	0.28	0.34
4.0	0.11	3.00
6.0	0.09	2.96
8.0	0.07	1.47
AUC (μg · h/mL)	0.99	12.39

Source: From Clayton, D. and Leslie, A., *J. Int. Med. Res.*, 9, 470, 1981.

erythromycin stearate for subject 7 is 0.99, whereas the AUC of erythromycin base is 12.39. Therefore, subject 7 has an extremely low relative bioavailability, which indicates that subject 7 is a potential outlying subject. For a further investigation, Table 8.2.2 presents hourly plasma erythromycin concentrations of the two formulations for subject 7. The extremely large AUC of the base formulation may be caused by extremely high plasma concentrations occurring at 4, 6, and 8 hours after administration of the drug. However, Clayton and Leslie (1981) did not discuss the possible causes of this extreme difference.

For evaluation of the second assumption of 8.1.2, the normal probability plot of studentized intra-subject residuals is used, which is given in Figure 8.2.2. The plot shows a quadratic trend that certainly argues against the normality assumption. Departure from linearity may be explained by the unusual studentized intra-subject residuals occurring in subjects 2, 7, and 14. Shapiro–Wilk's test gives a p-value of 0.028, which also leads to rejection of the normality assumption hypothesis of e_{ilk}.

Studentized inter-subject residuals can be used to examine the first normality assumption given in Equation 8.1.2. From Table 8.2.1, no substantial studentized inter-subject residuals were observed. The normal probability plot (Figure 8.2.3) exhibits a linear relationship between residuals and their corresponding normal scores, which is in favor of the normality assumption of S_{ik}. Shapiro–Wilk's test yields a p-value of 0.267. Therefore, we fail to reject the normality assumption hypothesis of S_{ik}. Because the normality assumption for e_{ijk} may not hold, Spearman's rank correlation coefficient between $\widetilde{e}_{i1k}$ and $\widetilde{S}_{ik}$ is calculated to evaluate the independence between S_{ik} and e_{ijk}. Spearman's rank correlation coefficient gives a value of -0.013 with a p-value of 0.958. Thus, there is no evidence to suggest that

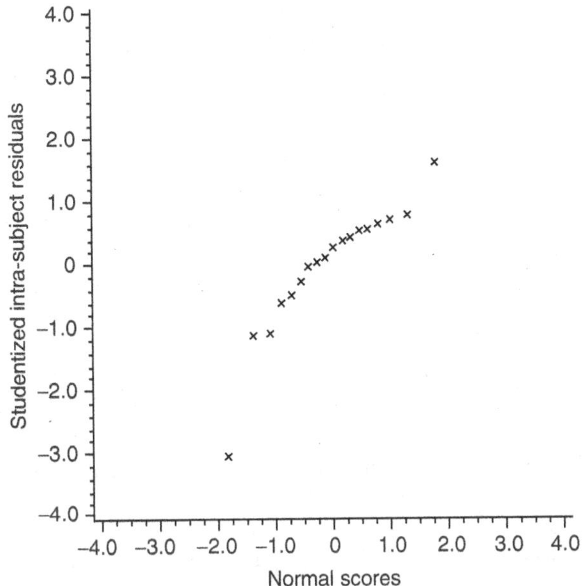

FIGURE 8.2.2: Normal probability plot of studentized intra-subject residuals. (From Liu, J.P. and Weng, C.S., *Stat. Med.*, 11, 881, 1992.)

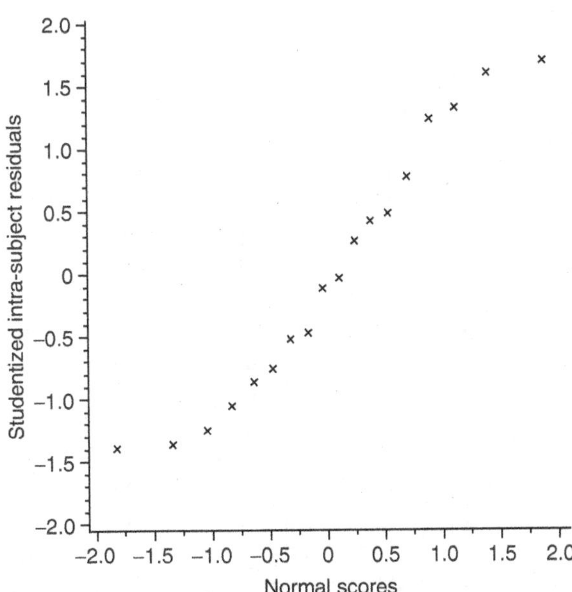

FIGURE 8.2.3: Normal probability plot of studentized inter-subject residuals. (From Liu, J.P. and Weng, C.S., *Stat. Med.*, 11, 881, 1992.)

assumption 3 of Equation 8.1.2 is not true. Therefore, based on raw AUC data, we are comfortable with all the assumptions in 8.1.2, except the normality assumption of e_{ijk}.

Log-Transformed Data

Similarly, we can examine the assumptions of 8.1.2 using intra-subject and inter-subject residuals based on log-transformed AUCs. Studentized intra-subject and inter-subject residuals are given in Table 8.2.3. The scatter plot of $\widehat{Y}_{ilk}$ versus $\widetilde{e}_{ilk}$ for log-transformed data is presented in Figure 8.2.4. From Figure 8.2.4, it can be seen that the pattern observed in the raw data disappears after log-transformation. This may indicate that the log-transformed model is more appropriate than the raw data model. However, subject 7 still has an unusually large studentized intra-subject residual (−2.750), which is outside the range of (−2, 2).

For evaluation of the first assumption of 8.1.2, both the normal probability plot for inter-subject residuals given in Figure 8.2.5 and the Shapiro–Wilk test (p-value = 0.903) suggest that S_{ik} follows a normal distribution. For assumption 2, the normal probability plot (Figure 8.2.6) for intra-subject studentized residuals shows a light departure from a straight line, which is probably due to the unusual residual of subject 7. The p-value from Shapiro–Wilk's test is given by 0.105, which

TABLE 8.2.3: Intra-subject and inter-subject residuals of log (AUC) for Clayton and Leslie's study at the first period.

Subject	Y_{ilk}	$\widehat{Y}_{ilk}$	$\widehat{e}_{ilk}$	$\widetilde{e}_{ilk}$	$Y_{i\cdot k}$	$\overline{Y}_{\cdot\cdot k}$	$\widehat{S}_{ik}$	$\widehat{S}_{ik}$
1	0.92	1.067	−0.143	−0.386	2.62	2.320	−0.304	−0.315
2	2.18	1.636	0.547	1.477	3.76	2.320	1.440	1.495
3	−0.24	0.043	−0.279	−0.753	0.58	2.320	−1.745	−1.812
4	0.52	0.315	0.204	0.551	1.12	2.320	−1.202	−1.249
5	1.94	1.757	0.182	0.491	4.00	2.320	1.682	1.747
6	0.05	0.369	−0.321	−0.865	1.23	2.320	−1.092	−1.135
7	−0.01	1.009	−1.019	−2.750	2.51	2.320	0.187	0.194
8	1.72	1.398	0.325	0.876	3.29	2.320	0.965	1.002
9	1.15	0.647	0.504	1.360	1.78	2.320	−0.538	−0.559
10	1.61	1.480	0.126	0.340	2.77	3.082	−0.316	−0.328
11	1.97	2.222	−0.257	−0.693	4.25	3.082	1.170	1.215
12	0.59	0.928	−0.334	−0.902	1.66	3.082	−1.420	−1.475
13	1.99	1.854	0.139	0.375	3.52	3.082	0.433	0.450
14	1.45	1.797	−0.350	−0.944	3.40	3.082	0.318	0.331
15	1.90	1.658	0.238	0.642	3.12	3.082	0.041	0.043
16	1.56	1.333	0.227	0.613	2.47	3.082	−0.609	−0.633
17	1.97	1.992	−0.023	−0.063	3.79	3.082	0.708	0.736
18	1.71	1.475	0.234	0.631	2.76	3.082	−0.326	−0.338

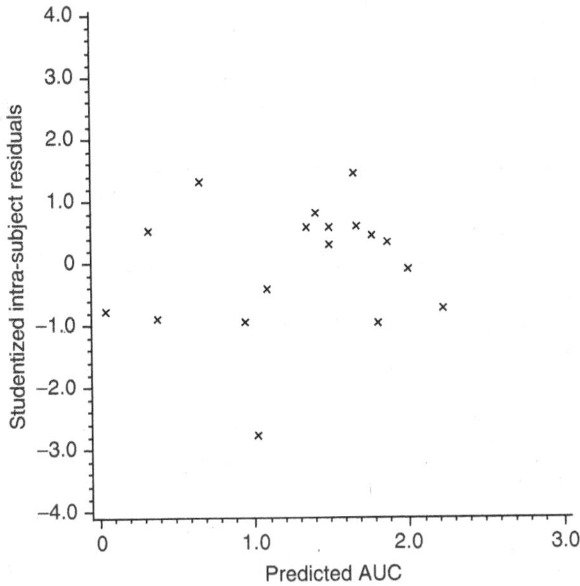

FIGURE 8.2.4: Predicted AUC versus studentized intra-subject residuals (log-transformed data).

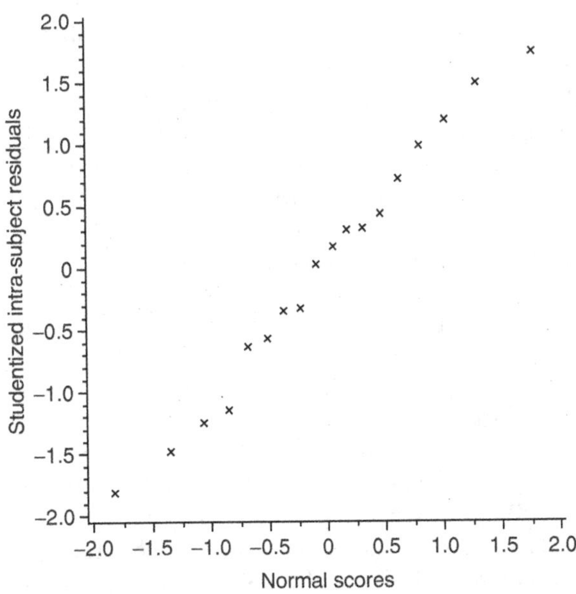

FIGURE 8.2.5: Normal probability plot of studentized inter-subject residuals (log-transformed data). (From Liu, J.P. and Weng, C.S., *Stat. Med.*, 11, 881, 1992.)

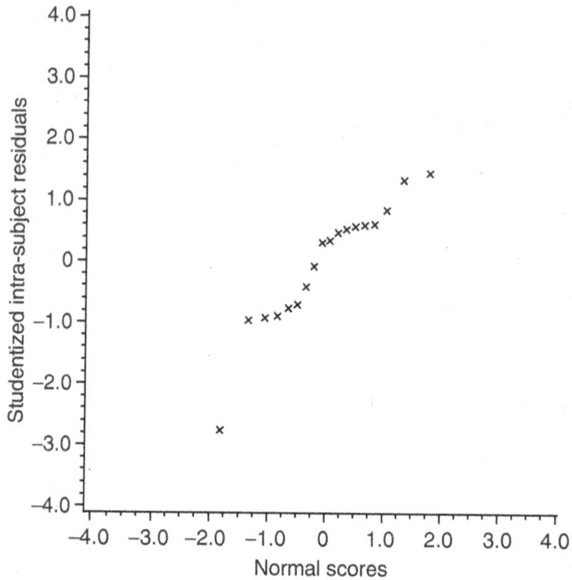

FIGURE 8.2.6: Normal probability plot of studentized intra-subject residuals (log-transformed data). (From Liu, J.P. and Weng, C.S., *Stat. Med.*, 11, 881, 1992.)

also indicates a slight deviation from the normality assumption of e_{ijk}. Independence between S_{ik} and e_{ijk} can be examined using either Pearson's correlation coefficient or Spearman's rank correlation coefficient. Both Pearson's correlation coefficient (0.211) and Spearman's rank correlation coefficient (0.214) failed to reject the hypothesis of independence (p-values $= 0.40$ and 0.39, respectively).

Note that (1) the signs of both correlation coefficients for the log-transformed data are positive, whereas correlation coefficients between $\widetilde{S}_{ik}$ and $\widetilde{e}_{i1k}$ are negative for the raw data; (2) the magnitudes of the two correlation coefficients for the log-transformed data are very close, whereas the magnitude of Spearman's rank correlation coefficient is much smaller than that of Pearson's correlation coefficient for raw data ($= -0.204$). This is because e_{ijk} of log-transformed AUCs may be normally distributed, whereas e_{ijk} of the raw AUCs are not.

It is possible that violation of the normality assumption of intra-subject variability is caused by the unusual AUCs for both stearate and base formulations observed on subject 7 in sequence 1. Therefore, we should repeat the same analyses with subject 7 deleted from the data set. These results are also summarized in Table 8.2.4 along with those obtained based on the complete data set. Because the results of the inter-subject residuals remain almost unchanged, only the normal probability plots of studentized intra-subject residuals are presented, which are given in Figure 8.2.7 for raw data and Figure 8.2.8 for log-transformed data. Figure 8.2.7 indicates little evidence of a normality assumption violation of e_{ijk} if subject 7 is excluded from the analysis. Shapiro–Wilk's test for normality also confirms this with a p-value of

TABLE 8.2.4: Summary of test results for normality assumptions.

	Shapiro–Wilk[a]		Pearson[b]		Spearman[c]	
Data Set	$\tilde{e}_{i1k}$	$\tilde{S}_{i1k}$	**Test**	***P***	**Test**	***P***
Raw AUC	0.028	0.267	−0.204	0.417	−0.013	0.958
Log (AUC)	0.105	0.903	0.211	0.400	0.214	0.395
Raw AUC[d]	0.657	0.276	0.054	0.836	0.098	0.708
Log (AUC)[d]	0.117	0.876	0.339	0.183	0.275	0.286

[a] *p*-Value of Shapiro–Wilk's test for normality.
[b] Pearson' correlation coefficient.
[c] Spearman's rank correlation coefficient.
[d] Results are obtained with deletion of subject 7.

0.657. For the log-transformed AUC, with and without subject 7, the normal probability plots are similar. The Shapiro–Wilk test also gives similar *p*-values, 0.117 (without subject 7) and 0.105 (with subject 7).

For raw data, with subject 7 deleted, both Pearson's and Spearman's correlation coefficients between studentized intra-subject and inter-subject residuals give *p*-values greater than 0.70. Although the independence assumption between e_{ijk} and S_{ik} seems to hold for log-transformed data without subject 7, the correlation coefficient magnitudes are much larger than those obtained based on the raw data. As

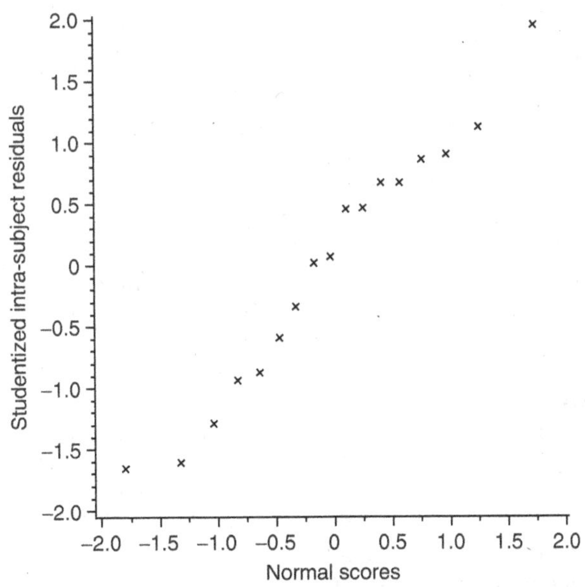

FIGURE 8.2.7: Normal probability plot of studentized intra-subject residuals without subject 7.

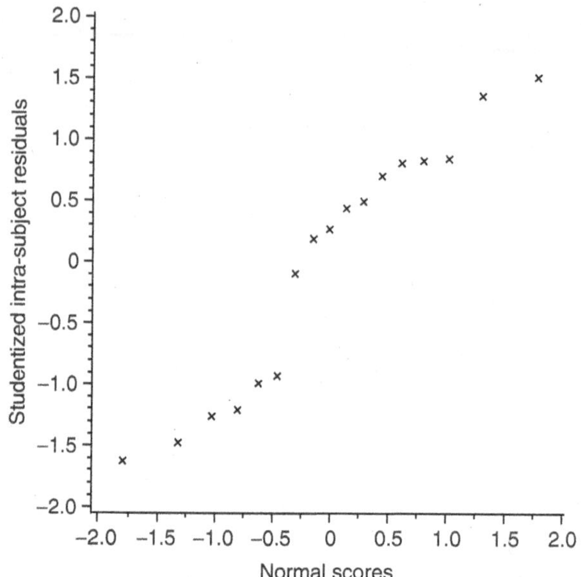

FIGURE 8.2.8: Normal probability plot of studentized intra-subject residuals (log-transformed data) without subject 7.

a result, if subject 7 is excluded, assumptions 8.1.2 hold for the raw data. In this case, the raw data model is an appropriate model for assessment of bioequivalence.

Table 8.2.5 provides estimates for inter-subject and intra-subject variabilities with and without subject 7. For the raw data, the estimate of intra-subject variability with subject 7 deleted reduces more than 55% from the estimate with subject 7 included, whereas the estimate of inter-subject variability without subject 7 increases more than 107% from the estimate including subject 7. The null hypothesis $H_0: \sigma_S^2 = 0$ is rejected at the 5% level if subject 7 is excluded from the analysis. Similar results are obtained for the log-transformed AUC. Consequently, inclusion and exclusion of the possible outlying subject has a tremendous influence on assessment of bioequivalence. Therefore, for the remainder of this chapter efforts are directed toward detection of potential outlying data.

TABLE 8.2.5: Summary of inter-subject and intra-subject variability of AUC data from Clayton and Leslie's study.

Data Set	$\widehat{\sigma}_e^2$	$\widehat{\sigma}_S^2$	*p*-Value
Raw AUC	5.992	1.459	0.218
Log (AUC)	0.309	0.106	0.153
Raw AUC[a]	2.669	2.964	0.015
Log (AUC)[a]	0.174	0.191	0.016

[a] Results are obtained with deletion of subject 7.

8.3 Definition of Outlying Observations

As indicated earlier, one of the problems commonly encountered in bioavailability studies is that the data set may contain some extremely large or small (i.e., outlying) observations. These observations may have an influence on the conclusion of bioequivalence. Basically, there are four different types of outliers:

1. Unexpected observations in the blood or plasma concentration–time curve
2. Extremely large or small observations within a given formulation
3. Unusual subjects who exhibit extremely high or low bioavailability relative to the reference formulation
4. Unusual subjects who have an extreme bioavailability to both formulations

For the first kind of outlier, Rodda (1986) indicated that unexpected observations in the plasma concentration–time curve usually have little effect on calculation of AUC and, consequently, have little effect on the comparison of bioavailbility. As an example let us consider the hourly plasma samples in Table 1.3.1. Suppose we observe an extremely high concentration at hour 16 (say 4.1). The concentration–time curve is plotted in Figure 8.3.1, which indicates that the concentration at hour 16 is a potential outlying data point. The AUC is recalculated in Table 8.3.1, which is given by 95.55. It can be seen that there is about 11.2% increase in AUC. However, contribution of this outlying concentration to the overall average is only 0.5% of 85.95 (original AUC = 11.2/24), if there are 24 subjects in the study.

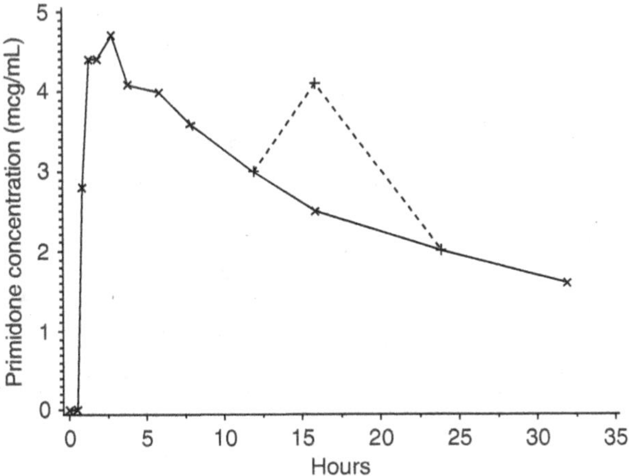

FIGURE 8.3.1: Primidone concentration–time curve: ×, raw data; +, unexpected primidone concentration of 16 hours.

TABLE 8.3.1: Calculation of AUC using the trapezoidal rule.

Blood Sample (i)	t_i	C_i	$(C_i + C_{i-1})/2$	$t_i - t_{i-1}$	$\frac{(C_i + C_{i-1})}{2(t_i - t_{i-1})}$
1	0.0	0.0	—	—	—
2	0.5	0.0	0.00	0.5	0.00
3	1.0	2.8	1.40	0.5	0.70
4	1.5	4.4	3.60	0.5	1.80
5	2.0	4.4	4.40	0.5	2.20
6	3.0	4.7	4.55	1.0	4.55
7	4.0	4.1	4.40	1.0	4.40
8	6.0	4.0	4.05	2.0	8.10
9	8.0	3.6	3.80	2.0	7.60
10	12.0	3.0	3.30	4.0	13.20
11	16.0	4.1	3.55	4.0	14.20
12	24.0	2.0	3.05	8.0	24.40
13	32.0	1.6	1.80	8.0	14.40

Note: AUC (0–32) = 95.55.

To illustrate outlying observations of a given formulation, let us again consider Clayton and Leslie's study. Figure 8.3.2 plots AUC versus subject for stearate and base formulations. It can be seen that the AUC of subject 7 has a potential outlying observation within the base formulation. This outlying observation within the base

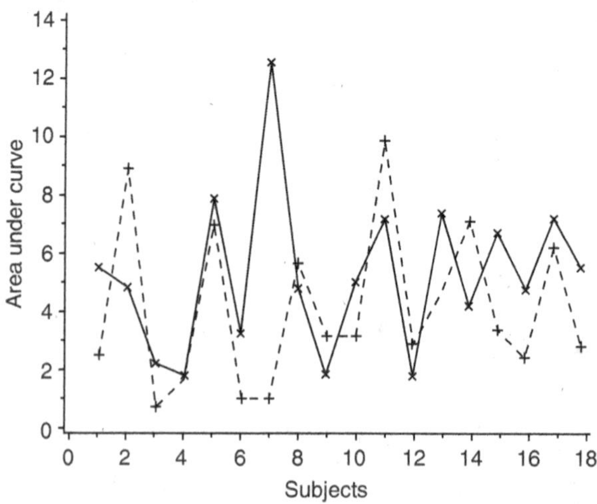

FIGURE 8.3.2: Distribution of AUC of stearate and base formulations: +, stearate formulation; ×, base formulation.

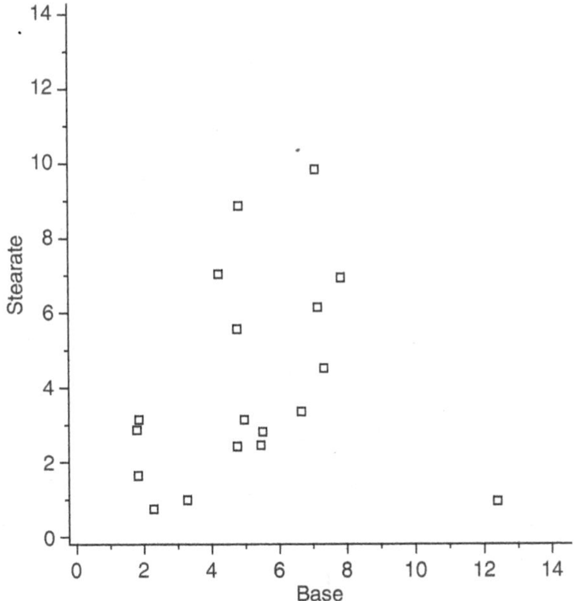

FIGURE 8.3.3: AUC of base formulations versus stearate formulations.

formulation certainly has an influence on the assessment of bioequivalence in average bioavailability because the average bioavailability is very sensitive to extreme values.

For the third kind of outlier, as indicated by Chow and Tse (1990a), an outlying subject may negate the conclusion of a bioequivalence study. Ki et al. (1995) referred this type of outliers as to Type A outliers. For a given set of data, a potential outlying subject can be examined by plotting the relative AUCs. For Clayton and Leslie's study, Figure 8.3.3 plots of AUCs of the stearate formulation versus the base formulation. An outlying subject can be detected by a relatively large deviation from the straight line $y=x$.

The last type of outliers is the subjects with extreme pharmacokinetic responses to both formulations. This type of outlier was identified as Type B oultiers by Ki et al. (1995). Although the magnitude of the relative bioavailability of test to reference formulation of Type B outlier may be similar to that of other subjects, Type B outliers increase the inter-subject variability. In addition, occurrence of Type B outliers may indicate that the underlying genetic mechanism for metabolism may be different from subjects to subjects and stratified randomization and its corresponding analysis should be considered.

It can be seen that Figures 8.3.2 and 8.3.3 are useful for a preliminary evaluation of potential outlying data. In the following section, statistical tests for detection of outlying subjects and observations within a given formulation are outlined.

8.4 Detection of Outlying Subjects

8.4.1 Likelihood Distance and Estimates Distance

For a $k \times k$ crossover design comparing f formulations of a drug product, model 8.1.1 can be rewritten as follows:

$$Y_{ijl} = \mu + S_i + F_j + P_l + e_{ijl}, \quad j, l = 1, \ldots, f; \quad i = 1, \ldots, N, \tag{8.4.1}$$

where

Y_{ijl} is the response variable on the ith subject in the lth period under the jth formulation
μ is the overall mean
F_j is the fixed effect of the jth formulation with $\Sigma_j F_j = 0$
P_l is the fixed effect of the lth period.

With $\Sigma_l P_l = 0$; S_i is the random effect of the ith subject, e_{ijl} is the error term. In the above model, it is assumed that $\{S_i\}$ and $\{e_{ijl}\}$ are independently and normally distributed with means 0 and variances σ_S^2 and σ_e^2, respectively.

For detection of an outlying subject, Chow and Tse (1990a) proposed two test procedures; namely, the likelihood distance (LD) and the estimates distance (ED) under the assumption that there are no period effects and formulation effects in model 8.4.1. Under assumption that there are no period and formulation effects, model 8.4.1 reduces to

$$Y_{ij} = \mu + S_i + e_{ij}, \quad j = 1, \ldots, f; \quad i = 1, \ldots, N. \tag{8.4.2}$$

Hence, the parameters of interest are μ, σ_S^2, and σ_e^2. Let $\boldsymbol{\theta} = (\theta_1, \theta_2, \theta_3)'$ where $\theta_1 = \mu, \theta_2 = \sigma_e^2$ and $\theta_3 = \sigma_e^2 + f\sigma_S^2$ The log-likelihood function is then given by

$$L(\theta) = \frac{-Nf}{2} \log 2\pi - \frac{N}{2} \log\left(\theta_2 \theta_3^{f-1}\right) - \frac{1}{2\theta_3} \sum_{i=i}^{N} \sum_{j=1}^{f} (Y_{ij} - \theta_1)^2$$
$$- \frac{f}{2}\left(\frac{1}{\theta_2} - \frac{1}{\theta_3}\right) \sum_{i=1}^{N} (\overline{Y}_i - \theta_1)^2. \tag{8.4.3}$$

The maximum likelihood estimator (MLE) $\widehat{\boldsymbol{\theta}}$ of θ is given by

$$\widehat{\theta}_1 = \overline{Y} = \frac{1}{Nf} \sum_{i=1}^{N} \sum_{j=1}^{f} Y_{ij},$$
$$\widehat{\theta}_2 = m_1,$$
$$\widehat{\theta}_3 = \frac{(N-1)m_2}{N}.$$

where

$$m_1 = \frac{1}{N(f-1)} \sum_{i=1}^{N} \sum_{j=1}^{f} (Y_{ij} - \overline{Y}_i)^2,$$

and

$$m_2 = \frac{f}{N-1} \sum_{i=1}^{N} (\overline{Y}_i - \overline{Y})^2.$$

It should be noted that although $\theta_3 \geq \theta_2$, it is possible that $\widehat{\theta}_3 < \widehat{\theta}_2$ [i.e., $(N-1)m_2 < Nm_1$]. In this case, the maximum likelihood estimators of θ_2 and θ_3 are modified as follows:

$$\widehat{\theta}_2 = \widehat{\theta}_3 = \frac{1}{Nf} \sum_{i=1}^{N} \sum_{j=1}^{f} (Y_{ij} - \overline{Y})^2,$$

which are obtained by maximizing $L(\theta)$ under the condition that $\theta_2 = \theta_3$. The LD test procedure is given by

$$\text{LD}_i(\widehat{\boldsymbol{\theta}}) = 2[L(\widehat{\boldsymbol{\theta}}) - L(\widehat{\boldsymbol{\theta}}_{(i)})], \tag{8.4.4}$$

where $\widehat{\boldsymbol{\theta}}_{(i)}$ denotes the MLE of θ with deletion of the ith subject. As N tends to infinity, it can be verified that $\text{LD}_i(\widehat{\boldsymbol{\theta}})$ is asymptotically distributed as a chi-square variable with 3 degrees of freedom. Thus we consider the ith subject as an outlying subject if

$$\text{LD}_i(\widehat{\boldsymbol{\theta}}) > \chi_3^2(\alpha),$$

where $\chi_3^2(\alpha)$ is the αth upper percentile point of a central chi-square distribution with 3 degrees of freedom.

A similar idea can also be applied to the estimates distance. We thus have

$$\text{ED}_i(\widehat{\boldsymbol{\theta}}) = f^2(\widehat{\boldsymbol{\theta}}_{(i)} - \widehat{\boldsymbol{\theta}})\widehat{\boldsymbol{\Sigma}}^{-1}(\widehat{\boldsymbol{\theta}}_{(i)} - \widehat{\boldsymbol{\theta}}), \tag{8.4.5}$$

where $\widehat{\boldsymbol{\Sigma}}$ is the estimate of

$$\boldsymbol{\Sigma} = \begin{bmatrix} \frac{\theta_3}{N} & 0 & 0 \\ 0 & \frac{2\theta_2^2}{N-1} & 0 \\ 0 & 0 & 2\theta_3^2 \end{bmatrix},$$

which can be obtained by substituting θ with $\widehat{\boldsymbol{\theta}}$.

Chow and Tse (1990a) showed that $\text{ED}_i(\widehat{\boldsymbol{\theta}})$ is distributed as a chi-square variable with 3 degrees of freedom as N tends to infinity. Therefore, we consider the ith subject as an outlying subject if

$$\text{ED}_i(\widehat{\boldsymbol{\theta}}) > \chi_3^2(\alpha).$$

Example 8.4.1

To illustrate the use of LD and ED test procedures, let us consider AUC data from Clayton and Leslie's study. Table 8.4.1 summarizes the MLEs of θ_1, θ_2, and θ_3 with each subject deleted and the corresponding LD and ED test results for both raw data and log-transformed data.

For raw data, it is obvious that estimates with subject 7 deleted differ substantially from the MLEs. This indicates that subject 7 is very influential in the estimation process. Furthermore, $\text{LD}_7(\widehat{\boldsymbol{\theta}}) = 9.203$ and $\text{ED}_7(\widehat{\boldsymbol{\theta}}) = 55.273$, and $\text{ED}_{11}(\widehat{\boldsymbol{\theta}}) = 8.091$ which are greater than $\chi^2_3(0.05) = 7.815$. Both LD and ED methods indicate that subject 7 is an outlier under model 8.4.1 at the 5% level of significance. However, ED method also indicates that subject 11 is an outlier based on the raw data.

For log-transformed data, the LD test procedure did not detect any outlying subject. The ED test procedure, however, indicates that subjects 3 and 7 are potential outlying subjects ($\text{ED}_3(\widehat{\boldsymbol{\theta}}) = 11.640$ and $\text{ED}_7(\widehat{\boldsymbol{\theta}}) = 39.072$, respectively).

An SAS Program for calculations of LD and ED procedures can be found in Lin et al. (1991).

8.4.2 Hotelling T^2

Liu and Weng (1991) proposed a procedure based upon the order statistics of the two-sample Hotelling T^2 to identify possible outlying subjects. A sequential step-down, closed testing procedure (Hochberg and Tamhane, 1987) is also introduced to detect multiple outlying subjects.

Under the assumption that there are no period effects and with further relaxation of the compound symmetry assumption for covariance structure of f responses observed on subject i, model 8.4.1 becomes

$$\begin{aligned} Y_{ij} &= \mu + F_j + \varepsilon_{ij} \\ &= \alpha_j + \varepsilon_{ij}, \end{aligned} \tag{8.4.6}$$

where

$i = 1, 2, \ldots, N$
$j = 1, 2, \ldots, f$
$\alpha_j = \mu + F_j$.

Let $\mathbf{Y}_i = (Y_{il}, \ldots, Y_{if})'$ be $f \times 1$ vector of the responses to f formulations observed on subject i. Thus, $\mathbf{Y}_i$ are f-dimensional multivariate normal (MVN) random vectors with mean vector $\boldsymbol{\alpha}$ and covariance matrix $\boldsymbol{\Lambda}$, where

$$\boldsymbol{\alpha} = (\boldsymbol{\alpha}_1, \ldots, \boldsymbol{\alpha}_f)',$$

and

$$\boldsymbol{\Lambda} = \text{Cov}(Y_{ij}, Y_{i'j'}) = \begin{cases} \sigma_j^2, & \text{if } i = i' \text{ and } j = j', \\ \sigma_{jj'}, & \text{if } i = i' \text{ and } j \neq j', \\ 0, & \text{otherwise.} \end{cases}$$

TABLE 8.4.1: Summary of estimation results.

I. Raw Data							
Subject[a]	$\hat{\theta}_{1(i)}$	$\hat{\theta}_{2(i)}$	$\hat{\theta}_{3(i)}$	$LD_i(\hat{\theta})$	P	$ED_i(\hat{\theta})$	P
1	4.714	6.096	8.745	0.032	0.999	0.603	0.896
2	4.546	5.875	8.210	0.078	0.994	1.378	0.711
3	4.859	6.290	7.564	0.267	0.966	4.380	0.223
4	4.846	6.352	7.738	0.214	0.975	3.642	0.303
5	4.513	6.327	7.870	0.171	0.982	2.964	0.397
6	4.822	6.210	8.009	0.122	0.989	2.135	0.545
7	4.555	2.530	8.296	9.203	0.027	55.273	0.000[b]
8	4.644	6.332	8.770	0.055	0.997	1.057	0.787
9	4.801	6.304	8.225	0.093	0.993	1.688	0.640
10	4.709	6.258	8.759	0.045	0.998	0.861	0.835
11	4.450	6.140	6.993	0.549	0.908	8.091	0.044
12	4.810	6.317	8.136	0.110	0.991	1.971	0.578
13	4.598	6.128	8.597	0.038	0.998	0.709	0.871
14	4.616	6.122	8.684	0.034	0.998	0.646	0.886
15	4.653	6.042	8.786	0.029	0.999	0.567	0.904
16	4.736	6.201	8.666	0.041	0.998	0.770	0.857
17	4.556	6.324	8.306	0.084	0.994	1.549	0.671
18	4.703	6.143	8.773	0.034	0.998	0.651	0.885
II. Log-Transformed Data							
Subject[a]	$\hat{\theta}_{1(i)}$	$\hat{\theta}_{2(i)}$	$\hat{\theta}_{3(i)}$	$LD_i(\hat{\theta})$	P	$ED_i(\hat{\theta})$	P
1	1.353	0.346	0.567	0.029	0.999	0.569	0.903
2	1.319	0.353	0.533	0.072	0.995	1.301	0.729
3	1.413	0.332	0.427	0.845	0.839	11.640	0.009
4	1.397	0.364	0.490	0.264	0.967	4.391	0.222
5	1.312	0.363	0.515	0.145	0.986	2.559	0.465
6	1.394	0.326	0.500	0.204	0.977	3.415	0.332
7	1.356	0.176	0.566	5.121	0.163	39.072	0.000[b]
8	1.333	0.363	0.557	0.059	0.996	1.123	0.772
9	1.377	0.356	0.541	0.060	0.996	1.105	0.776
10	1.348	0.358	0.567	0.044	0.998	0.844	0.839
11	1.305	0.361	0.493	0.239	0.971	3.978	0.264
12	1.381	0.357	0.534	0.076	0.995	1.385	0.709
13	1.326	0.357	0.547	0.055	0.997	1.017	0.797
14	1.330	0.356	0.552	0.047	0.997	0.882	0.830
15	1.338	0.351	0.562	0.033	0.998	0.635	0.888
16	1.357	0.352	0.566	0.034	0.998	0.644	0.886
17	1.318	0.363	0.531	0.098	0.992	1.783	0.619
18	1.349	0.351	0.567	0.033	0.998	0.635	0.888

[a] Deleted subject.
[b] p-Value < 0.001.

The hypothesis for outlying subjects caused by a location shift can be formulated as follows:

$$\begin{aligned} &\mathrm{H_0}\colon\ \mathbf{Y}_i \sim \mathrm{MVN}(\boldsymbol{\alpha}, \boldsymbol{\Lambda}), \quad \text{for all } i = 1, 2, \ldots, N, \\ \text{versus}\quad &\mathrm{H_a}\colon\ \mathbf{Y}_i \sim \mathrm{MVN}(\boldsymbol{\alpha} + \boldsymbol{\Delta}_i, \boldsymbol{\Lambda}) \quad \text{for at least one } i. \end{aligned} \tag{8.4.7}$$

The above hypothesis can be further decomposed into the following N subhypothesis:

$$\begin{aligned} &\mathrm{H}_{0i}\colon\ \mathbf{Y}_i \sim \mathrm{MVN}(\boldsymbol{\alpha}, \boldsymbol{\Lambda}) \\ \text{versus}\quad &\mathrm{H_a}i\colon\ \mathbf{Y}_i \sim \mathrm{MVN}(\boldsymbol{\alpha} + \boldsymbol{\Delta}_i, \boldsymbol{\Lambda}), \end{aligned} \tag{8.4.8}$$

where $i = 1, 2, \ldots, N$.

Note that $\mathrm{H_0} = \cap_i \mathrm{H}_{0i}$ and $\mathrm{H_a} = \cup_i \mathrm{H}_{ai}$. Therefore, the sequential step-down closed testing procedure introduced by Hochberg and Tamhane (1987) can be applied to subhypothesis Equation 8.4.8 for detection of possible multiple outlying subjects. Hypothesis Equation 8.4.8 can be tested using the two-sample Hotelling's T^2 statistics by comparing a sample that consists only of the ith subject with the sample of other $N-1$ subjects (Hawkins, 1980).

Let $\overline{\mathbf{Y}}$ and $\mathbf{A}$ be the sample mean and matrix of the sums of squares and cross products computed from $\mathbf{Y}_1, \ldots, \mathbf{Y}_N$, respectively. Also, let $\overline{\mathbf{Y}}_{(i)}$ and $\mathbf{A}_{(-i)}$ be the sample mean and matrix of the sum of squares and cross products computed from $N-1$ subjects with deletion of the ith subject. The two-sample Hotelling T^2 statistic for the ith subject is then given by

$$T_i^2 = \frac{(N-1)(N-2)}{N}(\mathbf{Y}_i - \overline{\mathbf{Y}}_{(-1)})'\mathbf{A}_{(-i)}^{-1}(\mathbf{Y}_i - \overline{\mathbf{Y}}_{(-i)}), \tag{8.4.9}$$

where $i = 1, 2, \ldots, N$.

Computation of T_i^2 can be simplified as

$$T_i^2 = \frac{(N-2)D_i^2}{\left[\dfrac{N-1}{N} - D_i^2\right]}, \tag{8.4.10}$$

where

$$D_i^2 = (\mathbf{Y}_i - \overline{\mathbf{Y}})'\mathbf{A}^{-1}(\mathbf{Y}_i - \overline{\mathbf{Y}}), \quad i = 1, 2 \ldots, N.$$

Note that Hotelling T^2 is invariant under any full-rank linear transformation. Consequently, the joint distribution of $\{T_i^2, i = 1, 2, \ldots, N\}$ is independent of the unknown parameters $\boldsymbol{\alpha}$ and $\boldsymbol{\Lambda}$. The testing procedure proposed by Liu and Weng (1991) is outlined as follows:

Let $T_{(1)}^2, \ldots, T_{(N)}^2$ be the order statistics of $T_1^2, \ldots, T_N^2$, and $\mathrm{H}_{0(i)}$ be the corresponding subhypothesis based on $T_{(i)}^2$. Also, let $(\mathbf{W}_1^2, \ldots, \mathbf{W}_N^2)$ be a vector of N Hotelling T^2 statistics computed from a sample of size N from an f-dimensional multivariate normal with mean $\mathbf{0}$ and covariance matrix $\mathbf{I}_f$. We start with the order subhypothesis $\mathrm{H}_{0(N)}$. Hypothesis $\mathrm{H}_{0(i)}$ is rejected if

$$P\left\{\max_{1 \le j \le i} W_j^2 > T_{(i)}^2\right\} < \alpha \tag{8.4.11}$$

provided that $H_{0(N)}$, $H_{0(N-1)}, \ldots, H_{0(i+1)}$ are rejected at the α level of significance, where $0 < \alpha < 1$.

Note that the joint distribution of order statistics of $\{T_i^2, i = 1, 2, \ldots, N\}$ is rather complicated. However, the sampling distribution of $T_{(i)}^2$ under $H_{0(i)}$ can be empirically evaluated by the Monte Carlo simulation using standard multivariate normal vectors because it is independent of $\boldsymbol{\alpha}$ and $\boldsymbol{\Lambda}$. Tables 8.4.2 and 8.4.3 give the 5% and 1% upper quantiles of the distribution of ordered T^2 statistics for $f = 2$, 3 and $N = 10(1)20$ and 20(5)50, which were obtained based on 3000 simulation samples.

The procedure for detection of a potential outlying subject proposed by Chow and Tse (1990a) is based on the asymptotic distribution of LD and ED. The disadvantage of Chow and Tse's procedure is that the sample size for a bioavailability study is sometimes too small to apply asymptotic distributions of LD and ED. In addition, evaluation of LD or ED involves simultaneous estimation of formulation average, inter-subject, and intra-subject variabilities. As an alternative, Liu and Weng (1991) suggested the use of the parametric bootstrap technique (Efron, 1982) for empirical evaluation of the sampling distribution of the order statistics of LD_i because the joint distribution of LD_i is not independent of the unknown parameters θ_1 θ_2, and θ_3. Chow and Tse's method can be further extended to detect possible multiple outlying subjects, which is stated as follows.

At each iteration, a sample of size N for f-dimensional multivariate normal random vectors with mean $\widehat{\boldsymbol{\theta}}_1 \mathbf{1}_f$ and covariance matrix $\widehat{\boldsymbol{\theta}}_2 \mathbf{I}_f + (\widehat{\boldsymbol{\theta}}_3 - \widehat{\boldsymbol{\theta}}_2) f^{-1} \mathbf{I}_f$ is generated, where $\mathbf{1}_f$ is an $f \times 1$ vector of 1s, $\mathbf{I}_f$ is an $f \times f$ identity matrix, and $\mathbf{J}_f$ is an $f \times f$ matrix of 1s. We can compute LD_i (or ED_i) according to Equation 8.4.4 or 8.4.5. Sampling distribution of the order statistics of LD_i (or ED_i) can then be obtained by iterating the process a large number of times (e.g., B times) and the same procedure in Equation 8.4.11 can be applied by replacing T^2 with LD_i (or ED_i).

Example 8.4.2

We again use AUC data from Clayton–Leslie's study to illustrate the above procedure for detection of possible outlying subjects. Table 8.4.4 gives likelihood distances, which were calculated based on model 8.4.2, and Hotelling T^2 statistics, which were obtained under model 8.4.6, for both raw and log-transformed AUC data.

For raw AUC data, as expected, subject 7 gives the maximum T^2 value of 28.738 with a p-value of 0.004. Therefore, we reject the order subhypothesis $H_{0(18)}$ at the 5% level of significance. We then proceed to test the subsequent order subhypothesis $H_{0(17)}$. Subject 11 yields the second largest $T^2[T_{(17)}^2 = 6.237]$ with a corresponding p-value of 0.38. Thus, we fail to reject $H_{0(17)}$ at the 5% level and the sequential testing procedure stops. On the basis of the empirical sampling distribution of the order statistics of Hotelling T^2, we conclude that subject 7 is an outlying subject. For use of likelihood distance, subject 7 also gives the maximum LD with a value of 9.203.

TABLE 8.4.2: α% upper quantiles of the ordered T^2 statistics.

Sample Size	$T^2_{(N)}$	$T^2_{(N-1)}$	$T^2_{(N-2)}$	$T^2_{(N-3)}$
For $f = 2$ and $\alpha = 0.05$				
10	22.67	9.01	5.25	3.72
11	21.80	8.97	5.46	3.88
12	20.16	9.03	5.55	4.05
13	18.83	9.12	5.70	4.32
14	18.67	9.03	6.03	4.46
15	18.55	9.30	6.09	4.63
16	17.92	9.11	6.22	4.73
17	17.15	9.34	6.34	4.90
18	17.32	9.25	6.43	5.04
19	16.88	9.33	6.48	5.18
20	16.47	9.49	6.71	5.20
25	16.21	9.61	6.96	5.70
30	15.79	9.83	7.39	6.09
35	16.33	10.05	7.77	6.43
40	16.29	10.27	8.00	6.74
45	16.12	10.37	8.29	6.95
50	15.86	10.57	8.40	7.17
For $f = 2$ and $\alpha = 0.01$				
10	40.26	12.04	6.44	4.35
11	36.38	12.23	6.64	4.59
12	32.37	11.67	6.79	4.69
13	29.65	11.98	7.11	4.97
14	28.68	11.37	7.16	5.20
15	28.32	11.63	7.17	5.25
16	25.96	11.49	7.30	5.50
17	26.07	12.47	7.53	5.57
18	24.99	11.79	7.58	5.82
19	22.73	12.01	7.74	5.83
20	25.14	11.59	7.87	5.98
25	22.51	11.98	8.03	6.49
30	21.96	11.89	8.69	6.82
35	21.90	12.17	8.97	7.14
40	20.84	12.21	9.20	7.65
45	20.73	12.67	9.31	7.70
50	19.67	12.17	9.61	7.90

As $9.203 > \chi^2_3(0.05) = 7.815$ according to Chow and Tse (1990a), subject 7 is also identified as an outlying subject. However, the p-value based on the empirical sampling distribution of $\text{LD}_{(18)}$, which was obtained from 3000 bootstrap samples, is 0.002.

TABLE 8.4.3: α% upper quantiles of the ordered T^2 statistics.

For $f = 3$ and $\alpha = 0.05$				
Sample Size	$T^2_{(N)}$	$T^2_{(N-1)}$	$T^2_{(N-2)}$	$T^2_{(N-3)}$
10	39.91	15.64	9.73	6.61
11	34.28	15.42	9.63	6.84
12	30.63	14.78	9.51	6.92
13	28.41	14.47	9.76	7.19
14	27.22	13.99	9.56	7.20
15	26.09	13.92	9.70	7.37
16	25.19	13.38	9.65	7.51
17	24.62	13.55	9.52	7.59
18	24.50	13.37	9.82	7.65
19	23.02	13.46	9.93	7.79
20	22.73	13.48	9.86	7.59
25	21.32	13.17	10.18	8.27
30	20.49	13.11	10.34	8.64
35	20.57	13.47	10.57	9.03
40	19.86	13.55	10.71	9.24
45	19.59	13.33	10.96	9.41
50	19.42	13.72	11.07	9.77
For $f = 3$ and $\alpha = 0.01$				
10	63.13	22.04	12.06	7.67
11	52.28	21.40	12.16	8.20
12	50.43	19.38	11.65	7.97
13	40.41	18.90	11.65	8.30
14	40.90	18.04	11.55	8.29
15	38.14	18.21	11.46	8.46
16	36.59	17.17	11.58	8.50
17	37.93	16.87	11.36	8.65
18	34.60	16.41	11.52	8.81
19	31.54	17.01	11.76	8.76
20	30.51	16.98	11.96	8.86
25	28.02	16.22	11.72	9.37
30	26.18	15.31	11.96	9.79
35	26.61	15.90	11.88	10.17
40	25.36	15.93	12.33	10.24
45	24.73	15.98	12.34	10.51
50	23.90	15.68	12.66	10.66

Source: From Liu, J.P. and Weng, C.S., *Stat. Med.*, 10, 1375, 1991.

TABLE 8.4.4: Hotelling T^2 and likelihood distances for AUC data from Clayton and Leslie's study.

	Raw Data		Log-Transformed Data	
Subject	T^2	**LD**	T^2	**LD**
1	0.403	0.032	0.327	0.029
2	4.222	0.078	2.163	0.072
3	2.629	0.267	5.452	0.845
4	2.329	0.214	3.511	0.264
5	1.898	0.171	1.650	0.145
6	1.695	0.122	2.678	0.204
7	28.738	9.203	17.545	5.121
8	0.395	0.055	0.571	0.059
9	1.749	0.093	3.388	0.060
10	0.118	0.045	0.029	0.044
11	6.237	0.549	2.677	0.239
12	1.860	0.110	3.593	0.076
13	0.647	0.038	0.795	0.055
14	1.703	0.034	1.414	0.047
15	0.444	0.029	0.494	0.033
16	0.369	0.041	0.167	0.034
17	0.957	0.084	1.119	0.098
18	0.267	0.034	0.206	0.033

Therefore, $H_{0(18)}$ is rejected at the 5% level. Similarly, $H_{0(17)}$ is not rejected because the p-value corresponding to the $LD_{(17)} = 0.549$ of subject 11 is 0.42. Hence, the sequential testing procedure stops and we conclude that subject 7 is an outlying subject.

For log-transformed AUC data, again subject 7 yields the maximum T^2 with a value of 17.545 which is greater than 17.32, the 5% upper quantile of $T^2_{(18)}$ (see Table 8.4.2). Therefore, $H_{0(18)}$ is rejected at the 5% level. Since $T^2_{(17)} = 5.452$ of subject 3 is less than 9.25, the 5% quantile of $T^2_{(17)}$, we fail to reject $H_{0(17)}$ at the 5% level. Consequently, the sequential testing procedure stops and we conclude that subject 7 is an outlying subject. For likelihood distance, subject 7 also gives the largest LD of 5.121. Because 5.121 is less than $\chi^2_3(0.05) = 7.815$, we cannot declare that subject 7 is an outlying subject according to the procedure proposed by Chow and Tse (1990a). However, the p-value evaluated from the empirical sampling distribution of $LD_{(18)}$ is 0.023, which suggests a rejection of $H_{0(18)}$ at the 5% level. The p-value corresponding to $LD_{(17)} = 0.845$ of subject 3 is 0.179. Therefore, the sequential testing procedure stops and we conclude that subject 7 is an outlying subject.

Inconsistency between the empirical sampling distribution of the order statistics and the asymptotic distribution of LD for log-transformed AUC data may occur because there are too few subjects in this study. A comparison between the 5% upper quantile of a χ^2 with 3 degrees of freedom and that of the empirical sampling distribution of LD strongly suggests that the empirical sampling distribution of LD is stochastically smaller than that of χ_3^2. This suggests that the empirical sampling distribution of LD should be used if the LD test procedure is considered for detection of a possible outlying subject.

8.5 Detection of Outlying Observations

8.5.1 Residual Approaches

Liu and Weng (1991) proposed a method for detection of potential outlying observations. Their procedure is based on residuals from the formulation means, which can be estimated under the following model:

$$\begin{aligned} Y_{ij} &= \mu + F_j + S_i + e_{ij} \\ &= \alpha_j + S_i + e_{ij}, \end{aligned} \tag{8.5.1}$$

where

$\alpha_j = \mu + F_j$

$i = 1, 2, \ldots, N$ (number of subjects)

$j = 1, 2, \ldots, f$ (number of formulations).

Model 8.5.1 is a reduced model of Equation 8.4.1 under the assumption of no period effects.

$$\text{Let } \overline{\mathrm{Y}}_i = (Y_{il}, \ldots, Y_{if})', \quad i = 1, \ldots, N; \quad \text{and} \quad \mathbf{Y} = (\mathbf{Y}_1', \ldots, \mathbf{Y}_N')'.$$

Under the assumption of model 8.4.1, $\mathbf{Y}$ is then an M-dimensional multivariate normal vector with mean vector $\mathbf{1}_\mathrm{N} \otimes \boldsymbol{\alpha}$ and covariance matrix $\mathbf{I}_\mathrm{N} \otimes \Sigma$, where $M = Nf$, $\otimes$ is the Kronecker product between two matrices $\boldsymbol{\alpha} = (\alpha_1, \ldots, \alpha_f)'$ and $\boldsymbol{\Sigma} = \sigma_\mathrm{e}^2 \mathbf{I}_f + \sigma_\mathrm{S}^2 \mathbf{J}_f$.

Define

$$\mathrm{MSF} = \frac{N}{f-1} \sum_{j=1}^{f} (\overline{Y}_{\cdot j} - \overline{Y}_{\cdot\cdot})^2,$$

$$\mathrm{MSB} = \frac{f}{N-1} \sum_{i=1}^{N} (\overline{Y}_{i\cdot} - \overline{Y}_{\cdot\cdot})^2,$$

and

$$\mathrm{MSE} = \frac{1}{(N-1)(f-1)} [\mathrm{SST} - (f-1)\mathrm{MSF} - (N-1)\mathrm{MSB}], \tag{8.5.2}$$

where

$$\text{SST} = \sum_{i=1}^{N} \sum_{j=1}^{f} (Y_{ij} - \overline{Y}_{\cdot\cdot})^2,$$

and

$$\overline{Y}_{\cdot j} = \frac{1}{N} \sum_{i=1}^{N} Y_{ij}, \quad \overline{Y}_{i\cdot} = \frac{1}{f} \sum_{j=1}^{f} Y_{ij},$$

and

$$\overline{Y}_{\cdot\cdot} = \frac{1}{Nf} \sum_{i=1}^{N} \sum_{j=1}^{f} Y_{ij}.$$

The restricted maximum likelihood estimators (Hocking, 1985) for α_j, σ_S^2, and σ_e^2 under model 8.5.1 are then given by

$$\begin{aligned} \widehat{\alpha}_j &= \overline{Y}_{\cdot j}, \\ \widehat{\sigma}_e^2 &= \text{MSE}, \\ \widehat{\sigma}_S^2 &= \frac{(\text{MSB} - \text{MSE})}{f}. \end{aligned} \qquad (8.5.3)$$

When MSB < MSE, $\widehat{\sigma}_S^2 = 0$, and

$$\widehat{\sigma}_e^2 = \frac{1}{f(N-1)} \sum_{i=1}^{N} \sum_{j=1}^{f} (Y_{ij} - \overline{Y}_{\cdot j})^2.$$

Therefore, consistent estimators for $\boldsymbol{\alpha}$ and $\boldsymbol{\Sigma}$ can be obtained as follows:

$$\begin{aligned} \widehat{\boldsymbol{\alpha}} &= (\overline{Y}_{\cdot 1}, \ldots, \overline{Y}_{\cdot f})', \\ \widehat{\boldsymbol{\Sigma}} &= \widehat{\sigma}_e^2 \mathbf{I}_f + \widehat{\sigma}_S^2 \mathbf{J}_f. \end{aligned} \qquad (8.5.4)$$

The vector of residuals from the formulation means is then given by

$$\begin{aligned} \mathbf{R} &= \mathbf{Y} - \mathbf{1}_N \otimes \widehat{\boldsymbol{\alpha}} \\ &= \left[\left(\mathbf{I}_N - \frac{1}{N} \mathbf{J}_N \right) \otimes \mathbf{I}_f \right] \mathbf{Y}. \end{aligned} \qquad (8.5.5)$$

$\mathbf{R}$ is distributed as an M-dimensional multivariate normal (singular) with mean $\mathbf{0}$ and covariance matrix

$$\text{Cov}(\mathbf{R}) = \left[\left(\mathbf{I}_N - \frac{1}{N} \mathbf{J}_N \right) \otimes \Sigma \right]. \qquad (8.5.6)$$

The studentized residuals from the formulation means are then given by

$$r_{ij} = \frac{Y_{ij} - \overline{Y}_{\times j}}{\left[\frac{N-1}{N}\left(\widehat{\sigma}_e^2 + \widehat{\sigma}_S^2\right)\right]^{1/2}}, \quad i = 1, 2, \ldots, N; \quad j = 1, 2, \ldots, f. \tag{8.5.7}$$

Define

$$z_m = r_{ij},$$

where

$$m = f(i-1) + j,$$

where

$i = 1, \ldots, N$
$j = 1, \ldots, f$
$m = 1, 2, \ldots, M.$

$\mathbf{Z} = (z_1, \ldots, z_m)'$ is then approximately distributed as a multivariate normal vector (singular, $M - f$) with mean vector $\mathbf{0}$ and covariance $\mathbf{V}$, where $\mathbf{V}$ is the M by M correlation matrix of $\mathbf{R}$ obtained from the estimated covariance matrix $\widehat{\mathbf{\Sigma}}$. If the possible outlying observations are due to a location shift and not due to dispersion, we can then express the hypothesis of outlying observations in terms of the means Δ_m of the distribution of z_m; namely,

$$\begin{aligned} &\text{H}_0\text{: } \Delta_m = 0 \quad \text{for all } m = 1, 2, \ldots, M, \\ \text{versus} \quad &\text{H}_\text{a}\text{: } \Delta_m \neq 0 \quad \text{for at least one } m. \end{aligned} \tag{8.5.8}$$

Under model 8.5.1 and H_0 in Equation 8.5.8, z_m are identically distributed as a standard normal variable. Hypothesis Equation 8.5.8 can be further decomposed into M subhypotheses

$$\begin{aligned} &\text{H}_{0m}\text{: } \Delta_m = 0 \\ \text{versus} \quad &\text{H}_{am}\text{: } \Delta_m \neq 0, \quad m = 1, \ldots, M. \end{aligned} \tag{8.5.9}$$

We can apply the sequential stepdown, closed testing procedure to these M subhypotheses for detection of possible outlying observations as presented in the following.

Let $|z|_{(1)}, \ldots, |z|_{(M)}$ be the order statistics of $|z_1|, \ldots, |z_M|$ and $\text{H}_{0(m)}$ be the corresponding ordered null subhypothesis, where $|z_M|$ is the absolute value of z_m. Also, let $(\mathbf{T}_1, \ldots, \mathbf{T}_M)'$ be an M-dimensional vector of the studentized residuals generated from the model 8.5.1. We then start with the ordered null subhypothesis $\text{H}_{0(M)}$. We reject $\text{H}_{0(m)}, m = M, M-1, \ldots, 1$, if

$$P\left\{\max_{1 \leq j \leq m} |T| > |z|_{(m)}\right\} < \alpha \tag{8.5.10}$$

provided that $H_{0(M)}, \ldots, H_{0(m+1)}$ are all rejected at the α level of significance. Because the exact joint distribution of the order statistics for $|z_1|, \ldots, |z_M|$ is somewhat complicated to obtain, Liu and Weng (1991) suggested the following parametric bootstrap procedure to evaluate the empirical sampling distribution of $|z|_{(m)}$ under $H_{0(m)}, m = M, M-1, \ldots, 1$.

At each iteration, a sample of size N for f-dimensional normal random vectors with mean $\widehat{\boldsymbol{\alpha}}$ and covariance matrix $\widehat{\boldsymbol{\Sigma}}$ are generated and studentized residuals $\mathbf{T}_1, \ldots, \mathbf{T}_M$ are calculated according to Equation 8.5.7. The empirical sampling distribution of $|z|_{(m)}$ can then be obtained by repeating this process many (e.g., B) times. The probability Equation 8.5.10 can then be evaluated by computing the proportion of the number of events that satisfy

$$P\left\{\max_{1 \leq j \leq m} |T| > z_{(m)}\right\}, \quad m = M, M-1, \ldots, 1.$$

Example 8.5.1

Under model Equation 8.27, the restricted MLE of σ_e^2 and σ_S^2 based on the AUC data [or log(AUC)] from Clayton and Leslie's study are given by 5.695 and 1.554 (0.302 and 0.133), respectively. Studentized residuals from the formulation means are given in Table 8.5.1 (for raw AUC) and Table 8.5.2 [for log(AUC)].

From Table 8.5.1, it can be seen that the maximum absolute studentized residual $|z|_{(36)}$ occurred at the AUC value of the erythromycin base formulation in subject 7 within sequence 1 with a value of 2.736. The p-value based on the empirical sampling distribution of $|z|_{(36)}$ from 3000 bootstrap samples is 0.15. Therefore, we fail to reject $H_{0(36)}$ at the 5% level of significance. Thus, the sequential testing procedure stops and we conclude that there are no outlying observations for the raw AUC data. Similarly, from Table 8.5.2, the empirical sampling distribution of $|z|_{(36)}$ for log-transformed AUC gives a p-value of 0.681 which leads to the same conclusion of no outlying observations.

Note that we are unable to identify any outlying observations according to the sequential testing procedure discussed in this section, although subject 7 in sequence 1 was identified as an outlying subject by either the two-sample Hotelling T^2 or likelihood distance. This inconsistency may be explained by the following reasons. First, model 8.5.1 proposed by Liu and Weng (1991) may not be adequate for Clayton and Leslie's data set. Second, the procedure proposed by Liu and Weng (1991) may not be able to detect outlying observations owing to differences in variabilities. Recall in Example 8.2.1 that intra-subject and inter-subject variabilities change more than 50% with deletion of subject 7. This indicates that subject 7 may be drawn from a population with different intra-subject or inter-subject variabilities than the rest of subjects in the study. Finally, the AUC of the two erythromycin formulations for subject 7 may differ, individually, from their respective formulation means. However, they are not extreme enough to be declared as outlying observations when considered

TABLE 8.5.1: Residuals from the formulation means (raw data).

Sequence	Subject	Formulation	AUC	Formulation Mean	Residual	Absolute Studentized Residual
1	1	Base	5.47	5.2311	0.2389	0.0913
1	1	Stearate	2.52	4.1167	−1.5967	0.6102
1	2	Base	4.84	5.2311	−0.3911	0.1495
1	2	Stearate	8.87	4.1167	4.7533	1.8167
1	3	Base	2.25	5.2311	−2.9811	1.1394
1	3	Stearate	0.79	4.1167	−3.3267	1.2714
1	4	Base	1.82	5.2311	−3.4111	1.3037
1	4	Stearate	1.68	4.1167	−2.4367	0.9313
1	5	Base	7.87	5.2311	2.6389	1.0086
1	5	Stearate	6.95	4.1167	2.8333	1.0829
1	6	Base	3.25	5.2311	−1.9811	0.7572
1	6	Stearate	1.05	4.1167	−3.0667	1.1721
1	7	Base	12.39	5.2311	7.1589	2.7361
1	7	Stearate	0.99	4.1167	−3.1267	1.1950
1	8	Base	4.77	5.2311	−0.4611	0.1762
1	8	Stearate	5.60	4.1167	1.4833	0.5669
1	9	Base	1.88	5.2311	−3.3511	1.2808
1	9	Stearate	3.16	4.1167	−0.9567	0.3656
2	10	Base	4.98	5.2311	−0.2511	0.0960
2	10	Stearate	3.19	4.1167	−0.9267	0.3542
2	11	Base	7.14	5.2311	1.9089	0.7296
2	11	Stearate	9.83	4.1167	5.7133	2.1836
2	12	Base	1.81	5.2311	−3.4211	1.3075
2	12	Stearate	2.91	4.1167	−1.2067	0.4612
2	13	Base	7.34	5.2311	2.1089	0.8060
2	13	Stearate	4.58	4.1167	0.4633	0.1771
2	14	Base	4.25	5.2311	−0.9811	0.3750
2	14	Stearate	7.05	4.1167	2.9333	1.1211
2	15	Base	6.66	5.2311	1.4289	0.5461
2	15	Stearate	3.41	4.1167	−0.7067	0.2701
2	16	Base	4.76	5.2311	−0.4711	0.1801
2	16	Stearate	2.49	4.1167	−1.6267	0.6217
2	17	Base	7.16	5.2311	1.9289	0.7372
2	17	Stearate	6.18	4.1167	2.0633	0.7886
2	18	Base	5.52	5.2311	0.2889	0.1104
2	18	Stearate	2.85	4.1167	−1.2667	0.4841

Source: From Clayton, D. and Leslie, A., *J. Int. Med. Res.*, 9, 470, 1981.

TABLE 8.5.2: Residuals from the formulation means (log-transformed data).

Sequence	Subject	Formulation	AUC	Formulation Mean	Residual	Absolute Studentized Residual
1	1	Base	1.6993	1.5209	0.1784	0.2783
1	1	Stearate	0.9243	1.1798	−0.2556	0.3987
1	2	Base	1.5769	1.5209	0.0560	0.0874
1	2	Stearate	2.1827	1.1798	1.0029	1.5646
1	3	Base	0.8109	1.5209	−0.7100	1.1077
1	3	Stearate	−0.2357	1.1798	−1.4155	2.2085
1	4	Base	0.5988	1.5209	−0.9221	1.4386
1	4	Stearate	0.5188	1.1798	−0.6610	1.0313
1	5	Base	2.0631	1.5209	0.5422	0.8459
1	5	Stearate	1.9387	1.1798	0.7589	1.1840
1	6	Base	1.1787	1.5209	−0.3422	0.5340
1	6	Stearate	0.0488	1.1798	−1.1310	1.7646
1	7	Base	2.5169	1.5209	0.9960	1.5539
1	7	Stearate	−0.0101	1.1798	−1.1899	1.8564
1	8	Base	1.5623	1.5209	0.0414	0.0647
1	8	Stearate	1.7228	1.1798	0.5429	0.8471
1	9	Base	0.6313	1.5209	−0.8896	1.3880
1	9	Stearate	1.1506	1.1798	−0.0293	0.0456
2	10	Base	1.6054	1.5209	0.0845	0.1319
2	10	Stearate	1.1600	1.1798	−0.0198	0.0309
2	11	Base	1.9657	1.5209	0.4448	0.6940
2	11	Stearate	2.2854	1.1798	1.1056	1.7249
2	12	Base	0.5933	1.5209	−0.9276	1.4472
2	12	Stearate	1.0682	1.1798	−0.1117	0.1742
2	13	Base	1.9933	1.5209	0.4724	0.7371
2	13	Stearate	1.5217	1.1798	0.3419	0.5334
2	14	Base	1.4469	1.5209	−0.0740	0.1154
2	14	Stearate	1.9530	1.1798	0.7732	1.2063
2	15	Base	1.8961	1.5209	0.3752	0.5854
2	15	Stearate	1.2267	1.1798	0.0469	0.0732
2	16	Base	1.5602	1.5209	0.0393	0.0614
2	16	Stearate	0.9123	1.1798	−0.2675	0.4174
2	17	Base	1.9685	1.5209	0.4476	0.6983
2	17	Stearate	1.8213	1.1798	0.6415	1.0008
2	18	Base	1.7084	1.5209	0.1875	0.2925
2	18	Stearate	1.0473	1.1798	−0.1325	0.2067

Source: From Clayton, D. and Leslie, A., *J. Int. Med. Res.*, 9, 470, 1981.

alone. On the other hand, the two-sample Hotelling T^2 and likelihood distance depend on the joint distribution of AUCs for both formulations. In other words, they take into account the magnitude of relative change for each subject. Therefore, subject 7 is identified as an outlying subject by both Hotelling T^2 and likelihood distance because the relative bioavailability or erythromycin stearate to erythromycin base for subject 7 is only 0.08.

8.5.2 Mean-Shift Model

Models 8.4.2 and 8.4.6 are employed to detect possible outlying subjects while model Equation 8.27 is used to identify potential outlying observations. Wang and Chow (2003) proposed a procedure to identify jointly the outlying subjects and observations in bioequivalence studies based on the mean-shift model proposed by Ferguson (1961) and Srikantan (1961), which is given as

$$Y_{ij} = \mu + S_i + F_j + \lambda_j \delta_{it} + e_{ij} \tag{8.5.11}$$

where $j = 1, \ldots, f$, $i = 1, \ldots, N$, and $\delta_{it} = 1$ if $t = i$ and 0 otherwise. On the basis of the mean-shift model, the hypothesis that subject i is an outlier subject can be formulated as

$$\begin{aligned} &\mathrm{H}_{0i}\colon \boldsymbol{\lambda} = (\lambda_1, \ldots, \lambda_{\mathrm{f}})' = 0, \\ \text{versus}\quad &\mathrm{H}_{ai}\colon \boldsymbol{\lambda} = (\lambda_1, \ldots, \lambda_f)' \neq 0, \quad \text{for} \quad i = 1, \ldots, N. \end{aligned} \tag{8.5.12}$$

Similar to the likelihood distance approach, let $\boldsymbol{\theta} = (\theta_1, \theta_2, \theta_3, \theta_4)'$, where

$$\theta_1 = \mu, \theta_2 = \mathbf{F} = (F_1, \ldots, F_f)', \quad \theta_3 = \sigma_{\mathrm{e}}^2,$$

and

$$\theta_4 = \sigma_{\mathrm{e}}^2 + f\sigma_{\mathrm{S}}^2.$$

The log-likelihood function is then given by

$$\begin{aligned} L(\boldsymbol{\theta}) = &\frac{-Nf}{2} \log 2\pi - \frac{N}{2} \log\left(\theta_4 \theta_3^{f-1}\right) - \frac{1}{2\theta_3} \sum_{i=i}^{N} \sum_{j=1}^{f} (Y_{ij} - F_j - \lambda_j \delta_{it})^2 \\ &- \frac{1}{2N}\left(\frac{1}{\theta_4} - \frac{1}{\theta_3}\right) \sum_{i=i}^{N} \left[\sum_{j=1}^{f} (Y_{ij} - F_j - \lambda_j \delta_{it})\right]^2. \end{aligned} \tag{8.5.13}$$

Let $e_i = (e_{i1}, \ldots, e_{if})'$ be the residual vector of subject i after fitting model Equation 8.5.11. The score test for hypothesis Equation 8.5.12 derived under likelihood function Equation 8.5.13 is given as

$$D_i = n(f-1)T_{i1n} + nT_{i2n}, \tag{8.5.14}$$

where

$$\begin{aligned} T_{i1N} &= \frac{(e_i - \bar{e}_i\mathbf{1})'(e_i - \bar{e}_i\mathbf{1})}{\sum_s (e_s - \bar{e}_s\mathbf{1})'(e_s - \bar{e}_s\mathbf{1})}, \\ T_{i2N} &= \frac{\bar{e}_i^2}{\sum_s \bar{e}_s^2}, \end{aligned} \tag{8.5.15}$$

and

$$\bar{e}_i = \frac{(\mathbf{1}'e_i)}{f}.$$

T_{i1n} is to detect whether subjects have an unusual high or low bioavailability for some formulations. On the other hand, T_{i2n} is a measure for the average pharmacokinetic response for subject i. As a result, T_{i1n} can be used to identify a specific pharmacokinetic measurement of a certain formulation for subject i is an outlying observation and T_{i2n} is to detect whether subject i as a whole is an outlying subject. In addition, T_{i1n} and T_{i2n} are independent beta random variables, i.e., $T_{i1n} \sim$ beta $[(f-1)/2, (N-1)(f-1)/2]$ and $T_{i2n} \sim \text{beta}[1/2, (N-1)/2]$. It follows that

$$\begin{aligned} D_i = n(f-1)T_{i1n} + nT_{i2n}, &\sim N(f-1)\text{beta}[(f-1)/2, (N-1)(f-1)/2] \\ &+ N\ \text{beta}[1/2, (N-1)/2]. \end{aligned} \tag{8.5.16}$$

With respect to hypothesis 8.5.12, subject i is declared as an outlier at the α significance level if $D_i = D_{(N)} = \max_{1<k<N} D_k$ is greater than the αth upper percentile of the distribution of the maximum of D_i. Table 8.5.3 provides the 10%, 5%, and 1% upper percentiles of the distribution of the maximum of D_i.

8.6 Discussion

In Section 8.2, we introduced the use of intra-subject and inter-subject residuals to verify the normality assumptions for model 8.1.1. Although the residual plot and the normal probability plot based on studentized residuals can provide useful information about the normality assumption, they are not rigorous statistical tests for normality. Further research on this topic is worthwhile.

TABLE 8.5.3: Upper percentiles of the distribution of the maximum of D_i.

N	10%	5%	1%
10	7.3914	8.0730	9.5967
11	7.5952	8.2866	9.9587
12	7.9641	8.7809	10.6040
13	8.1345	8.9709	10.7702
14	8.3541	9.2656	11.1475
15	8.5105	9.3900	11.1959
16	8.6748	9.5087	11.4840
17	8.8911	9.7756	11.6292
18	9.0721	10.0265	12.0951
19	9.2051	10.1734	12.4110
20	9.3347	10.3273	12.4644
25	9.8780	10.9030	13.1196
30	10.3645	11.5096	13.8076
35	10.6438	11.8797	14.5265
40	11.0180	12.1700	14.5265
45	11.3681	12.5030	14.9112
50	11.6866	12.8871	15.7853

For the model selection between the raw data model and the log-transformation model, one may compare residual plots for the raw AUC and the log-transformed AUC. When the two residual plots exhibit a similar pattern, it is difficult to determine which model is more appropriate. In this case, as an alternative, we may consider the following method. Suppose there are f formulations. We may apply Shapiro–Wilk's test to test normality for each formulation and the difference between any two formulations. In other words, a total of $f + f(f-1)/2$ tests are to be performed for each raw AUC and log (AUC). Based on the test results (i.e., p-values), we then select the model with the higher percentage of failure in rejection of the normality assumption hypothesis (p-values >0.05). Note that the above alternative provides a quick review for model selection between the raw data model and the log-transformed model which, however, does not directly address assumptions of S_{ik} and e_{ijk}.

In Sections 8.4 and 8.5, several statistical tests for detection of possible outlying subjects and outlying observations for an individual subject were reviewed. However, outliers are determined under an assumed statistical model. An outlier may indicate that the model is incorrect. In other words, an extreme value may be identified as an outlier under model A, but may not be concluded as an outlier under model B. However, model B may produce different outliers. Therefore, the treatment of a possible outlier in statistical analysis is critical. In bioavailability/bioequivalence studies, statistical analyses with and without the possible outlier may lead to a totally opposite conclusion for bioequivalence. Ramsay and Elkum (2005) performed a simulation study to compare the performance of likelihood distance, estimates distance, Hotelling T^2 procedure, and the mean-shift model method. Although the estimates distance method can inflate type I error, it is more powerful than the other three methods.

A report by a bioequivalence task force, which resulted from bioequivalence hearings conducted by the FDA in 1986, indicated that removal of certain subjects in a study because their data do not conform with the remaining data may affect validation of the study. One cannot determine whether the apparently nonconforming data result from laboratory error, data transcription, or other causes unrelated to bioequivalence. The above concerns certainly have built a case against data removal.

Both the FDA guidance on *General Considerations for Bioequivalence for Orally Administrated Drug Products* (FDA, 2003b) and guidance on *Statistical Approaches to Establishing Bioequivalence* (FDA, 2001) recommended that logarithmic transformation be applied to the pharmacokinetic responses AUC and C_{max}. Justification has been provided in the guidances. In addition, the FDA guidance on *Statistical Approaches to Establishing Bioequivalence* (FDA, 2001) also states that "Sponsors and/or applicants are not encouraged to test for normality of error distribution after log-transformation, nor should they use normality of error distribution as a justification for carrying out the statistical analysis on the original scale." Chapter 19 provides a comprehensive review and discussion about the FDA guidances, including logarithmic transformation and outlier detection.

Chapter 9

Optimal Crossover Designs for Two Formulations for Average Bioequivalence

9.1 Introduction

In previous chapters, most of our efforts were directed at the assessment of bioequivalence in average bioavailability for the standard 2×2 crossover design for comparing two formulations of a drug product. The standard two-sequence, two-period crossover, however, is not useful in the presence of carryover effects. In addition, it does not provide independent estimates of intra-subject variabilities. To account for these disadvantages, in practice, it is of interest to consider a higher-order crossover design. A *higher-order crossover design* is defined as a crossover design in which either the number of periods or the number of sequences is greater than the number of formulations to be compared. The most commonly used higher-order designs for comparing two formulations include a four-sequence, two-period design (or Balaam's design), a two-sequence, three-period design, and a four-period design with two or four sequences. Some of these designs were briefly described as designs A, B, and C in Section 2.5. In this chapter, statistical methods for assessing bioequivalence of average bioavailability from these experimental designs are discussed.

Consider the following general model for a higher-order crossover design:

$$Y_{ijk} = \mu + G_k + S_{ik} + P_j + F_{(j,k)} + C_{(j-1,k)} + e_{ijk}, \qquad (9.1.1)$$

where

$i = 1, 2, \ldots, n_k$

$j = 1, \ldots, J$, $k = 1, \ldots, K$

Y_{ijk}, μ, P_j, $F_{(j,k)}$, $C_{(j-1,k)}$, S_{ik}, and e_{ijk} are defined as those in model 2.5.1

G_k is the fixed effect of sequence k.

For Balaam's design, $K = 4$ and $J = 2$. For a two-sequence, three-period (or four-period) design, $K = 2$ and $J = 3$ (or $J = 4$). For a four-sequence, four-period design, $K = J = 4$. Note that, unlike model 2.5.1 for the standard two-sequence, two-period crossover design, G_k was included in the above model. This is because a higher-order crossover design can provide a statistical test for the sequence effect in the presence of the period effect, the direct formulation effect, and the carryover effect. The test for the sequence effect can be used to examine the success or failure of the randomization.

For assessment of equivalence in average bioavailability, as indicated in Chapter 4, Schuirmann's two one-sided tests procedure, the classic confidence interval approach, and Bayesian methods will essentially reach the same conclusion on bioequivalence. Therefore, in this chapter, we will focus on Schuirmann's two one-sided tests procedure and the classic confidence interval approach for assessing bioequivalence under a higher-order crossover design. Because both approaches depend on the direct formulation effect F, our primary emphasis will be placed on estimation of F and its variance.

In Sections 9.2 through 9.4, statistical analyses for assessing bioequivalence under Balaam's design, a two-sequence, three-period design, and a four-period design with two or four sequences are given. The use of log-transformation (or individual subject ratios) is outlined in Section 9.5. Sample size determination for equivalence in average bioavailability under higher-order crossover design is given in Section 9.6. A brief discussion is given in Section 9.7.

9.2 Balaam's Design

In this section, we first consider the following four-sequence and two-period design:

Balaam's design.

	Period	
Sequence	**I**	**II**
1	T	T
2	R	R
3	R	T
4	T	R

This design is usually referred to as Balaam's design (Balaam, 1968). It can be seen that if sequences 1 and 2 are omitted, then Balaam's design reduces to the standard two-sequence, two-period crossover design. Subjects in sequences 1 and 2 receive the same formulation twice, either the test formulation or the reference formulation, which allows us to estimate intra-subject variabilities.

Table 9.2.1 gives the expected values of the sequence-by-period means (i.e., $\overline{Y}_{j\cdot k}, j = 1, 2, 3, 4$ and $k = 1, 2$) where

$$\overline{Y}_{j\cdot k} = \frac{1}{n_k} \sum_{i=1}^{n_k} Y_{ijk}. \tag{9.2.1}$$

TABLE 9.2.1: Expected values of the sequence-by-period means for Balaam's design.

	Period	
Sequence	**I**	**II**
1	$\mu + G_1 + P_1 + F_T$	$\mu + G_1 + P_2 + F_T + C_T$
2	$\mu + G_2 + P_1 + F_R$	$\mu + G_2 + P_2 + F_R + C_R$
3	$\mu + G_3 + P_1 + F_R$	$\mu + G_3 + P_2 + F_T + C_R$
4	$\mu + G_4 + P_1 + F_T$	$\mu + G_4 + P_2 + F_R + C_T$

There are seven degrees of freedom associated with the eight sequence-by-period means, which can be decomposed as follows:

Source	Degrees of Freedom
Sequence effect	3
Formulation effect	1
Period effect	1
Carryover effect	1
Formulation-by-carryover interaction	1
Total	7

In model 9.1.1, however, we assume there is no formulation-by-carryover interaction. Therefore, the one degree of freedom is then combined with that of intra-subject residuals. The analysis of variance table for Balaam's design in terms of degrees of freedom is given in Table 9.2.2. From Table 9.2.2, it can be seen that Balaam's design allows us to estimate the direct formulation effect in the presence of the carryover effects. It also provides independent estimates of intra-subject variability σ_T^2 and σ_R^2. Note that unlike the standard two-sequence, two-period crossover design, the carryover effect under Balaam's design is not confounded with the sequence effect.

TABLE 9.2.2: Analysis of variance table for Balaam's design.

Source of Variation	Degrees of Freedom
Inter-subject	$n_1 + n_2 + n_3 + n_4 - 1$
Sequence	3
Residual	$n_1 + n_2 + n_3 + n_4 - 4$
Intra-subject	$n_1 + n_2 + n_3 + n_4$
Period	1
Formulation	1
Carryover	1
Residual	$n_1 + n_2 + n_3 + n_4 - 3$
Total	$2(n_1 + n_2 + n_3 + n_4) - 1$

9.2.1 Analysis of Average Bioavailability

Let d_{ik} be defined as in Equation 3.3.1; namely,

$$d_{ik} = \tfrac{1}{2}(Y_{i2k} - Y_{i1k}), \quad i = 1, 2, \ldots, n_k, \quad k = 1, 2, 3, 4. \tag{9.2.2}$$

Then, under normality assumptions and $\sigma_T^2 = \sigma_R^2 = \sigma_e^2$, the expected values and variances of the sample means of d_{ik} are given by

$$E(\bar{d}_{\cdot k}) = \begin{cases} \tfrac{1}{2}[(P_2 - P_1) + C_T], & k = 1, \\ \tfrac{1}{2}[(P_2 - P_1) + C_R], & k = 2, \\ \tfrac{1}{2}[(P_2 - P_1) + (F_T - F_R) + C_R], & k = 3, \\ \tfrac{1}{2}[(P_2 - P_1) - (F_T - F_R) + C_T], & k = 4, \end{cases} \tag{9.2.3}$$

and

$$\mathrm{Var}(\bar{d}_{\cdot k}) = \frac{1}{2n_k}\sigma_e^2. \tag{9.2.4}$$

It follows that

$$E(\bar{d}_{\cdot 3} - \bar{d}_{\cdot 4}) = F_T - F_R + \tfrac{1}{2}(C_R - C_T),$$

and

$$E(\bar{d}_{\cdot 2} - \bar{d}_{\cdot 1}) = \tfrac{1}{2}(C_R - C_T).$$

Consequently,

$$E[(\bar{d}_{\cdot 3} - \bar{d}_{\cdot 4}) - (\bar{d}_{\cdot 2} - \bar{d}_{\cdot 1})] = F_T - F_R = F.$$

Therefore, the best linear unbiased estimator for the direct formulation effect F after adjustment of the carryover effect is given by

$$\begin{aligned} \widehat{F}|C &= (\bar{d}_{\cdot 3} - \bar{d}_{\cdot 4}) - (\bar{d}_{\cdot 2} - \bar{d}_{\cdot 1}) \\ &= \tfrac{1}{2}\left[(\bar{Y}_{\cdot 23} - \bar{Y}_{\cdot 13}) - (\bar{Y}_{\cdot 24} - \bar{Y}_{\cdot 14}) - (\bar{Y}_{\cdot 22} - \bar{Y}_{\cdot 12}) + (\bar{Y}_{\cdot 21} - \bar{Y}_{\cdot 11})\right]. \end{aligned} \tag{9.2.5}$$

As $\bar{d}_{\cdot k}$, $k = 1, 2, 3, 4$, are independent of each other, the variance of $\widehat{F}|C$ can be obtained as follows:

$$\mathrm{Var}(\widehat{F}|C) = \frac{1}{2}\sigma_e^2\left(\frac{1}{n_1} + \frac{1}{n_2} + \frac{1}{n_3} + \frac{1}{n_4}\right). \tag{9.2.6}$$

Furthermore, as $F = F_T - F_R$ and $F_T + F_R = 0$, we have

$$F_T = \tfrac{1}{2}F \quad \text{and} \quad F_R = -\tfrac{1}{2}F.$$

Therefore, unbiased estimates for $\mu_T = \mu + F_T$ and $\mu_R = \mu + F_R$ are given by

$$\begin{aligned} \widehat{\mu}_T &= \overline{Y}... + \tfrac{1}{2}\,(\widehat{F}|C), \\ \widehat{\mu}_R &= \overline{Y}... - \tfrac{1}{2}(\widehat{F}|C), \end{aligned} \tag{9.2.7}$$

where

$$\overline{Y}... = \frac{1}{8}\sum_{k=1}^{4}\sum_{j=1}^{2}\overline{Y}_{\cdot jk},$$

which is an unbiased estimator for the overall mean μ. Therefore, the classic $(1 - 2\alpha) \times 100\%$ confidence interval for F or equivalently $\mu_T - \mu_R$, denoted by (L, U), is given by

$$(L,\ U) = \widehat{F}|C \pm t(\alpha, N-3)S\sqrt{\frac{1}{2}\left(\frac{1}{n_1} + \frac{1}{n_2} + \frac{1}{n_3} + \frac{1}{n_4}\right)}, \tag{9.2.8}$$

where $N = n_1 + n_2 + n_3 + n_4$, and S^2 is the intra-subject mean-squared error from the analysis of variance table that can be obtained by fitting model 9.1.1 using PROC GLM of SAS.

Thus, we claim the two formulations are bioequivalent if (L, U) is within the bioequivalent limits (θ_L, θ_U).

Similarly, Schuirmann's two one-sided tests procedure can be obtained as follows. We reject the interval hypothesis 4.3.1 and conclude bioequivalence at the α level of significance if

$$T_L = \frac{\widehat{F}|C - \theta_L}{S\sqrt{\frac{1}{2}\left(\frac{1}{n_1} + \frac{1}{n_2} + \frac{1}{n_3} + \frac{1}{n_4}\right)}} > t(\alpha,\ N-3),$$

and

$$T_U = \frac{\widehat{F}|C - \theta_U}{S\sqrt{\frac{1}{2}\left(\frac{1}{n_1} + \frac{1}{n_2} + \frac{1}{n_3} + \frac{1}{n_4}\right)}} < -t(\alpha,\ N-3). \tag{9.2.9}$$

Note that the p-value of Anderson and Hauck's procedure for interval hypotheses 4.3.1 can also be obtained by simply plugging T_L and T_U into either Equation 4.3.12 or Equation 4.3.13.

9.2.2 Inference for the Carryover Effect

Because $E[2(\bar{d}_{\cdot 1} - \bar{d}_{\cdot 2})] = C_T - C_R = C$, the following estimator is the best linear unbiased estimator for the carryover effect C after adjustment of formulation effect:

$$\begin{aligned}\widehat{C}|F &= 2(\bar{d}_{\cdot 1} - \bar{d}_{\cdot 2}) \\ &= [(\bar{Y}_{\cdot 21} - \bar{Y}_{\cdot 11}) - (\bar{Y}_{\cdot 22} - \bar{Y}_{\cdot 12})].\end{aligned} \quad (9.2.10)$$

The variance of $\widehat{C}|F$ is given by

$$\operatorname{Var}(\widehat{C}|F) = 2\sigma_e^2\left(\frac{1}{n_1} + \frac{1}{n_2}\right). \quad (9.2.11)$$

Hence, unlike the standard two-sequence, two-period crossover design, the variance of the estimate of the carryover effect is a function that involves only the intra-subject variability. Therefore, we reject the null hypothesis of equal carryover effects given in 3.2.4 at the α level of significance if

$$|T_C| > t(\alpha/2, n_1 + n_2 + n_3 + n_4 - 3), \quad (9.2.12)$$

where

$$T_C = \frac{\widehat{C}|F}{S\sqrt{2\left(\frac{1}{n_1} + \frac{1}{n_2}\right)}}. \quad (9.2.13)$$

If we fail to reject the null hypothesis $H_0\colon C_T = C_R$, we may drop the carryover effect from the model. In this case, the best linear unbiased estimator of F can be obtained based only on sequence-by-period means from the last two sequences; that is,

$$\begin{aligned}\widehat{F} &= \bar{d}_{\cdot 3} - \bar{d}_{\cdot 4} \\ &= \tfrac{1}{2}[(\bar{Y}_{\cdot 23} - \bar{Y}_{\cdot 13}) - (\bar{Y}_{\cdot 24} - \bar{Y}_{\cdot 14})].\end{aligned}$$

The variance of $\widehat{F}$ under the assumption of equal carryover effects is given by

$$\mathrm{Var}(\widehat{F}) = \frac{1}{2}\sigma_e^2\left(\frac{1}{n_3} + \frac{1}{n_4}\right).$$

Therefore, bioequivalence in average bioavailability can be assessed by using either $(1 - 2\alpha) \times 100\%$ confidence interval or Schuirmann's two one-sided tests procedure, which are given as follows:

$$(L, U) = \widehat{F} \pm t(\alpha, N-2)S\sqrt{\frac{1}{2}\left(\frac{1}{n_3} + \frac{1}{n_4}\right)},$$

$$T_L = \frac{\widehat{F} - \theta_L}{S\sqrt{\frac{1}{2}\left(\frac{1}{n_3} + \frac{1}{n_4}\right)}} > t(\alpha, N-2), \quad \text{and}$$

$$T_U = \frac{\widehat{F} - \theta_U}{S\sqrt{\frac{1}{2}\left(\frac{1}{n_1} + \frac{1}{n_2}\right)}} < -t(\alpha, N-2)$$

where S^2 is the intra-subject mean-squared error obtained from the model without the carryover effect.

9.2.3 Assessment of Intra-Subject Variabilities

In Section 9.2.1, for assessment of bioequivalence of average bioavailability, we assume the intra-subject variability is the same from formulation to formulation, $\left(\text{i.e.}, \sigma_T^2 = \sigma_R^2 = \sigma_e^2\right)$. Under the assumption of equal carryover effects, statistical methods for assessing bioequivalence were derived based on data from sequences 3 and 4. In practice, the intra-subject variabilities may differ from formulation to formulation; namely,

$$\mathrm{Var}(e_{ijk}) = \begin{cases} \sigma_T^2 & \text{for the test formulation,} \\ \sigma_R^2 & \text{for the reference formulation.} \end{cases} \tag{9.2.14}$$

In this case, the confidence interval and the two one-sided tests procedure are still valid. This can be seen by the fact that the estimate of the formulation effect F depends only on the period differences from sequences 3 and 4, which has a variance of $\left(\sigma_T^2 + \sigma_R^2\right)/4$ for both sequences. One advantage of Balaam's design is that, under assumption of equal carryover effects, data collected from sequences 1 and 2 can be used to assess equivalence of intra-subject variabilities by testing hypothesis Equation 7.3 for equivalence in variances.

Let SSD_1 and SSD_2 be sums of squares for period differences of sequences 1 and 2, respectively; that is,

$$SSD_k = \sum_{i=1}^{n_k} (d_{ik} - \overline{d}_{\cdot k})^2, \quad k = 1, 2, \tag{9.2.15}$$

where

$$\bar{d}_{\cdot k} = \frac{1}{n_k} \sum_{i=1}^{n_k} d_{ik}, \quad k = 1, 2.$$

Note that SSD_1 and SSD_2 are independent, and

$$2SSD_1 \sim \sigma_T^2 \chi^2(n_1 - 1),$$
$$2SSD_2 \sim \sigma_R^2 \chi^2(n_2 - 1).$$

Therefore,

$$\widehat{\sigma_T^2} = \frac{2SSD_1}{n_1 - 1} \quad \text{and} \quad \widehat{\sigma_R^2} = \frac{2SSD_2}{n_2 - 1},$$

are independent and unbiased estimators of σ_T^2 and σ_R^2, respectively. We reject the interval hypothesis 7.2.3 and conclude equivalence of intra-subject variabilities at the α level of significance if

$$F = \widehat{\sigma_T^2}/\widehat{\sigma_R^2} > \delta_1 F(\alpha, n_1 - 1, n_2 - 1),$$

and

$$F = \widehat{\sigma_T^2}/\widehat{\sigma_R^2} < \delta_2 F(1 - \alpha, n_1 - 1, n_2 - 1), \tag{9.2.16}$$

where $0 < \delta_1 < 1 < \delta_2$ are lower and upper equivalence limits and $F(a, v_1, v_2)$ is the upper αth quantile of an F distribution with v_1 and v_2 degrees of freedom.

The lower and upper limits of the classic $(1 - 2\alpha) \times 100\%$ confidence interval for σ_T^2/σ_R^2 are given by

$$\begin{aligned} L &= \frac{\widehat{\sigma_T^2}/\widehat{\sigma_R^2}}{F(\alpha, n_1 - 1, n_2 - 1)}, \quad \text{and} \\ U &= \left(\widehat{\sigma_T^2}/\widehat{\sigma_R^2}\right) F(\alpha, n_2 - 1, n_1 - 1). \end{aligned} \tag{9.2.17}$$

Because $F(1 - \alpha, n_1 - 1, n_2 - 1) = (F[\alpha, n_2 - 1, n_1 - 1])^{-1}$, (L, U) is within (δ_1, δ_2) if and only if, Equation 9.2.16 holds. Thus, the confidence interval approach is operationally equivalent to the two one-sided tests procedure for determination of equivalence of intra-subject variabilities.

Example 9.2.1

To illustrate Balaam's design, we consider AUC data given in Table 9.2.3. This study was designed to compare a test formulation with a reference formulation using Balaam's design with 24 normal subjects, who were assigned to each of the four

TABLE 9.2.3: AUC data for Balaam's design.

Sequence	Subject	Period I	Period II
1: TT	1	280	482
	2	219	161
	3	230	99
	4	229	260
	5	494	274
	6	112	171
2: RR	7	205	221
	8	349	420
	9	285	288
	10	266	247
	11	161	175
	12	240	248
3: RT	13	325	225
	14	374	439
	15	416	372
	16	243	119
	17	248	269
	18	345	334
4: TR	19	177	290
	20	174	224
	21	235	271
	22	380	340
	23	308	270
	24	269	249

sequences (TT, RR, RT, and TR) at random. The sequence-by-period means are given in Table 9.2.4. The intra-subject mean-squared error S^2 from the analysis of variance table, which is obtained by fitting model Equation 9.1.1 using PROC GLM of SAS, is 3827.79. Table 9.2.5 summarizes the results of Schuirmann's two one-sided tests

TABLE 9.2.4: Sequence-by-period means for AUC data in Table 9.2.3.

Sequence	Period I	Period II
1	260.67	241.17
2	251.00	266.50
3	325.17	293.00
4	257.17	274.00

Note: $S^2 = 16.67$.

TABLE 9.2.5: Summary of results for AUC data in Table 9.2.3.

Carryover	$\hat{F}$	Test Statistic[a]	p-Value	90% CI[b]
Yes	−42.0	$T_L = 0.46$	0.325	(−103.5, 19.5)
		$T_U = -2.81$	0.005	(64.6%, 106.7%)
No	−24.5	$T_L = 1.29$	0.105	(−67.4, 18.4)
		$T_U = -3.25$	0.002	(76.2%, 106.5%)

[a] The ±20 rule was applied by assuming $\mu_R = \hat{\mu}_R = 292.08$.

[b] CI, confidence interval, which was expressed in terms of $\hat{\mu}_R = \hat{\mu} - \frac{1}{2}\hat{F} = 292.08$ in presence of carryover effect, and $\hat{\mu}_R = 283.3$ in absence of carryover effect.

procedure and the 90% confidence interval based on the ±20 rule with $\widehat{\mu}_R$ assumed to be the true μ_R. In the presence of the carryover effect, from Equation 9.2.5, we have

$$\widehat{\mu} = \overline{Y}... = 271.08 \quad \text{and} \quad \widehat{F}|C = -42.0$$

Thus, estimates for the test and reference formulations means are given by

$$\widehat{\mu}_T = 250.08 \quad \text{and} \quad \widehat{\mu}_R = 292.08$$

The estimate of the carryover effect $\widehat{C}|F$ is 35 with a standard error of 50.52, which leads to a p-value of 0.496. Hence, we conclude there is no carryover effect. Furthermore, it can be verified that estimates of F, μ_T, and μ_R in the absence of unequal carryover effects are 24.5, 258.83, and 283.33, respectively. From Table 9.2.5, it can be seen that the interval approach and the two one-sided tests procedure lead to the same conclusion of bioinequivalence regardless of the presence of the carryover effect.

For testing the equivalence of intra-subject variabilities, estimates of σ_T^2 and σ_R^2 are given by 11188.94 and 448.55. The 90% confidence interval for σ_T^2/σ_R^2 based upon Equation 9.2.17 is (494%, 12597%), which indicates that the two formulations are not equivalent in intra-subject variabilities.

9.3 Two-Sequence Dual Design

In this section, we consider the following two-sequence, three-period design, which consists of the dual sequences TRR and RTT.

Two-sequence dual design.

	Period		
Sequence	**I**	**II**	**III**
1	T	R	R
2	R	T	T

This design is an extra period design, which is also known as the two-sequence dual design. The two-sequence dual design is balanced in the sense that each

TABLE 9.3.1: Expected values of the sequence-by-period means for the two-sequence dual design.

	Period		
Sequence	**I**	**II**	**III**
1	$\mu + G_1 + P_1 + F_T$	$\mu + G_1 + P_2 + F_R + C_T$	$\mu + G_1 + P_3 +$ $F_R + C_R$
2	$\mu + G_2 + P_1 + F_R$	$\mu + G_2 + P_2 + F_T + C_R$	$\mu + G_2 + P_3 +$ $F_T + C_T$

formulation follows other formulations, including itself, the same number of times. One advantage of this design is that it allows us to estimate the intra-subject variabilities because each subject receives either the test formulation or the reference formulation twice.

Table 9.3.1 provides the expected values of the sequence-by-period means. The analysis of variance table in terms of degrees of freedom is given in Table 9.3.2. There are a total of six sequence-by-period means with five degrees of freedom, which can be decomposed as follows:

Source	**Degrees of Freedom**
Sequence effect	1
Formulation effect	1
Period effect	2
Carryover effect	1
Total	5

Therefore, this design allows us to estimate the direct formulation effect in the presence of the carryover effect. In addition, statistical inference for the carryover effect can be obtained based on estimates of intra-subject variabilities. Under

TABLE 9.3.2: Analysis of variance table for the two-sequence dual design.

Source of Variation	**Degrees of Freedom**
Inter-subject	$n_1 + n_2 - 1$
Sequence	1
Residual	$n_1 + n_2 - 2$
Intra-subject	$2(n_1 + n_2)$
Period	2
Formulation	1
Carryover	1
Residual	$2(n_1 + n_2 - 2)$
Total	$3(n_1 + n_2) - 1$

normality assumption of Equation 8.1.2 for S_{ik} and e_{ijk}, the two-sequence dual design is optimal for estimation of the direct formulation effect and the carryover effect among all two-sequence and three-period designs (Cheng and Wu, 1980; Kershner and Federer, 1981; Laska et al., 1983; Lasserre, 1991; Jones and Kenward, 2003).

9.3.1 Analysis of Average Bioavailability

Under the two-sequence dual design, similar to the standard two-sequence, two-period design, the classic confidence interval for the direct formulation effect F and Schuirmann's two one-sided tests procedure for assessing bioequivalence can be derived similarly.

Let $\mathbf{Y}_{ik} = (\mathbf{Y}_{i1k}, \mathbf{Y}_{i2k}, \mathbf{Y}_{i3k})'$ be the vector of the three responses observed on subject i in sequence k. The assumption of compound symmetry requires that the covariance matrix of $\mathbf{Y}_{ik}$ has the following structure:

$$\text{Var}(\mathbf{Y}_{ik}) = \begin{bmatrix} \sigma_e^2 + \sigma_S^2 & \sigma_S^2 & \sigma_S^2 \\ \sigma_S^2 & \sigma_e^2 + \sigma_S^2 & \sigma_S^2 \\ \sigma_S^2 & \sigma_S^2 & \sigma_e^2 + \sigma_S^2 \end{bmatrix}. \tag{9.3.1}$$

Then, under the normality assumptions stated in Equation 8.1.2, the best linear unbiased estimator for the direct formulation effect, $F = F_T - F_R$, is the following linear contrast of sequence-by-period means (Kershner and Federer, 1981; Jones and Kenward, 2003):

$$\widehat{F} = \tfrac{1}{4}\left[\left(2\overline{Y}_{\cdot 11} - \overline{Y}_{\cdot 21} - \overline{Y}_{\cdot 31}\right) - \left(2\overline{Y}_{\cdot 12} - \overline{Y}_{\cdot 22} - \overline{Y}_{\cdot 32}\right)\right]. \tag{9.3.2}$$

The expected value and variance of $\widehat{F}$ are given respectively as

$$E(\widehat{F}) = F_T - F_R, \tag{9.3.3}$$

and

$$\text{Var}(\widehat{F}) = \frac{3}{8}\sigma_e^2\left(\frac{1}{n_1} + \frac{1}{n_2}\right). \tag{9.3.4}$$

Furthermore, an unbiased estimator for the overall mean μ can be obtained as

$$\overline{Y}_{\ldots} = \frac{1}{6}\sum_{k=1}^{2}\sum_{j=1}^{3}\overline{Y}_{j\cdot k}. \tag{9.3.5}$$

As $F = F_T - F_R$ and $F_T + F_R = 0$, we have

$$F_{\text{T}} = \tfrac{1}{2}F \quad \text{and} \quad F_{\text{R}} = -\tfrac{1}{2}F.$$

Therefore, unbiased estimates for $\mu_{\text{T}} = \mu + F_{\text{T}}$ and $\mu_{\text{R}} = \mu + F_{\text{R}}$ are given by

$$\widehat{\mu}_{\text{T}} = \overline{Y}_{\ldots} + \tfrac{1}{2}\widehat{F},$$

and

$$\widehat{\mu}_{\text{R}} = \overline{Y}_{\ldots} - \tfrac{1}{2}\widehat{F}. \tag{9.3.6}$$

The classic $(1 - 2\alpha) \times 100\%$ confidence interval for F, denoted by (L, U), is given by

$$(L, U) = \widehat{F} \pm t[\alpha, 2(n_1 + n_2 - 2)]S\sqrt{\left(\frac{3}{8}\right)\left(\frac{1}{n_1} + \frac{1}{n_2}\right)}. \tag{9.3.7}$$

As a result, we conclude the two formulations are bioequivalent if the interval (L, U) is within the bioequivalent limits, $(\theta_{\text{L}}, \theta_{\text{U}})$.

Similarly, Schuirmann's two one-sided tests procedure can be obtained based on the following two t statistics. We reject interval hypotheses 4.3.1 and conclude bioequivalence at the α level of significance if

$$T_{\text{L}} = \frac{\widehat{F} - \theta_{\text{L}}}{S\sqrt{\left(\frac{3}{8}\right)\left(\frac{1}{n_1} + \frac{1}{n_2}\right)}} > t[\alpha, 2(n_1 + n_2 - 2)],$$

and

$$T_{\text{U}} = \frac{\widehat{F} - \theta_{\text{U}}}{S\sqrt{\left(\frac{3}{8}\right)\left(\frac{1}{n_1} + \frac{1}{n_2}\right)}} < -t[\alpha, 2(n_1 + n_2 - 2)]. \tag{9.3.8}$$

Note that, the p-value of Anderson and Hauck's procedure for interval hypotheses 4.3.1 can be obtained by simply plugging T_{L} and T_{U} into either Equation 4.3.12 or 4.3.13.

9.3.2 Inference for the Carryover Effect

Jones and Kenward (2003) indicated that under normality assumptions given in 8.1.2, the best linear unbiased estimator for the carryover effect $C = C_{\text{T}} - C_{\text{R}}$ can be obtained by the following linear contrast of sequence-by-period means (also see Kershner and Federer, 1981):

$$\widehat{C} = \tfrac{1}{2}[(\overline{Y}_{\cdot 21} - \overline{Y}_{\cdot 31}) - (\overline{Y}_{\cdot 22} - \overline{Y}_{\cdot 32})]. \tag{9.3.9}$$

Under the two-sequence dual design, it can be verified that the cross products of the coefficients in linear contrasts between $\widehat{F}$ in Equation 9.3.3 and $\widehat{C}$ in Equation 9.3.9 is 0. This indicates that $\widehat{C}$ is independent of $\widehat{F}$. Therefore, $\widehat{F}$ remains the same, regardless of presence or absence of unequal carryover effects. The variance of $\widehat{C}$ is given by

$$\text{Var}(\widehat{C}) = \frac{1}{2}\sigma_e^2\left(\frac{1}{n_1} + \frac{1}{n_2}\right). \tag{9.3.10}$$

On the basis of Equations 9.3.9 and 9.3.10, we reject the null hypothesis Equation 3.2.4 of equal carryover effects at the α level of significance if

$$|T_C| > t[\alpha/2, 2(n_1 + n_2 - 2)], \tag{9.3.11}$$

where

$$T_C = \frac{\widehat{C}}{S\sqrt{\frac{1}{2}\left(\frac{1}{n_1} + \frac{1}{n_2}\right)}}.$$

9.3.3 Intra-Subject Contrasts

When the covariance of $\mathbf{Y}_{ik}$ does not follow the structure of compound symmetry defined in Equation 9.19, we can still assess bioequivalence of average bioavailability based on a two-sample t test provided that $\text{Var}(\mathbf{Y}_{i1}) = \text{Var}(\mathbf{Y}_{i2})$. When the assumption of compound symmetry of $\text{Var}(\mathbf{Y}_{ik})$ is violated, the model 9.1.1 becomes

$$Y_{ijk} = \mu + G_k + P_j + F_{(j,k)} + C_{(j-1,k)} + e^*_{ijk}, \tag{9.3.12}$$

where $(\mathbf{e}^*_{ik} = (\mathbf{e}^*_{i1k}, \mathbf{e}^*_{i2k}, \mathbf{e}^*_{i3k})'$ is distributed with mean 0 and covariance matrix Σ for $i = 1, 2, \ldots, n_k$; $k = 1, 2$.

Define the following intra-subject contrasts:

$$d_{ik} = \tfrac{1}{4}[2Y_{i1k} - Y_{i2k} - Y_{i3k}], \quad i = 1, 2, \ldots, n_k, \quad k = 1, 2. \tag{9.3.13}$$

The expected values and variance of d_{ik} are given by

$$E(d_{ik}) = \begin{cases} \frac{1}{2}(F_T - F_R) + \frac{3}{4}P_1 & k = 1, \\ -\frac{1}{2}(F_T - F_R) + \frac{3}{4}P_1 & k = 2, \end{cases} \tag{9.3.14}$$

$$\text{Var}(d_{ik}) = \sigma_d^2 = \mathbf{c}'\Sigma\mathbf{c}, \tag{9.3.15}$$

where $\mathbf{c}' = (0.5, -0.25, -0.25)$ and Σ is the common covariance matrix of $\mathbf{Y}_{ik}$.

Because $\{d_{i1}\}$ and $\{d_{i2}\}$ are two independent samples with common variance σ_d^2, the two one-sided tests procedure and the nonparametric methods discussed in Chapter 4 can be directly applied to assess bioequivalence of average bioavailability. Let $\bar{d}_{\cdot k}$ and SSD be the sample means and pooled sum of squares of d_{ik}, where

$$\bar{d}_{\cdot k} = \frac{1}{n_k}\sum_{i=1}^{n_k} d_{ik},$$

and

$$\text{SSD} = \sum_{k=1}^{2}\sum_{i=1}^{n} k(d_{ik} - \bar{d}_{\cdot k})^2. \tag{9.3.16}$$

Then, unbiased estimates for F and σ_d^2 can be obtained as

$$\hat{F} = \bar{d}_{\cdot 1} - \bar{d}_{\cdot 2},$$

and

$$\hat{\sigma}_d^2 = \frac{\text{SSD}}{(n_1 + n_2 - 2)}. \tag{9.3.17}$$

Note that, although $\hat{F}$ obtained from the difference in sample means of intra-subject contrasts between sequences 1 and 2 is the same as that of Equation 9.3.2, $\hat{\sigma}_d^2$ is not the same as S^2 obtained from the analysis of variance table. Moreover, the associated degrees of freedom for $\hat{\sigma}_d^2$ is $(n_1 + n_2 - 2)$ rather than $2(n_1 + n_2 - 2)$. The loss of degrees of freedom is the cost for relaxation of the assumption of compound symmetry for covariance matrix of $\mathbf{Y}_{ik}$.

On the basis of the intra-subject contrasts, $d_{ik}, i = 1, 2, \ldots, n_k$; $k = 1, 2$, a $(1 - 2\alpha) \times 100\%$ confidence interval for F, denoted by (L_d, U_d), is given by

$$(L_d, U_d) = \bar{d} \pm t(\alpha, n_1 + n_2 - 2)\hat{\sigma}_d\sqrt{\frac{1}{n_1} + \frac{1}{n_2}}. \tag{9.3.18}$$

Therefore, we conclude bioequivalence if (L_d, U_d) is within the bioequivalent limits (θ_L, θ_U). For Schuirmann's two one-sided tests procedure, similarly, we would reject the interval hypothesis given in 4.3.1 at the α level if

$$T_L = \frac{\widehat{F} - \theta_L}{\widehat{\sigma}_d\sqrt{\frac{1}{n_1} + \frac{1}{n_2}}} > t(\alpha, n_1 + n_2 - 2),$$

and

$$T_U = \frac{\widehat{F} - \theta_U}{\widehat{\sigma}_d\sqrt{\frac{1}{n_1} + \frac{1}{n_2}}} < -t(\alpha, n_1 + n_2 - 2). \tag{9.3.19}$$

Similarly, the p-value of Anderson and Hauck's procedure can also be obtained by plugging T_L and T_U into either Equation 4.3.12 or 4.3.13.

When the normality assumptions given in 8.1.2 are seriously in doubt, nonparametric methods described in Section 4.5.1 can be applied directly based on the intra-subject contrasts, d_{ik}, $i = 1, 2, \ldots, n_k$; $k = 1, 2$. For example, for the Wilcoxon–Mann–Whitney two one-sided tests procedure, we simply plug the intra-subject contrasts into b_{hik} in Equation 4.5.2, where $i = 1, 2, \ldots, n_k$; $k = 1, 2$; $h = L, U$. To construct a distribution-free confidence interval based on Hodges–Lehmann's estimator discussed in Section 4.5.2, we simply plug d_{ik} into the computation of all pairwise differences of $D'_{i,i'}$, which are defined in Section 4.5.2. In addition, the distribution-free confidence interval approach is equivalent to the Wilcoxon–Mann–Whitney two one-sided tests procedure.

9.3.4 Assessment of Intra-Subject Variabilities

As mentioned earlier, in practice, the intra-subject variabilities may differ from formulation to formulation. In this case, we have

$$\text{Var}(e_{ijk}) = \begin{cases} \sigma_T^2 & \text{if } j = 1 \text{ and } k = 1, \text{ or } j = 2, 3 \text{ and } k = 2, \\ \sigma_R^2 & \text{if } j = 1 \text{ and } k = 2, \text{ or } j = 2, 3 \text{ and } k = 1. \end{cases} \tag{9.3.20}$$

If S_{ik} are i.i.d. with mean 0 and variance σ_S^2, then covariance matrices of $\mathbf{Y}_{ik}$ for sequence 1 and sequence 2 are given by

$$\text{Var}(\mathbf{Y}_{i1}) = \begin{bmatrix} \sigma_T^2 + \sigma_S^2 & \sigma_S^2 & \sigma_S^2 \\ \sigma_S^2 & \sigma_R^2 + \sigma_S^2 & \sigma_S^2 \\ \sigma_S^2 & \sigma_S^2 & \sigma_R^2 + \sigma_S^2 \end{bmatrix},$$

and

$$\text{Var}(\mathbf{Y}_{i2}) = \begin{bmatrix} \sigma_R^2 + \sigma_S^2 & \sigma_S^2 & \sigma_S^2 \\ \sigma_S^2 & \sigma_T^2 + \sigma_S^2 & \sigma_S^2 \\ \sigma_S^2 & \sigma_S^2 & \sigma_T^2 + \sigma_S^2 \end{bmatrix}. \tag{9.3.21}$$

Hence,

$$\mathrm{Var}(d_{ik}) = \begin{cases} \frac{1}{8}\left(2\sigma_T^2 + \sigma_R^2\right) & \text{if } k = 1, \\ \frac{1}{8}\left(\sigma_T^2 + 2\sigma_R^2\right) & \text{if } k = 2. \end{cases} \tag{9.3.22}$$

As a result, if $\sigma_T^2 \neq \sigma_R^2$, the variances of d_{i1} and d_{i2} are not the same. Consequently, the procedures discussed in the previous section based on either the two-sample t test or Wilcoxon–Mann–Whitney rank sum test are no longer valid. Therefore, unlike the standard two-sequence, two-period crossover design, the two-sequence dual design requires a much stronger assumption of $\sigma_T^2 = \sigma_R^2 = \sigma_e^2$. This assumption is not generally true. However, it can be examined by testing the following hypothesis:

$$\begin{aligned} \mathrm{H_0}\colon\ & \sigma_T^2 = \sigma_R^2 \\ \text{versus}\quad \mathrm{H_a}\colon\ & \sigma_T^2 \neq \sigma_R^2. \end{aligned} \tag{9.3.23}$$

Define the following intra-subject contrasts:

$$g_{ik} = (Y_{i2k} - Y_{i3k}), \quad i = 1, 2, \ldots, n_k, \quad k = 1, 2. \tag{9.3.24}$$

Then, under covariance structure of Equation 9.3.21, unbiased estimates for σ_T^2 and σ_R^2 can be obtained as follows:

$$\widehat{\sigma_T^2} = \frac{1}{2(n_1 - 1)} \sum_{i=1}^{n_1} (g_{i1} - \bar{g}_{\cdot 1})^2,$$

and

$$\widehat{\sigma_R^2} = \frac{1}{2(n_2 - 1)} \sum_{i=1}^{n_2} (g_{i2} - \bar{g}_{\cdot 2})^2, \tag{9.3.25}$$

where

$$\bar{g}_{\cdot k} = \frac{1}{n_k} \sum_{i=1}^{n_k} g_{ik}.$$

Let $\widehat{\sigma_1^2} = \max\left(\widehat{\sigma_T^2}, \widehat{\sigma_R^2}\right)$, $\widehat{\sigma_2^2} = \min\left(\widehat{\sigma_T^2}, \widehat{\sigma_R^2}\right)$ and v_1 and v_2 be the corresponding degrees of freedoms. We then reject $\mathrm{H_0}$ of Equation 9.3.23 at the α level if

$$F_v = \widehat{\sigma_1^2}/\widehat{\sigma_2^2} > F(\alpha/2, v_1, v_2). \tag{9.3.26}$$

A $(1 - \alpha) \times 100\%$ confidence interval for σ_T^2/σ_R^2, denoted by (L_F, U_F), can then be obtained, where

$$L_F = \frac{\widehat{\sigma}_T^2/\widehat{\sigma}_R^2}{F(\alpha/2, n_1 - 1, n_2 - 1)},$$

and

$$U_F = (\widehat{\sigma}_T^2/\widehat{\sigma}_R^2)F(\alpha/2, n_2 - 1, n_1 - 1). \tag{9.3.27}$$

Note that, under normality assumptions, the intra-subject contrasts d_{ik} are independent of g_{ik}. It follows that $\widehat{\sigma}_T^2$ and $\widehat{\sigma}_R^2$ are not only independent of each other, but are also independent of $\widehat{F}$ and S^2 given in Equation 9.3.8. Consequently, test statistics T_L and T_U in Equation 9.3.8 are independent of F_v.

As indicated earlier, for the standard two-sequence, two-period crossover design, Schuirmann's two one-sided tests procedure is still valid when the intra-subject variabilities differ from formulation to formulation. This, however, is not true for the two-sequence dual design. Therefore, it is recommended that a preliminary test of the hypotheses given in 9.3.23 for equality of intra-subject variabilities be carried out before the assessment of bioequivalence is performed.

Example 9.3.1

To illustrate the methods discussed in this section, consider the example of a two-sequence dual crossover experiment that was conducted with 18 subjects to compare two formulations of a drug product. In the design, 9 subjects were randomly assigned to sequence 1 (TRR) and 9 other subjects were randomly assigned to sequence 2 (RTT). Table 9.3.3 lists AUC data for each subject. The sequence-by-period means are given in Table 9.3.4. The intra-subject mean-squared error, $S^2 = 16.67$, which is obtained by fitting model 9.1.1 using PROC GLM of SAS. From Equations 9.3.2 and 9.3.5, we have

$$\widehat{F} = 0.674 \quad \text{and} \quad \widehat{\mu} = \overline{Y}... = 34.009.$$

Hence, estimates for the test and reference formulation means are given by

$$\widehat{\mu}_T = \widehat{\mu} + \tfrac{1}{2}\widehat{F} = 34.346,$$

and

$$\widehat{\mu}_R = \widehat{\mu} - \tfrac{1}{2}\widehat{F} = 33.672.$$

The intra-subject contrasts d_{ik} and $\frac{1}{2}g_{ik}$ are given in Table 9.3.3. It can be verified that $\widehat{\sigma}_d^2$, computed from the intra-subject contrasts d_{ik}, is 6.86. Table 9.3.5 summarizes the results of Schuirmann's two one-sided tests procedures as well as the confidence interval based on the ± 20 rule with μ_R assumed to be $\widehat{\mu}_R = 33.672$. The results indicate that all procedures reach the same conclusion for bioequivalence of average bioavailability.

TABLE 9.3.3: AUC data and intra-subject contrasts.

Sequence	Subject	Period I	Period II	Period III	d_{ik}	$\frac{1}{2}g_{ik}$
1. TRR	2	32.14	42.55	36.08	−3.5875	3.235
	5	51.85	47.37	56.50	−0.0425	−4.565
	6	34.28	30.70	33.60	1.0650	−1.450
	8	27.48	27.87	33.54	−1.6125	−2.835
	10	17.32	18.93	19.05	−0.8350	−0.060
	11	31.61	24.93	28.21	2.5200	−1.640
	13	39.26	37.36	45.09	−0.9825	−3.685
	17	47.55	40.00	36.00	4.7750	2.000
	18	36.15	35.20	33.26	0.9600	0.970
2. RTT	1	26.79	27.23	31.60	−1.3125	−2.185
	3	26.71	30.81	26.39	−0.9450	2.210
	4	28.70	40.74	30.49	−3.4575	5.125
	7	35.01	45.85	43.86	−4.9225	0.995
	9	30.98	34.57	30.18	−0.6975	2.195
	12	57.70	54.39	44.35	4.1650	5.020
	14	27.87	30.02	27.00	−0.3200	1.510
	15	31.03	25.77	29.65	1.6600	−1.940
	16	27.67	21.61	25.64	2.0225	−2.015

TABLE 9.3.4: Sequence-by-period means for AUC data in Table 9.3.3.

Sequence	Period I	Period II	Period III
1	35.29	33.88	35.70
2	32.50	34.55	32.13

Note: $S^2 = 16.67$.

TABLE 9.3.5: Summary of results for AUC data in Table 9.3.2.

Method and Assumption	Test Statistic[a]	p-Value	90% CI
Two one-sided tests	$T_L = 6.29$	<.0001	(−1.32, 2.67)
Compound symmetry	$T_U = -5.14$	<.0001	(96.07%, 107.93%)[b]
Two one-sided tests	$T_L = 6.00$	<.0001	(−1.48, 2.83)
$\mathrm{Var}(Y_{ik}) = \Sigma$	$T_U = -4.91$	<.0001	(95.60%, 108.40%)[b]
Wilcoxon–Mann–Whitney			
Two one-sided tests	$W_L = 80$	<.05	(−1.65, 2.84)
$\mathrm{Var}(Y_{ik}) = \Sigma$	$W_U = 3$	<.05	(95.12%, 108.43%)[b]

[a] The ±20 rule was applied by assuming $\mu_R = \hat{\mu}_R = 33.67$.

[b] CI, confidence interval, which was expressed in terms of $\hat{\mu}_R = \hat{\mu} - 1/2\hat{F} = 33.67$.

For testing the equality of intra-subject variabilities, estimates of σ_T^2 and σ_R^2 are obtained based on the intra-subject contrasts g_{ik} as follows:

$$\widehat{\sigma_T^2} = 14.13 \quad \text{and} \quad \widehat{\sigma_R^2} = 15.94.$$

Hence, $F_v = 1.13$ with a p-value of 0.87. Therefore, we fail to reject the null hypothesis of equal intra-subject variability at the 5% level of significance. Because $F(0.025, 8, 8) = 4.03$, the lower and upper limits of the 95% confidence interval for σ_T^2/σ_R^2 are given by

$$L_F = \frac{14.13/15.94}{4.03} = 0.22, \quad \text{and}$$
$$U_F = (14.13/15.94)(4.03) = 3.57.$$

9.4 Optimal Four-Period Designs

In this section, we focus on estimation of the direct formulation effect for two four-period designs, namely, the two-sequence, four-period design and the four-sequence, four-period design. We will derive statistical methods for assessment of bioequivalence of average bioavailability under the general model 9.1.1, with the normality assumptions of Equation 8.1.2 for each of these four-period designs.

9.4.1 Two-Sequence, Four-Period Design

The two-sequence, four-period design, which is made of sequences of TRRT and RTTR, is summarized as follows:

Two-sequence, four-period design.

	Period			
Sequence	**I**	**II**	**III**	**IV**
1	T	R	R	T
2	R	T	T	R

It can be seen that if the last period is omitted, the two-sequence, four-period design reduces to the two-sequence dual design.

Table 9.4.1 lists expected values of the sequence-by-period means. The analysis of variance table in terms of degrees of freedom is given in Table 9.4.2. Similar to the two-sequence dual design, the two-sequence, four-period design can be used to assess bioequivalence of average bioavailability in the presence of the carryover effect. Moreover, it can also provide estimates of intra-subject variabilities.

Under the assumption of compound symmetry of $\text{Var}(Y_{ik})$ and normality assumptions given in 8.1.2, the best linear unbiased estimator for the formulation effect after adjustment for the carryover effect is given by

TABLE 9.4.1: Expected values of the sequence-by-period means for the two-sequence, four-period design.

	Period			
Sequence	**I**	**II**	**III**	**IV**
1	$\mu + G_1 + P_1 + F_T$	$\mu + G_1 + P_2 + F_R + C_T$	$\mu + G_1 + P_3 + F_R + C_R$	$\mu + G_1 + P_4 + F_T + C_R$
2	$\mu + G_2 + P_1 + F_R$	$\mu + G_2 + P_2 + F_T + C_R$	$\mu + G_2 + P_3 + F_T + C_T$	$\mu + G_2 + P_4 + F_R + C_T$

$$\widehat{F}|C = \frac{1}{20}\left[(6\overline{Y}_{\cdot 11} - 3\overline{Y}_{\cdot 21} - 7\overline{Y}_{\cdot 31} + 4\overline{Y}_{\cdot 41}) - (6\overline{Y}_{\cdot 12} - 3\overline{Y}_{\cdot 22} - 7\overline{Y}_{\cdot 32} + 4\overline{Y}_{\cdot 42})\right]. \tag{9.4.1}$$

On the basis of Equation 9.4.1, it can be verified that the variance of $\widehat{F}|C$ is given by

$$\mathrm{Var}(\widehat{F}|C) = \frac{11}{40}\sigma_e^2\left(\frac{1}{n_1} + \frac{1}{n_2}\right). \tag{9.4.2}$$

Since $\overline{Y}_{\dots}$ is an unbiased estimator of the overall mean μ, unbiased estimates for μ_T and μ_R can be obtained as follows:

$$\widehat{\mu}_T = \overline{Y}_{\dots} + \tfrac{1}{2}(\widehat{F}|C),$$

and

$$\widehat{\mu}_R = \overline{Y}_{\dots} - \tfrac{1}{2}(\widehat{F}|C).$$

TABLE 9.4.2: Analysis of variance table for the two-sequence, four-period design.

Source of Variation	Degrees of Freedom
Inter-subject	$n_1 + n_2 - 1$
Sequence	1
Residual	$n_1 + n_2 - 2$
Intra-subject	$3(n_1 + n_2)$
Period	3
Formulation	1
Carryover	1
Residual	$3(n_1+n_2)-5$
Total	$4(n_1 + n_2) - 1$

The classic $(1-2\alpha)\times 100\%$ confidence interval is then given by

$$(L, U) = \widehat{F}|C \pm t[\alpha, 3(n_1+n_2)-5]S\sqrt{\frac{11}{40}\left(\frac{1}{n_1}+\frac{1}{n_2}\right)}. \qquad (9.4.3)$$

Therefore, we conclude bioequivalence if (L, U) is within the bioequivalent limits (θ_L, θ_U).

Similarly, a two one-sided tests procedure can be obtained from the following two t statistics. We reject the null interval hypothesis given in 4.3.1 and conclude bioequivalence if

$$T_L = \frac{\widehat{F}|C - \theta_L}{S\sqrt{\frac{11}{40}\left(\frac{1}{n_1}+\frac{1}{n_2}\right)}} > t[\alpha, 3(n_1+n_2)-5],$$

and

$$T_U = \frac{\widehat{F}|C - \theta_U}{S\sqrt{\frac{11}{40}\left(\frac{1}{n_1}+\frac{1}{n_2}\right)}} < -t[\alpha, 3(n_1+n_2)-5]. \qquad (9.4.4)$$

Note that if the covariance matrix of the four responses observed on a subject does not follow the structure of compound symmetry, but is the same for all subjects in both sequences, then the method derived for the two-sequence dual design in the previous section can also be applied. Define the following intra-subject contrasts:

$$d_{ik} = \tfrac{1}{20}[6Y_{i1k} - 3Y_{i2k} - 7Y_{i3k} + 4Y_{i4k}], \quad i = 1, 2, \ldots, n_k, \quad k = 1, 2. \qquad (9.4.5)$$

Then, $\bar{d} = \bar{d}_{\cdot 1} - \bar{d}_{\cdot 2}$ is an unbiased estimator of F. Therefore, the confidence interval in Equation 9.4.3 and the two one-sided tests procedure in Equation 9.4.4 can be easily carried out by substituting $\widehat{F}|C$, and $t[\alpha, 3(n_1+n_2)-5]$ with $\bar{d}$, $\widehat{\sigma}_d$, and $t(\alpha, n_1+n_2-2)$, where

$$\widehat{\sigma}_d^2 = \frac{1}{n_1+n_2-2}\sum_{k=1}^{2}\sum_{i=1}^{n_k}(d_{ik} - \bar{d}_{\cdot k})^2$$

with (n_1+n_2-2) degrees of freedom.

When the normality assumptions given in 8.1.2 are questionable, nonparametric methods based upon d_{ik} can be directly applied to obtain the Wilcoxon–Mann–Whitney two one-sided test statistics and a distribution-free confidence interval as described in Section 9.3.3.

It should be noted that if the intra-subject variability differs from formulation to formulation, statistical inference for F may not be valid. This can be seen from the fact that

$$\mathrm{Var}(d_{ik}) = \begin{cases} \frac{1}{400}\left[52\sigma_{\mathrm{T}}^2 + 58\sigma_{\mathrm{R}}^2\right], & \text{if } k = 1, \\ \frac{1}{400}\left[52\sigma_{\mathrm{R}}^2 + 58\sigma_{\mathrm{T}}^2\right], & \text{if } k = 2. \end{cases} \quad (9.4.6)$$

In other words, random samples $\{d_{1k}\}$ and $\{d_{2k}\}$ do not have the same variance, although, the difference in variances is rather small.

As indicated earlier, the two-sequence, four-period design allows us to assess the carryover effect. The best linear unbiased estimator for the carryover effect can be obtained by the following linear contrasts of sequence-by-period means:

$$\widehat{C}|F = \frac{1}{5}\left[(\overline{Y}_{\cdot 11} + 2\overline{Y}_{\cdot 21} - 2\overline{Y}_{31} - \overline{Y}_{\cdot 41}) - (\overline{Y}_{\cdot 12} + 2\overline{Y}_{\cdot 22} - 2\overline{Y}_{\cdot 32} - \overline{Y}_{\cdot 42})\right]. \quad (9.4.7)$$

The variance of $\widehat{C}|F$ is then given by

$$\mathrm{Var}(\widehat{C}|F) = \frac{2}{5}\sigma_{\mathrm{e}}^2\left(\frac{1}{n_1} + \frac{1}{n_2}\right). \quad (9.4.8)$$

Therefore, the null hypothesis of equal carryover effects in Equation 3.2.4 is rejected at the α level of significance if

$$|T_{\mathrm{C}}| > t[\alpha/2, 3(n_1 + n_2) - 5], \quad (9.4.9)$$

where

$$T_{\mathrm{C}} = \frac{\widehat{C}|F}{S\sqrt{\frac{2}{5}\left(\frac{1}{n_1} + \frac{1}{n_2}\right)}}. \quad (9.4.10)$$

If we fail to reject the null hypothesis $\mathrm{H}_0\colon C_{\mathrm{T}} = C_{\mathrm{R}}$, we might drop the carryover effect from the model. In this case, the best linear unbiased estimator for F can be expressed by the following linear contrasts of sequence-by-period means:

$$\widehat{F} = \frac{1}{4}\left[(\overline{Y}_{\cdot 11} - \overline{Y}_{\cdot 21} - \overline{Y}_{\cdot 31} + \overline{Y}_{\cdot 41}) - (\overline{Y}_{\cdot 12} - Y_{\cdot 22} - \overline{Y}_{\cdot 32} + \overline{Y}_{\cdot 42})\right]. \quad (9.4.11)$$

The variance of $\widehat{F}$ under the assumption of equal carryover effects is given by

$$\mathrm{Var}(\widehat{F}) = \frac{1}{4}\sigma_{\mathrm{e}}^2\left(\frac{1}{n_1} + \frac{1}{n_2}\right). \quad (9.4.12)$$

Note that the precision of $\widehat{F}$ improves only by a very small fraction compared with that of $\widehat{F}|C$. The associated degrees of freedom using $\widehat{F}$ for evaluation of bioequivalence based on either the confidence interval or the two one-sided tests procedure is $3(n_1 + n_2) - 4$.

In absence of unequal carryover effects, the confidence interval and the two one-sided tests procedure are still valid, even when $\sigma_T^2 \neq \sigma_R^2$. To demonstrate this, we note that $\widehat{F}$ is the difference of the sample means of the following intra-subject contrasts between sequences 1 and 2:

$$d_{ik} = \frac{1}{4}[Y_{i1k} - Y_{i2k} - Y_{i3k} - Y_{i4k}], \quad i = 1, 2, \ldots, n_k; \quad k = 1, 2. \tag{9.4.13}$$

It can be verified that the variance of d_{ik} is given by

$$\text{Var}(d_{ik}) = \frac{1}{8}\left(\sigma_T^2 + \sigma_R^2\right), \tag{9.4.14}$$

which is the same for both sequences.

In addition, because each subject receives the test formulation and the reference formulation twice, estimates of σ_T^2 and σ_R^2 are available. Therefore, hypothesis 7.2.3 for equivalence in variabilities can be tested using these estimates. Define the following intra-subject contrasts:

$$D_{1ik} = (Y_{i1k} - Y_{i4k}),$$

and

$$D_{2ik} = (Y_{i2k} - Y_{i3k}), \tag{9.4.15}$$

where

$i = 1, 2, \ldots, n_k$
$k = 1, 2.$

Then, under normality assumptions of Equation 8.1.2, the vector $\mathbf{D} = (\mathrm{D}_{1ik}, \mathrm{D}_{2ik})'$ follows a bivariate normal distribution with mean vector and covariance matrix given as follows, respectively.

$$\boldsymbol{\mu}_\mathrm{D} = \begin{cases} (P_1 - P_4 - C_\mathrm{R}, \quad P_2 - P_3 + C_\mathrm{T} - C_\mathrm{R})', & \text{if } k = 1, \\ (P_1 - P_4 - C_\mathrm{T}, \quad P_2 - P_3 + C_\mathrm{R} - C_\mathrm{T})', & \text{if } k = 2, \end{cases}$$

$$\boldsymbol{\Sigma}_\mathrm{D} = \begin{cases} \begin{bmatrix} 2\sigma_T^2 & 0 \\ 0 & 2\sigma_R^2 \end{bmatrix}, & \text{if } k = 1, \\ \begin{bmatrix} 2\sigma_T^2 & 0 \\ 0 & 2\sigma_T^2 \end{bmatrix}, & \text{if } k = 2. \end{cases}$$

Because the covariance between D_{1ik} and D_{2ik} is 0, it follows that D_{1ik} and D_{2ik} are independent. Therefore, based on D_{1ik} and D_{2ik}, independent estimates for σ_T^2 and σ_R^2 can be derived as follows.

THEOREM 9.4.1

Let

$$\widehat{\sigma}_{\mathrm{T}}^{2}=\frac{1}{2(n_1+n_2-2)}\left[\sum_{i=1}^{n_1}(D_{1i1}-\overline{D}_{1\cdot 1})^2+\sum_{i=1}^{n_2}(D_{2i2}-\overline{D}_{2\cdot 2})^2\right], \tag{9.4.16}$$

and

$$\widehat{\sigma}_{\mathrm{R}}^{2}=\frac{1}{2(n_1+n_2-2)}\left[\sum_{i=1}^{n_1}(D_{2i1}-\overline{D}_{2\cdot 1})^2+\sum_{i=1}^{n_2}(D_{1i2}-\overline{D}_{1\cdot 2})^2\right],$$

where

$$\overline{D}_{h\cdot k}=\frac{1}{n_k}\sum_{i=1}^{n_k}D_{nik},\quad h=1,2,\quad k=1,2.$$

Then $\widehat{\sigma}_{\mathrm{T}}^{2}$ and $\widehat{\sigma}_{\mathrm{R}}^{2}$, which are independent, are unbiased estimators of σ_{T}^{2} and σ_{R}^{2}, respectively.

PROOF

1. Independence

Let $\mathbf{Y}_{ik}=(\mathbf{Y}_{i1k},\ldots,\mathbf{Y}_{i4k})'$, $\mathbf{Y}_k=(\mathbf{Y}'_{1k},\ldots,\mathbf{Y}'_{n_k k})'$, and $D_{hk}=(D_{h1k},\ldots,D_{hn_k k})$, $i=1,2,\ldots,n_k$; $h=1,2$; $k=1,2$. The covariance matrices of Y_k are given by

$$\mathrm{Cov}(\mathbf{Y}_k)=\mathbf{I}_{n_k}\otimes(\boldsymbol{\Gamma}_h+\sigma_{\mathrm{S}}^2\mathbf{J}_{n_k}),\quad h=1,2,\quad k=1,2.$$

where

$$\Gamma_h=\begin{cases}\mathrm{diag}\left(\sigma_{\mathrm{T}}^2,\sigma_{\mathrm{R}}^2,\sigma_{\mathrm{R}}^2,\sigma_{\mathrm{T}}^2\right), & \text{if } h=1,\\ \mathrm{diag}\left(\sigma_{\mathrm{R}}^2,\sigma_{\mathrm{T}}^2,\sigma_{\mathrm{T}}^2,\sigma_{\mathrm{R}}^2\right), & \text{if } h=2,\end{cases}$$

and where $\mathrm{diag}(a_1,a_2,a_3,a_4)$ is a 4×4 diagonal matrix with diagonal elements a_1,a_2,a_3, and a_4. Then,

$$\mathrm{SSD}_{hk}=\sum_{k=1}^{n_k}(D_{hik}-\overline{D}_{h\cdot k})^2,\quad h=1,2,\quad k=1,2.$$

can be expressed in terms of $\mathbf{Y}_k$ as

$$\text{SS}D_{hk} = \mathbf{Y}_k'[\mathbf{I}_{n_k} \otimes \mathbf{C}_h]\left[\mathbf{I}_{n_k} - \frac{1}{n_k}\mathbf{J}_{n_k}\right][\mathbf{I}_{n_k} \otimes \mathbf{C}_h']\mathbf{Y}_k,$$

where $\mathbf{I}_{n_k}$ is the $n_k \times n_k$ identity matrix $\mathbf{J}_{n_k}$ is the $n_k \times n_k$ matrix of 1, and

$$\mathbf{C}_h = \begin{cases} (1,0,0,-1)', & \text{if } h = 1, \\ (0,1,-1,0)', & \text{if } h = 2. \end{cases}$$

It follows that $\text{SS}D_{hk}$, $h = 1,2;\ k = 1,2$ are mutually independent owing to the fact that $\text{SS}D_{h1}$ and $\text{SS}D_{h2}$ are independent and

$$\begin{aligned} &[\mathbf{I}_{n_k} \otimes \mathbf{C}_1]\left[\mathbf{I}_{n_k} - \frac{1}{n_k}\mathbf{J}_{n_k}\right][\mathbf{I}_{n_k} \otimes \mathbf{C}_1'][\mathbf{I}_{n_k} \otimes (\mathbf{\Gamma}_h + \sigma_S^2\mathbf{J}_{n_k})], \\ &[\mathbf{I}_{n_k} \otimes \mathbf{C}_2]\left[\mathbf{I}_{n_k} - \frac{1}{n_k}\mathbf{J}_{n_k}\right][\mathbf{I}_{n_k} \otimes \mathbf{C}_2'] = \mathbf{0}. \end{aligned}$$

Since

$$\widehat{\sigma_T^2} = \frac{1}{2(n_1 + n_2 - 2)}[\text{SS}D_{11} + \text{SS}D_{22}],$$

and

$$\widehat{\sigma_R^2} = \frac{1}{2(n_1 + n_2 - 2)}[\text{SS}D_{12} + \text{SS}D_{21}],$$

the results follows.

2. Unbiasedness
It is sufficient to show that $\widehat{\sigma_T^2}$ is an unbiased estimator for σ_T^2. The result follows from the fact that

$$\begin{aligned} \text{SS}D_{11} &\sim 2\sigma_T^2\chi^2(n_1 - 1), \\ \text{SS}D_{22} &\sim 2\sigma_T^2\chi^2(n_2 - 1), \end{aligned}$$

and $\text{SS}D_{11}$ is independent of $\text{SS}D_{22}$.

On the basis of $\widehat{\sigma_T^2}$ and $\widehat{\sigma_R^2}$, the classic $(1 - 2\alpha) \times 100\%$ confidence interval for σ_T^2/σ_T^2 and the two one-sided tests procedure for equivalence in variabilities can then be obtained by simply plugging σ_T^2 and σ_R^2 and $v_1 = v_2 = (n_1 + n_2 - 2)$ into Equations 9.2.16 and 9.2.17, respectively.

Note that although the above procedure is still valid in the presence of unequal carryover effects, $\hat{\sigma}_T^2$ and $\hat{\sigma}_R^2$ are independent of each other, and they are independent of $\hat{F}$ given in Equation 9.4.11, they are not independent of $\hat{F}|C$ in Equation 9.4.1. Therefore, in the presence of unequal carryover effects, statistical procedures for average bioavailability are not independent of those for variability of bioavailability.

Example 9.4.1

To illustrate statistical methods for assessment of bioequivalence of average bioavailability for the two-sequence, four-period design, let us consider the data set published by Ryde et al. (1991). The two-sequence, four-period crossover experiment was conducted to compare the tablets (test) and the capsules (reference) formulations of a prodrug of olsalazine (OLZ) for local bioavailability of *N*-acetyl-5-aminosalicyclic acid (ac-5-ASA) in the colon.

In essence, this study consists of two standard two-sequence, two-period designs. This study was originally started with a standard two-sequence and two-period crossover design in 10 healthy volunteers (study A). There was a 1 month washout between periods. However, owing to a very large variability in study A, it is decided to repeat the study using the same subjects 6 months after completion of study A. The same randomization codes and drug batches were used, but the order of formulations was reversed (study B). It should be noted that (1) subject 5 did not participate in study B; (2) one subject, who is not identified in the paper, by mistake, received the formulations in the same order as study A; and (3) no assignment of sequence was given in the paper. For the purpose of illustration, we assign subjects 1 through 5 to sequence 1 and subjects 6 through 10 to sequence 2, where sequences 1 and 2 are TRRT and RTTR, respectively. Subject 5 is not included in all analyses. We assume that all subjects followed their sequence of formulations. The AUC data of ac-5-ASA are given in Table 9.4.3. Table 9.4.4 summarizes test results for average

TABLE 9.4.3: AUC data of ac-5-ASA.

		Study A		Study B	
Sequence	**Subject**	**Period I**	**Period II**	**Period III**	**Period IV**
TRRT[a]	1	106.3	36.4	94.7	58.9
	2	149.2	107.1	104.6	119.4
	3	134.8	155.1	132.5	122.0
	4	108.1	84.9	33.2	24.8
	5	92.3	98.5	—	—
RTTR	6	85.0	92.8	81.9	59.5
	7	64.1	112.8	70.4	55.2
	8	15.3	30.1	22.3	17.5
	9	77.4	67.6	72.9	48.9
	10	102.0	106.1	67.9	70.4

Source: From Ryde et al., *Biopharm. Drug Dispos.*, 12, 233, 1991.

[a] T = tablets; R = capsules.

bioavailability by the methods discussed in this section as well as those by study A and study B alone.

Under the two-sequence, four-period design, test results suggest that the tablet formulation is not equivalent to the capsule formulation in average bioavailability based on the ±20 rule. The results are similar regardless of the presence of the carryover effect. This is because the carryover effect is not significant ($\widehat{C}|F = 0.697$ with a p-value of 0.934). Under study A, the results also indicate that the two formulations are not bioequivalent. However, under study B, the results are in favor of bioequivalence under the assumption of equal carryover effects. One possible explanation for the inconsistency between test results from study A and study B is that intra-subject variabilities are different between studies. Study B has an estimate of 128.92 for σ_e^2, which is less than one-third that from study A ($\sigma_e^2 = 443.71$). Since $\widehat{\sigma}_e^2$ for study A is much larger than that of study B, it is doubtful that the assumption of compound symmetry for covariance matrix is satisfied for this data set. Therefore, we suggest that the nonparametric methods be used. The estimated CVs for study A, study B, and the combined study (A + B) under both the assumption of unequal and equal carryover effects are 26%, 16%, 25.5%, and 25.0%, respectively.

For assessment of intra-subject variabilities, estimates of σ_T^2 and σ_R^2 computed from Equation 9.61 are 316.20 and 524.61, respectively. On the basis of Equation 9.18, the 90% confidence interval for σ_T^2/σ_R^2 is (15.90%, 228.44%). Therefore, if $\delta_L = 80\%$ and $\delta_U = 120\%$, the two formulations are not bioequivalent in variability. Readers can easily verify that σ_T^2 and σ_R^2 are not equivalent in either study A or B by using Equations 7.38 and 7.39.

9.4.2 Four-Sequence, Four-Period Design

The following four-sequence, four-period design, which was previously described as design C in Section 2.5, is now presented.

TABLE 9.4.4: Summary of test results for AUC data in Table 9.4.3.

Data Set	Carryover	Methods	μ_T	μ_R	F	90% CI[a]
Combined[b]	Yes	ANOVA	87.62	76.63	10.99	(98.94, 129.73)
		t	87.62	76.63	10.99	(101.86, 126.82)
		Wilcoxon	—	—	10.61	(99.26, 127.60)
	No	ANOVA	87.71	76.55	11.16	(100.24, 128.93)
		t	87.71	76.55	11.16	(102.04, 127.13)
		Wilcoxon	—	—	11.16	(96.34, 128.45)
Study A	No	ANOVA	103.24	82.34	20.73	(102.42, 148.41)
		Wilcoxon	—	—	21.05	(96.70, 155.15)
Study B	No	ANOVA	72.18	70.78	1.40	(87.56, 116.40)
		Wilcoxon	—	—	2.88	(85.45, 121.19)

[a] In percentage of $\hat{\mu}_R$.

[b] The combination of study A and study B, which results in a two-sequence dual design.

Four-sequence, four-period design

Sequence	Period I	II	III	IV
1	T	T	R	R
2	R	R	T	T
3	T	R	R	T
4	R	T	T	R

The above four-period, four-sequence design is, in fact, made of two Balaam's designs. The first two periods are exactly the same as those of Balaam's design, whereas the other two periods are the mirror image of Balaam's design, with reversed treatments.

Table 9.4.5 provides the expected values of the sequence-by-period means. The analysis of variance table in terms of degrees of freedom is summarized in Table 9.4.6. Again, the four-sequence, four-period design provides estimates of intra-subject variabilities that can be used to assess the carryover effects. The direct formulation effect can be estimated in the presence of the carryover effect. The best linear unbiased estimator for the formulation effect can be found by the following linear contrasts of sequence-by-period means:

$$\begin{aligned}\widehat{F} = \frac{1}{8}[&(\overline{Y}_{\cdot 11} + \overline{Y}_{\cdot 21} - \overline{Y}_{\cdot 31} - \overline{Y}_{\cdot 41}) \\ &- (\overline{Y}_{\cdot 12} + \overline{Y}_{\cdot 22} - \overline{Y}_{\cdot 32} - \overline{Y}_{\cdot 42}) \\ &+ (\overline{Y}_{\cdot 13} - \overline{Y}_{\cdot 23} - \overline{Y}_{\cdot 33} + \overline{Y}_{\cdot 43}) \\ &- (\overline{Y}_{\cdot 14} - \overline{Y}_{\cdot 24} - \overline{Y}_{\cdot 34} + \overline{Y}_{\cdot 44})]. \end{aligned} \tag{9.4.17}$$

TABLE 9.4.5: Expected values of the sequence-by-period means for the four-sequence, four-period design.

Sequence	Period I	II	III	IV
1	$\mu + G_1 + P_1 + F_T$	$\mu + G_1 + P_2 + F_T + C_T$	$\mu + G_1 + P_3 + F_R + C_T$	$\mu + G_1 + P_4 + F_R + C_R$
2	$\mu + G_2 + P_1 + F_R$	$\mu + G_2 + P_2 + F_R + C_R$	$\mu + G_2 + P_3 + F_T + C_R$	$\mu + G_2 + P_4 + F_T + C_T$
3	$\mu + G_3 + P_1 + F_T$	$\mu + G_3 + P_2 + F_R + C_T$	$\mu + G_3 + P_3 + F_R + C_R$	$\mu + G_3 + P_4 + F_T + C_R$
4	$\mu + G_4 + P_1 + F_R$	$\mu + G_4 + P_2 + F_T + C_R$	$\mu + G_4 + P_3 + F_T + C_T$	$\mu + G_4 + P_4 + F_R + C_T$

TABLE 9.4.6: Analysis of variance table for the four-sequence, four-period design.

Source of Variation	Degrees of Freedom
Inter-subject	$n_1 + n_2 + n_3 + n_4 - 1$
Sequence	3
Residual	$n_1 + n_2 + n_3 + n_4 - 4$
Intra-subject	$3(n_1 + n_2 + n_3 + n_4)$
Period	3
Formulation	1
Carryover	1
Residual	$3(n_1 + n_2 + n_3 + n_4) - 5$
Total	$4(n_1 + n_2 + n_3 + n_4) - 1$

It can be verified that, under normality assumptions 8.1.2, $\widehat{F}$ is independent of the estimate of the carryover effect. Therefore, the estimate of F remains the same regardless of the presence or absence of unequal carryover effects. The variance of $\widehat{F}$ is given by

$$\mathrm{Var}(\widehat{F}) = \frac{1}{16}\sigma_e^2\left(\frac{1}{n_1} + \frac{1}{n_2} + \frac{1}{n_3} + \frac{1}{n_4}\right). \tag{9.4.18}$$

In a similar manner, assessment of bioequivalence of average bioavailability can then be carried out with degrees of freedom of $3(n_1 + n_2 + n_3 + n_4) - 5$ and S^2 from the analysis of variance table. It can also be verified that the confidence interval approach and the two one-sided tests procedure under the four-sequence, four-period design are still valid when $\sigma_T^2 \neq \sigma_R^2$.

For assessment of intra-subject variabilities, define the following intra-subject contrasts:

$$\begin{aligned} D_{1ik} &= (Y_{i1k} - Y_{i2k}) \quad \text{if } k = 1, 2, \\ D_{2ik} &= (Y_{i3k} - Y_{i4k}) \quad \text{if } k = 1, 2, \\ D_{3ik} &= (Y_{i1k} - Y_{i4k}) \quad \text{if } k = 3, 4, \\ D_{4ik} &= (Y_{i2k} - Y_{i3k}) \quad \text{if } k = 3, 4. \end{aligned} \tag{9.4.19}$$

Then, based on the same argument in the proof of Theorem 9.4.1, it can be verified that $\widehat{\sigma}_T^2$ and $\widehat{\sigma}_R^2$ are independent and unbiased estimators of σ_T^2 and σ_R^2, respectively, where

$$\begin{aligned} \widehat{\sigma}_T^2 = \frac{1}{2(N-4)}\Bigg[&\sum_{i=1}^{n_1}(D_{1i1} - \overline{D}_{1\cdot 1})^2 + \sum_{i=1}^{n_2}(D_{2i2} - \overline{D}_{2\cdot 2})^2 \\ &+ \sum_{i=1}^{n_3}(D_{3i3} - \overline{D}_{3\cdot 3})^2 + \sum_{i=1}^{n_4}(D_{4i4} - \overline{D}_{4\cdot 4})^2\Bigg], \end{aligned}$$

and

$$\widehat{\sigma}_{\mathrm{R}}^2 = \frac{1}{2(N-4)}\left[\sum_{i=1}^{n_1}(D_{2i1}-\overline{D}_{2\cdot 1})^2 + \sum_{i=1}^{n_2}(D_{1i2}-\overline{D}_{1\cdot 2})^2 + \sum_{i=1}^{n_3}(D_{4i3}-\overline{D}_{4\cdot 3})^2 + \sum_{i=1}^{n_4}(D_{3i4}-\overline{D}_{3\cdot 4})^2\right], \tag{9.4.20}$$

and

$$\overline{D}_{h\cdot k} = \frac{1}{n_k}\sum_{i=1}^{n_k} D_{hik}, \quad h = 1,\, 2, 3, 4, \quad k = 1, 2, 3, 4.$$

Therefore, the $(1-2\alpha)\times 100\%$ confidence interval for $\sigma_{\mathrm{T}}^2/\sigma_{\mathrm{R}}^2$ and the two one-sided tests procedure for equivalence in variabilities can be obtained by plugging $\widehat{\sigma}_{\mathrm{T}}^2$ and $\widehat{\sigma}_{\mathrm{R}}^2$ into Equations 9.2.17 and 9.2.16 with degrees of freedoms $2(n_1+n_2+n_3+n_4-4)$ and $2(n_1+n_2+n_3+n_4-4)$, respectively. It should be noted that $\widehat{\sigma}_{\mathrm{T}}^2$ and $\widehat{\sigma}_{\mathrm{R}}^2$ are independent of $\widehat{F}$ given in Equation 9.4.17.

9.5 Transformation and Individual Subject Ratios

As indicated in Chapter 6, when the responses are skewed, a log-transformation is often considered to remove the skewness and achieve an additive model with relatively homogeneous variance. In addition, the FDA 2001 guidance on statistical approaches as well as the 2003 FDA guidance on general considerations requires the log-transformation for $C_{\max}$ and AUC. Let X_{ijk} be the responses and $Y_{ijk} = \log(X_{ijk})$. Suppose Y_{ijk} follows the additive model 9.1.1 with normality assumptions and structure of compound symmetry of covariance matrix. Then, the relative average bioavailability on the original scale for an individual subject can be measured by some individual subject ratios. Therefore, in this section, we will focus on estimation of a ratio of bioavailabilities [i.e., $\delta = \exp(F)$] on the original scale between the two formulations defined in Equation 6.3.1 under Balaam's design, the two-sequence dual design, and the four-sequence, four-period design.

9.5.1 Balaam's Design

Let $r_{ik} = X_{i2k}/X_{i1k}$, $i = 1, 2, \ldots, n_k$; $k = 1, 2, 3, 4$, be the period ratio as defined in Equation 6.4.2. Then, the maximum likelihood estimate of $\delta = \exp(F)$ is given by

$$\widehat{\delta}_{\text{ML}} = \exp(\widehat{F}/C)$$
$$= \frac{\left(\prod_{i=1}^{n_1} r_{i1}\right)^{1/2n_1} \left(\prod_{i=1}^{n_3} r_{i3}\right)^{1/2n_3}}{\left(\prod_{i=1}^{n_2} r_{i2}\right)^{1/2n_2} \left(\prod_{i=1}^{n_4} r_{i4}\right)^{1/2n_4}}. \tag{9.5.1}$$

Therefore, the minimum variance unbiased estimator of δ is given by

$$\widehat{\delta}_{\text{MVUE}} = \widehat{\delta}_{\text{ML}} \cdot \Phi_f[-m\text{SS}], \tag{9.5.2}$$

where $f = n_1 + n_2 + n_3 + n_4 - 3$, $m = (1/n_1 + 1/n_2 + 1/n_3 + 1/n_4)$, SS = SSE/2, and SSE is the intra-subject residual sum of squares obtained from the analysis of variance table.

9.5.2 Two-Sequence Dual Design

Under the two-sequence dual design, consider the following ratios:

$$r_{ik} = \left[\frac{X_{i1k}^2}{(X_{i2k})(X_{i3k})}\right]^{1/4}, \quad i = 1, 2, \ldots, n_k, \quad k = 1, 2. \tag{9.5.3}$$

It can be verified that r_{ik} is independently distributed as a univariate lognormal distribution with mean and median given as

$$E(r_{ik}) = \begin{cases} \exp\left\{\frac{1}{2}F + \frac{3}{4}P_1 + \frac{3}{16}\sigma_e^2\right\} & \text{if } k = 1, \\ \exp\left\{-\frac{1}{2}F + \frac{3}{4}P_1 + \frac{3}{16}\sigma_e^2\right\} & \text{if } k = 2, \end{cases} \tag{9.5.4}$$

and

$$\text{Med}(r_{ik}) = \begin{cases} \exp\left\{\frac{1}{2}F + \frac{3}{4}P_1\right\} & \text{if } k = 1, \\ \exp\left\{\frac{1}{2}F + \frac{3}{4}P_1\right\} & \text{if } k = 2. \end{cases}$$

Hence,

$$\delta = \frac{E(r_{i1})}{E(r_{i2})} = \frac{\text{Med}(r_{i1})}{\text{Med}(r_{i2})} = \exp(F), \tag{9.5.5}$$

which is the ratio of bioavailabilities on the original scale between the two formulations defined in Equation 6.3.1. The maximum likelihood estimator of δ is $\exp(\widehat{F})$, which always overestimates δ. The minimum variance unbiased estimator of δ is given by

$$\delta_{\text{MVUE}} = \widehat{\delta}_{\text{ML}} \cdot \Phi_f[-m\text{SS}], \tag{9.5.6}$$

where $f = 2(n_1 + n_2 - 2)$, $m = (1/n_1 + 1/n_2)$, and $\text{SS} = 3\text{SSE}/8$, where SSE is the sum of squares error obtained from the analysis of variance table.

On the other hand, if after a log-transformation, Y_{ijk} follows model 9.3.12 with a common error covariance matrix Σ, then the minimum variance unbiased estimator of δ is given by

$$\widehat{\delta}_{\text{MVUE}} = \widehat{\delta}_{\text{ML}} \cdot \Phi_f[-m\text{SS}D], \tag{9.5.7}$$

where $f = n_1 + n_2 - 2$ and $\text{SS}D$ is as defined in Equation 9.3.16.

9.5.3 Four-Sequence, Four-Period Design

Under the four-sequence, four-period design, the maximum likelihood estimator of δ is given by

$$\begin{aligned}\widehat{\delta}_{\text{ML}} &= \exp(\widehat{F}) \\ &= \frac{\left[\dfrac{X_{i11} \cdot X_{i21}}{X_{i31} \cdot X_{i41}}\right]^{1/8n_1} \left[\dfrac{X_{i13} \cdot X_{i43}}{X_{i23} \cdot X_{i33}}\right]^{1/8n_3}}{\left[\dfrac{X_{i12} \cdot X_{i22}}{X_{i32} \cdot X_{i42}}\right]^{1/8n_2} \left[\dfrac{X_{i14} \cdot X_{i44}}{X_{i24} \cdot X_{i34}}\right]^{1/8n_4}}.\end{aligned} \tag{9.5.8}$$

Therefore, the minimum variance unbiased estimator of δ is given by

$$\widehat{\delta}_{\text{MVUE}} = \widehat{\delta}_{\text{ML}} \cdot \Phi_f[-m\text{SS}], \tag{9.5.9}$$

where $f = 3(n_1 + n_2 + n_3 + n_4) - 5$, $m = 3(1/n_1 + 1/n_2 + 1/n_3 + 1/n_4)$, $\text{SS} = \text{SSE}/16$, and SSE is the intra-subject residual sum of squares obtained from the ANOVA table.

9.6 Sample Size for Higher-Order Crossover Designs

In Section 9.5, we considered sample size determination for standard two-sequence, two-period crossover design based on interval hypotheses. For higher-order crossover designs comparing two formulations of the same drug products or two drug products, similar formulae can be derived (Chen et al., 1997).

Because the power curves of Schuirmann's two one-sided tests procedure are symmetric about zero, we present only the equations for the case where $\theta \geq 0$. Let n_i, the number of subjects in each sequence i, have the same value n, and F_v denote the cumulative distribution function of the t distribution with v degrees of freedom. Then the power function, $P_k(\theta)$, of Schuirmann's tests at the α nominal level for design (k) is the following:

$$P_k(\theta) = F_{\nu_k}\left(\left[(\Delta - \theta)/\left(\mathrm{CV}\sqrt{b_k/n}\right)\right] - t[\alpha, \nu_k]\right) - F_{\nu_k}\left(t[\alpha, \nu_k] - \left[(\Delta + \theta)/\left(\mathrm{CV}\sqrt{b_k/n}\right)\right]\right) \quad \text{for } k = 1, 2, 3, 4,$$

where

$\nu_1 = 4n - 3$
$\nu_2 = 4n - 4$
$\nu_3 = 6n - 5$
$\nu_4 = 12n - 5$
$b_1 = 2$
$b_2 = 3/4$
$b_3 = 11/20$
$b_4 = 1/4$.

Hence, the exact equation for determination of n required to achieve a $1 - \beta$ power at the α nominal level for each design (k) when $\theta = 0$ is the following:

$$n \geq b_k[t(\alpha, \nu_k) + t(\beta/2, \nu_k)]^2[\mathrm{CV}/\Delta]^2 \quad \text{for } k = 1, 2, 3, 4,$$

and if $\theta > 0$ the approximate formula for n is

$$n \geq b_k[t(\alpha, \nu_k) + t(\beta, \nu_k)]^2[\mathrm{CV}/(\Delta - \theta)]^2 \quad \text{for } k = 1, 2, 3, 4.$$

For the multiplicative model, we consider (0.8, 1.25) as the bioequivalence limit for μ_T/μ_R, which is denoted by δ and μ_T and μ_R are the median bioavailabilities of the test and reference formulations. Similarly, the sample size n required to achieve a $1 - \beta$ power at the α nominal level for each corresponding design (k) after the logarithmic transformation is determined by the following equations:

$$n \geq b_k[t(\alpha, \nu_k) + t(\beta/2, \nu_k)]^2[\mathrm{CV}/\log 1.25]^2 \quad \text{if } \delta = 1,$$
$$n \geq b_k[t(\alpha, \nu_k) + t(\beta, \nu_k)]^2[\mathrm{CV}/(\log 1.25 - \log \delta)]^2 \quad \text{if } 1 < \delta < 1.25,$$

and

$$n \geq b_k[t(\alpha, \nu_k) + t(\beta, \nu_k)]^2[\mathrm{CV}/(\log 0.8 - \log \delta)]^2 \quad \text{if } 0.8 < \delta < 1,$$

where

log denotes the natural logarithm
β is the probability of a type II error
$\mathrm{CV} = \sqrt{\exp(\sigma^2) - 1}$, the coefficient of variation in the multiplicative model
σ^2 is the residual (within-subject) variance on the log-scale.

TABLE 9.6.1: Number of subjects for Schuirmann's two one-sided tests procedure at $\Delta = 0.2$ and the 5% nominal level in Balaam's design.

		θ			
Power (%)	**Coefficient of Variation (%)**	**0%**	**5%**	**10%**	**15%**
80	10	20	24	52	200
	12	28	36	76	288
	14	36	48	100	392
	16	48	60	132	508
	18	60	76	164	644
	20	72	92	200	796
	22	88	108	244	960
	24	104	132	288	1144
	26	120	152	336	1340
	28	136	176	392	1556
	30	156	200	448	1784
	32	180	228	508	2028
	34	200	256	576	2292
	36	224	288	644	2568
	38	252	320	716	2860
	40	276	356	796	3168
90	10	24	36	72	276
	12	36	48	104	400
	14	48	64	136	540
	16	60	80	180	704
	18	76	104	224	892
	20	92	124	276	1100
	22	108	152	336	1328
	24	128	180	400	1584
	26	152	208	468	1856
	28	172	244	540	2152
	30	200	276	620	2472
	32	224	316	704	2808
	38	284	400	892	3556
	38	316	444	992	3960
	40	352	492	1100	4388

However, because the degrees of freedom are usually unknown, an easy way to find the sample size is to enumerate n.

Tables 9.6.1 through 9.6.4 present the required total number of subjects N_k for the additive model under each design (k) to achieve either an 80% or 90% power for θ from 0% to 15% by increments of 5% as well as CVs from 10% to 40% by increments of 2%, where

TABLE 9.6.2: Number of subjects for Schuirmann's two one-sided tests procedure at $\Delta = 0.2$ and the 5% nominal level in two-sequence dual design.

Power (%)	Coefficient of Variation (%)	θ 0%	5%	10%	15%
80	10	6	6	12	38
	12	6	8	16	56
	14	8	10	20	74
	16	10	12	26	96
	18	12	16	32	122
	20	14	18	38	150
	22	18	22	46	182
	24	20	26	56	216
	26	24	30	64	252
	28	28	34	74	292
	30	30	38	86	336
	32	34	44	96	382
	34	38	50	108	430
	36	44	56	122	482
	38	48	62	136	538
	40	54	68	150	596
	10	6	8	14	54
	12	8	10	20	76
	14	10	14	28	102
	16	12	16	34	134
	18	16	20	44	168
	20	18	24	54	208
	22	22	30	64	250
	24	26	34	76	298
	26	30	40	88	350
	28	34	46	102	404
	30	38	54	118	464
	32	44	60	134	528
	34	48	68	150	596
	36	54	76	168	668
	38	60	84	188	744
	40	66	94	208	824

$$N_1 = 4n, \quad N_2 = 2n, \quad N_3 = 2n, \quad N_4 = 4n.$$

Tables 9.6.5 through 9.6.8 present the required total number of subjects $N_k (k = 1, 2, 3, 4)$ for the multiplicative model to achieve either an 80% or 90% power for δ from 0.85 to 1.20 by increments of 0.05 as well as CV_ms from 10% to 40% by increments of 2%.

TABLE 9.6.3: Number of subjects for Schuirmann's two one-sided tests procedure at $\Delta = 0.2$ and the 5% nominal level in four-period design with two sequences.

Power (%)	Coefficient of Variation (%)	θ 0%	5%	10%	15%
80	10	4	4	8	28
	12	6	6	12	40
	14	6	8	14	54
	16	8	10	18	72
	18	10	12	24	90
	20	12	14	28	110
	22	14	16	34	134
	24	16	18	40	158
	26	18	22	48	186
	28	20	26	54	214
	30	22	28	62	246
	32	26	32	72	280
	34	28	36	80	316
	36	32	40	90	354
	38	36	46	100	394
	40	40	50	110	436
90	10	4	6	12	40
	12	6	8	16	56
	14	8	10	20	76
	16	10	12	26	98
	18	12	16	32	124
	20	14	18	40	152
	22	16	22	48	184
	24	18	26	56	218
	26	22	30	66	256
	28	24	34	76	296
	30	28	40	86	340
	32	32	44	98	388
	34	36	50	110	438
	36	40	56	124	490
	38	44	62	138	546
	40	50	68	152	604

9.7 Discussion

As indicated earlier, for assessment of bioequivalence in average bioavailability between two formulations of a drug product, the standard two-sequence, two-period crossover design is often considered. In Chapter 4, under the assumption of no

TABLE 9.6.4: Number of subjects for Schuirmann's two one-sided tests procedure at $\Delta = 0.2$ and the 5% nominal level in four-period design with four sequences.

Power (%)	Coefficient of Variation (%)	θ 0%	5%	10%	15%
80	10	4	4	8	28
	12	4	8	12	40
	14	8	8	16	52
	16	8	8	20	64
	18	8	12	24	84
	20	12	12	28	100
	22	12	16	32	124
	24	16	20	40	144
	26	16	20	44	168
	28	20	24	52	196
	30	20	28	60	224
	32	24	32	64	256
	34	28	36	72	288
	36	32	40	84	324
	38	32	44	92	360
	40	36	48	100	400
90	10	4	8	12	36
	12	8	8	16	52
	14	8	12	20	68
	16	8	12	24	92
	18	12	16	32	112
	20	12	16	36	140
	22	16	20	44	168
	24	20	24	52	200
	26	20	28	60	236
	28	24	32	68	272
	30	28	36	80	312
	32	32	40	92	352
	34	32	48	100	400
	36	36	52	112	448
	38	40	56	128	496
	40	44	64	140	552

carryover effects, we have introduced several statistical methods for this assessment. When the carryover effect is present, the standard two-sequence, two-period crossover design may not be useful because it does not provide an estimate of the formulation effect in the presence of the carryover effect. In addition, it does not provide independent estimates for intra-subject variabilities, which can be used to

TABLE 9.6.5: Number of subjects for Schuirmann's two one-sided tests procedure at the 5% nominal level for the (0.8, 1.25) bioequivalence range in the case of the multiplicative model in Balaam's design.

Power (%)	Coefficient of Variation (%)	δ 0.85	0.90	0.95	1.00	1.05	1.1	1.15	1.2
80	10	140	40	20	16	20	32	76	300
	12	196	56	28	24	28	48	104	432
	14	268	72	36	32	36	64	144	584
	16	348	96	48	40	44	80	184	764
	18	440	120	56	48	56	100	236	964
	20	540	148	72	60	68	124	288	1192
	22	656	176	84	72	84	152	348	1440
	24	780	208	100	84	96	176	412	1712
	26	912	244	116	96	112	208	484	2008
	28	1060	284	136	112	132	240	560	2332
	30	1216	324	156	128	148	276	644	2676
	32	1380	368	176	144	172	312	732	3044
	34	1560	416	196	164	192	352	824	3436
	36	1748	464	220	180	216	396	924	3852
	38	1948	520	244	204	240	440	1032	4288
	40	2156	572	272	224	264	488	1140	4752
90	10	192	52	28	20	28	44	104	416
	12	272	76	36	28	36	64	144	596
	14	368	100	48	40	48	84	196	808
	16	480	132	64	48	60	112	256	1056
	18	608	164	80	60	76	140	324	1336
	20	748	200	96	72	92	172	396	1648
	22	904	244	116	88	112	208	480	1992
	24	1076	288	136	104	132	244	572	2372
	26	1264	336	160	120	156	288	668	2784
	28	1464	392	184	140	180	332	776	3228
	30	1680	448	212	160	208	380	892	3704
	32	1912	508	240	180	236	432	1012	4212
	34	2160	576	272	204	264	488	1144	4756
	36	2420	644	304	228	296	548	1280	5332
	38	2696	716	340	256	328	608	1428	5940
	40	2988	792	376	284	364	676	1580	6580

establish equivalence in intra-subject variabilities. In this case, as an alternative, a higher-order crossover design is usually preferred because it allows us (1) to estimate the formulation effect when the carryover effect is present, (2) to estimate intra-subject variabilities, (3) to draw inference on the carryover effect, and (4) to establish equivalence in variability of bioavailability. The FDA 2001 guidance on statistical

TABLE 9.6.6: Number of subjects for Schuirmann's two one-sided tests procedure at the 5% nominal level for the (0.8, 1.25) bioequivalence range in the case of the multiplicative model in the two-sequence dual design.

Power (%)	Coefficient of Variation (%)	δ 0.85	0.90	0.95	1.00	1.05	1.1	1.15	1.2
80	10	28	8	6	6	6	8	16	58
	12	38	12	6	6	6	10	22	82
	14	52	14	8	8	8	14	28	110
	16	66	18	10	8	10	16	36	144
	18	84	24	12	10	12	20	46	182
	20	102	28	14	12	14	24	56	224
	22	124	34	18	14	16	30	66	272
	24	148	40	20	16	20	34	78	322
	26	172	46	24	20	22	40	92	378
	28	200	54	26	22	26	46	106	438
	30	228	62	30	26	30	52	122	502
	32	260	70	34	28	34	60	138	572
	34	294	80	38	32	38	68	156	646
	36	328	88	42	36	42	76	174	722
	38	366	98	48	40	46	84	194	806
	40	406	108	52	44	50	92	216	892
90	10	36	12	6	6	6	10	20	78
	12	52	16	8	8	8	14	28	112
	14	70	20	10	8	10	18	38	152
	16	92	26	14	10	12	22	50	200
	18	116	32	16	12	16	28	62	252
	20	142	38	20	16	18	34	76	310
	22	170	46	22	18	22	40	92	374
	24	204	56	26	20	26	48	108	446
	26	238	64	32	24	30	54	126	522
	28	276	74	36	28	34	64	146	606
	30	316	86	40	32	40	72	168	696
	32	360	96	46	36	46	82	192	792
	34	406	108	52	40	50	92	216	892
	36	454	122	58	44	56	104	242	1000
	38	506	136	64	50	62	116	268	1114
	40	562	150	72	54	70	128	298	1236

approaches recommends the higher-order design (TRTR, RTRT) and (TRT, RTR) for evaluation of individual bioequivalence. These designs are further reviewed and compared in Chapter 11. Although a higher-order crossover possesses some desirable statistical properties, one should be aware of some practical problems that may be encountered when a higher-order crossover design is used. For a higher-order

TABLE 9.6.7: Number of subjects for Schuirmann's two one-sided tests procedure at the 5% nominal level for the (0.8, 1.25) bioequivalence range in the case of the multiplicative model in the four-period design with two sequences.

Power (%)	Coefficient of Variation (%)	δ 0.85	0.90	0.95	1.00	1.05	1.1	1.15	1.2
80	10	20	6	4	4	4	6	12	42
	12	28	8	6	4	6	8	16	60
	14	38	12	6	6	6	10	20	82
	16	48	14	8	6	8	12	26	106
	18	62	18	10	8	8	16	34	134
	20	76	22	10	10	10	18	40	164
	22	92	26	12	10	12	22	48	200
	24	108	30	14	12	14	26	58	236
	26	126	34	18	14	16	30	68	278
	28	146	40	20	16	20	34	78	322
	30	168	46	22	18	22	38	90	368
	32	190	52	26	20	24	44	102	420
	34	216	58	28	24	28	50	114	474
	36	242	66	32	26	30	56	128	530
	38	268	72	34	28	34	62	142	590
	40	298	80	38	32	38	68	158	654
90	10	28	8	6	4	4	8	16	58
	12	38	12	6	6	6	10	22	82
	14	52	14	8	6	8	12	28	112
	16	68	18	10	8	10	16	36	146
	18	84	24	12	10	12	20	46	184
	20	104	28	14	12	14	24	56	228
	22	126	34	18	14	16	30	68	276
	24	150	40	20	16	20	34	80	328
	26	174	48	24	18	22	40	94	384
	28	202	54	26	20	26	46	108	444
	30	232	62	30	24	30	54	124	510
	32	264	72	34	26	34	60	140	580
	34	298	80	38	30	38	68	158	656
	36	334	90	42	32	42	76	178	734
	38	372	100	48	36	46	84	198	818
	40	412	110	52	40	52	94	218	906

crossover design with more than two periods, the consequences are not only that it may be very time consuming to complete the study, but also that it may increase the number of dropouts. Besides, as indicated in Chapter 2, it may not be desirable to draw too many blood samples from each subject owing to medical concerns. On the other hand, if the higher-order crossover design has more than two sequences, it may

TABLE 9.6.8: Number of subjects for Schuirmann's two one-sided tests procedure at the 5% nominal level for the (0.8, 1.25) bioequivalence range in the case of the multiplicative model in the four-period design with four sequences.

	Coefficient of	δ							
Power (%)	Variation (%)	0.85	0.90	0.95	1.00	1.05	1.1	1.15	1.2
80	10	20	8	8	8	8	8	12	40
	12	28	8	8	8	8	8	16	56
	14	36	12	8	8	8	12	20	76
	16	44	12	8	8	8	12	24	96
	18	56	16	8	8	8	16	32	124
	20	68	20	12	8	12	16	40	152
	22	84	24	12	12	12	20	44	184
	24	100	28	16	12	16	24	52	216
	26	116	32	16	16	16	28	64	252
	28	136	36	20	16	20	32	72	292
	30	152	44	20	20	20	36	84	336
	32	176	48	24	20	24	40	92	384
	34	196	56	28	24	28	48	104	432
	36	220	60	28	24	28	52	116	484
	38	244	68	32	28	32	56	132	540
	40	272	72	36	32	36	64	144	596
90	10	24	8	8	8	8	8	16	52
	12	36	12	8	8	8	12	20	76
	14	48	16	8	8	8	12	28	104
	16	64	20	12	8	8	16	36	136
	18	80	24	12	8	12	20	44	168
	20	96	28	16	12	12	24	52	208
	22	116	32	16	12	16	28	64	252
	24	136	40	20	16	20	32	72	300
	26	160	44	24	16	20	36	84	348
	28	184	52	24	20	24	44	100	404
	30	212	60	28	24	28	48	112	464
	32	240	64	32	24	32	56	128	528
	34	272	72	36	28	36	64	144	596
	36	304	84	40	32	40	72	164	668
	38	340	92	44	36	44	80	180	744
	40	376	100	48	36	48	88	200	824

increase the chance of errors occurring in the randomization schedules. Richardson and Flack (1996) and Chow and Shao (1997) proposed several methods for treatment of missing values occurring from two-sequence, three-period design. However, more research is needed for managing missing values in higher-order crossover designs (see also Pong and Chow, 1996 and Shao et al., 1995).

TABLE 9.7.1: Distribution of degrees of freedom with 24 subjects.

	Design				
Source	**2 × 2[a]**	**4 × 2[b]**	**2 × 3[c]**	**2 × 4[d]**	**4 × 4[e]**
Inter-subject	23	23	23	23	23
Sequence	1	3	1	1	3
Residual	22	20	22	22	20
Intra-subject	24	24	48	72	72
Period	1	1	2	3	3
Formulation	1	1	1	1	1
Carryover	—[f]	1	1	1	1
Residual	22	21	44	67	67
Total	47	47	71	95	95

[a] 2 × 2 is the standard two-sequence, two-period design.
[b] 4 × 2 is the Balaam's design.
[c] 2 × 3 is the two-sequence dual design.
[d] 2 × 4 is the two-sequence, four-period design.
[e] 4 × 4 is the four-sequence, four-period design.
[f] The carryover effect is confounded with the sequence effect.

In this chapter, we have introduced several higher-order crossover designs. To compare their relative advantages and disadvantages in evaluation of average bioequivalence with the standard two-sequence, two-period crossover design, we summarize the distribution of degrees of freedoms for each study in Table 9.7.1 assuming that there are 24 subjects. From Table 9.7.1, it can be seen that for the standard 2×2 crossover design, the carryover effect is confounded with the sequence effect, which cannot be separated in the analysis. The 4×2 crossover design (i.e., Balaam's design) allows us to estimate the carryover effect independently. The degrees of freedom for the intra-subject residuals for the 2×2 design and the 4×2 design are 22 and 21, respectively. Therefore, there is little difference in testing power. For a 2×2 design, if we add one period (or two periods), the design becomes a 2×3 design (or a 2×4 design). It can be seen that the degrees of freedom for the intra-subject residuals increases from 22 to 44 (or 22 to 67). Here, although the testing power will certainly increase significantly, the overall effects associated with the addition of extra periods should be examined carefully. For the comparison between a 2×4 design and a 4×4 design, there is no difference except for testing of the sequence effect. On the basis of the above argument, we suggest that the relative gain and loss caused by the increase of additional period or sequence (or subject) be examined before a decision is made.

In the previous section, we briefly introduced the use of log-transformation for a higher-order crossover design. As an alternative, Chow et al. (1991) proposed a general approach using individual subject ratios under a multiplicative model. However, this method does not provide statistical inference for the carryover effect. More discussion on a higher-order crossover design can be found in Chow and Liu (1992).

Chapter 10

Assessment of Bioequivalence for More Than Two Formulations

10.1 Introduction

In Chapter 9, we introduced statistical methods for the assessment of average bioequivalence under a higher-order crossover design for comparing two formulations of a drug product. The statistical methods depend on the estimation of the direct formulation effect and its variance. The analysis of a higher-order crossover design for comparing two formulations is quite straightforward because there are only two formulations to be compared regardless of how many sequences or periods in the design. In practice, however, it is often of interest to compare more than two (e.g., three or four) formulations of the same drug in a bioavailability/bioequivalence study. In this case, a standard highway (or higher-order) crossover design is usually considered. For example, for comparing three formulations, we may consider a standard three-sequence, three-period crossover design. The analysis for assessing average bioequivalence, however, is much more complicated because there are three pairs of formulation effects to be compared and the variance of these pairs of formulation effects may differ from one another. Moreover, a standard crossover design may not be useful when the carryover effect is present.

To overcome the disadvantages that a standard crossover design may have, as indicated in Chapter 2, variance-balanced designs are usually recommended because (1) it possesses the property of equal variances for each pairwise average differences among formulations; (2) it provides an estimate for each pairwise average difference in the presence of the carryover effect. A variance-balanced design allows us to estimate each pairwise average difference with the same degree of precision and provides analyses for assessing average bioequivalence in the presence of carryover effects. The most common variance-balanced design used for comparing three or four formulations in bioavailability/bioequivalence studies is the so-called Williams design. The Williams designs for comparing three or four formulations were briefly described earlier in Chapter 2. In this chapter, statistical methods for assessment of average bioequivalence under a Williams design are discussed.

Frequently, pharmaceutical companies may be interested in comparing a large number of formulations in a bioavailability study. For this, a complete standard highway (or higher-order) crossover design may not be of practical interest because (1) it is too time consuming to complete the study; (2) it is not desirable to draw many blood samples from each subject; (3) a subject is more likely to drop out when he or she is required to return frequently for evaluations. In addition, a complete higher-order crossover design may increase the chance of making errors in the randomization schedules, which has an influence on valid statistical inference. To accommodate these concerns, Westlake (1973, 1974) suggested that a balanced incomplete block design be used when comparing a large number of formulations. Several methods for constructing a balanced incomplete block design have been introduced earlier in Chapter 2. In the absence of carryover effects, a balanced incomplete block design is also a variance-balanced design. In this chapter, statistical methods for assessment of average bioequivalence under a balanced incomplete block design is also discussed.

Section 10.2 describes a statistical model and methods like the confidence interval and the two one-sided tests procedure for a general $K \times J$ crossover design are derived. The application of these methods to the two Williams designs and an incomplete balanced block design is given in Sections 10.3 and 10.4, respectively. A brief discussion is presented in the Section 10.5.

10.2 Assessment of Average Bioavailability with More Than Two Formulations

In this section, statistical methods for assessment of bioequivalence of average bioavailability under a $K \times J$ (i.e., K-sequence and J-period) crossover design for comparing $t(t > 2)$ formulations are discussed. Again, we focus only on the confidence interval approach and Schuirmann's two one-sided tests procedure.

10.2.1 Statistical Model and Assumptions

Consider the following statistical model for a K-sequence and J-period crossover design comparing $t(t > 2)$ formulations

$$Y_{ijk} = \mu + G_k + S_{ik} + P_j + F_{(j,k)} + C_{(j-1,k)} + e_{ijk}, \tag{10.2.1}$$

where

$i = 1, 2, \ldots, n_k$
$j = 1, 2, \ldots, J$
$k = 1, 2, \ldots, K$
Y_{ijk}, μ, G_k, S_{ik}, P_k, $F_{(j,k)}$, $C_{(j-1,k)}$, and e_{ijk} are as defined in model 9.1.1.

The assumptions for the fixed effects, compound symmetry, and normality of inter-subject and intra-subject variabilities were outlined in model 9.1.1.

For assessment of bioequivalence in average bioavailability under model 10.2.1, the parameters of interest are (1) the unknown formulation means; (2) pairwise differences in formulation means (or direct formulation effects); and (3) pairwise first-order carryover effects. The unknown population mean for the hth formulation is defined as

$$\mu_h = \mu + F_h, \quad h = 1, 2, \ldots, t. \tag{10.2.2}$$

Pairwise differences in formulation means (or direct formulation effects) are defined as

$$\theta_{hh'} = F_h - F_{h'}, \quad 1 \leq h \neq h' < t. \tag{10.2.3}$$

Similarly, pairwise first-order carryover effects are given by

$$\lambda_{hh'} = C_h - C_{h'}, \quad 1 \leq h \neq h' < t. \tag{10.2.4}$$

From estimates of μ_h and $\theta_{hh'}$ and the estimates of their variance, the confidence interval approach and Schuirmann's two one-sided tests procedure for assessing average bioequivalence among formulations can be derived. Furthermore, statistical inference for the carryover effects can also be drawn based on estimates of $\lambda_{hh'}$.

For estimation of $\theta_{hh'}$ and $\lambda_{hh'}$ there are unbiased estimators, which can be obtained by ordinary least squares (OLS) method based on model 10.2.1. The unbiased estimators, which can be expressed as a linear contrast of sequence by period means, are given as

$$\mathscr{L}a = \sum_{k=1}^{K} \sum_{j=1}^{J} C_{ajk} \overline{Y}_{\cdot jk}, \quad a = 1, 2, \ldots, \frac{t!}{2!(t-2)!} \tag{10.2.5}$$

Since

$$\sum_{j=1}^{J} C_{ajk} = \sum_{k=1}^{K} C_{ajk} = 0.$$

under assumptions of normality and $\sigma_h^2 = \sigma_e^2$ for $h = 1, 2, \ldots, t$, the variance of $\mathscr{L}a$ is given by

$$\mathrm{Var}(\mathscr{L}a) = \sigma_e^2 \sum_{k=1}^{K} \left[\frac{1}{n_k}\right] \sum_{j=1}^{J} C_{ajk}^2. \tag{10.2.6}$$

Note that when $n_k = n$ for $k = 1, 2, \ldots, K$, the above variance reduces to

$$\mathrm{Var}(\mathscr{L}a) = \frac{\sigma_e^2}{n} \sum_{k=1}^{K} \sum_{j=1}^{J} C_{ajk}^2. \tag{10.2.7}$$

For Equations 10.2.5 and 10.2.6, the $(1-2\alpha)\times 10\%$ confidence interval and Schuirmann's two one-sided tests procedure can be obtained to assess bioequivalence between the hth formulation and the h'th formulation.

10.2.2 Confidence Interval and Two One-Sided Tests Procedure

An unbiased estimator of the overall mean is the arithmetic average of sequence-by-period means; namely,

$$\widehat{\mu} = \frac{1}{JK}\sum_{j=1}^{J}\sum_{k=1}^{K}\overline{Y}_{\cdot jk\cdot}$$

Let $\widehat{F}_h$ be the OLS unbiased estimate of F_h. Then, the population means μ_h, $h = 1, 2, \ldots, t$, can be estimated unbiasedly by

$$\widehat{\mu}_h = \widehat{\mu} + \widehat{F}_h.$$

The OLS unbiased estimates for $\theta_{hh'}$ are then given by

$$\begin{aligned}\theta_{hh'} &= \widehat{\mu}_h - \widehat{\mu}_{h'} \\ &= \widehat{F}_h - \widehat{F}_{h'}, \quad 1 \le h \ne h' \le t.\end{aligned} \tag{10.2.8}$$

Therefore, the $(1-2\alpha)\times 100\%$ confidence interval for $\theta_{hh'}$ is given by

$$[L(\theta_{hh'}),\ U(\theta_{hh'})] = \theta_{hh'} \pm t(\alpha, \nu)\left[S^2\sum_{k=1}^{K}\frac{1}{n_k}\sum_{j=1}^{J}C_{ajk}^2\right]^{1/2}, \tag{10.2.9}$$

where S^2 is the intra-subject mean squared error, with ν degrees of freedom, obtained from the analysis of variance table. Under model 10.2.1, S^2 is an unbiased estimator of σ_e^2. Hence, we conclude that the hth formulation and the h'th formulation are bioequivalent in average bioavailability if $[L(\theta_{hh'}), U(\theta_{hh'})]$ is within bioequivalent limits (θ_L, θ_U).

Similarly, for the two one-sided tests procedure, we would reject the interval hypothesis 4.3.1 and conclude bioequivalent at the α level of significance if

$$T_L = \frac{\widehat{\theta}_{hh'} - \theta_L}{\left[S^2\sum_{k=1}^{K}\frac{1}{n_k}\sum_{j=1}^{J}C_{ajk}^2\right]^{1/2}} > t(\alpha, \nu),$$

and

$$T_U = \frac{\widehat{\theta}_{hh'} - \theta_U}{\left[S^2\sum_{k=1}^{K}\frac{1}{n_k}\sum_{j=1}^{J}C_{ajk}^2\right]^{1/2}} < -t(\alpha, \nu). \tag{10.2.10}$$

Note that p-values of Anderson and Hauck's procedure for interval hypotheses 4.3.1 can also be obtained by simply plugging T_{L} and T_{U} into either Equation 4.3.12 or Equation 4.3.13.

Although the primary hypothesis of interest is to evaluate the equality of carryover effects, confidence interval for the carryover effect can also be obtained in a similar manner.

10.2.3 Log-Transformation

When the responses are skewed, a log-transformation may be considered to remove the skewness and achieve model 10.2.1 with relatively homogeneous variance. In this case, a parameter of interest is given by

$$\begin{aligned}\delta_{hh'} &= \exp(\theta_{hh'}) = \exp(F_h - F_{h'})\\ &= \frac{\exp(\mu + F_h)'}{\exp(\mu + F_{h'})} \quad 1 \leq h \neq h' \leq t.\end{aligned}$$

Under normality assumptions and $\sigma_h^2 = \sigma_e^2$ for $h = 1,2,\ldots,\ t$, the maximum likelihood estimate of $\delta_{hh'}$ can be obtained by simply replacing the maximum likelihood estimate of $\theta_{hh'}$ with $\widehat{\theta}_{hh'}$ in the above expression; that is,

$$\widehat{\delta}_{hh'} = \exp(\widehat{\theta}_{hh'}).$$

The minimum variance unbiased estimator of $\delta_{hh'}$ is then given by

$$\widehat{\delta}_{hh'} = \exp(\widehat{\theta}_{hh'}) \bullet \Phi_f[-m\mathrm{SSE}], \tag{10.2.11}$$

where $\widehat{\theta}_{hh'}$ is the OLS unbiased estimate of $\theta_{hh'}$ on the log scale, SSE in the intra-subject sum of squares from the analysis of variance table with degrees of freedom $f = \nu$, and

$$m = \sum_{k=1}^{K} \frac{1}{n_k} \sum_{j=1}^{J} C_{ajk}^2.$$

10.2.4 Variance-Balanced Designs

For assessment of bioequivalence of average bioavailability, as indicted earlier, the confidence interval approach and the two one-sided tests procedure depend on the estimation of the formulation effects (or difference in formulation means) and their variances. For comparing more than two formulations, there are several possible pairs of differences in formulation means. For example, there are three possible pairwise differences among formulation means (i.e., formulation

1 versus formulation 2; for formulation 2 versus formulation 3; formulation 1 versus formulation 3). In this case, it is desirable to estimate these pairwise formulation effects with the same degrees of precision. In other words, it is desirable that there is a common variance for each pair of formulation effect. A design with this property is known as a variance-balanced design. Therefore, an ideal crossover design for comparing more than two formulations is a design that can minimize this common variance. Such a design can lead to the best precision within the class of variance-balanced designs. An example of a variance-balanced design is the so-called Williams design, which is further discussed in the Section 10.3.

For a variance-balanced design, the quantity

$$\nu_a = \sum_{k=1}^{K} \sum_{j=1}^{J} C_{ajk}^2$$

is the same for all pairwise formulation effects. In the case where $n_k = n$ for $k = 1, 2, \ldots, K$, the $(1 - 2\alpha) \times 100\%$ confidence interval for $\theta_{hh'}$ given in Equation 10.9 reduces to

$$[L(\theta_{hh'}),\ U(\theta_{hh'})] = \widehat{\theta}_{hh'} \pm t(\alpha,\ \nu)\left[S^2 \frac{\nu_a}{n}\right]^{1/2}. \tag{10.2.12}$$

The two one-sided tests procedure given in Equation 10.2.10 become

$$T_{\mathrm{L}} = \frac{\widehat{\theta}_{hh'} - \theta_{\mathrm{L}}}{\left[S^2 \frac{\nu_a}{n}\right]^{1/2}} > t(\alpha,\ \nu),$$

and

$$T_{\mathrm{U}} = \frac{\widehat{\theta}_{hh'} - \theta_{\mathrm{U}}}{\left[S^2 \frac{\nu_a}{n}\right]^{1/2}} < -t(\alpha,\ \nu). \tag{10.2.13}$$

Note that the p-values of Anderson and Hauck's procedure for interval hypotheses 4.3.1 can also be obtained by simply plugging T_{L} and T_{U} into either Equation 4.3.12 or Equation 4.3.13.

Similarly, the minimum variance unbiased estimator of $\delta_{hh'}$ under a multiplicative model is given by

$$\widehat{\delta}_{hh'} = \exp(\widehat{\theta}_{hh'}) \bullet \Phi_f\left[-\frac{\nu_a}{n}\mathrm{SSE}\right]. \tag{10.2.14}$$

When $n_k = n$ for all k, under the structure of Williams design, ν_a for the ordinary least squares unbiased estimate of $\lambda_{hh'}$ are the same for all $1 \leq h \neq h' \leq t$. Therefore, the Williams designs are not only variance-balanced designs for the direct formulation effects, but are also for the carryover effects.

10.3 Analyses for Williams Designs

In Sections 10.3.1 and 10.3.2, we focus on statistical analysis for assessment of average bioequivalence under a Williams design for comparing three and four formulations.

10.3.1 Williams Designs with Three Formulations

A Williams design for comparing three formulations is a variance-balanced design, which consists of six sequences and three periods (see Table 2.5.4). For the sake of convenience, we summarize a Williams a design with three formulations as follows:

Williams design with three formulations.

	Period		
Sequence	**I**	**II**	**III**
1	R	T_2	T_1
2	T_1	R	T_2
3	T_2	T_1	R
4	T_1	T_2	R
5	T_2	R	T_1
6	R	T_1	T_2

Under model 10.2.1, Tables 10.3.1 and 10.3.2 provide the expected values of sequence-by-period means and analysis of variance table in terms of degrees of freedom, respectively. As can be seen from Table 10.3.2, there are $2(N-3)$ degrees of freedom for the intra-subject mean squared error, where $N = \Sigma_{k=1}^{6} n_k$. For estimation of the three formation effects, F_h, $h = 1, 2, 3$ we need to find C_{ajk}, the coefficient of linear contrasts of sequence-by-period means. From Table 10.3.1, the C_{ajk} for each formulation effect can be obtained. Table 10.3.3 lists C_{ajk} for the unbiased ordinary least squares estimators of F_h, $h = 1, 2, 3$. Therefore, the three population formulation means μ_h, $h = 1, 2, 3$, can be estimated unbiasedly by the sum of $\overline{Y}\ldots$ and the linear contrasts of sequence-by-period means with the coefficients given in Table 10.3.3.

To establish bioequivalence of average bioavailability between formulations h and h', $1 \leq h \neq h' \leq t$, the confidence interval given in Equation 10.2.9 and Schuirmann's two one-sided tests procedure given in Equation 10.2.10 can be used. For this purpose, Tables 10.3.4 and 10.3.5 list the coefficients of linear contrasts for the unbiased ordinary least squares estimates of $\theta_{hh'}$ in the presence and absence of

TABLE 10.3.1: Expected values of the sequence-by-period means for the Williams design with three formulations.

Sequence	Period I	Period II	Period III
1	$\mu + G_1 + P_1 + F_R$	$\mu + G_1 + P_2 + F_2 + C_R$	$\mu + G_1 + P_3 + F_1 + C_2$
2	$\mu + G_2 + P_1 + F_1$	$\mu + G_2 + P_2 + F_R + C_1$	$\mu + G_2 + P_3 + F_2 + C_R$
3	$\mu + G_3 + P_1 + F_2$	$\mu + G_3 + P_2 + F_1 + C_2$	$\mu + G_3 + P_3 + F_R + C_1$
4	$\mu + G_4 + P_1 + F_1$	$\mu + G_4 + P_2 + F_2 + C_1$	$\mu + G_4 + P_3 + F_R + C_2$
5	$\mu + G_5 + P_1 + F_2$	$\mu + G_5 + P_2 + F_R + C_2$	$\mu + G_5 + P_3 + F_1 + C_R$
6	$\mu + G_6 + P_1 + F_R$	$\mu + G_6 + P_2 + F_1 + C_R$	$\mu + G_6 + P_3 + F_2 + C_1$

TABLE 10.3.2: Analysis of variance table for the Williams design with three formulations.

Source of Variation	Degrees of Freedom[a]
Inter-subject	$N^b - 1$
Sequence	5
Residual	$N - 6$
Intra-subject	$2N$
Period	2
Formulation	2
Carryover	2
Residual	$2(N - 3)$
Total	$3N - 1$

[a] Degrees of freedom for the intra-subject residual is $2(N - 2)$ if carryover effects are not included in the model.
[b] $N = n_1 + n_2 + n_3 + n_4 + n_5 + n_6$.

TABLE 10.3.3: Coefficients for estimates of formulations F_R, F_1, and F_2 in the Williams design with three formulations (adjusted for carryover effects).

	F_R Period			F_1 Period			F_2 Period		
Sequence	I	II	III	I	II	III	I	II	III
1	3	0	−3	−1	−2	3	−2	2	0
2	−2	2	0	3	0	−3	−1	−2	3
3	−1	−2	3	−2	2	0	3	0	−3
4	−1	−2	3	3	0	−3	−2	2	0
5	−2	2	0	−1	−2	3	3	0	−3
6	3	0	−3	−2	2	0	−1	−2	3

Note: Coefficients are multiplied by 24.

TABLE 10.3.4: Coefficients for estimates of pairwise formulation effects in the Williams design with three formulations (adjusted for carryover effects).

	$\theta_{1R} = F_1 - F_R$				$\theta_{2R} = F_2 - F_R$				$\theta_{21} = F_2 - F_1$			
	Period				Period				Period			
Sequence	1	2	3	$\Sigma_j C_{ajk}^2$	1	2	3	$\Sigma_j C_{ajk}^2$	1	2	3	$\Sigma_j C_{ajk}^2$
1	−4	−2	6	$56/(24)^2$	−5	2	3	$38/(24)^2$	−1	4	−3	$26/(24)^2$
2	5	−2	−3	$38/(24)^2$	1	−4	3	$26/(24)^2$	−4	−2	6	$56/(24)^2$
3	−1	4	−3	$26/(24)^2$	4	2	−6	$56/(24)^2$	5	−2	−3	$38/(24)^2$
4	4	2	−6	$56/(24)^2$	−1	4	−3	$26/(24)^2$	−5	2	3	$38/(24)^2$
5	1	−4	3	$26/(24)^2$	5	−2	−3	$38/(24)^2$	4	2	−6	$56/(24)^2$
6	−5	2	3	$38/(24)^2$	−4	−2	6	$56/(24)^2$	1	−4	3	$26/(24)^2$
Variance[a]				$\frac{5}{12n}\sigma_e^2$				$\frac{5}{12n}\sigma_e^2$				$\frac{5}{12n}\sigma_e^2$

Note: Coefficients are multiplied by 24.

[a] Variance when $n = n_k$ for $1 \leq k \leq 6$.

TABLE 10.3.5: Coefficients for estimates of pairwise formulation effects in the Williams design with three formulations (in absence of unequal carryover effects).

	$\theta_{1R} = F_1 - F_R$				$\theta_{2R} = F_2 - F_R$				$\theta_{21} = F_2 - F_1$			
	Period				Period				Period			
Sequence	**1**	**2**	**3**	$\Sigma_j C_{ajk}{}^2$	**1**	**2**	**3**	$\Sigma_j C_{ajk}{}^2$	**1**	**2**	**3**	$\Sigma_j C_{ajk}{}^2$
1	−1	0	1	1/18	−1	1	0	1/18	0	1	−1	1/18
2	1	−1	0	1/18	0	−1	1	1/18	−1	0	1	1/18
3	0	1	−1	1/18	1	0	−1	1/18	1	−1	0	1/18
4	1	0	−1	1/18	0	1	−1	1/18	−1	1	0	1/18
5	0	−1	1	1/18	1	−1	0	1/18	1	0	−1	1/18
6	−1	1	0	1/18	−1	0	1	1/18	0	−1	1	1/18
Variance[a]				$\frac{1}{3n}\sigma_e^2$				$\frac{1}{3n}\sigma_e^2$				$\frac{5}{12n}\sigma_e^2$

Note: Coefficients are multiplied by 6.

[a] Variance when $n = n_k$ for $1 \leq k \leq 6$.

TABLE 10.3.6: Coefficients for estimates of carryover effects in the Williams design with three formulations (adjusted for formulation effects).

	$\lambda_{1R} = C_1 - C_R$				$\lambda_{2R} = C_2 - C_R$				$\lambda_{21} = C_2 - C_1$			
	Period				Period				Period			
Sequence	**1**	**2**	**3**	$\Sigma_j C_{ajk}^2$	**1**	**2**	**3**	$\Sigma_j C_{ajk}^2$	**1**	**2**	**3**	$\Sigma_j C_{ajk}^2$
1	0	−2	2	4/32	−1	−2	3	7/32	−1	0	1	1/32
2	1	2	−3	7/32	1	0	−1	1/32	0	−2	2	4/32
3	−1	0	1	1/32	0	2	−2	4/32	1	2	−3	7/32
4	0	2	−2	4/32	−1	0	1	1/32	−1	−2	3	7/32
5	1	0	−1	1/32	1	2	−3	7/32	0	2	−2	4/32
6	−1	−2	3	7/32	0	−2	2	4/32	1	0	−1	1/32
Variance[a]				$\frac{3}{4n}\sigma_e^2$				$\frac{3}{4n}\sigma_e^2$				$\frac{5}{12n}\sigma_e^2$

Note: Coefficients are multiplied by 8.

[a] Variance when $n = n_k$ for $1 \leq k \leq 6$.

unequal carryover effects, respectively. Based on these coefficients, the confidence interval and the two one-sided tests can be easily carried out.

To draw statistical inference on the carryover effect, the coefficients for estimates of pairwise carryover effects, $\lambda_{hh'}$, $1 \leq h \neq h' \leq t$, given in Table 10.3.6 are useful. Note that Tables 10.3.3 through 10.3.6 are obtained by the following steps:

Step 1 Set up the design matrix for the 6×3 Williams design.

Step 2 Find $(\mathbf{X}'\mathbf{X})^{-1}\mathbf{X}'$, where $\mathbf{X}$ is the 6×3 Williams design matrix. We then obtain $\widehat{F}_R$ using the constraint

$$\widehat{F}_1 + \widehat{F}_2 + \widehat{F}_R = 0$$

The coefficients of $\widehat{F}_1$ and $\widehat{F}_2$ are the element of $(\mathbf{X}'\mathbf{X})^{-1}\mathbf{X}'$ which are given in Table 10.3.3.

Step 3 The estimates of $\theta_{ij} = F_i - F_j$, $R < i \neq j \leq 2$ can be obtained by the difference of the corresponding coefficients between $\widehat{F}_1$ and $\widehat{F}_j$. The estimates of θ_{ij} are given in Tables 10.3.4 and 10.3.5.

Step 4 The estimates $\lambda_{ij} = C_i - C_j$, $R \leq i \neq j \leq 2$ can be similarly obtained and one given in Table 10.3.6.

10.3.2 Williams Design with Four Formulations

A Williams design for comparing four formulations, which consists of four sequences and four periods (see Table 2.5.7), is summarized as follows:

Williams design with three formulations.

	Period			
Sequence	**I**	**II**	**III**	**IV**
1	R	T_3	T_1	T_2
2	T_1	R	T_2	T_3
3	T_2	T_1	T_3	R
4	T_3	T_2	R	T_1

Tables 10.3.7 and 10.3.8 give the expected values of the sequence-by-period means and the analysis of variance table for the degrees of freedom. Coefficients of the linear contrasts for the unbiased ordinary least squares estimates of F_h, $\theta_{hh'}$, and $\lambda_{hh'}$, $1 \leq h \neq h' \leq t$, are given in Tables 10.3.9 through 10.3.12. Note that a Williams design with three formulations compares three pairs of formulations, whereas there are a total of six pairs of formulations to be compared for a Williams design with four formulations. The degrees of freedom for the intra-subject means squared error is $3(N-3)$, where $N = \Sigma_{k=1}^{4} n_k$. From the coefficients given in Tables 10.3.9 through 10.3.12,

TABLE 10.3.7: Expected values of the sequence-by-period means for the Williams design with four formulations.

	Period			
Sequence	**I**	**II**	**III**	**IV**
1	$\mu + G_1 + P_1 + F_R$	$\mu + G_1 + P_2 + F_3 + C_R$	$\mu + G_1 + P_3 + F_1 + C_3$	$\mu + G_1 + P_4 + F_2 + C_1$
2	$\mu + G_2 + P_1 + F_1$	$\mu + G_2 + P_2 + F_R + C_1$	$\mu + G_2 + P_3 + F_2 + C_R$	$\mu + G_2 + P_4 + F_3 + C_2$
3	$\mu + G_3 + P_1 + F_2$	$\mu + G_3 + P_2 + F_1 + C_2$	$\mu + G_3 + P_3 + F_3 + C_1$	$\mu + G_3 + P_4 + F_R + C_3$
4	$\mu + G_4 + P_1 + F_3$	$\mu + G_4 + P_2 + F_2 + C_3$	$\mu + G_4 + P_3 + F_R + C_2$	$\mu + G_4 + P_4 + F_1 + C_R$

average bioequivalence between formulation h and h' can be evaluated using either the confidence interval Equation 10.2.9 or the two one-sided tests Equation 10.2.10.

Example 10.3.1

To illustrate the methods discussed in previous sections, we use the AUC data from a study discussed in Purich (1980). This study was conducted with 12 normal subjects to establish bioequivalence among two formulations of 100 mg beta-blocker tablets (domestic and European) and a solution (reference). There was a 7 day washout between treatment periods. No assignment of sequence and period was given in Purich's paper. Thus, for the purpose of illustration, we assign subjects 1 and 2 to sequence 1; 3 and 4 to sequence 2; 5 and 6 to sequence 3; 7 and 8 to sequence 4; 9 and 10 to sequence 5; 11 and 12 to sequence 6. Table 10.3.13 gives the AUC data after

TABLE 10.3.8: Analysis of variance table for the Williams design with four formulations.

Source of Variation	Degrees of Freedom[a]
Inter-subject	$N^b - 1$
Sequence	3
Residual	$N - 4$
Intra-subject	$3N$
Period	3
Formulation	3
Carryover	3
Residual	$3(N - 3)$
Total	$4N - 1$

[a] Degrees of freedom for the intra-subject residual is $3(N - 2)$ if carryover effects are not included in the model.

[b] $N = n_1 + n_2 + n_3 + n_4$.

TABLE 10.3.9: Coefficients for estimates of formulations F_R, F_1, F_2, and F_3 in the Williams design with four formulations (adjusted for carryover effects).

	F_R Period				F_1 Period				F_2 Period				F_3 Period			
Sequence	**1**	**2**	**3**	**4**	**1**	**2**	**3**	**4**	**1**	**2**	**3**	**4**	**1**	**2**	**3**	**4**
1	8	0	−4	−4	−3	−4	7	0	−2	−3	−3	8	−3	7	0	4
2	−3	7	0	−4	8	0	−4	−4	−3	−4	7	0	−2	−3	−3	8
3	−2	−3	−3	8	−3	7	0	−4	8	0	−4	−4	−3	−4	7	0
4	−3	−4	7	0	−2	−3	−3	−8	−3	7	0	−4	8	0	−4	−4

Note: The coefficients are multiplied by 40.

TABLE 10.3.10: Coefficients for estimates of pairwise formulations effects in the Williams design with four formulations (adjusted for carryover effects).

	$\theta_{2R} = F_1 - F_R$					$\theta_{2R} = F_2 - F_R$				
	Period					Period				
Sequence	**1**	**2**	**3**	**4**	$\Sigma_j C_{ajk}^2$	**1**	**2**	**3**	**4**	$\Sigma_j C_{ajk}^2$
1	−11	−4	11	4	$274/(40)^2$	−10	−3	1	12	$254/(40)^2$
2	11	−7	−4	0	$186/(40)^2$	0	−11	7	4	$186/(40)^2$
3	−1	10	3	−12	$254/(40)^2$	10	3	−1	−12	$254/(40)^2$
4	1	1	−10	8	$166/(40)^2$	0	11	−7	−4	$186/(40)^2$
Variance[a]					$\frac{11}{20n}\sigma_e^2$					$\frac{11}{20n}\sigma_e^2$

	$\theta_{3R} = F_3 - F_R$					$\theta_{21} = F_2 - F_1$				
	Period					Period				
Sequence	**1**	**2**	**3**	**4**	$\Sigma_j C_{ajk}^2$	**1**	**2**	**3**	**4**	$\Sigma_j C_{ajk}^2$
1	−11	7	4	0	$186/(40)^2$	1	1	−10	8	$166/(40)^2$
2	1	−10	−3	12	$254/(40)^2$	−11	−4	11	4	$274/(40)^2$
3	−1	−1	10	−8	$166/(40)^2$	11	−7	−4	0	$186/(40)^2$
4	11	4	−11	−4	$274/(40)^2$	−1	10	3	−12	$254/(40)^2$
Variance[a]					$\frac{11}{20n}\sigma_e^2$					$\frac{11}{20n}\sigma_e^2$

(*continued*)

TABLE 10.3.10 (continued): Coefficients for estimates of pairwise formulations effects in the Williams design with four formulations
(adjusted for carryover effects).

	$\theta_{31} = F_3 - F_1$					$\theta_{32} = F_3 - F_2$				
	Period					Period				
Sequence	**1**	**2**	**3**	**4**	$\Sigma_j C^2_{ajk}$	**1**	**2**	**3**	**4**	$\Sigma_j C^2_{ajk}$
1	0	11	−7	−4	$186/(40)^2$	−1	10	3	−12	$254/(40)^2$
2	−10	−3	1	12	$254/(40)^2$	1	1	−10	8	$166/(40)^2$
3	0	−11	7	4	$186/(40)^2$	−11	−4	11	4	$274/(40)^2$
4	10	3	−1	−12	$254/(40)^2$	11	−7	−4	0	$186/(40)^2$
Variance[a]					$\frac{11}{20n}\sigma^2_e$					$\frac{11}{20n}\sigma^2_e$

Note: Coefficients are multiplied by 40.
[a] Variance when $n = n_k$ for $1 \leq k \leq 4$.

TABLE 10.3.11: Coefficients for estimates of carryover effects in the Williams design with four formulations (adjusted for formulation effects).

	$\lambda_{1R} = C_1 - C_R$					$\lambda_{2R} = C_3 - C_R$				
	Period					Period				
Sequence	**1**	**2**	**3**	**4**	$\Sigma_j C^2_{ajk}$	**1**	**2**	**3**	**4**	$\Sigma_j C^2_{ajk}$
1	−1	−4	1	4	$34/(10)^2$	0	−3	1	2	$14/(10)^2$
2	1	3	−4	0	$26/(10)^2$	0	−1	−3	4	$26/(10)^2$
3	−1	0	3	−2	$14/(10)^2$	0	3	−1	−2	$14/(10)^2$
4	1	1	0	−2	$6/(10)^2$	0	1	3	−4	$26/(10)^2$
Variance[a]					$\frac{4}{5n}\sigma^2_e$					$\frac{4}{5n}\sigma^2_e$

	$\lambda_{3R} = C_3 - C_R$					$\lambda_{21} = C_2 - C_1$				
	Period					Period				
Sequence	**1**	**2**	**3**	**4**	$\Sigma_j C^2_{ajk}$	**1**	**2**	**3**	**4**	$\Sigma_j C^2_{ajk}$
1	−1	−3	4	0	$26/(10)^2$	1	1	0	−2	$6/(10)^2$
2	1	0	−3	2	$14/(10)^2$	−1	−4	1	4	$34/(10)^2$
3	−1	−1	0	2	$6/(10)^2$	1	3	−4	0	$26/(10)^2$
4	1	4	−1	−4	$34/(10)^2$	−1	0	3	−2	$14/(10)^2$
Variance[a]					$\frac{4}{5n}\sigma^2_e$					$\frac{4}{5n}\sigma^2_e$

(*continued*)

TABLE 10.3.11 (continued): Coefficients for estimates of carryover effects in the Williams design with four formulations (adjusted for formulation effects).

	$\lambda_{31} = C_3 - C_1$					$\lambda_{32} = C_3 - C_2$				
	Period					Period				
Sequence	**1**	**2**	**3**	**4**	$\Sigma_j C^2_{ajk}$	**1**	**2**	**3**	**4**	$\Sigma_j C^2_{ajk}$
1	0	1	3	−4	$26/(10)^2$	−1	0	3	−2	$14/(10)^2$
2	0	−3	1	2	$14/(10)^2$	1	1	0	−2	$6/(10)^2$
3	0	−1	−3	4	$26/(10)^2$	−1	−4	1	4	$34/(10)^2$
4	0	3	1	−2	$14/(10)^2$	1	3	−4	0	$26/(10)^2$
Variance[a]					$\frac{4}{5n}\sigma_e^2$					$\frac{4}{5n}\sigma_e^2$

Note: Coefficients are multiplied by 10.
[a] Variance when $n = n_k$ for $1 \leq k \leq 4$.

TABLE 10.3.12: Coefficients for estimates of pairwise formulation effects in the Williams design with four formulations (in absence of unequal carryover effects).

	$\theta_{1R} = F_1 - C_R$					$\theta_{2R} = F_2 - F_R$				
	Period					Period				
Sequence	**1**	**2**	**3**	**4**	$\Sigma_j C^2_{ajk}$	**1**	**2**	**3**	**4**	$\Sigma_j C^2_{ajk}$
1	−1	0	1	0	1/8	−1	0	0	1	1/8
2	1	−1	0	0	1/8	0	−1	1	0	1/8
3	0	1	0	−1	1/8	1	0	0	−1	1/8
4	0	0	−1	1	1/8	0	1	−1	0	1/8
Variance[a]					$\frac{11}{20n}\sigma^2_e$					$\frac{11}{20n}\sigma^2_e$
	$\theta_{3R} = F_3 - F_R$					$\theta_{21} = F_2 - F_1$				
	Period					Period				
Sequence	**1**	**2**	**3**	**4**	$\Sigma_j C^2_{ajk}$	**1**	**2**	**3**	**4**	$\Sigma_j C^2_{ajk}$
1	−1	1	0	0	1/8	0	0	−1	1	1/8
2	0	−1	0	1	1/8	−1	0	1	0	1/8
3	0	0	1	−1	1/8	1	−1	0	0	1/8
4	1	0	−1	0	1/8	0	1	0	−1	1/8
Variance[a]					$\frac{1}{2n}\sigma^2_e$					$\frac{1}{2n}\sigma^2_e$

(continued)

TABLE 10.3.12 (continued): Coefficients for estimates of pairwise formulation effects in the Williams design with four formulations (in absence of unequal carryover effects).

	$\theta_{31} = F_3 - F_R$					$\theta_{32} = F_3 - F_2$				
	Period					**Period**				
Sequence	**1**	**2**	**3**	**4**	$\Sigma_j C^2_{ajk}$	**1**	**2**	**3**	**4**	$\Sigma_j C^2_{ajk}$
1	0	1	−1	0	1/8	0	1	0	−1	1/8
2	−1	0	0	1	1/8	0	0	−1	1	1/8
3	0	−1	1	0	1/8	−1	0	1	0	1/8
4	1	0	0	−1	1/8	1	−1	0	0	1/8
Variance[a]					$\frac{1}{2n}\sigma^2_e$					$\frac{1}{2n}\sigma^2_e$

Note: Coefficients are multiplied by 4.

[a] Variance when $n = n_k$ for $1 \leq k \leq 4$.

TABLE 10.3.13: AUC data from a study by Purich.

		Period		
Sequence[a]	**Subject**	**I**	**II**	**III**
(R, T_2, T_1)	1	5.68	4.21	6.83
	2	3.60	5.01	5.78
(T_1, R, T_2)	3	3.55	5.07	4.49
	4	7.31	7.42	7.86
(T_2, T_1, R)	5	6.59	7.72	7.26
	6	9.68	8.91	9.04
(T_1, T_2, R)	7	4.63	7.23	5.06
	8	8.75	7.59	4.82
(T_2, R, T_1)	9	7.25	7.88	9.02
	10	5.00	7.84	7.79
(R, T_1, T_2)	11	4.63	6.77	5.72
	12	3.87	7.62	6.74

Source: From Purich, E., *Drug Absorption and Disposition: Statistical Considerations*, American Pharmaceutical Association, Academy of Pharmaceutical Sciences, Washington, DC, 1980, 115–137.

Note: R, solution; T_1, domestic tablet; and T_2, European tablet.

rearrangement of reference and period according to the Williams design for comparing three formulations. The sequence-by-period means are given in Table 10.3.14. Table 10.3.15 provides estimates of three formulation means both in the presence and absence of carryover effects. Test results (without adjustment for significance level) for assessing bioequivalence of average bioavailability are summarized in Table 10.3.16.

The carryover effects are not statistically significant from 0 (p-value = 0.32). Both the confidence interval approach and the two one-sided tests procedure reach the same conclusion on bioequivalence regardless of the presence of the carryover effect. According to the ± 20 rule, the European 100 mg tablet is equivalent to the solution for

TABLE 10.3.14: Sequence by period means of Purich's data.

	Period		
Sequence	**I**	**II**	**III**
1	4.640	4.610	6.305
2	4.530	6.245	6.175
3	8.135	8.315	8.150
4	6.690	7.410	4.940
5	6.125	7.860	8.405
6	4.250	7.195	6.230

TABLE 10.3.15: Estimates of formulation effects for Purich's data.

Carryover Effects	Solution	Domestic	European
Yes	5.67	7.24	6.30
No	6.01	7.06	6.45

average bioavailability; but the domestic tablet is not equivalent to the European table or to the solution for average bioavailability.

10.3.3 Heterogeneity of Intra-Subject Variabilities

For assessment of average bioequivalence in the Williams designs with three formulations or four formulations, we assume that $\sigma_h^2 = \sigma_e^2$ for all h. In practice, this is not always true. However, when the intra-subject variabilities differ from formulation to formulation, bioequivalence of average bioavailability can still be established using a Williams design, provided that there are no carryover effects, which is a reasonable assumption when there is a sufficient length of washout between periods.

In the following, statistical methods for the comparison of test formulation 1 with the reference formulation in a Williams design with four formulations will be derived when the heterogeneity of intra-subject variabilities is present. The method can be easily applied to compare any other pair of formulations in any Williams design.

When the intra-subject variabilities are different, the covariance matrix of the vector of four responses

TABLE 10.3.16: Summary of test results for Purich's data.

Comparison	Carryover	Tests[a]	p-Value	90% CI
T_1 versus R[b]	Yes	$T_L = 5.08$	<0.001	(0.43, 2.11)
		$T_U = 0.16$	0.56	(107.20%, 135.41%)
	No	$T_L = 5.12$	<0.001	(0.29, 1.80)
		$T_U = -0.37$	0.36	(104.75%, 129.92%)
T_2 versus R	Yes	$T_L = 3.14$	0.003	(−0.51, 1.18)
		$T_U = -1.77$	0.047	(94.47%, 119.68%)
	No	$T_L = 3.73$	0.001	(−0.32, 1.19)
		$T_U = -1.75$	0.047	(92.62%, 119.79%)
T_1 versus T_2	Yes	$T_L = 4.39$	<0.001	(0.097, 1.78)
		$T_U = -0.53$	0.30	(101.63%, 129.83%)
	No	$T_L = 4.13$	<0.001	(−0.15, 1.37)
		$T_U = -1.35$	0.096	(97.54%, 122.72%)

[a] Calculations were based upon ±20 rule and estimate of solution formation mean which is 5.97 in the presence of carryover effects and is 6.01 in the absence of carryover effects.

[b] R, solution; T_1, domestic table; and T_2, European tablet.

$$Y_{ik} = (Y_{i1k}, Y_{i2k}, Y_{i3k}, Y_{i4k})',$$

which are observed on subject i in the sequence k, is given by

$$\text{Var}(\mathbf{Y}_{ik}) = \mathbf{\Gamma}_k + \sigma_S^2 \mathbf{J}_4, \quad i = 1, 2, \ldots, nk, \quad k = 1, 2, 3,$$

where $\mathbf{J}_4$ is a 4×4 matrix of 1 and

$$\mathbf{\Gamma}_k = \begin{cases} \text{diag}\left(\sigma_R^2, \sigma_3^2, \sigma_1^2, \sigma_2^2\right), & \text{if } k = 1, \\ \text{diag}\left(\sigma_1^2, \sigma_R^2, \sigma_2^2, \sigma_3^2\right), & \text{if } k = 2, \\ \text{diag}\left(\sigma_2^2, \sigma_2^2, \sigma_3^2, \sigma_R^2\right), & \text{if } k = 3, \\ \text{diag}\left(\sigma_3^2, \sigma_2^2, \sigma_R^2, \sigma_1^2\right), & \text{if } k = 4, \end{cases} \tag{10.3.1}$$

and diag(a_1, a_2, a_3, a_4) is a 4×4 diagonal matrix with diagonal elements a_1, a_2, a_3, and a_4. Define the period differences as the following intra-subject contrasts

$$d_{ik} = \begin{cases} \frac{1}{4}[Y_{i31} - Y_{i11}], & \text{if } k = 1, \\ \frac{1}{4}[Y_{i12} - Y_{i22}], & \text{if } k = 2, \\ \frac{1}{4}[Y_{i23} - Y_{i43}], & \text{if } k = 3, \\ \frac{1}{4}[Y_{i44} - Y_{i34}], & \text{if } k = 4. \end{cases} \tag{10.3.2}$$

Then, under normality assumptions, d_{ik} are independently normally distributed with the common variance

$$\text{Var}(d_{ik}) = \frac{1}{16}\left(\sigma_1^2 + \sigma_R^2\right), \tag{10.3.3}$$

and the means

$$E(d_{ik}) = \begin{cases} \frac{1}{4}[(F_1 - F_R) + (P_3 - P_1)], & \text{if } k = 1, \\ \frac{1}{4}[(F_1 - F_R) + (P_1 - P_2)], & \text{if } k = 2, \\ \frac{1}{4}[(F_1 - F_R) + (P_2 - P_4)], & \text{if } k = 3, \\ \frac{1}{4}[(F_1 - F_R) + (P_4 - P_3)], & \text{if } k = 4. \end{cases} \tag{10.3.4}$$

Let $\overline{d}_{\cdot k}$ be the mean of d_{ik} for sequence i and $\overline{d}$ be the sum of $\overline{d}_{\cdot k}$; that is

$$\overline{d} = \sum_{k=1}^{4} \overline{d}_{\cdot k} = \sum_{k=1}^{4} \frac{1}{n_k} \sum_{i=1}^{n_k} d_{ik}. \tag{10.3.5}$$

Then $\bar{d}$ is normally distributed with mean $\theta_{1R} = F_1 - F_R$ and variance

$$\text{Var}(\bar{d}) = \frac{1}{16}\left(\sigma_1^2 + \sigma_R^2\right)\sum_{k=1}^{4}\frac{1}{n_k}.$$

Therefore, $\bar{d}$ is an unbiased estimator of θ_{1R}, and an unbiased estimator of $\frac{1}{16}(\sigma_1^2 + \sigma_R^2)$ is given by

$$S_d^2 = \frac{1}{N-4}\sum_{k=1}^{4}\sum_{i=1}^{n_k}(d_{ik} - \bar{d}_{\cdot k})^2, \tag{10.3.6}$$

which is distributed as $\frac{1}{N-4}\chi^2(N-4)$. Since S_d^2 is independent of $\bar{d}$, the statistic

$$T_d = \frac{\bar{d}}{\left[S_d^2\sum_{k=1}^{4}\frac{1}{n_k}\right]^{1/2}}$$

has a central t distribution with $N-4$ degrees of freedom. Given $\bar{d}$ and S_d^2, assessment of bioequivalence of average bioavailability can be established using either Equation 10.2.8 for the confidence interval approach or Equation 10.2.9 for the two one-sided tests procedure. From the above methods, it can be seen that the heterogeneity of intra-subject variabilities causes a decrease in degrees of freedom from $3(N-3)$ to $(N-4)$ or a loss in precision. This is because we use only the information from those periods when test formulation 1 and the reference formulation are administered.

For assessment of bioequivalence of intra-subject variabilities between a test formulation and the reference formulation in a Williams design, the test procedure for hypotheses 7.5.2 described in Section 7.5 can be directly applied. The procedure is outlined in the following.

Let R_{iRk} and R_{iT_1k} be the respective residuals from the sequence-by-period means corresponding to the periods of sequence k where test formulation 1 and the reference formulation are administered. We first calculate

$$\begin{aligned} V_{ik} &= R_{iT_1k} - R_{iRk}, \\ U_{Lik} &= R_{iT_1k} + \delta_L R_{iRk}, \\ U_{Uik} &= R_{iT_1k} + \delta_U R_{iRk}, \end{aligned} \tag{10.3.7}$$

where

$i = 1, 2, \ldots, n_k$
$k = 1, 2, 3, 4.$

Then, compute Pearson's (Spearman's) correlation coefficients $\widehat{\rho}_L(\tilde{\rho}_L)$ between V_{ik} and U_{Lik} and $\widehat{\rho}_U(\tilde{\rho}_U)$ between V_{ik} and U_{Uik}, as described in Chapter 7. If normality assumptions are satisfied, test formulation 1 and the reference formulation are considered to be bioequivalent in intra-subject variabilities at the α level of significance if

$$t_L = \frac{\hat{\rho}_L}{\left[\frac{1-\hat{\rho}_L^2}{N-5}\right]^{1/2}} > t(\alpha, N-5),$$

and

$$t_U = \frac{\hat{\rho}_U}{\left[\frac{1-\hat{\rho}_U^2}{N-5}\right]^{1/2}} < -t(\alpha, N-5). \tag{10.3.8}$$

On the other hand, if the normality assumptions are in doubt, nonparametric test procedure such as Spearman's rank correlation coefficient can be used. We conclude bioequivalence if

$$\tilde{\rho}_L > r_S(\alpha, N-4),$$

and

$$\tilde{\rho}_U < -r_S(\alpha, N-4), \tag{10.3.9}$$

where $r_S(\alpha, N-4)$ is the αth upper quantile of distribution of Spearnman's rank correlation coefficient based upon the $N-4$ observations.

To illustrate the use of the above methods, we use Purich's data, which was described in Example 10.3.1. Test results for assessment of intra-subject variabilities are summarized in Table 10.3.17. The results indicate that all three formulations are not equivalent to each other intra-subject variability.

TABLE 10.3.17: Summary of intra-subject variabilities test results for Purich's data.

		Correlation	
Comparison[a]	**Hypotheses**[b]	**Pearson (*p*-Value)**	**Spearman (*p*-Value)**
T_1 versus R	$\rho_L > 0$	0.55 (0.98)	0.61 (0.05)
	$\rho_U < 0$	0.47 (0.85)	0.55 (>0.05)
T_2 versus R	$\rho_L > 0$	0.45 (0.15)	0.38 (>0.05)
	$\rho_U < 0$	0.36 (0.79)	0.38 (>0.05)
T_1 versus T_2	$\rho_L > 0$	−0.12 (0.60)	−0.03 (>0.05)
	$\rho_U < 0$	−0.21 (0.33)	−0.17 (>0.05)

[a] R = solution; T_1 = domestic tablets; and T_2 = European tablets.
[b] Based upon hypotheses Equation 7.3 with equivalent limits ±20%.

10.4 Analysis for Balanced Incomplete Block Design

In Chapter 2, several balanced incomplete block designs (BIBD) were constructed for comparing four and five formulations. These designs include four formulations with two or three periods and five formulations with two, three, as four periods. For the analyses of these balanced incomplete block designs, statistical methods introduced in Section 10.2 can be directly applied. Therefore, in this section, for the purpose of illustration, we focus on a balanced incomplete block design for comparing four formulations with three periods. Other balanced incomplete block designs can be treated similarly. The balanced incomplete block design for comparing four formulations with three periods is summarized as

Balanced incomplete block design for three formulations with three periods.

Sequence	Period I	Period II	Period III
1	T_1	T_2	T_3
2	T_2	T_3	R
3	T_3	R	T_1
4	R	T_1	T_2

From this design, one can see that only subjects in sequences 2, 3, and 4 receive the reference formulation. In other words, comparison within each subject between a test formulation and the reference formulation can be made only by using data from these sequences. There are a total of six pairs of formulations to be compared.

Tables 10.4.1 and 10.4.2 give the expected values of the sequence-by-period means and the analysis of variance table for the distribution of the degrees of

TABLE 10.4.1: Expected values of the sequence-by-period means for BIBD with four formulations and three periods.

Sequence	Period I	Period II	Period III
1	$\mu + G_1 + P_1 + F_1$	$\mu + G_1 + P_2 + F_2 + C_1$	$\mu + G_1 + P_3 + F_3 + C_2$
2	$\mu + G_2 + P_1 + F_2$	$\mu + G_2 + P_2 + F_3 + C_2$	$\mu + G_2 + P_3 + F_R + C_3$
3	$\mu + G_3 + P_1 + F_3$	$\mu + G_3 + P_2 + F_R + C_3$	$\mu + G_3 + P_3 + F_1 + C_R$
4	$\mu + G_4 + P_1 + F_R$	$\mu + G_4 + P_2 + F_1 + C_R$	$\mu + G_4 + P_3 + F_2 + C_1$

TABLE 10.4.2: Analysis of variance table for the BIBD with four formulations and three periods.

Source of Variation	Degrees of Freedom[a]
Inter-subject	$N^{b} - 1$
Sequence	3
Residual	$N - 4$
Intra-subject	2N
Period	3
Formulation	3
Carryover	3
Residual	$2(N - 4)$
Total	$3N - 1$

[a] Degrees of freedom for the intra-subject residual is $2N - 5$ if carryover effects are not included in the model.
[b] $N = n_1 + n_2 + n_3 + n_4$.

freedom. Coefficients of the linear contrasts for the unbiased ordinary least squares estimates of F_h, $\theta_{hh'}$, and $\lambda_{hh'}$, $1 \leq h \neq h' \leq 4$, are given in Table 10.4.3 through 10.4.6. The degrees of freedom for the intra-subject mean squared error is $2(N - 4)$, where $N = n_1 + n_1 + n_3 + n_4$. From the coefficients give in Tables 10.4.3 through 10.4.6, bioequivalence of average bioavailability between formulation h and h' can be evaluated using either the confidence interval Equation 10.2.9 or the two one-sided tests Equation 10.2.10.

From Table 10.4.5, it can be seen that when there are no carryover effects, the balanced incomplete block design is a variance-balanced design. However, in the presence of carryover effect, this is not true, as indicated in Table 10.4.4. This suggests that, in the interest of having the property of variance-balanced, a sufficient length of washout should be given between dosing periods to wear off the possible carryover effects.

Note that the p-values of Anderson and Hauck's procedure for interval hypothesis 4.3.1 can also be obtained by simply plugging T_L and T_U of Equation 10.2.10 into either Equation 4.3.12 or Equation 4.3.13.

TABLE 10.4.3: Coefficients for estimates of formulations F_R, F_1, F_2, and F_3 in the BIBD with four formulations and three periods (adjusted for carryover effects).

	F_R Period			F_1 Period			F_2 Period			F_3 Period		
Sequence	**1**	**2**	**3**	**1**	**2**	**3**	**1**	**2**	**3**	**1**	**2**	**3**
1	−2	3	−1	6	−3	−3	−2	1	3	−2	1	1
2	−2	1	1	−2	3	−1	6	−3	−3	−2	−1	3
3	−2	−1	3	−2	1	1	−2	3	−1	6	−3	−3
4	6	−3	−3	−2	−1	3	−2	1	1	−2	3	1

Note: The coefficients are multiplied by 8.

TABLE 10.4.4: Coefficients for estimates for pairwise formulation effects in BIBD with four formulations and three periods (adjusted for carryover effects).

	$\theta_{1R} = F_1 - F_R$				$\theta_{2R} = F_2 - F_R$			
	Period				Period			
Sequence	**1**	**2**	**3**	$\Sigma_j C^2_{ajk}$	**1**	**2**	**3**	$\Sigma_j C^2_{ajk}$
1	8	−6	−2	$104/(8)^2$	0	−4	4	$32/(8)^2$
2	0	2	−2	$8/(8)^2$	8	−4	−4	$96/(8)^2$
3	0	2	−2	$8/(8)^2$	0	4	−4	$32/(8)^2$
4	−8	2	6	$104/(8)^2$	−8	4	4	$96/(8)^2$
Variance[a]				$\frac{7}{2n}\sigma_e^2$				$\frac{4}{n}\sigma_e^2$

	$\theta_{3R} = F_3 - F_R$				$\theta_{21} = F_2 - F_1$			
	Period				Period			
Sequence	**1**	**2**	**3**	$\Sigma_j C^2_{ajk}$	**1**	**2**	**3**	$\Sigma_j C^2_{ajk}$
1	0	−2	2	$8(8)^2$	−8	2	6	$104/(8)^2$
2	0	−2	2	$8/(8)^2$	8	−6	−2	$104/(8)^2$
3	8	−2	−6	$104/(8)^2$	0	2	−2	$8/(8)^2$
4	−8	6	2	$104/(8)^2$	0	2	−2	$8/(8)^2$
Variance[a]				$\frac{7}{2n}\sigma_e^2$				$\frac{7}{2n}\sigma_e^2$

	$\theta_{31} = F_3 - F_1$				$\theta_{32} = F_3 - F_2$			
	Period				Period			
Sequence	**1**	**2**	**3**	$\Sigma_j C^2_{ajk}$	**1**	**2**	**3**	$\Sigma_j C^2_{ajk}$
1	−8	4	4	$96/(8)^2$	0	2	−2	$8/(8)^2$
2	0	−4	4	$32/(8)^2$	−8	2	6	$104/(8)^2$
3	8	−4	−4	$96/(8)^2$	−8	−6	−2	$104/(8)^2$
4	0	4	−4	$32/(8)^2$	0	2	−2	$8/(8)^2$
Variance[a]				$\frac{4}{n}\sigma_e^2$				$\frac{7}{2n}\sigma_e^2$

Note: Coefficients are multiplied by 8.
[a] Variance when $n = n_k$ for $1 \leq k \leq 4$.

10.5 Discussion

In this chapter, bioequivalence in average bioavailability was assessed based on statistical inference on the difference in formulation means under an additive model 10.2.1. When comparing more than two formulations, Locke (1984) provided a

TABLE 10.4.5: Coefficients for estimates of pairwise formulation effects in BIBD with four formulations and three periods (in absence of unequal carryover effects).

	$\theta_{1R} = F_1 - F_R$				$\theta_{2R} = F_2 - F_R$			
	Period				Period			
Sequence	**1**	**2**	**3**	$\Sigma_j C^2_{ajk}$	**1**	**2**	**3**	$\Sigma_j C^2_{ajk}$
1	2	−1	−1	$6/(8)^2$	−1	2	−1	$6/(8)^2$
2	1	1	−2	$6/(8)^2$	3	0	−3	$18/(8)^2$
3	0	−3	3	$18/(8)^2$	1	−2	1	$6/(8)^2$
4	−3	3	0	$18/(8)^2$	−3	0	3	$18/(8)^2$
Variance[a]				$\frac{3}{4n}\sigma^2_e$				$\frac{3}{4n}\sigma^2_e$

	$\theta_{3R} = F_3 - F_R$				$\theta_{21} = F_2 - F_1$			
	Period				Period			
Sequence	**1**	**2**	**3**	$\Sigma_j C^2_{ajk}$	**1**	**2**	**3**	$\Sigma_j C^2_{ajk}$
1	−1	−1	2	$6(8)^2$	−3	3	0	$18/(8)^2$
2	0	3	−3	$18/(8)^2$	2	−1	−1	$6/(8)^2$
3	3	−3	0	$18/(8)^2$	1	1	−2	$6/(8)^2$
4	−2	1	1	$6/(8)^2$	0	−3	3	$18/(8)^2$
Variance[a]				$\frac{3}{4n}\sigma^2_e$				$\frac{3}{4n}\sigma^2_e$

	$\theta_{31} = F_3 - F_1$				$\theta_{32} = F_3 - F_2$			
	Period				Period			
Sequence	**1**	**2**	**3**	$\Sigma_j C^2_{ajk}$	**1**	**2**	**3**	$\Sigma_j C^2_{ajk}$
1	−3	0	3	$18/(8)^2$	0	−3	3	$18/(8)^2$
2	−1	2	−1	$6/(8)^2$	−3	3	0	$18/(8)^2$
3	3	0	−3	$18/(8)^2$	2	−1	−1	$6/(8)^2$
4	1	−2	1	$6/(8)^2$	1	1	−2	$6/(8)^2$
Variance[a]				$\frac{3}{4n}\sigma^2_e$				$\frac{3}{4n}\sigma^2_e$

Note: Coefficients are multiplied by 8.
[a] Variance when $n = n_k$ for $1 \leq k \leq 4$.

procedure for assessment of bioequivalence based on the ratio of formulation means under the same additive model, which requires a rather weak assumption for covariance matrix. This procedure is basically a generalization of the exact confidence interval based on Fieller's theorem discussed in Section 4.2.3.

When comparing more than two formulations in study, multiple comparisons are usually made. For example, for comparing three formulations, there are a total of three comparisons, namely, formulations 1 versus 2; formulations 1 versus 3; and

TABLE 10.4.6: Coefficients for estimates for carryover effects in BIBD with four formulations and three periods (adjusted for formulation effects).

	$\lambda_{1R} = C_1 - C_R$				$\lambda_{2R} = C_2 - C_R$			
	Period				Period			
Sequence	1	2	3	$\Sigma_j C^2_{ajk}$	1	2	3	$\Sigma_j C^2_{ajk}$
1	4	0	−4	$32/(4)^2$	4	−4	0	$32/(4)^2$
2	−4	4	0	$32/(4)^2$	0	4	−4	$32/(4)^2$
3	0	0	0	$0/(4)^2$	−4	4	0	$32/(4)^2$
4	0	−4	4	$32/(4)^2$	0	−4	4	$32/(4)^2$
Variance[a]				$\frac{6}{n}\sigma^2_e$				$\frac{8}{n}\sigma^2_e$

	$\lambda_{3R} = F_3 - F_R$				$\lambda_{21} = F_2 - F_1$			
	Period				Period			
Sequence	1	2	3	$\Sigma_j C^2_{ajk}$	1	2	3	$\Sigma_j C^2_{ajk}$
1	4	−4	0	$32/(4)^2$	0	−4	4	$32/(4)^2$
2	0	0	0	$0/(4)^2$	4	0	−4	$32/(4)^2$
3	0	4	−4	$32/(4)^2$	−4	4	0	$32/(4)^2$
4	−4	0	4	$32/(4)^2$	0	0	0	$0/(4)^2$
Variance[a]				$\frac{6}{n}\sigma^2_e$				$\frac{6}{n}\sigma^2_e$

	$\lambda_{31} = F_3 - F_1$				$\lambda_{32} = F_3 - F_2$			
	Period				Period			
Sequence	1	2	3	$\Sigma_j C^2_{ajk}$	1	2	3	$\Sigma_j C^2_{ajk}$
1	0	−4	4	$32/(4)^2$	0	0	0	$0/(4)^2$
2	4	−4	0	$32/(4)^2$	0	−4	4	$32/(4)^2$
3	0	4	−4	$32/(4)^2$	4	0	−4	$32/(4)^2$
4	−4	4	0	$32/(4)^2$	−4	4	0	$32/(4)^2$
Variance[a]				$\frac{8}{n}\sigma^2_e$				$\frac{6}{n}\sigma^2_e$

Note: Coefficients are multiplied by 4.
[a] Variance when $n = n_k$ for $1 \leq k \leq 4$.

formulations 2 versus 3. Here, whether the overall type I error rate should be adjusted is a question interest. It is our feeling that if the purpose of the study is to establish equivalence between each test formulation and the reference formulation and it is stated in the study protocol, then the adjustment of the significance level is not warranted. However, some comparisons are not specified in advanced in the protocol and are carried out after the study, then appropriate adjustment of overall type I error rate is necessary.

Suppose we are interested in comparing k test formulations, T_i, $i = 1, 2, \ldots, k$, and reference formulation R. The assessment of bioequivalence basically involves either (1) T_i versus R for all i, or (2) T_i versus T_j for $i \neq j$, or (3) pairwise comparison among T_i, $i = 1, 2, \ldots, k$ and R. For the first case, the method described in this chapter can be applied directly. For case (2), since the reference formulation R is not involved, the conclusion of bioequivalence may depend on which formulation (i.e., T_i or T_j) is used as the reference formulation. For example, it is possible that T_1 is bioequivalent to T_2, which is treated as the reference formulation, and T_3 is bioequivalent to T_2. However, T_1 may not be bioequivalent to T_3. This may be partially explained by the fact that T_2 is not used as the reference formulation when comparing T_1 and T_3. In this case, it is suggested that the formulation to be used as the reference formulation be specified in the protocol with appropriate adjustment of overall type I error rate if necessary.

For comparing more than two formulations, as indicated either, a Williams design or a balanced incomplete block design is usually considered. As discussed in previous sections, a Williams design is not only a variance-balanced design for the formulation effect but also a variance-balanced design for the carryover effect. In other words, it is a variance-balanced design, regardless of the presence or absence of the carryover effect. On the other hand, although the balanced incomplete block design is a variance-balanced design when there are no carryover effects, it is not a variance-balanced design in the presence of carryover effect. Moreover, the degree of freedom for the mean squared error for the balanced incomplete block design is smaller than that of the Williams design. For example, for comparing four formulations, the degrees of freedom for the balanced incomplete block design is $2(N-4)$, whereas the degrees of freedom for the Williams design is $3(N-3)$. When there are no carryover effects, the variance for the balance incomplete block design is much larger than that of the Williams design; that is,

$$\frac{3}{4n}\sigma_e^2$$

$$\text{versus} \quad \frac{1}{2n}\sigma_e^2.$$

In the presence of the carryover effect, the variance for the balanced incomplete block design is even larger. Although the Williams design possesses some good properties, it does require the number of periods at least to be equal to the number of formulations being compared, whereas the balanced incomplete block design does not have this limitation. When there are many formulations to be compared, a balanced incomplete design may be preferred because it can be carried out on a small number of periods. Therefore to choose between a Williams design and a balanced block design for comparing more than two formulations, the relative gain and between the two designs should be taken into consideration.

The statistical procedures for evaluation of average bioequivalence for multiple formulations are derived under normality assumption described in Section 10.2.1 for a Williams design or a balanced incomplete block design. When normality assumption is in serious doubt, Bellavance and Tardif (1995) provide a nonparametric procedure for a Williams design with three formulations. Their method is based on obtaining unbiased estimates of the effects within each replication of six subjects and transforming the analysis of the original design into one randomized block design so that well-known Wilcoxon rank sum test can be applied.

Part III

Population and Individual Bioequivalence

Chapter 11

Population and Individual Bioequivalence

11.1 Introduction

For physicians and patients, bioequivalent drug products can and should be used interchangeably to achieve a similar therapeutic effect. As mentioned in Chapter 1, therefore, bioequivalence studies, in fact, serve as surrogates for clinical trials in evaluation of therapeutic equivalence in efficacy and safety between the innovator product and its generic copies. However, when a physician has the possibility of administering a generic drug product, he or she needs to consider the anticipated therapeutic effect that may be obtained from the patient. If a new patient has just begun a drug regimen, the physician does not have any informations about the patient's therapeutic response to any of the different formulation that he or she could prescribe. As a result, the only relevant information that the physician could have is the comparison of the marginal distributions for some pharmacokinetic responses or metric between the generic and innovator drug product from a population of subjects. If the marginal distributions follow an approximate normal distribution, the equivalence can be evaluated through inferences on population parameters, such as average and intra-subject variability. This concept, as indicated in Chapter 1, is referred to as the population bioequivalence (PBE). Given the information about population parameters, the physician can determine whether to prescribe an innovator drug product or its generic copies to a new patient who just begins to receive the drug regime. Prescribability, therefore, is the interchangeability for the new patient.

On the other hand, suppose a patient with a chronic disease, such as hypertension or diabetes, has been well controlled under long-term administration of an innovator drug product. In other words, the concentration of its active ingredients has been titrated to an efficacious and safety level within the patient's individual therapeutic window. After the patent of the innovator drug product has expired and its generic copies become available, in the United States, many states have generic substitution laws requiring that pharmacists dispense the cheapest formulation unless the physician specifies that no substitution of the generic product is allowed (Hauck and Anderson, 1992). However, for the patients already receiving the long-term administration of a formulation, the physician now has the information about patient's response to that formulation. To ensure the similar efficacy and safety by the generic switch, the concentration of the active ingredient for the generic drug product must still be within the patient's same therapeutic window established by the innovator's drug product. This concept is then referred to as switchability that requires bioequivalence within the same patient.

Chow and Liu (1995) defined switchability as the switch to an alternative drug product from a drug product within the same subject for whom the concentration has been titrated to a steady efficacious and safe level. On the other hand, Hauck (1996a) gave a definition of switchability such that a patient who is presently on one formulation can be switched to another formulation and retained essentially the same (or better) efficacy and safety profile. Switchability, therefore, is exchangeability within the same subject. To assure drug switchability, it is suggested that bioequivalence be assessed within the same individuals. This concept of bioequivalence is known as *individual bioequivalence* (IBE). From both definitions of switchability, individual bioequivalence not only assesses the closeness of the distributions of a patient's pharmacokinetic responses under repeated administration between the generic and the innovator's drug products, but also evaluates whether both distributions lie within the therapeutic window established by the innovator's drug product.

Statistical procedures for evaluation of average bioequivalence were introduced in Chapters 4 and 9, respectively, for the standard two-sequence, two-period crossover, and higher-order crossover designs. On the other hand, Chapters 7 and 9, under the assumption of compound symmetry for the covariance matrix, described various methods for assessment of equivalence in intra-subject variability under either 2×2 or higher-order designs. Schuirmann's two one-sided tests approach for average bioequivalence can be used jointly with the procedures for evaluation for equivalence in variability for assessment of PBE. Since this approach first evaluates ABE and bioequivalence in variability separately and then uses the intersection–union test (IUT) principle (Berger, 1982) to combine the individual results for assessment of PBE, it is called disaggregate criteria. However, the FDA statistical guidance on bioequivalence issued in 2001 uses a criterion that integrates average and variability into a single summary measure. It is then referred to as an aggregate criterion for PBE. On the basis of the same concept, aggregate criteria are suggested in the FDA statistical guidance for evaluation of IBE.

A general two-stage model for pharmacokinetic metrics or responses is introduced and limitations of average bioequivalence are illustrated through concepts of prescribability and switchability in Section 11.2. In Section 11.3 merits of IBE are provided and desirable features for bioequivalence criteria are given relative to improving the drawbacks suffered by ABE. Section 11.4 provides difference measures for describing the discrepancy of pharmacokinetic metrics between the test and reference formulations. Concepts of disaggregate and aggregate criteria are also introduced in this section. Different criteria for evaluation of population and individual bioequivalence, based on probability measures for discrepancy, are given in Section 11.5. Various moment-based aggregate criteria for population and individual bioequivalence are provided in Section 11.6. Interrelations among different criteria are explored in Section 11.7. Design issues for assessment of PBE and IBE are given in Section 11.8. Determination of population and individual bioequivalence limits are reviewed in Section 11.9. Final remarks and comments on selection of criteria and design for assessment of PBE and IBE are provided in Section 11.10.

11.2 Limitation of Average Bioequivalence

Let Y_{ijk} be the original or logarithmic transformation of the pharmacokinetic metric or response of interest for the kth repeated administration under the jth formulation for the ith subject, $k = 1, \ldots, K$; $i = 1, \ldots, N$; and $j = \mathrm{T}$, and R. Following the notations used by Sheiner (1992), and Hauck and Anderson (1994) and for illustration of concepts, a two-stage mixed-effects model without considerations of nuisance parameters, such as sequence or period effects, imposed by the design is assumed for Y_{ijk}. Within (conditional on) each subject, Y_{ijk} is independently distributed with mean μ_{ij} and variance σ^2_{iWj}; $i = 1, \ldots, N$; and $j = \mathrm{T}$ and R. μ_{ij} and intra-subject variability σ^2_{iWj} are referred as subject-specific average bioavailability and intra-subject variability of the distribution obtained from the jth formulation of the ith subject, $i = 1, \ldots, N$; and $j = \mathrm{T}$ and R. In this model, not only average bioavailability but also intra-subject variability are assumed to be different from subject to subject. The distribution of subject-specific average bioavailability $\boldsymbol{\mu}_{ik} = (\mu_{i\mathrm{T}}, \mu_{i\mathrm{R}})'$ is assumed to have a mean vector $\boldsymbol{\mu}$ and variance-covariance matrix $\boldsymbol{\Sigma}_{\mathrm{B}}$, where

$$\boldsymbol{\mu} = (\mu_{\mathrm{T}}, \mu_{\mathrm{R}})', \tag{11.2.1}$$

$$\boldsymbol{\Sigma}_{\mathrm{B}} = \begin{pmatrix} \sigma^2_{\mathrm{BT}} & \rho\sigma_{\mathrm{BT}}\sigma_{\mathrm{BR}} \\ \rho\sigma_{\mathrm{BT}}\sigma_{\mathrm{BR}} & \sigma^2_{\mathrm{BR}} \end{pmatrix}, \tag{11.2.2}$$

where μ_j is the population average and $\sigma^2_{\mathrm{B}j}$ is the inter-subject variability for the jth formulation, ρ is the correlation of subject-specific averages between the test and reference formulations $\mu_{i\mathrm{T}}$, and $\mu_{i\mathrm{R}}$; $k = 1, \ldots, K$; $i = 1, \ldots, N$.

The above model can also be reformulated as follows:

$$Y_{ijk} = \mu_j + b_{ij} + e_{ij}, \tag{11.2.3}$$

where

b_{ij} is the mean deviation from the population average μ_j of the jth formulation for the ith subject

e_{ij} is the intra-subject variability from the individual subject's response on repeated administrations of the jth formulation

Conditional on the ith subject

$$\begin{aligned} E_{\mathrm{I}}(Y_{ijk}) &= \mu_{ij} \\ &= \mu_j + b_{ij}, \end{aligned} \tag{11.2.4}$$

and b_{ij} and e_j are independent of each other, where E_{I} denotes the expectation conditional on the ith subject.

Furthermore,

$$E(b_{ij}) = E(e_{ij}) = E_I(e_{ij}) = 0,$$

and

$$V(e_j) = \sigma^2_{iWj}.$$

For the ith subject, b_{iT} and b_{iR} are correlated with each other by correlation coefficient ρ. It follows that the covariance matrix of $(b_{iT}, b_{iR})'$ is the same as that of $\boldsymbol{\mu}_{ik}$, which is given in Equation 11.2.2. Therefore, the marginal distribution of $\boldsymbol{Y}_{ik} = (Y_{iTk}, Y_{iRk})'$ has the average vector $\boldsymbol{\mu} = (\mu_T, \mu_R)'$ and covariance matrix $\boldsymbol{\Sigma} = \boldsymbol{\Sigma}_B + \boldsymbol{\Sigma}_W$, where $\boldsymbol{\Sigma}_B$ is given in Equation 11.2.2 and $\boldsymbol{\Sigma}_W$ is a 2×2 diagonal matrix with σ^2_{iWT} and σ^2_{iWR} on its diagonal.

Under normality assumption, within each subject, bioequivalence can be assessed through the difference in average bioavailability and intra-subject variability, that is,

$$\begin{aligned} \mu_{iD} &= \mu_{iT} - \mu_{iR}, \\ \delta_{id} &= \sigma^2_{iWT} - \sigma^2_{iWR} \ \left(\text{or } \sigma^2_{iWT}/\sigma^2_{iWR}\right). \end{aligned}$$

If distributions of the test and reference formulations are close enough, then the absolute value of μ_{iD} and δ_{id} should be very small. In addition, if the distribution of the test formulation is within the therapeutic window established by the reference formulation for the ith subject, then test formulation can be claimed to be bioequivalent to the reference formulation for the ith subject. However, the distributions of the test and reference formulations for the pharmacokinetic metric can be different from subject to subject and therapeutic window might also vary among subjects. Hence, μ_{iD} and δ_{id} are different from subject to subject. For the sake of simplicity, throughout this book, for each formulation, the intra-subject variability is assumed to be the same among all subjects (i.e., $\sigma^2_{iWT} = \sigma^2_{WT}$ and $\sigma^2_{iWR} = \sigma^2_{WR}$, $i = 1, \ldots, N$). On the other hand, following the two-stage mixed-effects model and formulation in Equation 11.2.3, $\mu_{iD} = \mu_{iT} - \mu_{iR} = b_{iT} - b_{iR}$, has a population mean $\mu_D = \mu_T - \mu_R$ and variance

$$\begin{aligned} V(\mu_{iD}) &= V(\mu_{iT} - \mu_{iR}) \\ &= V(b_{iT} - b_{iR}) \\ &= \sigma^2_{BT} + \sigma^2_{BR} - 2\rho\sigma_{BT}\sigma_{BR} \\ &= (\sigma_{BT} - \sigma_{BR})^2 + 2(1 - \rho)\sigma_{BT}\sigma_{BR}. \end{aligned} \tag{11.2.5}$$

Because $V(\mu_{iD})$ measures the homogeneity of $\mu_{iT} - \mu_{iR}$ across all subjects, it is also referred as the variance of subject-by-formulation interaction and is denoted as σ^2_D. If $\sigma^2_D = 0$, all differences in subject-specific averages will be equal to $\mu_T - \mu_R$ for all subjects.

	A	B	C	D	E	F
	R T	R T	R T	R T	R T	R T
$(\mu_T - \mu_R)^2$	0	+	0	0	0	+
σ_D^2	0	0	+	(+)	(+)	(+)
$\sigma_{WT}^2 - \sigma_{WR}^2$	0	0	0	+	−	−
Average BE	√	×	√	√	√	×
Individual BE	√	×	×	×	√	√

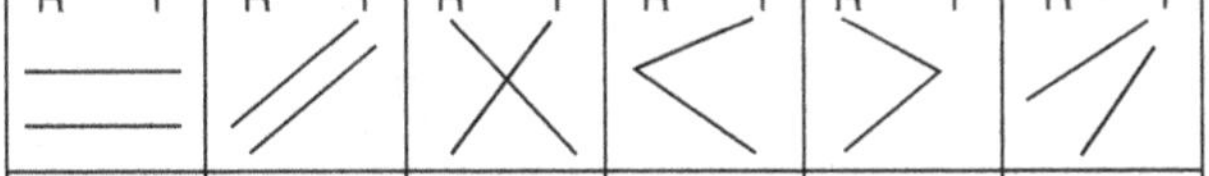

FIGURE 11.2.1: Schematic contrast of the responses by two subjects to the intake of reference (R) and test (T) formulations. The effects of the difference between the mean responses $[(\mu_T - \mu_R)^2]$, subject × formulation interaction (σ_D^2), and the deviation between the intra-individual variance ($\sigma_{WT}^2 - \sigma_{WR}^2$) are illustrated. These sources of variation can be absent (0), positive (+) or, when comparing the intra-subject variances, negative (−). Under each condition, either the acceptance (√) or rejection (×) of average and individual bioequivalence is indicated. (From Endrenyi, L. and Midha, K.K., *Eur. J. Pharm. Sci.*, 6, 271, 1998.)

One can evaluate bioequivalence from a viewpoint of quality control for generic drug products. Difference in population averages $\mu_T - \mu_R$, difference (or ratio) in population intra-subject variability $\sigma_{WT}^2 - \sigma_{WR}^2$, and subject-by-formulation interaction σ_D^2 can be considered as three characteristics representing the quality assurance for the generic drug product. Endrenyi and Midha (1998) use the results of some pharmacokinetic metrics from two subjects to provide a graphic illustration about the relation among three characteristics, which is reproduced in Figure 11.2.1. Six different situations are considered in Figure 11.2.1. Panel A of Figure 11.2.1 illustrates a rare circumstance for which two formulations are identical. Therefore, it is the ideal situation when there is no difference in population averages, no intra-subject variability, and no subject-by-formulation interaction. This scenario occurs very rarely, even for reference formulation versus reference formulation itself. Panel B of Figure 11.2.1 provides a circumstance for which there is a difference in population averages, but no difference in intra-subject variability and no subject-by-formulation interaction. The difference in population averages in panel C is negative for subject 1 and positive for subject 2. However, the population averages and intra-subject variability for both formulations are the same. This is a typical situation in which even if there is no difference in either population averages or intra-subject variability, subject-by-formulation interaction may and can exist. Panels D and E demonstrate the situation for which there is no difference in population averages, but a difference in intra-subject variability and subject-by-formulation interaction exists. The last panel provides the worst scenario for which differences in population average and intra-subject variability, and subject-by-formulation interaction exist.

From Figure 11.2.1, population averages of reference and test formulations are equal in panels A, C, D, and E. Except for panel A, however, differences in intra-subject variability and subject-by-formulation interaction exist. Under the situation for panel A, $\sigma_{\mathrm{WT}}^2 = \sigma_{\mathrm{WR}}^2 = \sigma_{\mathrm{e}}^2$, from Table 5.4.1, sample size should be at least 70 when intra-subject CV is 40%. Therefore, for highly variable drugs, even for comparison of the reference formulation with itself, average bioequivalence cannot be demonstrated with the usual sample size of 20–40 subjects (see also Benet and Goyan, 1995). From Equation 11.2.5, homogeneity of difference in subject-specific averages occurs only if inter-subject variability is the same for both tests and reference formulations and there is a perfect correlation between $\mu_{i\mathrm{T}}$ and $\mu_{i\mathrm{R}}$. It follows that $\sigma_{\mathrm{BT}}^2 = \sigma_{\mathrm{BR}}^2 = \sigma_{\mathrm{S}}^2$, $\rho = 1$ and covariance matrix of $\boldsymbol{Y}_{ik}$ becomes

$$\Sigma = \begin{pmatrix} \sigma_{\mathrm{WT}}^2 + \sigma_{\mathrm{S}}^2 & \sigma_{\mathrm{S}}^2 \\ \sigma_{\mathrm{S}}^2 & \sigma_{\mathrm{WR}}^2 + \sigma_{\mathrm{S}} \end{pmatrix}, \tag{11.2.6}$$

which is the same covariance of the two pharmacokinetic metrics of the same subject obtained under the standard 2×2 crossover design given in Equation 2.5.5. As a result, the standard 2×2 crossover design selected by most pharmaceutical companies and regulatory agencies around the world for evaluation of average bioequivalence cannot be used for inference about the subject-by-formulation interaction.

The FDA has published the data of AUC and $C_{\max}$ from 12 studies with 34 analytes on its Web site (FDA, 1998). Table 11.2.1 provides characteristics of these drug products. Some of these studies are conducted in normal volunteers and some in a targeted patient population. The sponsors employed higher-order (replicate) designs described in Chapter 9, with three or four periods. Patnaik (1996) reported some results of the estimated variance components, such as reference intra-subject variability σ_{WR}^2, the ratio of test to reference intra-subject variability $\sigma_{\mathrm{WT}}^2/\sigma_{\mathrm{WR}}^2$, and the variance of the subject-by-formulation interaction σ_{D}^2. The results are summarized in Table 11.2.2. From Table 11.2.2, the intra-subject variability is greater than 20% for 24 and 53% of 34 reference drug products under study, respectively, for AUC and $C_{\max}$. On the other hand, the range of the ratio of test to reference intra-subject variability is from 0.5 to 2.0 and from 0.6 to 1.7, respectively, for AUC and

TABLE 11.2.1: Characteristics of the drug products in FDA database.

Drug Number	Drug Class	Dose Form
1	Antianxiety agent	Immediate-release
2	Calcium channel blocking agent	Extended-release
$3(a-f)$	Hormone therapy	Immediate-release
4	Antidepressant agent	Immediate-release
5	Antiinflammatory agent	Immediate-release
7	β-Adrenergic blocking agent	Immediate-release
8	β-Adrenergic blocking agent	Immediate-release
$13(a-c)$	Antihypertensive agent	Patch
$14(a-d)$	MAO inhibitor	Immediate-release
$17(a-c)$	Antihypertensive agent	Patch

Source: Chen, M.L., Individual bioequivalence criterion. Presented at the meeting of the Advisory Committee for Pharmaceutical Sciences, Gaitherburg, Maryland, August 15–16, 1996.

TABLE 11.2.2: Summary of results for variance components.

PK Response	ISV (Ref.) > 0.2	ISV Ratio (Test/Ref.) Range	Subject-by-Formulation Interaction > 0.15
AUC	8/34 (24%)	0.5–2.0	8/34 (24%)
$C_{\max}$	18/34 (53%)	0.6–1.7	10/34 (29%)

Source: Patnaik, R.N., Individual bioequivalence: pharmacokinetic data—replicated designs. Presented at the Meeting of the Advisory Meeting for Pharmaceutical Science, Holiday Inn, Gaithersburg, MD, August 15, 1996.

Note: ISV, intra-subject variability; ref., reference.

$C_{\max}$. In addition, the subject-by-formulation interaction for AUC is greater than 0.15 for 24% of the reference drug products. For $C_{\max}$, the proportion is 29%. These results show that moderate to high intra-subject variability is observed for a fair amount of reference products, especially for $C_{\max}$, with a proportion greater than 50%. About one-fourth of the drugs investigated demonstrate the magnitude of σ_D greater than 0.15. A value of σ_D greater than 0.15 implies that approximately 14% of the differences in subject-specific averages lie outside the average bioequivalence limits of (ln 0.8, ln 1.25). Chen et al. (2000) also reported similar results with focus on only the studies with two-sequence, four-period replicate design from the same data set on the FDA Web site. From Patnaik (1996) and Chen et al. (2000) average bioequivalence alone seems inadequately to address switchability.

As indicated in Chen (1997), the average bioequivalence focuses only on the comparison in population averages of a bioavailability metric between the test and reference formulations. As illustrated in Figures 11.2.2 through 11.2.5, equivalence in average does not guarantee equivalence in intra-subject variability and closeness

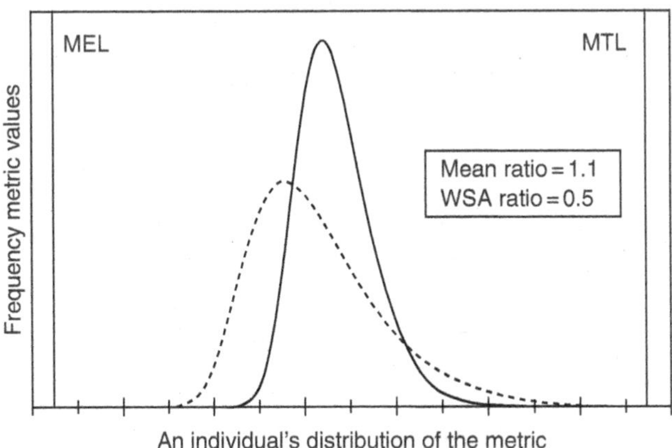

FIGURE 11.2.2: Individual distribution of the bioavailability metrics: wide individual therapeutic window. MEL, minimum effective level; MTL, maximum tolerable level; WSV, within-subject (intra-subject) variability. (From Hauck, W.W., Individual bioequivalence: Concepts. Presented at the Meeting of the Advisory Meeting for Pharmaceutical Science, Holiday Inn, Gaithersburg, Maryland, August 15, 1996b.)

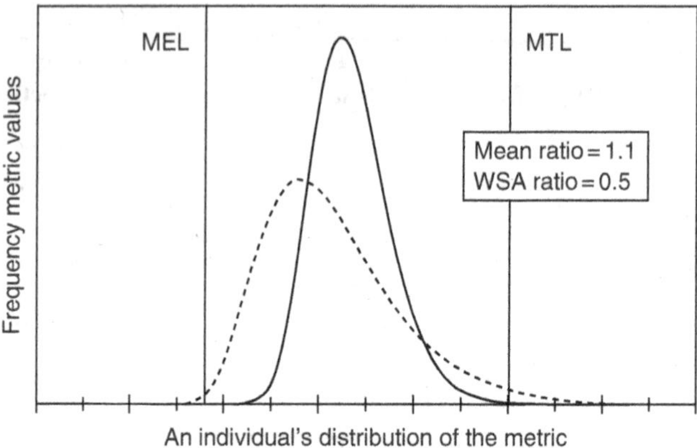

FIGURE 11.2.3: Individual distribution of the bioavailability metrics: narrow individual therapeutic window. MEL, minimum effective level; MTL, maximum tolerable level; WSV, within-subject (intra-subject) variability. (From Hauck, W.W., Individual bioequivalence: Concepts. Presented at the Meeting of the Advisory Meeting for Pharmaceutical Science, Holiday Inn, Gaithersburg, Maryland, August 15, 1996b.)

of the distributions of pharmacokinetic responses between the test and reference formulations. In addition, as mentioned in Chapter 7, for the standard 2 × 2 crossover design, average bioequivalence can be evaluated even when the intra-subject variabilities of test and reference formulations are different. As a result, during evaluation of average bioequivalence both pharmaceutical companies and regulatory

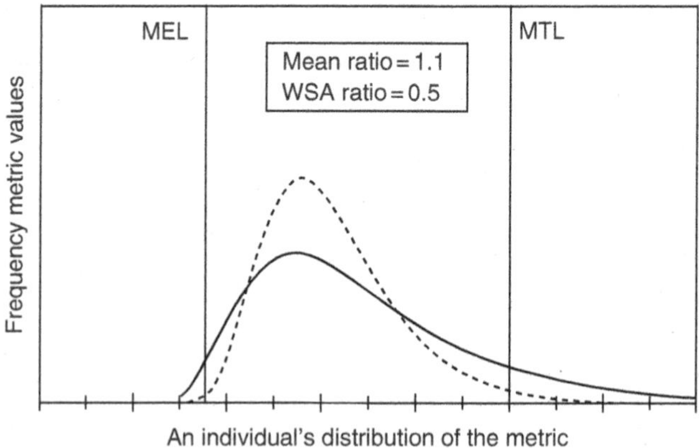

FIGURE 11.2.4: Individual distribution of the bioavailability metrics: narrow individual therapeutic window and increased variability of the test formulation. MEL, minimum effective level; MTL, maximum tolerable level; WSV, within-subject (intra-subject) variability. (From Hauck, W.W., Individual bioequivalence: Concepts. Presented at the Meeting of the Advisory Meeting for Pharmaceutical Science, Holiday Inn, Gaithersburg, Maryland, August 15, 1996b.)

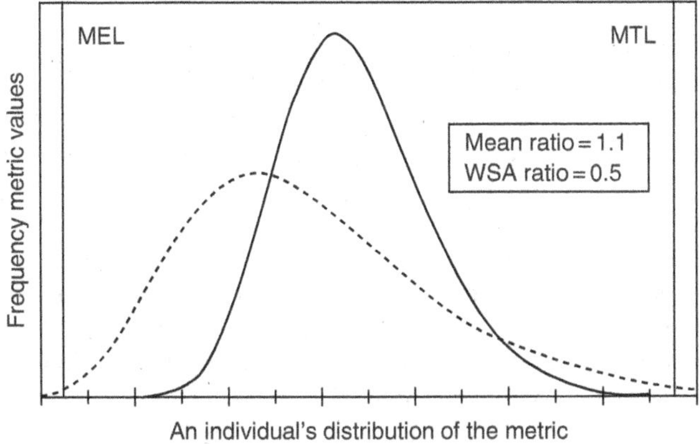

FIGURE 11.2.5: Individual distribution of the bioavailability metrics: narrow individual therapeutic window and highly variable drug products. MEL, minimum effective level; MTL, maximum tolerable level; WSV, within-subject (intra-subject) variability. (From Hauck, W.W., Individual bioequivalence: Concepts. Presented at the Meeting of the Advisory Meeting for Pharmaceutical Science, Holiday Inn, Gaithersburg, Maryland, August 15, 1996b.)

agencies often ignore the comparison between intra-subject variabilities. Furthermore, average bioequivalence fails to take into account the variation of difference in subject-specific average bioavailability between the test and reference formulations across subjects. As a result, Patnaik et al. (1997) and Chen et al. (2000) asserted that average bioequivalence can be used either for evaluation of prescribability for new patients or for switchability for patients already receiving long-term administration of medications.

11.3 Merits of Individual Bioequivalence and Desirable Features of Bioequivalence Criteria

From the above discussion, average bioequivalence can guarantee neither prescribability nor switchability. Therefore, assessment of bioequivalence has to take these two concepts into consideration. Both concepts compare not only distributions of pharmacokinetic responses between the test and reference formulations, but also need to verify whether the distributions are within the therapeutic window for the administrated medications. A therapeutic window is defined as an interval of bioavailability metric or pharmacokinetic response such as $AUC_{(0-\infty)}$ in which the drug is efficacious and safe. The lower and upper limits of a therapeutic window are referred to the minimally effective level (MEL) and maximally tolerated level (MTL).

The MEL is defined as the lowest level of the pharmacokinetic response such that the drug still maintains effectiveness (also see Liu and Chow, 2005a,b for minimum therapeutic effective dose and median effective dose, respectively). The highest level of the bioavailability metric, for which the safety of the drug is still preserved, is referred to as the MTL. The MEL and MTL of therapeutic windows vary from drug to drug. If the difference between MTL and MEL of a drug is large, then it is said to have a wide therapeutic window. A drug has a narrow therapeutic window if the interval is small. Small changes in pharmacokinetic response for a drug with a narrow therapeutic window can lead to marked changes in pharmacodynamic response (Benet and Goyan, 1995).

The relation between the distribution and therapeutic window lies not only in the average, but also in the variability of the pharmacokinetic response, as illustrated in Figures 11.2.2 through 11.2.5. In general, as suggested at Bio-International'89 and Bio-International'92, a drug product is classified as a highly variable drug if its intra-subject variability is greater than 30% (Blume and Midha, 1993a,b). The probability that the distribution of a drug falls in the wide therapeutic window is generally higher than that of a drug with a narrow therapeutic window. In other words, the distribution of the pharmacokinetic responses to a drug with a wide therapeutic window can allow a much larger variability than that of the drug with a narrow window. As a result, it is more difficult to demonstrate bioequivalence for the drug with a narrow therapeutic window than for the drug with a wide therapeutic window. Ideally, the bioequivalence limit, therefore, should be determined by the expected average, subject-by-formulation interaction, variability of the pharmacokinetic response, and therapeutic window of the drug.

For prescribability, assessment of bioequivalence is on a population basis. In other words, because the physician prescribes a drug product to a patient for the first time, the comparison between distributions and verification of enclosure of distribution inside the therapeutic window is performed through a population of subjects. Therefore, the therapeutic window is assumed to be the same for each of the subjects in the population. On the other hand, switchability evaluates the exchangeability of generic copies of an innovator's drug product within the same patient whose concentration has been titrated to an efficacious and safety level within the individual therapeutic window. As a result, not only the distribution of the pharmacokinetic responses, but also the therapeutic window can vary from individual to individual.

Again, Figures 11.2.2 through 11.2.5 illustrate the concepts of switchability, distribution, and therapeutic window. As can be seen in these figures, even though the two distributions to test and reference formulations are different, as long as the distribution of the generic copy lies within the patient's individual therapeutic window, the generic copy can be considered individually bioequivalent to the innovator's reference (Hauck, 1996b). The situation for a drug with a narrow therapeutic window, however, is different, because even the distribution of the pharmacokinetic responses of the test formulation might not be totally within the therapeutic window. As a result, even though the distribution of the pharmacokinetic responses for the test formulation may be close to that of the reference product, it may not be bioequivalent to the reference formulation because it is not within the individual therapeutic window established by the reference product. Therefore, on

TABLE 11.3.1: Classification of drugs.

Class	ITW	ISV	Example
A	Narrow	High	Cyclosporine
B	Narrow	Low	Theophylline
C	Wide	Low to moderate	Most drugs
D	Wide	High	Chlorpromazine or topical corticosteroids

Source: From Chen, M.L., Individual bioequivalence. Invited presentation at International Workshop: Statistical and Regulatory Issues on the Assessment of Bioequivalence. Dusseldorf, Germany, October 19–20, 1995; Patnaik, R.N., Lesko, L.J., Chen, M.L., Williams, R.L., and the FDA Individual Bioequivalence Working Group, *Clin. Pharmacokinet.*, 33, 1, 1997.

Note: ITW, individual therapeutic window; ISV, intra-subject variability.

assessment of individual bioequivalence for assurance of switchability, one needs to consider both individual distributions and therapeutic windows, which can be different from subject to subject.

From the individual therapeutic window and intra-subject variability, the FDA classifies drugs (Chen, 1997; Patnaik et al., 1997) into four categories that are given in Table 11.3.1. Most drugs fall into the class of wide therapeutic windows, with low to medium intra-subject variability. Drugs such as cyclosporine have a narrow therapeutic window and high intra-subject variability. Theophylline belongs to the narrow therapeutic window class, but with a low intra-subject variability. Examples for the drug with a wide therapeutic window and high intra-subject variability are topical corticosteroids and chlorpromazine.

For the limitation of average bioequivalence, consideration of individual therapeutic windows, and the objective of interchangeability, Chen (1995) summarized the merits of individual bioequivalence as follows:

- Comparison of both averages and variances
- Considerations of subject-by-formulation interaction
- Assurance of switchability
- Provision of flexible bioequivalence criteria for different drugs based on their therapeutic windows
- Provision of reasonable bioequivalence criteria for drugs with highly intra-subject variability
- Encouragement or reward of pharmaceutical companies to manufacture a better formulation

To achieve the objective of exchangeability among bioequivalent pharmaceutical products, the criteria for assessment of bioequivalence must possess certain important properties. Chen (1995, 1997) outlined the desirable characteristics of bioequivalence

TABLE 11.3.2: Desirable features of bioequivalence criteria.

Comparison of both averages and variances
Assurance of switchability
Encouragement or reward of pharmaceutical companies to manufacture a better formulation
Control of type I error rate (consumer's risk) at 5%
Allowance for determination of sample size
Admission of the possibility of sequence and period effects as well as missing values
User-friendly software application for statistical methods
Provision of easy interpretation for scientists and clinicians
Minimization of increased cost for conducting bioequivalence studies

Source: From Chen, M.L., *J. Biopharm. Stat.*, 7, 5, 1997.

criteria proposed by the FDA, which is provided in Table 11.3.2. In addition, to address the issues of intra-subject variability and subject-by-formulation interaction and to ensure switchability, valid statistical procedures, both estimation and hypothesis testing, should be developed from the criteria to control the consumer's risk at the prespecific nominal level (e.g., 5%). In addition, the statistical methods developed from the criteria should be able to provide sample size determination; to take into consideration the nuisance design parameters, such as period or sequence effects; and to develop user-friendly computer software. The most critical characteristics for any proposed criteria will be their interpretation to scientists and clinicians and the cost of conducting bioequivalence studies to provide inference for the criteria.

11.4 Measures of Discrepancy

Average, intra-subject variability, and subject-by-formulation interaction are three characteristics for assessment of bioequivalence of a generic product with the innovator reference. As a result, criteria for evaluation of either population or individual bioequivalence are functions of these parameters. For example, the criterion for average bioequivalence adopted by most regulatory agencies is formulated on the logarithmic scale for some pharmacokinetic measure such as AUC or $C_{\max}$ in the alternative hypothesis of Equation 4.3.1

$$\theta_L < \mu_T - \mu_R \le \theta_U.$$

If $-\theta_L = \theta_U = \Delta$, then the criterion for average bioequivalence becomes

$$(\mu_T - \mu_R)^2 \le \Delta^2. \tag{11.4.1}$$

On the other hand, the criterion for the intra-subject variability can be formulated either as a close interval as in Equation 7.2.2 or Equation 7.2.3, or as an open-end interval as Equation 7.7.1.

$$\sigma_{\mathrm{WT}}^2 - \sigma_{\mathrm{WR}}^2 < \delta, \tag{11.4.2}$$

where δ is the allowable upper limit for the test intra-subject variability over the reference intra-subject variability.

In addition, a possible criterion for subject-by-formulation interaction can also be formulated in terms of its variance as

$$\sigma_{\mathrm{D}}^2 < \gamma, \tag{11.4.3}$$

where γ is the allowable upper limit for the variance of subject-by-formulation interaction.

Bioequivalence can then be claimed if each of three criteria from Equations 11.4.1 through 11.4.3 are met. Because this approach first evaluates differences in averages, intra-subject variability, and variance of subject-by-formulation interaction separately, it is then referred as to the disaggregate criterion. If the criterion is a single summary measure composed of $(\mu_{\mathrm{T}} - \mu_{\mathrm{R}})^2$, $\sigma_{\mathrm{WT}}^2 - \sigma_{\mathrm{WR}}^2$, and σ_{D}^2 it is called the aggregate criterion.

$\mu_{\mathrm{T}} - \mu_{\mathrm{R}}$, $\sigma_{\mathrm{WT}}^2 - \sigma_{\mathrm{WR}}^2$, and σ_{D}^2 are the characteristics resulting from comparing distributions of pharmacokinetic responses, $Y_{i\mathrm{T}k}$ and $Y_{i\mathrm{R}}$. Criteria for assessment of bioequivalence, therefore, should be derived from some measures of discrepancy of pharmacokinetic responses between the test and reference formulations, or between the same reference formulations. To illustrate the concept, we drop all subscripts of Y except for those of formulations. Let $d(Y_j; Y_{j'})$ denote some measure of the expected discrepancy between pharmacokinetic responses Y_j and $Y_{j'}$, $j, j' = \mathrm{T, R}$. There are many indices for measuring the expected discrepancy between Y_j and $Y_{j'}$. Schall and Luus (1993) proposed the moment-based and probability-based measures for the expected discrepancy. The moment-based measure suggested by Schall and Luus (1993) is based on the expected mean-squared differences

$$d(Y_j; Y_{j'}) = \begin{cases} E(Y_{\mathrm{T}} - Y_{\mathrm{R}})^2 & \text{if } j = \mathrm{T} \text{ and } j' = \mathrm{R} \\ E(Y_{\mathrm{R}} - Y'_{\mathrm{R}})^2 & \text{if } j = \mathrm{R} \text{ and } j' = \mathrm{R}. \end{cases} \tag{11.4.4}$$

For some prespecific positive number r, one of probability-based measures for the expected discrepancy is given as (Schall and Luus, 1993)

$$d(Y_j; Y_{j'}) = \begin{cases} P\{|Y_{\mathrm{T}} - Y_{\mathrm{R}}| < r\} & \text{if } j = \mathrm{T} \text{ and } j' = \mathrm{R} \\ P\{|Y_{\mathrm{R}} - Y'_{\mathrm{R}}| < r\} & \text{if } j = \mathrm{R} \text{ and } j' = \mathrm{R}. \end{cases} \tag{11.4.5}$$

$d(Y_{\mathrm{T}}; Y_{\mathrm{R}})$ measures the expected discrepancy for some pharmacokinetic metrics between test and reference formulations, and $d(Y_{\mathrm{R}}; Y'_{\mathrm{R}})$ provides the expected discrepancy between the repeated administrations of the reference formulation. The role of $d(Y_{\mathrm{R}}; Y'_{\mathrm{R}})$ in formulation of bioequivalence criteria is to serve as a control.

The rationale is that the reference formulation should be bioequivalent to itself. Therefore, for the moment-based measures, if the test formulation is indeed bioequivalent to the reference formulation, then $d(Y_T; Y_R)$ should be very close to $d(Y_R, Y'_R)$. It follows that if the criteria are functions of the difference (or ratio) between $d(Y_T; Y_R)$ and $d(Y_R; Y'_R)$, bioequivalence is concluded if they are smaller than some prespecific limit. On the other hand, for probability-based measures, if the test formulation is indeed bioequivalent to the reference formulation, as compared with $d(Y_R; Y'_R)$, $d(Y_T; Y_R)$ should be relatively large. As a result, bioequivalence is concluded if the criteria based on the probability-based measure are greater than some prespecified limit.

11.5 Probability-Based Criteria

As mentioned in Chapter 1, the 75/75 decision rule is an early attempt by the FDA to determine individual bioequivalence. For the standard 2×2 crossover design, according to this rule, individual bioequivalence is claimed if on the original scale, at least 75% of individual subject's ratios fall within the limits (0.75, 1.25). However, the 75/75 rule cannot control the type I error rate at the prespecified nominal level if the variability of the test formulation is larger than that of the reference formulation (Haynes, 1981; Metzler and Huang, 1983; Thiyagarajan and Dobbins, 1987). Anderson and Hauck (1990) reformulated the concept of 75/75 rule as an individual equivalence ratio (IER) on the original scale as

$$-r' < \frac{\mu'_{iT}}{\mu'_{iR}} < r', \tag{11.5.1}$$

where

μ'_{iT} and μ'_{iR} are the subject-specific average of the test and reference formulations on the original scale

$r' = \exp(r)$, and exp is the natural exponentiation

Therefore, the measures of the expected discrepancy can also be based on the subject-specific averages $d(\mu'_{iT}; \mu'_{iR})$ The probability-based measures derived from the expected discrepancy on the original and logarithmic scale are equivalent because a logarithm is a monotonic function of any positive number and

$$\begin{aligned} P_{\text{TIER}} &= P\{-r' < \mu'_{iT}/\mu'_{iR} < r'\} \\ &= P\{|\mu_{iT} - \mu_{iR}| < r\} \\ &= P\{-r < \mu_{iT} - \mu_{iR} < r\}. \end{aligned} \tag{11.5.2}$$

The individual bioequivalence of a generic drug product to the innovator's product is concluded if P_{TIER} is greater than the minimum proportion of the population (in which the two formulations must be bioequivalent to call the two formulations individual bioequivalent, MINP; Anderson and Hauck, 1990). Anderson and Hauck (1990) also proposed a binomial test that is referred to as the test for individual equivalence ratio (TIER) for assessment of individual bioequivalence.

Define

$$\begin{aligned} P_{\mathrm{TR}} &= d(Y_{\mathrm{T}};\, Y_{\mathrm{R}}) \\ &= P\{|Y_{\mathrm{T}} - Y_{\mathrm{R}}| < r\}, \end{aligned} \tag{11.5.3}$$

and

$$\begin{aligned} P_{\mathrm{RR}} &= d(Y_{\mathrm{R}};\, Y'_{\mathrm{R}}) \\ &= P\{|Y_{\mathrm{R}} - Y'_{\mathrm{R}}| < r\}. \end{aligned} \tag{11.5.4}$$

Schall and Luus (1993) and Schall (1995) proposed alternative criteria based on the probability-based measures of the expected discrepancy:

$$\begin{aligned} P_{\mathrm{d}} &= d(Y_{\mathrm{T}};\, Y'_{\mathrm{R}}) - d(Y_{\mathrm{R}};\, Y'_{\mathrm{R}}) \\ &= P_{\mathrm{TR}} - P_{\mathrm{RR}} \\ &= P\{|Y_{\mathrm{T}} - Y_{\mathrm{R}}| < r\} - P\{|Y_{\mathrm{R}} - Y'_{\mathrm{R}}| < r\}, \end{aligned} \tag{11.5.5}$$

or

$$\begin{aligned} P_r &= \frac{d(Y_{\mathrm{T}};\, Y_{\mathrm{R'}})}{d(Y_{\mathrm{R}};\, Y'_{\mathrm{R}})} \\ &= \frac{P_{\mathrm{TR}}}{P_{\mathrm{RR}}} \\ &= \frac{P\{|Y_{\mathrm{T}} - Y_{\mathrm{R}}| < r\}}{P\{|Y_{\mathrm{R}} - Y'_{\mathrm{R}}| < r\}}. \end{aligned} \tag{11.5.6}$$

Schall (1995) suggested $r = c\sqrt{2}\sigma_{\mathrm{WR}}$ for individual bioequivalence, and $r = c\sqrt{2}\sigma_{\mathrm{TR}}$ for population bioequivalence, where $\sigma^2_{\mathrm{TR}} = \sigma^2_{\mathrm{BR}} + \sigma^2_{\mathrm{WR}}$.

Bioequivalence is claimed if $P_{\mathrm{d}}(P_r)$ is sufficiently larger than some prespecified lower limit, say $\pi_{\mathrm{d}}(\pi_r)$. The general formulation for the hypothesis based on the probability-based criteria is then given as

$$\begin{aligned} &H_0\colon\ P_{\mathrm{d}}(P_r) < \pi_{\mathrm{d}}(\pi_r) \\ \text{versus}\quad &H_{\mathrm{a}}\colon\ P_{\mathrm{d}}(P_r) > \pi_{\mathrm{d}}(\pi_r), \end{aligned} \tag{11.5.7}$$

where $\pi_{\mathrm{d}}(\pi_r)$ is the minimum proportion of the population in which the two formulations must be bioequivalent to call the two formulations bioequivalent.

Because

$$E(Y_T - Y_R) = \theta,$$
$$E(Y_R - Y'_R) = 0,$$
$$V(Y_T - Y_R) = \sigma^2_{WR} + \sigma^2_{WT} + \sigma^2_D,$$

and

$$V(Y_R - Y'_R) = 2\sigma^2_{WR},$$

therefore, if normality is assumed for Y_T and Y_R, it follows that

$$\begin{aligned} P_{RR} &= \Phi\{c\sqrt{2}\sigma_{WR}/\sqrt{2}\sigma_{WR}\} - \Phi\{-c\sqrt{2}\sigma_{WR}/\sqrt{2}\sigma_{WR}\} \\ &= \Phi\{c\} - \Phi\{-c\}. \end{aligned}$$

As a result, P_{RR} is a constant under the normality assumption, for example, $P_{RR} = 0.68$ when $c = 1$. In other words, when pharmacokinetic responses approximately follow a normal distribution, bioequivalence can be evaluated through P_{TR} only. For population bioequivalence because $V(Y_T - Y_R) = \sigma^2_{TR} + \sigma^2_{TT}$, then

$$P_{TR} = \Phi\left\{\frac{(r-\theta)}{\sqrt{\sigma^2_{TR} + \sigma^2_{TT}}}\right\} - \Phi\left\{\frac{(-r-\theta)}{\sqrt{\sigma^2_{TR} + \sigma^2_{TT}}}\right\}, \qquad (11.5.8)$$

where

$$\sigma^2_{TT} = \sigma^2_{BT} + \sigma^2_{WT},$$

and

$$\sigma^2_{TR} = \sigma^2_{WR} + \sigma^2_{BR}.$$

On the other hand, for individual bioequivalence, P_{TR} becomes

$$P_{TR} = \Phi\left\{\frac{(r-\theta)}{\sqrt{\sigma^2_{WR} + \sigma^2_{WT} + \sigma^2_D}}\right\} - \Phi\left\{\frac{(-r-\theta)}{\sqrt{\sigma^2_{WR} + \sigma^2_{WT} + \sigma^2_D}}\right\}.$$

For ideal situation of perfect individual bioequivalence when $\mu_T - \mu_R = 0$, $\sigma^2_D = 0$ and $\sigma^2_{WR} = \sigma^2_{WT}$, and for $P_{TR} \geq 0.9$, Hauck and Anderson (1994) suggest that c be 1.645 so that $r = 2.326\sigma_{WR}$.

P_{TIER} can also be expressed in terms of P_r in Equation 11.5.6 without the additional normality assumption. As indicated in the above, P_{TIER} is defined in terms of subject-specific averages, $E_{\text{I}}(Y_{i\text{T}})$ and $E_{\text{I}}(Y_{i\text{R}})$. It follows that P_{RR} becomes

$$\begin{aligned} P_{\text{RR}} &= d[E_{\text{I}}(Y_{i\text{R}});\ E_{\text{I}}(Y'_{i\text{R}})] \\ &= P\{|E_{\text{I}}(Y_{i\text{R}}) - E_{\text{I}}(Y'_{i\text{R}})| < r\} \\ &= P\{|\mu_{i\text{R}} - \mu_{i\text{R}}| < r\} \\ &= 1, \end{aligned}$$

and P_r in Equation 11.5.6 turns out to be P_{TIER} and $P_{\text{d}} = P_{\text{TIER}} - 1$.

11.6 Moment-Based Criteria

The concept of formulation of bioequivalence criteria is to compare the difference in bioavailability metrics of the test and reference formulations with that of the reference versus reference itself. The FDA guidance on *Statistical Approaches to Establishing Bioequivalence* (FDA, 2001), therefore, suggests use of the difference ratio (DR) as a formulation for the bioequivalence criteria:

$$\text{DR} = \frac{\text{Difference between test and reference formulations}}{\text{Difference between two formulations}}. \tag{11.6.1}$$

For inter-subject differences $Y_{\text{T}} - Y_{\text{R}}$ and $Y_{\text{R}} - Y'_{\text{R}}$ the moment-based measures become

$$\begin{aligned} d(Y_{\text{T}};\ Y_{\text{R}}) &= E(Y_{\text{T}} - Y_{\text{R}})^2 \\ &= (\mu_{\text{T}} - \mu_{\text{R}})^2 + \sigma_{\text{TR}}^2 + \sigma_{\text{TT}}^2 \\ &= \theta^2 + \sigma_{\text{TR}}^2 + \sigma_{\text{TT}}^2, \end{aligned} \tag{11.6.2}$$

and

$$\begin{aligned} d(Y_{\text{R}};\ Y'_{\text{R}}) &= E(Y_{\text{R}} - Y'_{\text{R}})^2 \\ &= 2\sigma_{\text{TR}}^2. \end{aligned}$$

Therefore, the difference ratio in Equation 11.6.1 becomes the population difference ratio (PDR) as

$$\text{PDR} = \left[\frac{(\theta^2 + \sigma_{\text{TR}}^2 + \sigma_{\text{TT}}^2)}{2\sigma_{\text{TR}}^2}\right]^{1/2}. \tag{11.6.3}$$

On the other hand, for intra-subject differences, $d(Y_T;\, Y_R)$ and $d(Y_R;\, Y'_R)$ are given respectively as

$$\begin{aligned} d(Y_T;\, Y_R) &= E(Y_T - Y_R)^2 \\ &= (\mu_T - \mu_R)^2 + \sigma_D^2 + \sigma_{WT}^2 + \sigma_{WR}^2 \\ &= \theta^2 + \sigma_D^2 + \sigma_{WT}^2 + \sigma_{WR}^2, \end{aligned} \tag{11.6.4}$$

and

$$\begin{aligned} d(Y_R;\, Y'_R) &= E(Y_R - Y'_R)^2 \\ &= 2\sigma_{WR}^2. \end{aligned}$$

As a result, the difference ratio in Equation 14.6.1 becomes the individual difference ratio (IDR) as

$$\text{IDR} = \left[\frac{(\theta^2 + \sigma_D^2 + \sigma_{WT}^2 + \sigma_{WR}^2)}{2\sigma_{WR}^2}\right]^{1/2}. \tag{11.6.5}$$

Various moment-based criteria have been proposed (Sheiner, 1992; Schall and Luus, 1993; Holder and Hsuan, 1993; FDA, 2001). All these criteria are different, but all are functions of the difference ratio. Schall and Luus (1993) considered the difference of the expected squared difference in pharmacokinetic responses between the test and reference formulations with that between two repeated administrations of reference formulations.

$$\begin{aligned} M_I &= d(Y_T;\, Y_R) - d(Y_R;\, Y'_R) \\ &= E(Y_T - Y_R)^2 - E(Y_R - Y'_R)^2. \end{aligned}$$

For inter-subject differences $Y_T - Y_R$ and $Y_R - Y'_R$, the criterion proposed by Schall and Luus (1993) for evaluation of population bioequivalence is given as

$$M_{PI} = \theta^2 + \sigma_{TT}^2 - \sigma_{TR}^2. \tag{11.6.6}$$

On the other hand, for intra-subject differences $Y_T - Y_R$ and $Y_R - Y'_R$, Schall and Luus (1993) proposed the following criterion for assessment of individual bioequivalence:

$$M_{II} = \theta^2 + \sigma_D^2 + \sigma_{WT}^2 - \sigma_{WR}^2. \tag{11.6.7}$$

For individual bioequivalence, Sheiner (1992) proposed the following criterion:

$$M_{I2} = \frac{E(Y_T - Y_R)^2 - (1/2)E(Y_R - Y_R')^2}{(1/2)E(Y_R - Y_R')^2} = \frac{\left(\theta^2 + \sigma_D^2 + \sigma_{WT}^2\right)}{\sigma_{WR}^2}. \quad (11.6.8)$$

The 2001 FDA guidance (FDA, 2001) suggested another formulation for evaluation for bioequivalence that is a hybrid of formulations proposed by Sheiner (1992) and Schall and Luus (1993). For the FDA formulation, the numerator is the same formulation M_1 as proposed by Schall and Luus (1993) and is scaled by the same denominator as that suggested by Sheiner (1992):

$$M_3 = \frac{E(Y_T - Y_R)^2 - E(Y_R - Y_R')^2}{(1/2)E(Y_R - Y_R')^2}. \quad (11.6.9)$$

It follows that the moment-based criterion for assessment of population bioequivalence proposed by the draft FDA guidance is given as

$$M_{P3} = \frac{\left(\theta^2 + \sigma_{TT}^2 - \sigma_{TR}^2\right)}{\sigma_{TR}^2}. \quad (11.6.10)$$

For evaluation of individual bioequivalence, the FDA guidance (2001) proposed the following moment-based criterion:

$$M_{I3} = \frac{\left(\theta^2 + \sigma_D^2 + \sigma_{WT}^2 - \sigma_{WR}^2\right)}{\sigma_{WR}^2}. \quad (11.6.11)$$

Other moment-based criteria have been also suggested, and they are also functions of difference in population average, subject-by-formulation interaction, and intra-subject variability. For example, the moment-based criterion proposed by Holder and Hsuan (1993) is given as

$$M_{I4} = \theta^2 + \sigma_D^2, \quad (11.6.12)$$

On the other hand, Ekbohm and Melander (1989) proposed the ratio of the variance of the subject-by-formulation interaction to the sum of the test and reference intra-subject variability as another criterion for evaluation of exchangeability among different formulations

$$M_{I5} = \frac{\sigma_D^2}{\left(\sigma_{WT}^2 + \sigma_{WR}^2\right)}. \quad (11.6.13)$$

M_{I4} proposed by Holder and Hsuan (1993) can also be derived using the concept of the expected discrepancy. However, M_{I4} is M_{I1} where the expected discrepancy in

Equation 11.6.2 is defined in terms of subject-specific averages, rather than the subject-observed pharmacokinetic responses:

$$\begin{aligned} M_{I4} &= d[E_I(Y_{iT}); E_I(Y_{iR})] - d[E_I(Y_{iR}); E_I(Y'_{iR})] \\ &= E[E_I(Y_{iT}) - E_I(Y_{iR})]^2 - E[E_I(Y_{iR}) - E_I(Y'_{iR})]^2 \\ &= \theta^2 + \sigma_D^2 + 0. \end{aligned}$$

For the moment-based criteria, bioequivalence is concluded if $M_I(M_P)$ is sufficiently smaller than some prespecified lower limit, say $\Delta_I(\Delta_P)$. As a result, the general formulations for the hypothesis based on moment-based criteria are given as

$$\begin{aligned} &\text{H}_0\text{: } M_I(M_P) \geq \Delta_I(\Delta_P) \\ \text{versus } &\text{H}_a\text{: } M_I(M_P) < \Delta_I(\Delta_P). \end{aligned} \tag{11.6.14}$$

Although various aggregate moment-based criteria have been proposed for evaluation of individual bioequivalence, these different criteria are related to or are functions of each other. Define

$$\begin{aligned} \lambda_1 &= \frac{\theta^2}{\sigma_{WR}^2} \\ &= \frac{(\mu_T - \mu_R)^2}{\sigma_{WR}^2}, \\ \lambda_2 &= \frac{\sigma_D^2}{\sigma_{WR}^2}, \end{aligned} \tag{11.6.15}$$

and

$$\lambda_3 = \frac{\sigma_{WT}^2}{\sigma_{WR}^2}.$$

λ_1, λ_2, and λ_3, in fact, represent three characteristics of the generic drug product; population average, variance of subject-by-formulation interaction, and the test intra-subject variability, all scaled by the intra-subject variability of the reference formulation.

Instead of assessment by a single summary quantity, individual bioequivalence, therefore, can be evaluated by each of the following hypotheses for individual moments (Liu and Chow, 1996a; Liu, 1998):

1. Average

$$\begin{aligned} &\text{H}_{0a}\text{: } \mu_T - \mu_R \geq \sqrt{\lambda'_{10}}, \quad \text{or} \quad \mu_T - \mu_R \leq -\sqrt{\lambda'_{10}} \\ \text{versus } &\text{H}_{aa}\text{: } -\sqrt{\lambda'_{10}} < \mu_T - \mu_R \leq \sqrt{\lambda'_{10}}. \end{aligned}$$

2. Subject-by-formulation interaction

$$\begin{aligned} &H_{0i}:\ \sigma_D^2 \geq \lambda'_{20} \\ \text{versus}\quad &H_{0i}:\ \sigma_D^2 < \lambda'_{20}. \end{aligned} \tag{11.6.16}$$

3. Intra-subject variability

$$\begin{aligned} &H_{0v}:\ \sigma_{WT}^2/\sigma_{WR}^2 \geq \lambda_{30} \\ \text{versus}\quad &H_{0v}:\ \sigma_{WT}^2/\sigma_{WR}^2 < \lambda_{30}, \end{aligned}$$

where
$\lambda'_{10} = \lambda_{10}\sigma_{WR}^2$
$\lambda'_{20} = \lambda_{20}\sigma_{WR}^2$
λ_{10}, λ_{20}, and λ_{30} are the upper limits specified for λ_1, λ_2, and λ_3

By application of the intersection–union test (IUT) principle (Berger, 1982), individual bioequivalence is concluded at the α-nominal significance level if, and only if, all three hypotheses are also rejected at the same α-level. Because this approach to assessment of individual bioequivalence evaluates each characteristic individually, it is, therefore, called as disaggregate moment-based criterion. On the other hand, the criteria, M_{I1}, M_{I2}, M_{I3} proposed by Schall and Luus (1993), Sheiner (1992), and FDA (2001), respectively, are a single composite measure of λ_1, λ_2, and λ_3. As a result, they are referred to as *aggregate criteria*. The hypothesis for average can also be formulated as

$$H_{0a}:\ (\mu_T - \mu_R)^2 \geq \lambda'_{10} \quad \text{or} \quad (\mu_T - \mu_R)^2 < \lambda'_{10} \tag{11.6.17}$$

Although the hypothesis for average is equivalent to that expressed in hypotheses 11.6.17, procedures for inference based on these two hypotheses may be different. The hypothesis for average is for the first moment, as represented in the average difference between the test and reference formulations. On the other hand, the inference for the hypotheses 11.6.17 is for the second moment of the squared average difference.

Figure 11.6.1 illustrates the relation of the parameter spaces on the hypotheses between aggregate and disaggregate criteria. For disaggregate criteria, the parameter space formed by the hypotheses 11.6.16 is a cuboid in the first quadrant of the three-dimensional space spanned by λ_1, λ_2, and λ_3. The boundary of the cuboid is determined by the prespecified upper allowable limits for average, subject-by-formulation interaction, and intra-subject variability, λ_{10}, λ_{20}, and λ_{30}. The complement of this cuboid is the parameter space for the null hypothesis of the disaggregate approach. On the other hand, for example, the aggregate criterion, M_{I3}, is a hyperplane that separates the three-dimensional space into the two parameter spaces, each corresponding to null and alternative hypotheses 11.6.14. If the prespecific upper allowable limit is determined λ_{10}, λ_{20}, and λ_{30}, then the hyperplane M_{I3} goes through the point $(\lambda_{10}, \lambda_{20}, \lambda_{30} - 1)$.

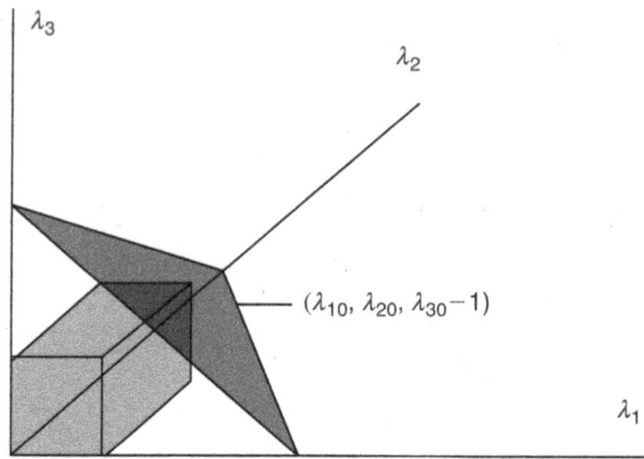

FIGURE 11.6.1: Relation of parameter spaces between the aggregate and disaggregate criteria.

11.7 Relations among Criteria

From Equations 11.6.7 through 11.6.11 aggregate moment-based criteria for individual bioequivalence, M_{I1}, M_{I2}, M_{I3}, are a summary measure of λ_1, λ_2, and λ_3. As a result, the relation among the criteria suggested by the FDA guidance (2001) for individual bioequivalence and those proposed by Sheiner (1992) and Schall and Luus (1993) can be examined through the following equation:

$$\begin{aligned} M_{I3} &= \lambda_1 + \lambda_2 + \lambda_3 - 1 \\ &= M_{I2} - 1 \\ &= \frac{M_{I1}}{\sigma^2_{WR}}. \end{aligned} \tag{11.7.1}$$

When $\sigma^2_{WR} = \sigma^2_{WT}$, $M_{I1} = M_{I4}$. As a result, if the test and reference intra-subject variability are the same, the moment-based criterion proposed by Schall and Luus (1993) is the same as that suggested by Holder and Hsuan (1993).

On the other hand, the relation among M_{I1}, M_{I2}, and M_{I3} can also be investigated by the individual difference ratio given in Equation 11.6.5. Recall that the square of IDR is

$$\mathrm{IDR}^2 = \frac{\left(\theta^2 + \sigma^2_D + \sigma^2_{WT} + \sigma^2_{WR}\right)}{2\sigma^2_{WR}}.$$

It can be easily shown that

TABLE 11.7.1: Relation among moment-based criteria for individual bioequivalence.

Criteria	Individual Components	IDR²
M_{I1} (Schall and Luus, 1993)	$\sigma^2_{WR}(\lambda_1 + \lambda_2 + \lambda_3 - 1)$	$2\sigma^2_{WR}(\text{IDR}^2 - 1)$
M_{I2} (Sheiner, 1992)	$\lambda_1 + \lambda_2 + \lambda_3$	$2\text{IDR}^2 - 1$
M_{I3} (FDA, 2001)	$\lambda_1 + \lambda_2 + \lambda_3 - 1$	$2(\text{IDR}^2 - 1)$

Note: $M_{I1} = \theta^2 + \sigma^2_D + \sigma^2_{WT} - \sigma^2_{WR} = M_{I4}$ (if $\sigma^2_{WT} = \sigma^2_{WR}$); $M_{I2} = (\theta^2 + \sigma^2_D + \sigma^2_{WT})/\sigma^2_{WR}$; $M_{I3} = (\theta^2 + \sigma^2_D + \sigma^2_{WT} - \sigma^2_{WR})/\sigma^2_{WR}$; $\lambda_1 = \theta^2/\sigma^2_{WR}$; $\lambda_2 = \sigma^2_D/\sigma^2_{WR}$; $\lambda_3 = \sigma^2_{WT}/\sigma^2_{WR}$; IDR, individual difference ratio.

$$\begin{aligned}
\text{IDR}^2 &= \frac{\left(\theta^2 + \sigma^2_D + \sigma^2_{WT} - \sigma^2_{WR} + 2\sigma^2_{WR}\right)}{2\sigma^2_{WR}} \\
&= \frac{M_{I3}}{2 + 1} \\
&= \frac{M_{I1}}{2\sigma^2_{WR} + 1} \\
&= \frac{\left(\theta^2 + \sigma^2_D + \sigma^2_{WT} + \sigma^2_{WR}\right)}{2\sigma^2_{WR}} \\
&= \frac{(M_{I2} + 1)}{2}.
\end{aligned}$$

The relation among various moment-based criteria for evaluation of individual bioequivalence is summarized in Table 11.7.1.

The normal distribution is uniquely determined by the first two moments; therefore, if the pharmacokinetic responses follow approximately a normal distribution, then probability- and moment-based criteria should be equivalent. Here we focus on the criteria for evaluation of individual bioequivalence. The relation between probability- and moment-based criteria for population bioequivalence can be similarly established. From the two-stage model described in Section 11.2, the marginal distribution of $Y_T - Y_R$ follows a normal distribution, with mean $\mu_T - \mu_R$ and variance $\sigma^2_I = \sigma^2_D + \sigma^2_{WT} + \sigma^2_{WR}$. Note the following relation:

$$\begin{aligned}
M_{I3} + 2 &= M_{I2} + 1 \\
&= \frac{(\mu_T - \mu_R)^2 + \left(\sigma^2_D + \sigma^2_{WT} + \sigma^2_{WR}\right)}{\sigma^2_{WR}}.
\end{aligned} \tag{11.7.2}$$

Recall that

$$\begin{aligned}
\sigma^2_D &= \sigma^2_{BT} + \sigma^2_{BR} - 2\rho\sigma_{BT}\sigma_{BR} \\
&= (\sigma_{BT} - \sigma_{BR})^2 + 2(1 - \rho)\sigma_{BT}\sigma_{BR}.
\end{aligned}$$

Let $\sigma_{BT} = c_B\sigma_{BR}$ and $\sigma_{WT} = c_W\sigma_{WR}$ Then σ_I^2, M_{I2}, and M_{I3} can be reformulated as follows:

$$\begin{aligned}
\sigma_I^2 &= \left(1 + c_W^2\right)\sigma_{WR}^2 + \left[(c_B - 1)^2 + 2c_B(1 - \rho)\right]\sigma_{BR}^2, \\
M_{I2} &= \left\langle\left\{\theta^2 + \left[(c_B - 1)^2 + 2c_B(1 - \rho)\right]\sigma_{BR}^2\right\}/\sigma_{WR}^2\right\rangle + c_W^2, \\
M_{I3} &= \left\langle\left\{\theta^2 + \left[(c_B - 1)^2 + 2c_B(1 - \rho)\right]\sigma_{BR}^2\right\}/\sigma_{WR}^2\right\rangle + \left(c_W^2 - 1\right).
\end{aligned} \quad (11.7.3)$$

Individual bioequivalence can then be evaluated by P_{TR} defined in Equation 11.5.3 as

$$P_{TR} = P\{-r < Y_T - Y_R < r\}.$$

The corresponding hypothesis based on P_{TR} is given as

$$\begin{aligned}
&\text{H}_0\text{: } P_{TR} \leq \pi_0 \\
\text{versus } &\text{H}_a\text{: } P_{TR} > \pi_0,
\end{aligned} \quad (11.7.4)$$

where π_0 is the MINP by Anderson and Hauck (1990).

Let $P_L = P\{Y_T - Y_R < r\}$ and $P_U = P\{Y_T - Y_R \geq r\}$. It follows that under the normality assumption, $P_{TR} = 1 - (P_L + P_U)$ and the hypothesis in Equation 11.7.4 can be further decomposed into two sets of one-sided hypotheses

$$\begin{aligned}
&\text{H}_{0L}\text{: } P_L \geq \omega_0 \\
\text{versus } &\text{H}_{aL}\text{: } P_L < \omega_0,
\end{aligned} \quad (11.7.5)$$

and

$$\begin{aligned}
&\text{H}_{0U}\text{: } P_U \geq \omega_0 \\
\text{versus } &\text{H}_{aU}\text{: } P_U < \omega_0,
\end{aligned}$$

where

$\pi_0 = 1 - 2\omega_0$

$\omega_0 \leq 0.5$

Because the marginal distribution of $Y_T - Y_R$ is approximately normal and is symmetric about $\theta = \mu_T - \mu_R$, then

$$\begin{aligned}
P_L &= P\{Y_T - Y_R \leq -r\} \\
&= \Phi\left[\frac{(-r - \theta)}{\sqrt{\left(\sigma_D^2 + \sigma_{WT}^2 + \sigma_{WR}^2\right)}}\right],
\end{aligned}$$

and

$$\begin{aligned}P_U &= P\{Y_T - Y_R \geq r\}\\ &= 1 - \Phi\left[\frac{(r-\theta)}{\sqrt{\left(\sigma_D^2 + \sigma_{WT}^2 + \sigma_{WR}^2\right)}}\right].\end{aligned}$$

Note that

$$\Phi^{-1}\Phi\left[\frac{(-r-\theta)}{\sqrt{\left(\sigma_D^2 + \sigma_{WT}^2 + \sigma_{WR}^2\right)}}\right] < -\Phi^{-1}(\omega_0)$$

$$\Leftrightarrow$$

$$-r < \theta - z(\omega_0)\sqrt{\left(\sigma_D^2 + \sigma_{WT}^2 + \sigma_{WR}^2\right)},$$

and

$$\Phi^{-1}\left\{1 - \Phi\left[\frac{(r-\theta)}{\sqrt{\left(\sigma_D^2 + \sigma_{WT}^2 + \sigma_{WR}^2\right)}}\right]\right\} > \Phi^{-1}(\omega_0)$$

$$\Leftrightarrow$$

$$r > \theta + z(\omega_0)\sqrt{\left(\sigma_D^2 + \sigma_{WT}^2 + \sigma_{WR}^2\right)},$$

where

$z(\omega_0) = \Phi^{-1}(\omega_0)$ is the ω_0th upper quantile of a standard normal distribution
Φ^{-1} is the inverse cumulative distribution function of a standard normal random variable

If follows that the hypotheses in Equation 11.7.5 can be reformulated in terms of the quantiles of the marginal distribution of $Y_T - Y_R$ as follows:

$$\begin{aligned}&H_{0L}: \theta - z(\omega_0)\sqrt{\left(\sigma_D^2 + \sigma_{WT}^2 + \sigma_{WR}^2\right)} \leq -r\\ \text{versus}\quad &H_{aL}: \theta - z(\omega_0)\sqrt{\left(\sigma_D^2 + \sigma_{WT}^2 + \sigma_{WR}^2\right)} > -r,\end{aligned} \tag{11.7.6}$$

and

$$\begin{aligned}&H_{0U}: \theta + z(\omega_0)\sqrt{\left(\sigma_D^2 + \sigma_{WT}^2 + \sigma_{WR}^2\right)} \geq r\\ \text{versus}\quad &H_{aU}: \theta + z(\omega_0)\sqrt{\left(\sigma_D^2 + \sigma_{WT}^2 + \sigma_{WR}^2\right)} < r.\end{aligned}$$

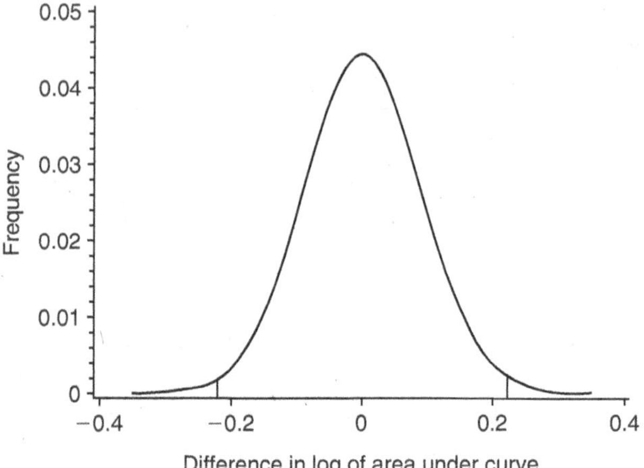

FIGURE 11.7.1: Relation between moment-based and probability-based criteria through the quantile of the distribution of the difference in bioavailabilities between the formulations.

As illustrated in Figure 11.7.1, the concept of this formulation of hypotheses follows. If the lower (upper) ω_0th quantile of the marginal distribution of $Y_T - Y_R$ is larger (smaller) than the lower (upper) limit $-r(r)$, the MINP, P_{TR}, is then at least π_0. Liu and Chow (1997b) have proposed similar formulation of hypotheses for individual bioequivalence when $\sigma_D^2 = 0$ and $\sigma_{WT}^2 = \sigma_{WR}^2$. Note that if $\omega_0 = 0.5$, $(\omega_0) = 0$, the hypotheses in Equation 11.7.6 become the usual two one-sided hypothesis for average bioequivalence in Equation 4.3.3.

From H_{aL}, we have

$$-\theta + z(\omega_0)\sqrt{\sigma_D^2 + \sigma_{WT}^2 + \sigma_{WR}^2} < r,$$

and from H_{aU}, we have

$$\theta + z(\omega_0)\sqrt{\sigma_D^2 + \sigma_{WT}^2 + \sigma_{WR}^2} < r.$$

As a result,

$$|\theta| + z(\omega_0)\sqrt{\omega_D^2 + \sigma_{WT}^2 + \sigma_{WR}^2} < r. \tag{11.7.7}$$

As suggested by Schall (1995), if $c\sqrt{2\sigma_{WR}}$ is selected for r, then the inequality of Equation 11.7.7 becomes

$$M_{I6} = \frac{\left[|\theta| + z(\omega_0)\sqrt{(\sigma_D^2 + \sigma_{WT}^2 + \sigma_{WR}^2)}\right]}{\sigma_{WR}} < c\sqrt{2}, \tag{11.7.8}$$

or

$$M_{I7} = \frac{\left\{\left[|\theta| + z(\omega_0)\sqrt{(\sigma_D^2 + \sigma_{WT}^2 + \sigma_{WR}^2)}\right] - \sigma_{WR}\right\}}{\sigma_{WR}} < c\sqrt{2} - 1.$$

For the ideal situation of perfect bioequivalence, as described in Section 11.5, c is selected as 1.645 such that

$$M_{I6} = \frac{\left[|\theta| + z(\omega_0)\sqrt{(\sigma_D^2 + \sigma_{WT}^2 + \sigma_{WR}^2)}\right]}{\sigma_{WR}} < 2.326 \qquad (11.7.9)$$

or,

$$M_{I7} = \frac{\left\{\left[|\theta| + z(\omega_0)\sqrt{(\sigma_D^2 + \sigma_{WT}^2 + \sigma_{WR}^2)}\right] - \sigma_{WR}\right\}}{\sigma_{WR}} < 1.326$$

As a result, under the normality assumption, the probability-based criteria P_{TR} can be converted into moment-based criteria M_{I6} and M_{I7} through the quantiles of the marginal distributions of $Y_T - Y_R$. Comparison of M_{I6} and M_{I7} with M_{I2} and M_{I3} yields the following observations (Hauck and Anderson, 1994):

- The moment-criteria M_{I6} and M_{I7} are very similar to M_{I2} and M_{I3} proposed by Sheiner (1992) and the FDA guidance (2001).
- M_{I6} and M_{I7} use the standard deviation of the reference intra-subject variability of σ_{WR} as the scale factor while M_{I2} and M_{I3} employ the variance σ_{WR}^2.
- For M_{I2} and M_{I3}, the weight for the variance is 1, whereas the weight for the standard deviation of $Y_T - Y_R$ is $z(\omega_0)$ for M_{I6} and M_{I7} which can vary according to the different values of π_0.
- The relation between M_{I6} and M_{I7} and probability-based criterion P_{TR} can be derived through the quantile of the marginal distribution of $Y_T - Y_R$. On the other hand, the implicit relation exists between the moment-based criteria, M_{I6} and M_{I7} and any probability-based criteria because $\pi_0 = 0.68$ for M_{I2} and M_{I3} with weight being 1.

11.8 Bioequivalence Limits

For the scaled moment-based criteria, such as Equations 11.6.8 through 11.6.11, because as illustrated in hypothesis 11.6.14, bioequivalence is concluded only if they are sufficiently smaller than some prespecified allowable limit. Because the selected scaled factor is the variance of the reference intra-subject variability, a serious consequence caused by the scaled version of the criteria and the formulation of hypothesis is the relaxation of bioequivalence requirements for highly variable drugs. In other words, bioequivalence is always concluded if the variability of the reference formulation is large. On the other hand, unnecessary conservative bioequivalence limits are posed for safe drug products with low intra-subject variability, such that it is almost impossible to claim bioequivalence. In other words, generic copies for the high-variability innovator's drug, such as cyclosporine, can easily pass bioequivalence testing for market approval, whereas it is very difficult to claim bioequivalence for the generic copies for the reference formulation with low variability. To overcome this drawback, the FDA guidance (2001) suggests the use of either the reference-scaled or constant-scaled moment-based criteria by a mixed-scaling approach. For individual bioequivalence, if the variance of the reference intra-subject variability is greater than some prespecified value, σ^2_{W0}, then use the moment-based criterion M_{I3}, defined in Equation 11.6.11, which is also referred to as the reference-scaled bioequivalence criterion. On the other hand, if the variance of the reference intra-subject variability is no greater than σ^2_{W0}, then use the following constant-scaled criterion:

$$M_{\mathrm{I3}} = \frac{\left(\theta^2 + \sigma^2_{\mathrm{D}} + \sigma^2_{\mathrm{WT}} - \sigma^2_{\mathrm{WR}}\right)}{\sigma^2_{\mathrm{W0}}}. \tag{11.8.1}$$

As a result, the individual bioequivalence criterion proposed in the FDA guidance (FDA, 2001) can be expressed as

$$M_{\mathrm{I3}} = \frac{\left(\theta^2 + \sigma^2_{\mathrm{D}} + \sigma^2_{\mathrm{WT}} - \sigma^2_{\mathrm{WR}}\right)}{\max\left\{\sigma^2_{\mathrm{W0}}, \sigma^2_{\mathrm{WR}}\right\}}. \tag{11.8.2}$$

Similarly, the criterion for assessment of population bioequivalence suggested in the FDA guidance (FDA, 2001) is given as

$$M_{\mathrm{P3}} = \frac{\left(\theta^2 + \sigma^2_{\mathrm{TT}} - \sigma^2_{\mathrm{TR}}\right)}{\max\left\{\sigma^2_{\mathrm{T0}}, \sigma^2_{\mathrm{TR}}\right\}}. \tag{11.8.3}$$

However, σ^2_{W0} is a prespecified known constant; therefore, the constant-scale criteria for population and individual bioequivalence are, in fact, equivalent to M_{I1} and M_{P1} proposed by Schall and Luus (1993). Recall that the relation between PDR and IDR, with their respective moment-based criteria M_{I3} and M_{P3}, is given as

$$\mathrm{PDR}^2 = \frac{M_{\mathrm{I3}}}{2+1},$$

and

$$\text{IDR}^2 = \frac{M_{P3}}{2+1}.$$

As a result, the FDA guidance suggested the value of 0.20 for both σ^2_{w0}. The rationale for selection of the value of 0.20 is outlined in the following. If the maximal allowable limit for IDR is set as 1.25 and we also assume that $\sigma^2_D = 0$, $\sigma^2_{WT} = \sigma^2_{WR}$, and the upper average bioequivalence limit log1.25 for θ, it follows that

$$\begin{aligned}\sigma_{w0} = \sigma_{T0} &= \sqrt{(0.2231)^2/\{2[(1.25)^2 - 1]\}} \\ &= 0.21 \\ &\approx 0.20.\end{aligned}$$

However, as indicated in the above, the choice of 0.2 for σ^2_{W0} is derived actually without consideration of the variance terms.

All probability-based and moment-based criteria are aggregate criteria that evaluate bioequivalence by a single summary measure. As indicated in Section 11.6, they are, however, functions of different components of each that represents a characteristic of quality assurance for the generic drug product. As a result, it is necessary to consider for each component its contribution to bioequivalence in determination of the bioequivalence limit. Here, we describe the concepts and procedure for selection of a bioequivalence limit for the aggregate criteria proposed in the FDA guidance (FDA, 2001).

Both aggregate criteria for evaluation of population and individual bioequivalence, M_{P3} and M_{I3}, proposed in the FDA guidance (FDA, 2001) can be expressed in the following form:

$$M = \frac{\text{average bioequivalence limit} + \text{variance allowance}}{\text{scaled variance}}.$$

The currently employed average bioequivalence limit of 80/125 in the FDA guidance for average bioequivalence (2003b) is assumed for both criteria. In other words, average bioequivalence limit $= [\log 1.25]^2 = (0.2231)^2 = 0.04977$ is assumed for determination of the limits for individual bioequivalence. Furthermore, the variance allowance of aggregate criterion M_{I3} for individual bioequivalence is the sum of two components. The first term σ^2_D measures the heterogeneity of differences in subject-specific averages and second term $\sigma^2_{WT} - \sigma^2_{WR}$ is the difference in intra-subject variability between the test and reference formulations. Because under the two-stage model assumed in Section 11.2, the differences in subject-specific averages follow a distribution with mean $\mu_T - \mu_R$ and variance σ^2_D, it follows that the magnitude of σ^2_D is associated with the proportion of the subjects whose differences in subject-specific averages, $\mu_{iT} - \mu_{iR}$, lie outside the current average bioequivalence range of (log0.8, log1.25). Suppose that there is no difference in population average, i.e., $\mu_T = \mu_R$ and $\sigma^2_D = 0.01839$, then under normal assumption, the proportion of the subjects whose subject-specific averages fall outside $(-0.2231,\ 0.2231)$ can be computed as $2[-\Phi(0.2231/\sqrt{0.01839})] = 2[1 - \Phi(0.2231/0.1356)] = 2[1 - \Phi(1.645)] = 0.1$. When $\sigma_D^2 = 0.03031$, the probability is $2[1-\Phi(1.28)] = 0.2$. If one allows 10%–20% of the subjects whose differences in subject-specific averages lie outside the current average bioequivalence interval of $(-0.2231,\ 0.2231)$, then the allowance for σ_D^2 ranges from approximately 0.02 to 0.03.

The allowance for difference in intra-subject variability suggested in the draft FDA guidance is 0.02 and scaled reference intra-subject variability σ_{W0}^2 is assumed to be 0.04. Accordingly, the individual bioequivalence limit (IBE) Δ_{I3}, for aggregate criterion M_{I3}, is given as

$$\begin{aligned}\Delta_{I3} &= \frac{[(\log 1.25)^2 + 0.02 + 0.02]}{0.04}\\ &= 2.2448\\ &\cong 2.25, \quad \text{for} \quad \sigma_D^2 = 0.02,\end{aligned} \tag{11.8.4}$$

and

$$\begin{aligned}\Delta_{I3} &= \frac{[(\log 1.25)^2 + 0.03 + 0.02]}{0.04}\\ &= 2.4948\\ &\cong 2.5, \quad \text{for } \sigma_D^2 = 0.03.\end{aligned}$$

For assessment of individual bioequivalence, from the relation M_{I1}, M_{I2}, and M_{I3}, individual bioequivalence limits for M_{I1} and M_{I2} can also be computed as follows:

$$\Delta_{I1} = \begin{cases} 0.09, & \text{for } \sigma_D^2 = 0.02\\ 0.1, & \text{for } \sigma_D^2 = 0.03.\end{cases} \tag{11.8.5}$$

and

$$\Delta_{I2} = \begin{cases} 3.25, & \text{for } \sigma_D^2 = 0.02\\ 3.5, & \text{for } \sigma_D^2 = 0.03.\end{cases}$$

11.9 Designs for Population and Individual Bioequivalence

Under the two-stage model assumed in Section 11.2, the mean and covariance matrix of the distribution of the paired pharmacokinetic responses observed from the ith subject $(Y_{iT},\ Y_{iR})'$, respectively, are $(\mu_T,\ \mu_R)'$, and

$$\sum = \begin{pmatrix} \sigma_{\mathrm{WT}}^2 + \sigma_{\mathrm{BT}}^2 & \rho\sigma_{\mathrm{BT}}\sigma_{\mathrm{BR}} \\ \rho\sigma_{\mathrm{BT}}\sigma_{\mathrm{BR}} & \sigma_{\mathrm{WR}}^2 + \sigma_{\mathrm{BR}}^2 \end{pmatrix}.$$

Therefore, the variance for the difference of the paired pharmacokinetic responses observed from the ith subject $Y_{i\mathrm{T}} - Y_{i\mathrm{R}}$ is then given as

$$\begin{aligned} V(Y_{i\mathrm{T}} - Y_{i\mathrm{R}})' &= \sigma_{\mathrm{WT}}^2 + \sigma_{\mathrm{BT}}^2 + \sigma_{\mathrm{WR}}^2 + \sigma_{\mathrm{BR}}^2 - 2\rho\sigma_{\mathrm{BT}}\sigma_{\mathrm{BR}} \\ &= \sigma_{\mathrm{TT}}^2 + \sigma_{\mathrm{TR}}^2 - 2\rho\sigma_{\mathrm{BT}}\sigma_{\mathrm{BR}}, \end{aligned} \qquad (11.9.1)$$

where $\sigma_{\mathrm{TT}}^2 = \sigma_{\mathrm{WT}}^2 + \sigma_{\mathrm{BT}}^2$ and $\sigma_{\mathrm{TR}}^2 = \sigma_{\mathrm{WR}}^2 + \sigma_{\mathrm{BR}}^2$ are the variances of the marginal distribution of $Y_{i\mathrm{T}}$ and $Y_{i\mathrm{R}}$, respectively.

If the correlation ρ is positive, then the variance of the difference will be smaller than the sum of the individual total variances of the marginal distribution. This can be accomplished through the crossover designs in which both test and reference formulations are administrated to the same subject during the different periods of the study. For example, under the model 2.5.1 for the standard 2×2 crossover design, the inference for average bioequivalence is based only on the intra-subject variability, where ρ is assumed to be 1 and $\sigma_{\mathrm{BT}}^2 = \sigma_{\mathrm{BR}}^2$. As a result, a more precise inference for average bioequivalence can be achieved by employment of the standard 2×2 crossover design. However, the aggregate criterion for population bioequivalence is a summary measure of the squared average difference and difference in total variances. Statistical procedures involve the inference for average and total variances and have nothing to do with the inferences for individual intra-subject, intra-subject variance, and the variance of subject-by-formulation interaction. As a result, the advantage for using crossover design over parallel designs no longer exists.

In addition to squared difference in population average, the test and reference intra-subject variances and the variance of subject-by-formulation interaction are also integral components in the aggregate criteria for evaluation of individual bioequivalence. Consequently, the higher-order designs for two formulations introduced in Chapter 9 should be employed to estimate these parameters. The FDA guidance (FDA, 2001) recommended the following four-period, two-sequence, two-formulation design for individual bioequivalence:

	Period			
Sequence	**I**	**II**	**III**	**IV**
1	Test	Reference	Test	Reference
2	Reference	Test	Reference	Test

An adequate washout period should be inserted between two periods of active treatments. For this design, each subject receives test and reference formulations twice. To eliminate lot-to-lot variability for unbiased estimation of intra-subject variability, the guidance also suggested that the same lots of the test and reference formulations be used for the repeated administrations. For the three-period designs, the FDA guidance recommends the following design:

	Period		
Sequence	**I**	**II**	**III**
1	Test	Reference	Test
2	Reference	Test	Reference

Other possible three- or four-period higher-order crossover designs are given in Table 11.9.1. Note that all higher-order crossover designs are made of a pair of dual sequences, and all three-period designs can be constructed from the corresponding four-period designs by elimination of the last period. Because each subject in the four-period higher-order designs receives both test and reference formulations twice, pharmacokinetic responses from all subjects can be used for estimating both test and reference intra-subject variances. However, only half of the subjects in the three-period higher-order crossover designs are for inference of the test intra-subject variance, and the other half for the reference intra-subject variance. In addition, more subjects might be needed for the three-period higher-order designs than for the four-period higher-order designs to accomplish the same power to conclude bioequivalence. As a result, although the total duration of the study is shorter for three-period higher-order crossover designs, the four-period higher-order crossover designs are still preferred for evaluation of individual bioequivalence. To avoid any ambiguities in estimating the individual parameters in the aggregate moment-based criteria, the FDA guidance also suggested use of the two-sequence designs only, unless there one suspects the possible existence of a carryover effect.

The FDA guidance (FDA, 2001) and Chen et al. (2000) compare the sample size required for the four-period higher-order design given in the above for individual bioequivalence with that for the standard 2×2 crossover design for average bioequivalence. The results are modified and summarized in Table 11.9.2 for the sample sizes required for 80% and 90% power, respectively, at the 5% nominal significance level. The sample sizes were computed for the two drug products with a difference in averages of 5%, no difference in intra-subject variability, no subject-by-formulation interaction, and $\sigma^2_{WO} = 0.04$. For evaluation of individual bioequivalence, the true value of M_{I3} for the alternative hypothesis in Figure 11.6.2 is equal to $(\log 1.05)^2/0.025 = 0.106$ when $CV = 15\%$. The other values can be found in Table 11.9.2. The null value for Δ_{I3} is approximately equal to 2.5 by specifying a total variance allowance of 0.05. The sample size for average bioequivalence based on the two one-sided tests procedure under the standard 2×2 crossover design is calculated according to Diletti et al. (1991).

From Table 11.9.2, the sample sizes increase as the intra-subject variability increases for both average and individual bioequivalence. As demonstrated in Figure 5.3.1, rejection region for average bioequivalence based on the confidence approach becomes smaller and smaller as the intra-subject variability increases. The sample

TABLE 11.9.1: Crossover design for individual bioequivalence.

Four-Period Higher-Order Crossover Design

Design A1

	Period			
Sequence	**I**	**II**	**III**	**IV**
1	Test	Reference	Test	Reference
2	Reference	Test	Reference	Test

Design A2

	Period			
Sequence	**I**	**II**	**III**	**IV**
1	Test	Reference	Reference	Test
2	Reference	Test	Test	Reference

Design A3

	Period			
Sequence	**I**	**II**	**III**	**IV**
1	Test	Test	Reference	Reference
2	Reference	Reference	Test	Test

Three-Period Higher-Order Crossover Design

Design B1

	Period		
Sequence	**I**	**II**	**III**
1	Test	Reference	Test
2	Reference	Test	Reference

Design B2

	Period		
Sequence	**I**	**II**	**III**
1	Test	Reference	Reference
2	Reference	Test	Test

Design B3

	Period		
Sequence	**I**	**II**	**III**
1	Test	Test	Reference
2	Reference	Test	Test

TABLE 11.9.2: Comparison of sample sizes required for the four-period higher-order design and the standard 2×2 crossover design.

Intra-subject Variability ($\sigma_{WR} = \sigma_{WT}$)	CV	M_{I3}	Power (%)	Individual Bioequivalence (IBE)	Average Bioequivalence (ABE)
0.15	15	0.106	80	10	6
			90	12	8
0.23	23	0.045	80	22	12
			90	30	16
0.30	31	0.026	80	28	20
			90	36	28
0.50	53	0.0095	80	28	54
			90	36	72

Source: From Guidance on Statistical Approaches to Establishing Bioequivalence, Center for Drug Evaluation and Research, U.S. Food and Drug Administration, Rockville, MD, 2001; Chen, M.L., Patnaik, R., Hauck, W.W., Schuirmann, D.J., Hysloip, T., and Williams, R., *Stat. Med.*, 19, 2821, 2000.

Note: The four-period higher-order design is (TRTR, RTRT) and the standard 2×2 crossover design is (RT, TR). Intra-subject variability is the standard deviation on the nature log scale, assuming $\sigma_{WR} = \sigma_{WT}$. CV is the coefficient of intra-subject variation on the original scale. The null value of Δ_{I3} is approximately 2.5.

size for concluding average bioequivalence, according to the two one-sided tests procedure, will continue to increase as the intra-subject variability increases. On the other hand, the sample size for concluding individual bioequivalence reaches a plateau when the intra-subject subject variability reaches beyond 0.3. This phenomenon is probably because the true value of M_{I3} is a decreasing function of the intra-subject variability owing to scaling by the reference intra-subject variability. The value of M_{I3} for the intra-subject standard deviation being 0.5 is only 9% of that when the intra-subject standard deviation is 0.15. The number of subjects needed for the four-period design for individual bioequivalence is more than twice that required for the standard 2×2 crossover design for average bioequivalence when the true reference intra-subject standard deviation is equal or less than 0.3. However, as shown in Table 11.9.2, aggregate moment-based criterion M_{I3} for evaluation of individual bioequivalence seems to require considerably fewer subjects for highly variable drug products with the intra-subject standard deviation greater than 0.3.

11.10 Discussion

Selection of criteria for evaluation of bioequivalence, as illustrated in the above, is a very complicated and difficult issue. Criteria should measure the closeness of the distributions of pharmacokinetic responses between test and reference formulations with respect to the therapeutic window of the drug product. As a result, various criteria have been proposed over the past decade, depending on the characteristics for describing the quality of the drug products, the manner of assessment of these characteristics, and representation of criteria. The characteristics of the drug products in evaluation of bioequivalence are difference in averages, variance of subject-by-formulation interaction, and difference (ratio) in test and reference intra-subject variability. Bioequivalence can be assessed by investigation of each characteristic individually, or by a composite index of these characteristics. The criteria derived from the former manner are referred to as disaggregate criteria, and those formulated from the later manner are called aggregate criteria. Except for the criterion in Equation 11.6.16, proposed by Liu and Chow (1996a) and Liu (1998), all criteria introduced in this chapter are aggregate criteria. In addition, scaling factors are used for some criteria, whereas other criteria are not scaled. However, the aggregate moment-based criteria, M_{I3} and M_{P3}, suggested in the 2001 FDA guidance use a mixed-scaling approach. On the other hand, the criteria can be represented as either a function of moments or probabilities for measuring the discrepancy in bioavailabilities between the test and reference formulations. Therefore, all criteria in this chapter can be classified into moment-based or probability-based criteria.

Recall that the aggregate moment-based criterion M_{I3} is given as

$$M_{I3} = \frac{\left[\theta^2 + \sigma_D^2 + \left(\sigma_{WT}^2 - \sigma_{WR}^2\right)\right]}{\max\left\{\sigma_{W0}^2, \sigma_{WR}^2\right\}}.$$

This is an aggregate function of λ_1, λ_2, and λ_3. As a result, the effect of one component can be offset by another. Chen (1996) and Hauck et al. (1996) reported the results from one actual data set of the FDA files (FDA, 1998). This is a study with 22 subjects that compared a test formulation with the reference formulation in a four-sequence, four-period crossover design. The intra-subject reference standard deviation on the natural logarithmic scale is 0.336, which translates to a coefficient of variation of 35% on the original scale. As a result, the reference drug is considered as a highly variable product. The ratio of average AUCs is 1.144, with a confidence interval of (1.025, 1.280). Therefore, according to the current unscaled average bioequivalence criterion, the test and reference formulations cannot be concluded average bioequivalent. On the other hand, the ratio of intra-subject standard deviation of test to the reference formulation is 0.522 (90% confidence interval: 0.395 to 0.862), a reduction in the subject variability nearly 50% by the test formulation. The upper limit of the 90% confidence interval for M_{I3}, obtained by 2000 bootstrap samples, is 1.312. As a result, individual bioequivalence can be concluded for either 2.25 or 2.5, the individual bioequivalence limits in Equation 11.8.4 suggested by the 2001 FDA guidance (FDA, 2001).

This example shows that a 14% increase in the average is offset by a 48% reduction in the variability. In addition, the test product passes individual bioequivalence, yet it fails average bioequivalence. This example demonstrates one serious drawback of aggregate criteria: individual bioequivalence can be concluded, even though the distributions of bioequivalence responses are totally different, i.e., different in both average and variability. Hauck et al. (1996) and Chen et al. (1999) argued that the sponsor of the generic drug product with a smaller intra-subject variability than the reference product should be rewarded because its product is a preferred product. However, the issue lies in whether the generic and reference products are, in fact, bioequivalent and are within the therapeutic window.

Liu (1998) provides an example for illustration of the above concept. Suppose that the average and variance of intra-subject variability of the log bioavailability in some metric form of an individual subject for an approved reference are 1.5 and 0.16, respectively. Because the standard deviation of the intra-subject variability on the log scale is 0.4, this is a highly variable drug product. Furthermore, assume that it has a narrow therapeutic range with the minimum effective level (MEL) of 1.1 and maximum tolerable level (MTL) of 1.9. Figure 11.10.1 shows that with such bioavailability, the individual has a 16% chance of being above the MDL and developing some undesirable adverse effects with possibly serious consequences. Suppose that a new generic formulation, for the same individual, delivers an average bioavailability of 1.8464 and a variance of intra-subject variability of 0.04. In other words, the bioavailability average increases 23% and standard deviation of intra-subject variability reduces 50%. For sake of illustration, there is no subject-by-formulation interaction, then M_{I3} is equal to 0, which will pass the current individual bioequivalence limit of either 2.25 or 2.5 suggested in the draft FDA guidance. However, the probability is almost 40% for the same individual that the bioavailability of the generic formulation is above the MTL. Although the generic and reference products are neither average bioequivalent nor individual bioequivalent, according to the aggregate criteria M_{I1} and M_{I3}, a generic drug product with an inequivalent, but a smaller test intra-subject variability, may still be declared individual bioequivalent because of masking and offsetting effects between individual contributions. Note that the increase in average and reduction in intra-subject variability in the above example are quite close to those reported by Chen (1996) and Hauck et al. (1996).

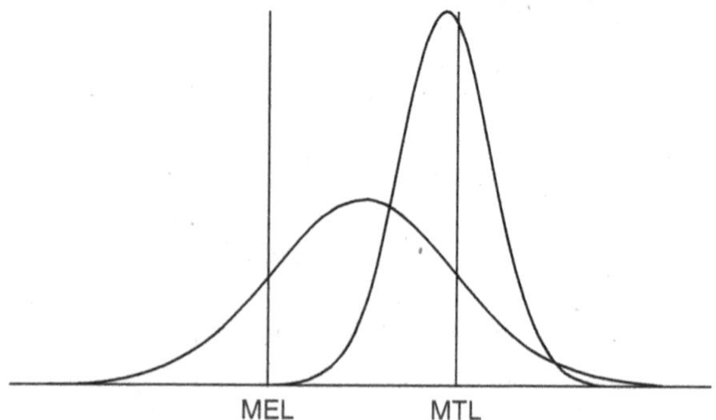

FIGURE 11.10.1: Relation between average intra-subject variability and therapeutic window. σ_D^2 is assumed to be 0. MEL, minimum effective level; MTL, maximum tolerable level. (From Liu, J.P., *Commun. Stat. Theo. Methods*, 27, 1433, 1998.)

TABLE 11.10.1: Tradeoff and between changes (in %) in average bioavailability and change in intra-subject variability.

	Reference Intra-subject Coefficient of Variation		
Change in CV (%)	**20%**	**30%**	**40%**
−15	10.9	16.4	21.8
−10	8.9	13.4	17.7
−5	6.4	9.4	12.3
5	−6.1	−8.8	−11.2
10	−8.6	−12.3	−15.5
15	−10.5	−15.0	−18.8

Source: From Endrenyi, L. and Hao, Y., *Int. J. Clin. Pharmacol. Ther. Toxicol.*, 36, 1, 1998.

Note: The entries are the difference in average bioavailability divided by the reference average bioavailability. Change in CV is the difference in intra-subject coefficient of variation divided by the reference intra-subject coefficient of variation.

Endrenyi and Hao (1998) also investigated the issue of mean-variability tradeoffs. They observed that the tradeoff in aggregate criteria is rather asymmetric. As illustrated in Table 11.10.1, the asymmetry in the tradeoff is twofold. First, a small change in intra-subject variability can elicit a substantial allowable change in average difference for concluding individual bioequivalence. For example, if the reference intra-subject coefficient of variation is 40%, a reduction of the test intra-subject coefficient of variation by only 5%–38% leads to an allowable increase of 12.3% in average difference for declaration of individual bioequivalence. This allowable increase in difference between averages can be considered as a benefit for the generic product with a smaller intra-subject variability. Second, the tradeoff might not be all beneficial to the generic product. If the same magnitude change in intra-subject variability is observed, but with a difference direction (i.e., the test intra-subject coefficient of variation is 42%), then the difference in averages must be shrunk by a 11.2% to claim individual bioequivalence. This, therefore, is a penalty for the sponsor who manufactures a more variable generic product.

Hauck et al. (1996) recommended the use of a single aggregate criterion over disaggregate approaches for evaluation of individual bioequivalence. They suggested that the negative influence of the average-variability tradeoff on the aggregate criteria be controlled by either modifying the effect of scaling in aggregate criteria, or by using different weights for individual components, λ_1, λ_2, and λ_3. A large value than the currently recommended one of 0.04 is suggested for the σ^2_{W0} so that the scaling effect will be less aggressive (Hauck et al., 1996). For the study on the FDA files discussed earlier, if a large value of σ^2_{W0}, say 0.09, is selected for the individual bioequivalence limit, then the test formulation cannot be claimed individually bioequivalent to the reference formulation because the upper limit of the 90% confidence interval of 1.312 is no longer smaller than either 1 or 1.1 for Δ_{I3}, respectively, for $\sigma^2_{\mathrm{D}} = 0.02$ or 0.03. On the other hand, different-weighted versions of the aggregate moment-based criteria M_3 are also proposed:

$$M_3' = \begin{cases} \{\theta^2 + c[\sigma_D^2 + (\sigma_{WT}^2 - \sigma_{WR}^2)]\}/\sigma_{WR}^2 & \text{(Hauck et al., 1996)} \\ \theta^2 + c_1\sigma_D^2 + c_2(\sigma_{WT}^2 - \sigma_{WR}^2)]/\sigma_{WR}^2 & \text{(Midha et al., 1997)}, \end{cases} \quad (11.10.1)$$

where c, c_1, and c_2 are positive real numbers smaller than 1.

However, the weighed version of the aggregate criteria is not consistent with the concept of difference ratio introduced in Section 11.6. In addition, selection of weights remains an issue to resolve. Consequently, the U.S. FDA guidance on the statistical approaches adopted the unweighed M_{P3} and M_{I3} for population and individual bioequivalence. To overcome the issue of offset between mean and variance, the FDA guidance on the statistical approaches also recommends that in addition to meeting the individual bioequivalence limit specified in 11.8, the observed geometric mean of the test to reference formulation should completed contained within 0.8 and 1.25.

The current criterion for evaluation of average bioequivalence is based on the unscaled difference in population average:

$$-\Delta < \mu_T - \mu_R < \Delta. \quad (11.10.2)$$

The current regulation in most countries uses ln 1.25 = 0.2231 for Δ when logarithms of $AUC_{(0-t\mathrm{last})}$ and $AUC_{(0-\infty)}$ are the bioequivalence metrics. The selection of equivalence limit of 0.2231 for average bioequivalence considers only the ratio (or difference) averages of the test to reference formulations. Supposedly, in addition to the ratio of averages, the reference intra-subject variability is taken into account for determination of the bioequivalence limit such that $\Delta = \Delta'\sigma_{WR}$. It follows that the criterion for average bioequivalence can be expressed as

$$(\mu_T - \mu_T)^2/\sigma_{WR}^2 < \Delta'. \quad (11.10.3)$$

This is a scaled criterion for average bioequivalence with the reference intra-subject variance as the scaled factor. The criterion in Equation 11.10.3 can be derived from aggregate moment-based criterion for individual bioequivalence M_{I3} by assuming that there is no subject-by-formulation interaction and equal intra-subject variability for both formulations. On the other hand, if selection of equivalence limit r in P_d of Equation 11.5.5, P_r of Equation 11.5.6, and in the hypotheses formulated as the quantile of the distribution in Equation 11.7.6, also take into consideration the reference intra-subject variability, probability-based criterion such as P_{TR} is also a scaled probability criterion (Schall, 1995; Hauck and Anderson, 1994).

As mentioned in Section 11.3, individual bioequivalence can be concluded as long as the distribution of the generic drug product lies within the subject's individual therapeutic window, although the distributions of test and reference formulations are different (Hauck, 1996a,b). In addition, the intra-subject reference variability is assumed to be related to the therapeutic window and is used as a scaled factor for taking the therapeutic window into account in the formulation of the individual bioequivalence criteria. Conceptually, considerations of a therapeutic window for evaluation of bioequivalence are sound. However, quantification of a therapeutic window is a rather formidable task. A therapeutic window for any drug product is determined by the clinical efficacy and safety endpoints. The relation between bioequivalence metrics, through the doses of the drug product, with clinical and safety endpoints are rather complicated and difficult to characterize. In addition, most drug products have a wide therapeutic window, with low to moderate intra-subject variability. As a result, average bioequivalence should be sufficient to evaluate interchangeability between the test and reference formulations for most drug products because of these characteristics. The situation is different for those drug products with either a narrow therapeutic window or a high intra-subject variability. For these drug products, a small change in pharmacokinetic responses of the generic drug might lead to a marked increase in the proportion of its distribution outside the therapeutic window established by the reference drug product owing to either the higher intra-subject variability or a narrow therapeutic window. Given that most subjects fall into the therapeutic window established by the reference product, equivalence of the distributions between the test and reference products guarantees the generic distribution inside the therapeutic window. For the drugs with a narrow therapeutic window or a higher intra-subject variability, establishment of the closeness of the distributions between the test and reference formulations, therefore, is much more important than examination of the distribution of the generic drug product lying inside the therapeutic window.

Midha et al. (1997) investigated the influence of scaling on concluding bioequivalence. For average bioequivalence, they considered the unscaled and scaled versions, given in Equations 11.10.2 and 11.10.3, respectively. Aggregate moment-based criterion M_{I3} in Equation 11.8.2 and its numerator are the scaled and unscaled criteria for assessment of individual bioequivalence. In addition, unweighed and weighed versions of M_{I3}, with weights 0.5 for both σ_D^2 and $(\sigma_{WT}^2 - \sigma_{WR}^2)$, are also examined. Their results show that, in general, for both average and individual bioequivalence, the unscaled criteria are more conservative than the scaled criteria. In addition, in two of the three data sets considered in their study, the scaled individual bioequivalence criterion appears too liberal in concluding individual bioequivalence. They also suggested that when the intra-subject variabilities of the two formulations are not identical, but are similar, the scaled individual bioequivalence criterion is very sensitive to which formulation—test or reference—has the higher variance. Their results also show that weighting has little effect on scaled or unscaled criteria for individual bioequivalence. Subject by formulation exists in one of the three data sets in their study. However, test and reference formulations can be concluded as average bioequivalent by the usual unscaled criterion in Equation 11.10.2, but not as individual bioequivalence by the scaled criterion M_{I3}. The subject-by-formulation interaction, therefore, plays an important role in assessment of individual bioequivalence. See Polli and McLean (2001), Tothfalusi and Endrenyi (2003), and Karalis et al. (2004) for the more criteria based on scaled average bioequivalence and other recent proposed criteria of bioequivalence.

Endrenyi and Tothfalusi (1999) investigated the properties of the estimated variance of the subject-by-formulation interaction and prevalence of the interaction in the studies with higher-order crossover designs published by the FDA (1998).

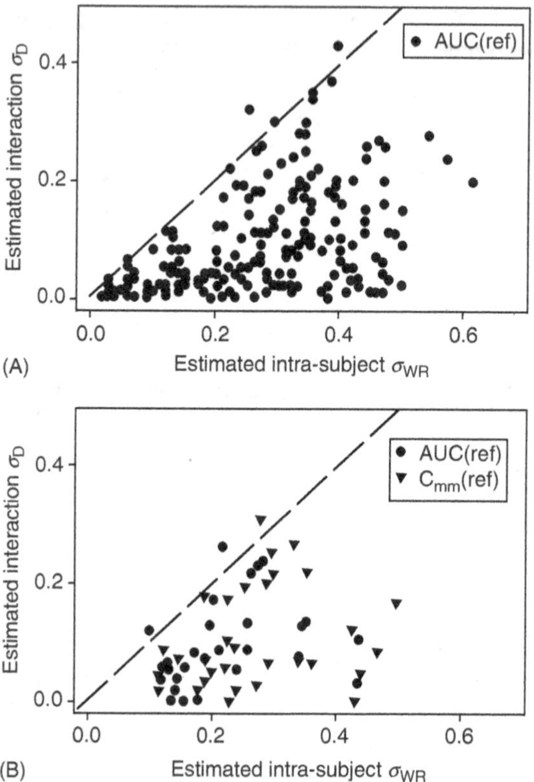

FIGURE 11.10.2: Relation between estimated σ_D and σ_{WR}. (From Endrenyi, L. and Tothfalusi, L., *Pharm. Res.*, 16, 186, 1999.)

They performed a simulation using a four-period crossover design for 24 subjects. They assume that the two formulations are, in fact, perfectly bioequivalent. In other words, $\mu_T = \mu_R$ and $\sigma_D^2 = 0$, and $\sigma_{WT}^2 = \sigma_{WR}^2$. Both σ_{WR}^2 and σ_D^2 are estimated by the method of restricted maximum likelihood (REML). The relationship between the estimated σ_{WR} and estimated σ_D, from the simulation (Figure 11.10.2) and from the FDA data sets (Figure 11.10.2) is given. Also recall that Patnaik et al. (1997), the FDA guidance on *Statistical Approaches* (2001), and Chen et al. (2000) proposed a value of 0.15 for σ_D, as the indicator beyond which the subject-by-formulation interaction may be considered to be important. From Figure 11.10.2, estimated σ_D is positively biased and the magnitude of the bias increased proportionally with the estimated σ_{WR}. In addition, they reported that the probability of an observed and estimated σ_D that exceeded 0.15 increases from 5%, to 25%, to 50%, when σ_{WR} increases from 0.15, to 0.20, to 0.30, respectively. Positive bias observed in the estimation of σ_D from the simulation is not surprising even when σ_D is assumed to be 0, because it is the consequence of the constraint being put on the estimated variance. What is surprising is that the results from the FDA data sets exhibit an almost identical pattern with those from the simulation. In other words, about one-quarter to one-third of estimated σ_D greater than the cutoff value of 0.15 in the FDA files (Patnaik, 1996; Chen et al., 2000) do not result from the true existence of the subject-by-formulation, rather more likely, from the higher values of the reference intra-subject variability. Endrenyi and Tothfalusi (1999) concluded that the FDA data files do not demonstrate a high prevalence of the subject-formulation-by-formulation interaction. Therefore, the higher-order designs are not needed when the intra-subject variability is small, and the use of such design is questionable even for highly variable drugs. Furthermore, as a final remark, it is wrong to conclude the existence of the subject-by-formulation interaction if the value of σ_D is numerically greater than a prespecified value such 0.15. The existence of the subject-by-formulation interaction must be evaluated through a formal statistical procedure, either by a confidence interval approach or the p-value obtained from the hypothesis-testing approach.

The concept of individual bioequivalence for ensuring the switchability between the generic and innovative drug products within the same individual is very attractive. However transition and implementation from the concept to regulatory practice for approval of generic drug products has not been easy. We have reviewed the advantages and drawbacks of aggregate and disaggregate criteria of individual bioequivalence. The major shortcoming of disaggregate criteria is too conservative. The consequence is that the sample size required based on disaggregate criteria is formidably large for any practical consideration. On the other hand, one of the major disadvantages of aggregate criteria is the masking effect by summary measures, which obscure their ultimate objective for evaluating the closeness of the marginal distributions of the test and reference formulations within the same subject. In addition, due to aggregate nature of the criteria, as shown in Chapter 12, inference based on aggregate criteria is rather complicated because of nuisance parameters, scaled factors, and unclear behavior of size and power. Consequently, although the FDA guidance on *Statistical Approaches to Bioequivalence* (FDA, 2001) describes the concept and statistical procedures for population and individual bioequivalence, the 2003 FDA guidance on general considerations for bioequivalence (FDA, 2003b), the EMEA guidance on bioequivalence (EMEA, 2001), and the WHO draft guideline (WHO, 2005) currently still require the evidence of average bioequivalence for approval of generic drug products.

Chapter 12

Statistical Procedures for Assessment of Population and Individual Bioequivalence

12.1 Introduction

The concept of individual bioequivalence was introduced in Chapter 11 to address the issue of switchability. Although its objective is very clear, no consensus has been reached for a precise definition of individual bioequivalence. As a result, under the two-stage mixed-effects model given in Equation 11.2.3, various similar or different criteria have been proposed for evaluation of individual bioequivalence. According to the distribution measures, they can be grouped as either moment-based or probability-based criteria. On the other hand, relative to the manner of assessment, criteria can be classified into aggregate or disaggregate criteria. All these criteria, however, are based on the same three characteristics for quality assurance of the generic drug product that include difference in average bioavailabilities, variance of the subject-by-formulation interaction, and difference in intra-subject variabilities.

For the disaggregate criteria, individual components are assessed separately for individual bioequivalence. Therefore, the estimates of averages, the variance of the subject by formulation, and intra-subject variabilities must be obtained from the pharmacokinetic responses generated under the higher-order design for inference of individual bioequivalence. On the other hand, because the aggregate criteria are a composite index of the three components, it is not necessary to estimate individual parameters for evaluation of individual bioequivalence. In addition, as already indicated in Chapter 11, most of aggregate criteria are rather complicated functions of difference in average bioavailabilities, variance of the subject-by-formulation interaction, and difference in intra-subject variability. To resolve the analytical difficulty, the 2001 FDA guidance recommends a linearized form of M_{I3} proposed by Hyslop et al. (2000) for inference of individual bioequivalence. Recently, McNally et al. (2003) applied the technique of generalized p-value based on generalized pivotal quantities (Tsui and Weerahandi, 1989; Weerahandi, 1995) directly to M_{I3}. Because inference of bioequivalence involves hypothesis testing as well as estimation, similar to average bioequivalence, most currently available statistical procedures for assessment of individual bioequivalence adopt the confidence interval (CI) approach.

From Chapter 11, the criteria for evaluation of population and individual bioequivalence, regardless of aggregate and disaggregate criteria, are formulated in a similar fashion. Therefore, analogous approaches were used for development of statistical methods for assessing population and individual bioequivalence. As a result, in this chapter, we focus on the statistical procedures proposed only for the inference of individual bioequivalence based on both the moment-based and probability-based criteria. The statistical methods for evaluation of individual bioequivalence discussed in this chapter can be directly extended to assessment of population bioequivalence. Procedures for estimating the parameters of the two-stage mixed-effects model described in Chapter 12 are illustrated through higher-order designs in Section 12.2. Section 12.3 reviews the procedures using the linearized criterion suggested by Hylsop et al. (2000). In addition, the inference of individual bioequivalence based on the disaggregate criteria suggested by Liu (1998) is also covered in Section 12.3. For other methods, see Schall and Luus (1993), Sheiner (1992), and Holder and Hsuan (1993). Methods for the criteria other than the aggregate and disaggregate criteria are also available. See, for example, Phillips (1993), Endrenyi (1994), and Kimanani and Potvin (1997). Section 12.4 reviews the procedures for probability-based criteria. Binomial test proposed by Hauck and Anderson and its parametric version suggested by Liu and Chow (1997b) for P_{TIER} is provided in this section. Section 12.4 also covers the method proposed by Schall (1995) for P_{TR} and the use of tolerance intervals for evaluation of individual bioequivalence (Esinhart and Chinchilli, 1994a). Section 12.5 reviews the generalized p-value approach for the evaluation of individual bioequivalence proposed by McNally et al. (2003). Final remarks are provided in Section 12.6. Numerical examples are used throughout this chapter to illustrate the application of various procedures.

12.2 Estimation Procedures

In this section, the procedures proposed by Chinchilli and Esinhart (1996) are illustrated by estimating the parameters of a two-stage mixed-effects model introduced in Section 12.2. Because each subject in the higher-order designs in Table 11.9.1 receives some formulation for more than once, they are also called the replicated crossover designs. Although the procedures proposed by Chinchilli and Esinhart (1996) can be applied to the situations in which subjects may receive different numbers of repeated administrations for different formulations, in this chapter we use Design A1 for the purpose of illustration of the procedures. Design A1 is also the replicated crossover design recommended in the 2001 FDA guidance on statistical approaches.

Let Y_{ijkl} be the original or logarithmic transformation of the bioavailability metric for the lth repeated administration of formulation j for subject i in sequence k, where $l = 1, 2$; $k = 1, 2$; $j = \mathrm{T, R}$; and $i = 1, \ldots, n_k$. Design A1 is uniform within both sequences and periods and each formulation occurs twice within each sequence. In addition, test formulation immediately precedes reference formulation three times and reference formulation immediately precedes test formulation three times. Therefore, it is also balanced for the first-order carryover effect. Following Chinchilli and Esinhart (1996), the model for a balanced crossover design used to describe Design A1 is given as follows:

$$Y_{ijkl} = \mu_j + \tau w_{jkl} + \xi_{jkl} + \omega_{ijk} + \varepsilon_{ijkl} \tag{12.2.1}$$

where

μ_j is the fixed population average for formulation j

ξ_{jkl} is the fixed effect for the lth replicated administration of formulation j within sequence k

ω_{ijk} is the random subject effect for subject i in sequence k receiving formulation j

ε_{ijkl} is the random error associated with the lth replicated administration of formulation j received by subject i within sequence k

τ is the common carryover effect

$w_{jkl} = 1$; if the lth replicated administration of formulation j within sequence k occurs after period 1 and equal zero; otherwise

Because Design A1 has two sequences and four periods, we can compute a total of eight sequence-by-period means. On the other hand, Model 12.2.1 assumes a total of eight location parameters that are population averages, μ_T and μ_R, the common carryover effect τ, and other five nuisance parameters ξ_{jkl}. As a result, there is one-to-one correspondence between eight sequence-by-period means and eight location parameters. Therefore, it is referred to as a saturated statistical model (Ratkowsky et al., 1993). To avoid overparameterization of model 12.2.1 and because ξ_{jkl} is the sequence-by-period interaction nested within formulation, the following two constraints are necessary to put on the nuisance parameters:

$$\sum_{(j,k,l)\in A}\sum \xi_{jkl} = 0 \quad \text{for} \quad j = \text{T and R}, \tag{12.2.2}$$

where $A = \{(j, k, l);\ w_{jkl} = 1 \text{ for each } j = \text{T, R};\ k = 1, 2;\ \text{and } l = 1, 2\}$.

Table 12.2.1 gives the expected values of the sequence-by-formulation means for Design A1. From Table 12.2.1, although there are a total of eight nuisance parameters, only five of them are not confounded with other fixed-effects parameters.

TABLE 12.2.1: Expected values of the sequence-by-period means for Design 11.9.1.1.

	Period			
Sequence	**I**	**II**	**III**	**IV**
1	$\mu_T + \xi_{T11}$	$\mu_R + \xi_{R11} + \tau$	$\mu_T + \xi_{T12} + \tau$	$\mu_R + \xi_{R12} + \tau$
2	$\mu_R - \xi_{T11}$	$\mu_T + \xi_{T21} + \tau$	$\mu_R + \xi_{T11} - \xi_{R11} - \xi_{R12} + \tau$	$\mu_T + \xi_{T11} + \xi_{T12} + \xi_{T21} + \tau$

Denote the 2×1 vector of random subject effects for subject i in sequence k as $\boldsymbol{\omega}'_{ik} = (\omega_{i\mathrm{T}k}, \omega_{i\mathrm{R}k}), i = 1, \ldots, n_k;\ k = 1, 2$. $\boldsymbol{\omega}_{ik}$ is assumed to be mutually independently distributed as a bivariate normal vector with mean $\mathbf{0}$ and covariance matrix $\boldsymbol{\Sigma}_\mathbf{B}$, where $\boldsymbol{\Sigma}_\mathbf{B}$ is defined in Equation 11.2.2. If $\sigma_{\mathrm{TR}} = \rho\sigma_{\mathrm{BT}}\sigma_{\mathrm{BR}}$, then $\boldsymbol{\Sigma}_\mathbf{B}$ becomes

$$\sum\nolimits_{\mathbf{B}} = \begin{pmatrix} \sigma^2_{\mathrm{BT}} & \sigma_{\mathrm{TR}} \\ \sigma_{\mathrm{TR}} & \sigma^2_{\mathrm{BR}} \end{pmatrix}. \tag{12.2.3}$$

Let $\boldsymbol{\mu}' = (\boldsymbol{\mu}_\mathrm{T}, \boldsymbol{\mu}_\mathrm{R})$ and $\boldsymbol{\mu}_{ik} = \boldsymbol{\mu} + \boldsymbol{\omega}_{ik}$. $\boldsymbol{\mu}_{ik}$, in fact, represent the subject-specific averages for subject i in sequence k, $i = 1, \ldots, n_k; k = 1, 2$. It follows that $\boldsymbol{\mu}_{ik}$ is mutually independently distributed as a bivariate normal vector with mean vector $\boldsymbol{\mu}$ and covariance matrix $\boldsymbol{\Sigma}_\mathbf{B}$. Random errors, ε_{ijkl}, are assumed to be mutually independently distributed as univariate normal distribution with mean 0 and variance σ^2_{wj}, for $l = 1, 2;\ k = 1, 2;\ j = \mathrm{T}, \mathrm{R}$; and $i = 1, \ldots, n_k$. The four observed pharmacokinetic responses for subject i in sequence k can be arranged in the order of test and reference formulations and by the order of administration in the 4×1 vector $\boldsymbol{Y}_{ik}$ as

$$\begin{aligned} \mathbf{Y}'_{ik} &= (\mathbf{Y}_{i\mathrm{T}k}, \mathbf{Y}_{i\mathrm{R}k}) \\ &= (Y_{i\mathrm{T}k1}, Y_{i\mathrm{T}k2} | Y_{i\mathrm{R}k1}, Y_{i\mathrm{R}k2}), \end{aligned} \tag{12.2.4}$$

$k = 1, 2;\ i = 1, \ldots, n_k$.

It follows that $\boldsymbol{Y}_{ik}$ are mutually independently distributed as a multivariate normal distribution with mean vector $\boldsymbol{X}_k\boldsymbol{\beta}$ and covariance matrix $\boldsymbol{\Omega}$, for $i = 1, \ldots, n_i; k = 1, 2$, where $\boldsymbol{X}_k$ is 4×8 design matrix of known constants $\boldsymbol{\beta}$ is the 8×1 vector of fixed-effects location parameters, and

$$\boldsymbol{\Omega} = \begin{pmatrix} \sigma^2_{\mathrm{BT}}J_2 + \sigma^2_{\mathrm{WT}}I_2 & \sigma_{\mathrm{TR}}J_2 \\ \sigma_{\mathrm{TR}}J_2 & \sigma^2_{\mathrm{BR}}J_2 + \sigma^2_{\mathrm{WR}}I_2 \end{pmatrix}, \tag{12.2.5}$$

where

J_2 is a 2×2 matrix of 1s
I_2 is a 2×2 identity matrix

Denote the sequence mean vector $\overline{\boldsymbol{Y}}_k$ as

$$\overline{\mathbf{Y}}_k = (1/n_k) \sum \mathbf{Y}_{ik},$$

and

$$\begin{aligned} \overline{\boldsymbol{Y}} &= (\overline{\boldsymbol{Y}}_1, \overline{\boldsymbol{Y}}_2), \\ \boldsymbol{X} &= (\boldsymbol{X}'_1, \boldsymbol{X}'_2), \\ \boldsymbol{\Gamma} &= \boldsymbol{\Omega} \otimes \boldsymbol{I}_2, \\ \boldsymbol{N} &= \boldsymbol{I}_4 \otimes \boldsymbol{n}, \end{aligned}$$

where $\boldsymbol{n}$ is a 2×2 diagonal matrix with n_1 and n_2 on the main diagonal.

Because model 12.2.1 is a saturated model with the number of location parameters corresponding to the number of sequence-by-period means, **X** is 8×8 matrix of full rank. It follows that the maximum likelihood (ML) or restricted maximum likelihood (REML) estimators of $\boldsymbol{\beta}$ can be obtained from the framework of mixed-effects linear model (Laird and Ware, 1982; Ware, 1985; Jennrich and Schluchter, 1986), respectively as

$$\begin{aligned}\widehat{\boldsymbol{\beta}}_{\text{ML}} &= \left(\boldsymbol{X}'\boldsymbol{N}\widehat{\Gamma}_{\text{ML}}^{-1}\,\boldsymbol{X}\right)^{-1}\left(\boldsymbol{X}'\boldsymbol{N}\widehat{\Gamma}_{\text{ML}}^{-1}\,\overline{\boldsymbol{Y}}\right) = \boldsymbol{X}^{-1}\overline{\boldsymbol{Y}},\\ \widehat{\boldsymbol{\beta}}_{\text{REML}} &= \left(\boldsymbol{X}'\boldsymbol{N}\widehat{\Gamma}_{\text{REML}}^{-1}\,\boldsymbol{X}\right)^{-1}\left(\boldsymbol{X}'\boldsymbol{N}\widehat{\Gamma}_{\text{REML}}^{-1}\,\boldsymbol{Y}\right) = \boldsymbol{X}^{-1}\overline{\boldsymbol{Y}},\end{aligned} \tag{12.2.6}$$

where $\widehat{\Gamma}_{\text{ML}}$ and $\widehat{\Gamma}_{\text{REML}}$ are the ML and REML estimators of $\boldsymbol{\Gamma}_{\text{ML}}$ and $\boldsymbol{\Gamma}_{\text{REML}}$, respectively.

In addition, the least squares (LS) estimator of β is given as

$$\begin{aligned}\widehat{\boldsymbol{\beta}}_{\text{LS}} &= \left(\sum\nolimits_{ki}\sum \boldsymbol{X}_j'\boldsymbol{X}_j\right)^{-1}\left(\sum\nolimits_{ki}\sum \boldsymbol{X}'\boldsymbol{Y}_{ik}\right)\\ &= (\boldsymbol{X}'\boldsymbol{N}\boldsymbol{X})^{-1}(\boldsymbol{X}'\boldsymbol{N}\boldsymbol{Y})\boldsymbol{X}^{-1}\boldsymbol{Y} = \boldsymbol{X}^{-1}\overline{\boldsymbol{Y}}.\end{aligned} \tag{12.2.7}$$

From Equations 12.2.6 and 12.2.7, under a saturated model, not only the closed-form solutions exist for ML and REML estimators of $\boldsymbol{\beta}$, but also they are the same and both reduce to the LS estimator. As a result, estimating process for $\boldsymbol{\beta}$ does not involve estimation of covariance matrix and the resulting estimator is a simple linear function of observed vector $\boldsymbol{Y}$. It follows that β is distributed as a multivariate normal distribution with mean vector $\boldsymbol{\beta}$ and covariance matrix $\boldsymbol{X}^{-1}\boldsymbol{N}^{-1}\boldsymbol{\Gamma}\boldsymbol{X}^{-1}$.

For evaluation of individual bioequivalence, it is necessary to obtain the estimators of the variance and covariance components in $\boldsymbol{\Omega}$. For general crossover design, iterative procedure is required to obtain the ML or REML estimators of $\boldsymbol{\Omega}$. However, Design A1–A3 described in Table 11.9.1 are uniform within sequence and both test and reference formulations occur exactly twice within each sequence. It follows that the closed-form solutions exist for variance and covariance components in Ω. For the two pharmacokinetic responses obtained from subject i receiving formulation j in sequence k, we can apply a full-rank transformation from $\boldsymbol{Y}_{ik}$ to the mean of the two pharmacokinetic responses and its corresponding orthogonal contrast, denoted as

$$\overline{Y}_{ijk\cdot} = (1/2)\sum Y_{ijkl},$$

and Y^*_{ijkl}, respectively.

Denote

$$\begin{aligned}\mathbf{Y}^*_{ik} &= (\boldsymbol{Y}_{ik}, \boldsymbol{Y}^*_{ik})'\\ &= (\overline{Y}_{iTk\cdot}, \overline{Y}_{iRk}|Y^*_{iTk1}, Y^*_{iRk1})'\\ i &= 1, \ldots, nk,\\ k &= 1, 2.\end{aligned} \tag{12.2.8}$$

Therefore, $\boldsymbol{Y}_{ik}^*$ consists of the sample subject-specific formulation means and their corresponding orthogonal contrast. Since $\boldsymbol{Y}_{ik}^*$ is a linear function of $\boldsymbol{Y}_{ik}$, it follows that $\boldsymbol{Y}_{ik}^*$ is distributed as a 4×1 normal random vector with mean vector $E(\boldsymbol{Y}_{ik}^*)$ and variance $V(Y_{ik}^*)$ where

$$
\begin{aligned}
E(Y_{ik}^*) &= [E(\overline{Y}_{iTk}), E(\overline{Y}_{iRk}) | E(Y_{iTkl}^*), E(Y_{iRkl}^*)]', \\
E(\overline{Y}_{ijk\cdot}) &= \mu_j + \tau w_{jk\cdot} + \xi_{jk\cdot}, \\
E(Y_{ijk1}^*) &= 2\varepsilon_{ijk}; \quad j = \text{T, R}; \quad k = 1, 2; \quad i = 1, \ldots, n_k, \\
V(Y_{ik}^*) &= \begin{pmatrix} \Lambda & 0 \\ 0 & \Gamma \end{pmatrix}.
\end{aligned}
\tag{12.2.9}
$$

$w_{jk}.$ and $\xi_{jk\cdot}$ are averages of w_{jkl} and ξ_{jkl}, respectively, $\boldsymbol{\Lambda} = \boldsymbol{\Sigma}_{\text{B}} + (1/2)\boldsymbol{\Gamma}$, and $\boldsymbol{\Gamma}$ is a 2×2 diagonal matrix with σ_{WT}^2 and σ_{WR}^2 on the main diagonal.

Because $\overline{Y}_{ijk\cdot}$ is the subject-specific means of the two repeated pharmacokinetic responses of subject i under administration of formulation j in sequence k, their difference

$$
d_{ik} = \overline{Y}_{iTk\cdot} - \overline{Y}_{iRk\cdot} \tag{12.2.10}
$$

in fact, is an estimate of the difference in subject-specific formulation averages

$$
\mu_{iTk} - \mu_{iRk} = (\mu_{\text{T}} + \tau w_{\text{T}k\cdot} + \zeta_{\text{T}k\cdot}) + (\mu_{\text{R}} + \tau w_{\text{R}k\cdot} + \zeta_{\text{R}k\cdot})
$$

Under the normality assumption, it follows that d_{ik} is distributed as a normal distribution with mean $\mu_{iTk} - \mu_{iRk}$ and variance

$$
\begin{aligned}
V(d_{ik}) &= \left[\sigma_{\text{BT}}^2 + \sigma_{\text{BR}}^2 - 2\sigma_{\text{TR}} + (1/2)\left(\sigma_{\text{WT}}^2 + \sigma_{\text{WR}}^2\right)\right] \\
&= \left[\sigma_{\text{D}}^2 + (1/2)\left(\sigma_{\text{WT}}^2 + \sigma_{\text{WR}}^2\right)\right].
\end{aligned}
\tag{12.2.11}
$$

As a result, the ML and REML estimators for $\mu_{\text{T}} - \mu_{\text{R}}$ can be obtained from individual difference in subject-specific formulation means, which is given as

$$
\overline{Y}_{\text{T}} - \overline{Y}_{\text{R}} \tag{12.2.12}
$$

where $\overline{Y}_j = (1/2)\sum \overline{Y}_{\cdot jk\cdot} = (1/2n_k)\sum\sum \overline{Y}_{ijk\cdot}, \quad j = \text{T, R}.$

Variance of $\overline{Y}_{\text{T}} - \overline{Y}_{\text{R}}$ is given as

$$
\begin{aligned}
V(\overline{Y}_{\text{T}} - \overline{Y}_{\text{R}}) &= [(1/4)][(1/n_1) + (1/n_2)] \times \left[\sigma_{\text{BT}}^2 + \sigma_{\text{BR}}^2 - 2\sigma_{\text{TR}} + (1/2)\left(\sigma_{\text{WT}}^2 + \sigma_{\text{WR}}^2\right)\right] \\
&= [(1/4)][(1/n_1) + (1/n_2)]\left[\sigma_{\text{D}}^2 + (1/2)\left(\sigma_{\text{WT}}^2 + \sigma_{\text{WR}}^2\right)\right].
\end{aligned}
\tag{12.2.13}
$$

From Equation 12.2.13, the REML of $\mu_{\text{T}} - \mu_{\text{R}}$ involves not only intra-subject variability, but also the variance of the subject-by-formulation interaction unless $\sigma_{\text{BT}}^2 = \sigma_{\text{BR}}^2$ and the correlation of the subject-specific averages between the test and reference formulations is 1.

From the covariance matrix of Y_{ik}^* in Equation 12.2.9, the formulation means of subject i in sequence k, $(\overline{Y}_{iTk\cdot}, \overline{Y}_{iRk\cdot})'$, are independent of their corresponding orthogonal contrasts $(Y^*_{iTkl}, Y^*_{iRkl})'$. As a result, estimation of Λ and of Γ can be performed separately. Let **S** denote the 2×2 matrix of sums of squares and cross-products computed from the sample subject-specific formulation means:

$$\mathbf{S} = \left(\left[\sum_k \sum_i (\overline{Y}_{ijk\cdot} - \overline{Y}_{\cdot jk\cdot})(\overline{Y}_{ijk\cdot} - \overline{Y}_{\cdot j'k\cdot})\right]\right),$$

where

$$\overline{Y}_{\cdot jk\cdot} = (1/n_k)\sum \overline{Y}_{ijk\cdot}.$$

It follows that the ML and REML estimators of $\mathbf{\Lambda}$ are given, respectively, as follows:

$$\widehat{\Lambda}_{\text{ML}} = (1/N)S,$$

and

$$\widehat{\Lambda}_{\text{REML}} = [1/(N-2)]S, \tag{12.2.14}$$

where $N = n_1 + n_2$.

On the other hand, the ML and REML estimators of intra-subject variabilities, $\sigma^2_{\text{W}j}$ are given, respectively, as

$$s^2_{\text{W}j,\text{ ML}} = (1/N)\left[\sum_k \sum_i (Y^*_{ijkl} - \overline{Y}^*_{\cdot jkl})^2\right], \tag{12.2.15}$$

and

$$s^2_{\text{W}j,\text{ REML}} = [1/(N-2)]\left[\sum\sum (\overline{Y}^*_{ijkl} - \overline{Y}^*_{\cdot jkl})\right],$$

where

$$\overline{Y}^*_{\cdot jkl} = (1/n_k)\sum Y^*_{ijkl}, \quad j = \text{T, R}.$$

From Equation 12.2.9, it follows that the ML and REML estimators of σ^2_{BT}, σ^2_{BR}, and σ^2_{TR} are given, respectively, as

$$\begin{aligned} s^2_{\text{B}j,\text{ML}} &= \widehat{\delta}^2_{\text{B}j,\text{ML}} - (1/2)s^2_{\text{W}j,\text{ML}}, \\ s_{\text{TR, ML}} &= \widehat{\delta}_{\text{TR, ML}}, \end{aligned} \tag{12.2.16}$$

and

$$\begin{aligned} s^2_{\text{B}j,\text{REML}} &= \widehat{\delta}^2_{\text{B}j,\text{REML}} - (1/2)s^2_{\text{W}j,\text{REML}}, \\ s_{\text{TR, REML}} &= \widehat{\delta}_{\text{TR, REML}}, \end{aligned}$$

where

$\widehat{\delta^2_{\mathrm{B}j,\,\mathrm{ML}}}$, $\widehat{\delta^2_{\mathrm{TR},\,\mathrm{ML}}}$, $\widehat{\delta^2_{\mathrm{B}j,\,\mathrm{REML}}}$, and $\widehat{\delta^2_{\mathrm{TR},\,\mathrm{REML}}}$ are the corresponding entries of $\widehat{\Lambda}_{\mathrm{ML}}$ and $\widehat{\Lambda}_{\mathrm{REML}}$, respectively

$j = \mathrm{T, R}$

Note that the REML estimators, $s^2_{\mathrm{B}j,\,\mathrm{REML}}$, $s^2_{\mathrm{W}j,\,\mathrm{REML}}$, and $s^2_{\mathrm{TR},\,\mathrm{REML}}$, are unbiased for $j = \mathrm{T, R}$. Therefore, an unbiased estimator for the variance of the subject-by-formulation interaction is given as

$$s^2_{\mathrm{D,\,REML}} = \left(s^2_{\mathrm{BT,\,REML}} + s^2_{\mathrm{BR,\,REML}} - 2s_{\mathrm{TR,\,REML}}\right). \tag{12.2.17}$$

Although for $j = \mathrm{T, R}$, $s^2_{\mathrm{B}j,\,\mathrm{REML}}$ are unbiased,

$$\Pr\left\{s^2_{\mathrm{B}j,\mathrm{REML}} < 0\right\} > 0,$$

and

$$\Pr\{s^2_{\mathrm{D,\,REML}} < 0\} > 0.$$

In addition, the REML unbiased estimator of $V(d_{ik})$ is given as

$$v(d_{ik}) = [1/(N-2)] \sum_k \sum_i (d_{ik} - \bar{d}_{\cdot k}), \tag{12.2.18}$$

where

$$\bar{d}_{\cdot k} = (1/n_k) \sum d_{ik},\ k = 1, 2.$$

As a result, the REML estimator of $V(\overline{Y}_{\mathrm{T}} - \overline{Y}_{\mathrm{R}})$ can be obtained as

$$v(\overline{Y}_{\mathrm{T}} - \overline{Y}_{\mathrm{R}}) = [(1/4)]\,[1/n_1) + (1/n_2)]\,[v(d_{ik})] \tag{12.2.19}$$

Under the normality assumption, $\overline{Y}_{\mathrm{T}} - \overline{Y}_{\mathrm{R}}$ is distributed as a normal random variable with population average $\mu_{\mathrm{T}} - \mu_{\mathrm{R}}$ and $(N-2)v(d_{ik})/V(d_{ik})$ follows a central chi-square distribution with $N-2$ degrees of freedom. It can be immediately shown that the statistic

$$T = (\overline{Y}_{\mathrm{T}} - \overline{Y}_{\mathrm{R}}) \Big/ \sqrt{v(\overline{Y}_{\mathrm{T}} - \overline{Y}_{\mathrm{R}})} \tag{12.2.20}$$

is distributed as a central t-distribution with $N-2$ degrees of freedom.

On the other hand, the variance of the difference in the orthogonal contrasts between the test and reference formulations for subject i in sequence k

$$d^*_{ik} = Y^*_{i\mathrm{T}k1} - Y^*_{i\mathrm{R}k1} \tag{12.2.21}$$

has a variance equal to sum of the test and reference intra-subject variability. It follows that an unbiased estimator for $\sigma_{\mathrm{WT}}^2 + \sigma_{\mathrm{WR}}^2$ is given as

$$v(d_{ik}^*) = [1/(N-2)] \sum_k \sum_i (d_{ik}^* - \bar{d}_{\cdot k}^*)^2,$$
$$\bar{d}_k^* = (1/n_k) \sum d_{ik}^*, \tag{12.2.22}$$

where $k = 1, 2$.

Again, under the normality assumption, $(N-2)v(d_{ik}^*)/V(d_{ik}^*)$ follows a central chi-square distribution with $N-2$ degrees of freedom. Furthermore, $v(d_{ik})$ and $v(d_{ik}^*)$ are independent. It follows that

$$2v(d_{ik})/v(d_{ik}^*) \sim \left[2\sigma_{\mathrm{D}}^2 + \left(\sigma_{\mathrm{WT}}^2 + \sigma_{\mathrm{WR}}^2\right)\right] / \left(\sigma_{\mathrm{WT}}^2 + \sigma_{\mathrm{WR}}^2\right) F(N-2, N-2), \tag{12.2.23}$$

where $F(N-2, N-2)$ is the central F distribution with $N-2$ and $N-2$ degrees of freedom. Therefore, inference for the variance of the subject-by-formulation interaction can be performed through the statistic $v(d_{ik})/v(d_{ik}^*)$.

12.3 Procedures for Moment-Based Criteria

For aggregate moment-based criteria introduced in Chapter 11, the general formulation of the hypothesis for evaluation of individual bioequivalence is given as

$$\mathrm{H_0}\colon\ M_{\mathrm{I}} \geq \Delta$$
$$\text{versus}\quad \mathrm{H_a}\colon\ M_{\mathrm{I}} < \Delta, \tag{12.3.1}$$

where Δ is some prespecified upper IBE limit.

Table 12.3.1 summarizes the five aggregate moment-based criteria with their respective upper IBE limits. Although evaluation of individual bioequivalence is formulated as a hypothesis-testing procedure, because it is, in fact, an estimation issue, individual bioequivalence is usually assessed by the confidence interval approach.

12.3.1 Procedures Based on the Linearized Form of M_{I3}

Although Table 12.3.1 lists five aggregate criteria, the 2001 FDA guidance on *Statistical Approaches to Establishing Bioequivalence* recommends the use of M_{I3} for assessment of individual bioequivalence. In this section, we therefore focus only on the inference procedures for assessment of individual bioequivalence based on M_{I3} proposed by Hyslop et al. (2000). In addition, the procedures discussed in this section assume that the logarithmic transformation has been performed to the

TABLE 12.3.1: Summary of aggregate moment-based criteria and respective IBE limits.

Aggregate IBE criteria	Value of σ_D^2	IBE Limits
$M_{I1} = \theta^2 + \sigma_D^2 + \sigma_{WT}^2 - \sigma_{WR}^2$	0.02	0.09
	0.03	0.10
$M_{I2} = \left(\theta^2 + \sigma_D^2 + \sigma_{WT}^2\right)/\sigma_{WR}^2$	0.02	3.25
	0.03	3.50
$M_{I3} = \dfrac{\left(\theta^2 + \sigma_D^2 + \sigma_{WT}^2 - \sigma_{WR}^2\right)}{\max\left(\sigma_{WR}^2, \sigma_{WO}^2\right)}$	0.02	2.25
	0.03	2.50
$M_{I4} = \theta^2 + \sigma_D^2$	0.02	0.07
	0.03	0.08
$M_{I5} = \sigma_D^2/\left(\sigma_{WT}^2 + \sigma_{WR}^2\right)$	0.02	0.2
	0.03	0.3

$\sigma_{WR}^2 = \sigma_{WO}^2 = 0.04$ and $\sigma_{WT}^2 - \sigma_{WO}^2 = 0.02$

bioavailability metrics and follows the normal distribution specified in Section 12.2. Under M_{I3}, hypothesis 12.3.1 becomes

$$\begin{aligned} &\text{H}_0\colon \left(\theta^2 + \sigma_D^2 + \sigma_{WT}^2 - \sigma_{WR}^2\right)/\sigma_{WR}^2 \geq \Delta_{I3} \\ \text{versus } &\text{H}_a\colon \left(\theta^2 + \sigma_D^2 + \sigma_{WT}^2 - \sigma_{WR}^2\right)/\sigma_{WR}^2 < \Delta_{I3}, \quad \text{if } \sigma_{WR}^2 > \sigma_{WO}^2, \end{aligned} \tag{12.3.2}$$

and

$$\begin{aligned} &\text{H}_0\colon \left(\theta^2 + \sigma_D^2 + \sigma_{WT}^2 - \sigma_{WR}^2\right)/\sigma_{WO}^2 \geq \Delta_{I3} \\ \text{versus } &\text{H}_a\colon \left(\theta^2 + \sigma_D^2 + \sigma_{WT}^2 - \sigma_{WR}^2\right)/\sigma_{WO}^2 < \Delta_{I3}, \quad \text{if } \sigma_{WR}^2 \leq \sigma_{WO}^2. \end{aligned} \tag{12.3.3}$$

Hypothesis 12.3.2 is expressed in terms of the reference-scaled criterion of M_{I3} while the constant-scaled criterion is used for hypothesis 12.3.3. For the reference-scaled criterion, the statement $(\theta^2 + \sigma_D^2 + \sigma_{WT}^2 - \sigma_{WR}^2)/\sigma_{WR}^2 \geq \Delta_{I3}$ is equivalent to $\theta^2 + \sigma_D^2 + \sigma_{WT}^2 - (1 + \Delta_{I3})\sigma_{WR}^2 \geq 0$. It follows that hypothesis 12.3.2 can be reformulated in terms of the linearized form of reference-scaled criterion as

$$\begin{aligned} &\text{H}_0\colon \theta^2 + \sigma_D^2 + \sigma_{WT}^2 - (1 + \Delta_{I3})\sigma_{WR}^2 \geq 0 \\ \text{versus } &\text{H}_a\colon \theta^2 + \sigma_D^2 + \sigma_{WT}^2 - (1 + \Delta_{I3})\sigma_{WR}^2 < 0. \end{aligned} \tag{12.3.4}$$

Similarly for the constant-scaled criterion, hypothesis 12.3.3 can be expressed as

$$\begin{aligned} &\text{H}_0\colon \theta^2 + \sigma_D^2 + \sigma_{WT}^2 - \sigma_{WR}^2 - \Delta_{I3}\sigma_{WO}^2 \geq 0 \\ \text{versus } &\text{H}_a\colon \theta^2 + \sigma_D^2 + \sigma_{WT}^2 - \sigma_{WR}^2 - \Delta_{I3}\sigma_{WO}^2 < 0. \end{aligned} \tag{12.3.5}$$

For both hypotheses 12.3.4 and 12.3.5, individual bioequivalence is concluded at the α significance level if the $100(1 - \alpha)\%$ upper confidence limit for the linearized version of M_{I3} is less than 0. Note that the linearized version of M_{I3} is a linear combination of variance components and coefficients of linear combinations are either positive or negative. Based on the results from Howe (1974), Graybill and Wang (1980), Ting et al. (1990), and Hyslop et al. (2000) propose a modified large-sample (MLS) upper confidence limit for the linearized version of M_{I3}. The general procedure for constructing an MLS upper confidence limit for a general linear combination of variances is outlined as below (Lee et al., 2004):

Denote η as a general linear combination of variance as

$$\begin{aligned}\eta &= \eta_1 + \cdots + \eta_p - \eta_{p+1} - \cdots - \eta_q \\ &= \sum_{i=1}^{p} \eta_i - \sum_{i=p+1}^{q} \eta_i,\end{aligned} \tag{12.3.6}$$

where

η_i are positive parameters of variances
$i = 1, \ldots, q$

Let $\widehat{\eta}_i$ be an approximately unbiased point estimator of η_i. In addition, $\widehat{\eta}_i$'s are independent chi-square random variables. Denote $\widetilde{\eta}_i$ as a $100(1-\alpha)\%$ upper confidence limit if the sign for η_i is positive and as a $100(1-\alpha)\%$ lower confidence limit if the sign for η_i is negative, $i = 1, \ldots, q$. It follows that an MLS $100(1-\alpha)\%$ upper confidence limit for η is given as

$$\widehat{\eta}_U = \left[\sum_{i=1}^{p} \widehat{\eta}_i - \sum_{i=p+1}^{q} \widehat{\eta}_i\right] + \sqrt{\sum_{i=1}^{q} (\widetilde{\eta}_i - \widehat{\eta}_i)^2}. \tag{12.3.7}$$

Because independent estimator of θ, σ_D^2, σ_{WT}^2, and σ_{WR}^2 may not exist under different replicated crossover design. Design A1 is used to illustrate the procedures. Recall that Design A1 is a two-sequence and four-period dual design in which the test and reference formulations are alternately administrated twice in both sequences.

Define

$$\begin{aligned}Z_{1ik} &= (Y_{iT11} - Y_{iR11} + Y_{iT12} - Y_{iR12})/2, \\ Z_{2ik} &= (Y_{iT11} - Y_{iT12})/\sqrt{2}, \\ Z_{3ik} &= Y_{iR11} - Y_{iR12}/\sqrt{2},\end{aligned} \tag{12.3.8}$$

where

$k = 1, 2$
$i = 1, \ldots, n_i$

Note that Z_{hik} are within-subject contrasts and the sums of cross-products of their coefficients are zero for all pairs of Z_{hij}, $h = 1, \ldots, 3$; and $j = 1, 2$. Consequently, the distributions of any functions based on Z_{ijk} are mutually independent. The expected values and variances of Z_{ijk} are given as

$$\begin{aligned}
E(Z_{1i1}) &= E(Z_{1i2}) = \mu_T - \mu_R = \theta, \\
E(Z_{2i1}) &= E(Z_{3i1}) = E(Z_{2i2}) = E(Z_{3i2}) = 0, \\
V(Z_{1i1}) &= V(Z_{1i2}) = \sigma_D^2 + \left(\sigma_{WT}^2 + \sigma_{WR}^2\right)/2 = \sigma_I^2, \\
V(Z_{2i1}) &= V(Z_{2i2}) = \sigma_{WT}^2, \\
V(Z_{3i1}) &= V(Z_{3i2}) = \sigma_{WR}^2.
\end{aligned} \tag{12.3.9}$$

Let $\overline{Z}_{hk}$ and s_{hk}^2 be the sample means and sample variances computed from the within-subject contrasts Z_{hik},

$$\begin{aligned}
\overline{Z}_{hk} &= \frac{1}{n_k}\sum_{j=1}^{n_i} Z_{hik}, \quad \text{and} \\
s_{hk}^2 &= \frac{1}{(n_k-1)}\sum_{j=1}^{n_i}(Z_{hik} - \overline{Z}_{hk})^2,
\end{aligned} \tag{12.3.10}$$

where

$h = 1, \ldots, 3$

$k = 1, 2$

Because Design A1 is a dual sequence design, unbiased estimators of θ, σ_I^2, σ_{WT}^2, and σ_{WR}^2 can be obtained using the methods for the two independent samples. It follows that unbiased estimators of θ, σ_I^2, σ_{WT}^2, and σ_{WR}^2 are given as

$$\begin{aligned}
\widehat{\theta} &= \frac{1}{2}(\overline{Z}_{11} + \overline{Z}_{12}), \\
s_I^2 &= \frac{(n_1-1)s_{11}^2 + (n_2-1)s_{12}^2}{(n_1+n_2-2)}, \\
s_{WT}^2 &= \frac{(n_1-1)s_{21}^2 + (n_2-1)s_{22}^2}{(n_1+n_2-2)}, \\
s_{WR}^2 &= \frac{(n_1-1)s_{31}^2 + (n_2-1)s_{32}^2}{(n_1+n_2-2)}.
\end{aligned} \tag{12.3.11}$$

$\widehat{\theta}$ follows a normal distribution with mean θ and variance $(1/n_1 + 1/n_2)\sigma_I^2$, and

$$\begin{aligned}
s_I^2 &\sim \sigma_I^2\chi^2_{(n_1+n_2-2)}/(n_1+n_2-2), \\
s_{WT}^2 &\sim \sigma_{WT}^2\chi^2_{(n_1+n_2-2)}/(n_1+n_2-2), \quad \text{and} \\
s_{WR}^2 &\sim \sigma_{WR}^2\chi^2_{(n_1+n_2-2)}/(n_1+n_2-2).
\end{aligned} \tag{12.3.12}$$

In addition, $\widehat{\theta}$, s_I^2, s_{WT}^2, and s_{WR}^2 are mutually independent.

The linearized form of the reference-scale criterion for hypothesis 12.3.4 is given as

$$\eta_{RS} = \theta^2 + \sigma_D^2 + \sigma_{WT}^2 - (1 + \Delta_{I3})\sigma_{WR}^2 \tag{12.3.13}$$

In η_{RS}, θ, σ_{WT}^2, and σ_{WR}^2 can be estimated unbiasedly and independently by $\widehat{\theta}$, s_{WT}^2, and s_{WR}^2 given in Equation 12.3.11. However, independent and unbiased estimators of σ_D^2 are quite difficult to derive even if it exists. As discussed in Section 11.2, the representation of the bioavailability metrics for evaluation of individual bioequivalence involves a two-stage mixed-effects model. At the first stage, the within-subject relative average bioavailability was estimated using the within-subject contrasts such as Z_{1i1} and Z_{1i2}. Then θ is estimated as the average of the within-subject relative average bioavailability. Therefore, the variance of $\widehat{\theta}$ includes the variance of the subject-by-formulation interaction σ_D^2 as well as the intra-subject variability σ_{WT}^2 and σ_{WR}^2. For example, for Design A1, the variance of $\widehat{\theta}$ is given

$$\begin{aligned} V(\widehat{\theta}) &= \left(\frac{1}{n_1} + \frac{1}{n_2}\right)\left(\sigma_D^2 + \frac{1}{2}\sigma_{WT}^2 + \frac{1}{2}\sigma_{WR}^2\right) \\ &= \sigma_I^2 \\ &= \sigma_{0.5,0.5}^2, \end{aligned} \tag{12.3.14}$$

where

$$\sigma_{a,b}^2 = \sigma_D^2 + a\sigma_{WT}^2 + b\sigma_{WR}^2.$$

From Equation 12.3.11, σ_I^2 can be unbiasedly estimated by s_I^2 which are independent of $\widehat{\theta}$, s_{WT}^2, and s_{WR}^2. The next step is to see whether η_{RS} can be expressed in terms of θ, σ_I^2, σ_{WT}^2, and σ_{WR}^2. Note that

$$\begin{aligned} \eta_{RS} &= \theta^2 + \sigma_D^2 + \sigma_{WT}^2 - (1 + \Delta_{I3})\sigma_{WR}^2 \\ &= \theta^2 + \sigma_D^2 + \tfrac{1}{2}\,\sigma_{WT}^2 + \tfrac{1}{2}\,\sigma_{WT}^2 + \tfrac{1}{2}\,\sigma_{WR}^2 - \tfrac{1}{2}\,\sigma_{WR}^2 - (1 + \Delta_{I3})\sigma_{WR}^2 \\ &= \theta^2 + \sigma_I^2 + \tfrac{1}{2}\,\sigma_{WT}^2 - \left(\tfrac{3}{2} + \Delta_{I3}\right)\sigma_{WR}^2 \\ &= \eta_1 + \eta_2 + \eta_3 - \eta_4, \end{aligned}$$

where

$$\begin{aligned} \eta_1 &= \theta^2, \\ \eta_2 &= \sigma_I^2, \\ \eta_3 &= \tfrac{1}{2}\,\sigma_{WT}^2, \\ \eta_4 &= \left(\tfrac{3}{2} + \Delta_{I3}\right)\sigma_{WR}^2. \end{aligned}$$

Therefore, under Design A1, the linearized form of the reference-scaled criterion M_{I3} can be decomposed into four parameters for which unbiased and independent estimators are obtained from the within-subject contrasts given in Equation 12.3.8. According to Equation 12.3.7, an MLS 100(1 − α)% upper confidence limit for η_{RS} can be constructed as

$$\widehat{\eta}_{URS} = A + \sqrt{B},$$

where

$$\begin{aligned}
A &= \widehat{\theta}^2 + s_I^2 + \tfrac{1}{2}s_{WT}^2 - \left(\tfrac{3}{2} + \Delta_{I3}\right)s_{WR}^2,\\
B &= B_1 + B_2 + B_3 + B_4,\\
B_1 &= \left\{\left[\left|\widehat{\theta}\right| + \frac{t(\alpha, n_1+n_2-2)}{2}\sqrt{\left(\frac{1}{n_1}+\frac{1}{n_2}\right)s_I^2}\right]^2 - \widehat{\theta}^2\right\}^2,\\
B_2 &= s_I^4\left[\frac{(n_1+n_2-2)}{\chi^2(1-\alpha, n_1+n_2-2)} - 1\right]^2,\\
B_3 &= \left(\frac{1}{2}s_{WT}^2\right)^2\left[\frac{(n_1+n_2-2)}{\chi^2(1-\alpha, n_1+n_2-2)} - 1\right]^2,\\
B_4 &= \left[\left(\frac{3}{2}+\Delta_{I3}\right)s_{WR}^2\right]^2\left[\frac{(n_1+n_2-2)}{\chi^2(\alpha, n_1+n_2-2)} - 1\right]^2,
\end{aligned} \tag{12.3.15}$$

$t(\alpha, n_1+n_2-2)$ and $\chi^2(\alpha, n_1+n_2-2)$ are the α upper percentiles of the central t-distribution and the central chi-square distribution with n_1+n_2-2 degrees of freedom.

The linearized version of the constant-scaled criterion for hypothesis 12.3.5 is given as

$$\begin{aligned}
\eta_{CS} &= \theta^2 + \sigma_D^2 + \sigma_{WT}^2 - \sigma_{WR}^2 - \Delta_{I3}\sigma_{WO}^2\\
&= \theta^2 + \sigma_I^2 + \tfrac{1}{2}\,\sigma_{WT}^2 - \tfrac{3}{2}\,\sigma_{WR}^2 - \Delta_{I3}\sigma_{WO}^2.
\end{aligned} \tag{12.3.16}$$

Similarly, an MLS 100(1 − α)% upper confidence limit for η_{CS} can be constructed as an

$$\widehat{\eta}_{UCS} = A' + \sqrt{B'},$$

where

$$\begin{aligned}
A' &= A_1 + A_2 + A_3 + A_4',\\
B' &= B_1 + B_2 + B_3 + B_4',\\
A_4' &= \tfrac{3}{2}\,s_{WR}^2 - \Delta_{I3}\sigma_{WO}^2,
\end{aligned} \tag{12.3.17}$$

and

$$B_4' = \left(\frac{3}{2}s_{\mathrm{WR}}^2\right)^2 \left[\frac{(n_1 + n_2 - 2)}{\chi^2(\alpha,\, n_1 + n_2 - 2)} - 1\right]^2.$$

The method using the linearized version of M_{I3} and the within-subject contrasts can be directly extended to the four-sequence and four-period designs in which each subject in each of the four sequences also receives the test and reference formulations twice.

Define

$$Z_{1ik} = (Y_{i\mathrm{T}11} - Y_{i\mathrm{R}11} + Y_{i\mathrm{T}12} - Y_{i\mathrm{R}12})/2$$

$$Z_{2ik} = (Y_{i\mathrm{T}11} - Y_{i\mathrm{T}12})/\sqrt{2},$$

$$Z_{3ik} = Y_{i\mathrm{R}11} - Y_{i\mathrm{R}12}/\sqrt{2},$$

where $k = 1, 2, \quad i = 1, \ldots, n_i$.

It follows that estimators of θ, σ_{I}^2, σ_{WT}^2, and σ_{WR}^2 are given as

$$\widehat{\theta} = \frac{1}{k}\sum_{k=1}^{4} \overline{Z}_{1k},$$

$$s_{\mathrm{I}}^2 = \frac{\sum_{k=1}^{4} (n_k - 1)s_{1k}^2}{\sum_{k=1}^{4} (n_k - 1)},$$

$$s_{\mathrm{WT}}^2 = \frac{\sum_{k=1}^{4} (n_k - 1)s_{2k}^2}{\sum_{k=1}^{4} (n_k - 1)},$$

and

$$s_{\mathrm{WR}}^2 = \frac{\sum_{k=1}^{4} (n_k - 1)s_{3k}^2}{\sum_{k=1}^{4} (n_k - 1)},$$

where $\overline{Z}_{hk}$ and s_{hk}^2 are computed according to Equation 12.3.10.

The MLS $100(1-\alpha)\%$ upper confidence limit for η_{RS} and η_{CS} can be constructed according to Equations 12.3.15 and 12.3.17 with the following modifications:

1. The estimator of the estimated variance of σ_I^2 is modified to

$$\hat{V}(\hat{\theta}) = \sum_{k=1}^{4} \frac{1}{n_i} s_I^2$$

2. The degrees of freedom used in Equations 12.3.15 and 12.3.17 are changed to $(n_1 + n_2 + n_3 + n_4 - 4)$.

Decomposition of the linearized version of M_{13} depends upon the variance of the within-subject contrasts for estimation of the formulation effect. For the two-sequence and four-period dual design such as Design A1, each subject receives the test and reference formulations twice, respectively. Therefore, the within-subject contrasts for estimation of θ are Z_{1i1} and Z_{1i2} with variance $\sigma^2_{0.5,0.5}$ given in Equation 12.3.14. For the two-sequence and three-period Design A4, recommended by the 2001 FDA guidance, the within-subject contrasts for θ are

$$Z_{1i1} = (Y_{iT11} + Y_{iT12})/2 - Y_{iR11}, \quad \text{for sequence} = 1$$

and

$$Z_{3i2} = (Y_{iR21} + Y_{iR22})/2 - Y_{iT21}, \quad \text{for sequence} = 2.$$

It follows that

$$\begin{aligned} V(Z_{1i1}) &= \sigma_D^2 + \tfrac{1}{2}\sigma_{WT}^2 + \sigma_{WR}^2 = \sigma_{0.5,1}^2 \quad \text{and} \\ V(Z_{3i2}) &= \sigma_D^2 + \sigma_{WT}^2 + \tfrac{1}{2}\sigma_{WR}^2 = \sigma_{1,0.5}^2, \end{aligned} \tag{12.3.18}$$

It turns out that for Design 11.9.1.4 the linearized form of M_{13} is reformulated as

$$\eta = \theta^2 + \tfrac{1}{2}\left(\sigma_{0.5,1}^2 + \sigma_{1,0.5}^2\right) + \tfrac{1}{4}\sigma_{WT}^2 - \tfrac{7}{4}\sigma_{WR}^2 - \Delta_{I3}\max\left(\sigma_{WR}^2, \sigma_{WO}^2\right) \tag{12.3.19}$$

From Equation 12.3.19, there are five unknown parameters to be estimated. In addition, all variance components can be estimated from the observations only of one sequence. For example, because the subjects in sequence 1 receive test formulation twice and reference formulation only once, σ_{WT}^2 can be only estimated from the PK responses of the subjects in sequence 1. These undesirable properties make Design B1, although recommended by the 2001 FDA guidance, very inefficient for evaluation of individual bioequivalence.

Chow et al. (2002a) showed that in terms of total number of observations, the two-sequence and three-period (2×3) extra-reference design (TRR, RTR) is more efficient than Design A1 (2×4) and Design B2 (2×3) recommended by the 2001 FDA guidance. The within-subject contrast for estimation of for θ is

$$Z_{3ik} = (Y_{i\mathrm{R}k1} + Y_{i\mathrm{R}k2})/2 - Y_{i\mathrm{T}k1}, \tag{12.3.20}$$

and its variance is given

$$V(Z_{3ik}) = \sigma_{\mathrm{D}}^2 + \sigma_{\mathrm{WT}}^2 + \tfrac{1}{2}\,\sigma_{\mathrm{WR}}^2 = \sigma_{1,0.5}^2, \quad \text{for } k = 1,2 \quad \text{and} \quad i = 1,\ldots,nk.$$

Therefore, the linearized version of M_{I3} under the 2×3 extra-reference design (TRR, RTR) is given as

$$\eta = \theta^2 + \sigma_{1,0.5}^2 - \tfrac{3}{2}\,\sigma_{\mathrm{WR}}^2 - \Delta_{\mathrm{I3}} \max\left(\sigma_{\mathrm{WR}}^2, \sigma_{\mathrm{WO}}^2\right). \tag{12.3.21}$$

For the 2×3 extra-reference design (TRR, RTR), there are only three parameters to be estimated in η and all observations from both sequences are used to estimate these three parameters. Therefore, the simulation results by Chow et al. (2002a) demonstrate that the 2×3 extra-reference crossover design is more powerful than the replicated crossover designs recommended by the 2001 FDA guidance. Table 12.3.2 provides a summary of the linearized criteria of M_{I3} under various replicated crossover designs.

Example 12.3.1

The FDA website reports results of the applications of M_{I3} to three data sets (FDA, 1998). One of the datasets is the AUC from a bioequivalence study that compares a test formulation and a reference formulation of verapamil in 23 normal volunteers using a four-sequence and four-period crossover design (TRTR, RTRT, TRRT, RTTR) (Esinhart and Chinchilli, 1994a,b; Chinchilli, 1996; Chinchilli and Esinhart, 1996). This data set was used by Hyslop et al. (2000) to illustrate their proposed methods for evaluation of individual bioequivalence. The data of the AUC on the original scale are given in Table 12.3.3. In this experiment, six subjects were randomly assigned to sequences TRTR, RTRT, TRRT whereas the sequence RTTR only has five subjects. It turns that the degree of freedom for calculating the 95% upper limit for the linearized version of M_{I3} is 19. The point estimators of θ, σ_{I}^2, σ_{WT}^2, and σ_{WR}^2 are $\widehat{\theta} = -0.0196$, $s_{\mathrm{I}}^2 = 0.05924$, $s_{\mathrm{WT}}^2 = 0.1271$, and $s_{\mathrm{WR}}^2 = 0.0745$. Since $s_{\mathrm{WR}} = 0.2729 > 0.2$, the reference-scaled criterion of M_{I3} is applied with $\Delta_{\mathrm{I3}} = 2.4948$ for evaluation of individual bioequivalence between the generic and innovator drug products of verapamil. The point estimator of the linearized form of the reference-scaled criterion of M_{I3} is

$$\begin{aligned}\widehat{\eta} = \mathrm{A} &= \widehat{\theta}^2 + s_{\mathrm{I}}^2 + \tfrac{1}{2}\,s_{\mathrm{WT}}^2 - \left(\tfrac{3}{2} + \Delta_{\mathrm{I3}}\right)s_{\mathrm{WR}}^2 \\ &= (-0.0196)^2 + 0.05924 + 0.1271/2 - (1.5 + 2.4948)0.0745 \\ &= -0.1744.\end{aligned}$$

TABLE 12.3.2: Summary of linearized criteria of M_{I3}.

Design	η	Number of Parameters	Degrees of Freedom for Variance Components
(TRT, RTR)	$\theta^2 + \frac{1}{2}(\sigma^2_{0.5,1} + \sigma^2_{1,0.5}) + \frac{1}{4}\sigma^2_{WT} - \frac{7}{4}\sigma^2_{WR} - \Delta_{I3}\max(\sigma^2_{WR}, \sigma^2_{W0})$	5	$n_1 - 1$ or $n_2 - 1$
(TRR, RTR)	$\theta^2 + \sigma^2_{1,0.5} - \frac{3}{2}\sigma^2_{WR} - \Delta_{I3}\max(\sigma^2_{WR}, \sigma^2_{W0})$	3	$n_1 + n_2 - 2$
(TRTR, RTRT)	$\theta^2 + \sigma^2_{0.5,0.5} + \frac{1}{2}\sigma^2_{WT} - \frac{3}{2}\sigma^2_{WR} - \Delta_{I3}\max(\sigma^2_{WR}, \sigma^2_{W0})$	4	$n_1 + n_2 - 2$
(TTRR, RRTT, TRTR, RTRT)	$\theta^2 + \sigma^2_{0.5,0.5} + \frac{1}{2}\sigma^2_{WT} - \frac{3}{2}\sigma^2_{WR} - \Delta_{I3}\max(\sigma^2_{WR}, \sigma^2_{W0})$	4	$n_1 + n_2 + n_3 + n_4 - 4$

Source: Chow, S.C., Shao, J., and Wang, H., *Stat. Med.*, 21, 629, 2002a.

TABLE 12.3.3: AUC of verapamil.

Subject	Sequence	Test 1	Test 2	Reference 1	Reference 2
10	TRTR	165.45	318.43	270.44	185.37
11	RTRT	318.44	233.51	299.59	594.41
12	TRRT	319.01	212.61	210.33	332.87
13	RTTR	548.33	502.86	418.94	655.63
14	TRTR	273.24	393.62	629.80	482.12
15	RTRT	154.97	176.62	279.47	263.47
16	TRRT	237.68	303.26	323.68	301.66
17	RTTR	600.59	522.57	318.14	314.21
18	TRTR	197.89	140.54	251.37	115.24
19	RTRT	192.85	144.20	390.48	275.97
20	TRRT	612.90	514.90	448.88	883.06
21	RTTR	240.80	343.65	156.62	191.39
22	TRTR	217.36	185.01	185.30	272.20
23	RTRT	469.05	297.56	407.60	482.65
24	TRRT	100.18	137.65	113.60	120.23
25	RTTR	54.19	151.00	66.86	82.30
26	TRTR	665.87	333.79	442.46	277.27
27	RTRT	281.96	178.56	351.88	293.22
28	TRRT	277.50	191.85	167.04	235.89
29	RTTR	511.24	447.99	240.68	303.57
30	TRTR	611.83	255.66	711.83	396.34
31	RTRT	203.73	284.17	125.98	294.89
32	TRRT	849.39	292.56	763.20	517.79

Source: From Chinchilli, V.M., *J. Biopharm. Stat.*, 6, 6, 1996.

Because $t(0.05, 19) = 1.7291$, $\chi^2(0.95, 19) = 10.1170$, and $\chi^2(0.05, 19) = 30.1435$, it follows that

$$B_1 = \left\{\left[|\widehat{\theta}| + \frac{t(0.05,\ 19)}{4}\sqrt{\left(\frac{1}{n_1}+\frac{1}{n_2}+\frac{1}{n_3}+\frac{1}{n_4}\right)s_I^2}\right]^2 - \widehat{\theta}^2\right\}^2$$

$$= \left\{\left[|-0.0196| + \frac{1.7291}{4}\sqrt{\left(\frac{1}{6}+\frac{1}{6}+\frac{1}{6}+\frac{1}{5}\right)0.05924}\right]^2 - (-0.0196)^2\right\}^2$$

$$= 0.000125,$$

$$B_2 = s_I^4\left[\frac{(n_1+n_2-2)}{\chi^2(1-\alpha, n_1+n_2-2)} - 1\right]^2$$

$$= (0.05924)^2\left[\frac{19}{10.1170} - 1\right]^2$$

$$= 0.002708,$$

$$B_3 = \left(\frac{1}{2}s_{\text{WT}}^2\right)^2\left[\frac{(n_1+n_2-2)}{\chi^2(1-\alpha, n_1+n_2-2)} - 1\right]^2$$
$$= (0.1271/2)^2\left[\frac{19}{10.1170} - 1\right]^2$$
$$= 0.003117,$$

and

$$B_4 = \left[\left(\frac{3}{2}+\Delta_{13}\right)s_{\text{WR}}^2\right]^2\left[\frac{(n_1+n_2-2)}{\chi^2(\alpha, n_1+n_2-2)} - 1\right]^2$$
$$= [(1.5+2.4948)0.0745]^2\left[\frac{19}{30.1435} - 1\right]^2$$
$$= 0.0121.$$

Then an MLS 95% upper confidence limit for η_{RS} is given as

$$\begin{aligned}\widehat{\eta}_{\text{RS}} &= -0.1744 + \sqrt{0.000125 + 0.00270 + 0.00312 + 0.0121} \\ &= -0.1744 + \sqrt{0.01805} \\ &= -0.1744 + 0.1344 \\ &= -0.0400.\end{aligned}$$

Because the 95% upper confidence limit of η_{RS} is less than 0, the test formulation can be concluded to be individual bioequivalent to the reference formulation at the 5% significance level.

12.3.2 Algorithm Based on Disaggregate Criteria

Recall that for disaggregate criteria individual bioequivalence is assessed through separate evaluation of difference in averages, subject-by-formulation interaction, and ratio of intra-subject variability by the three hypotheses in Equation 11.6.16:

1. Average

$$\begin{aligned}&\text{H}_{0a}\colon\ \mu_{\text{T}} - \mu_{\text{R}} \geq -\sqrt{\lambda'_{10}} \quad \text{or} \quad \mu_{\text{T}} - \mu_{\text{R}} \leq \sqrt{\lambda'_{10}} \\ \text{versus}\quad &\text{H}_{aa}\colon\ -\sqrt{\lambda'_{10}} < \mu_{\text{T}} - \mu_{\text{R}} < \sqrt{\lambda'_{10}}.\end{aligned}$$

2. Subject-by-formulation interaction

$$\begin{aligned}&\text{H}_{0I}\colon\ \sigma_{\text{D}}^2 \geq \lambda'_{20} \\ \text{versus}\quad &\text{H}_{aI}\colon\ \sigma_{\text{D}}^2 < \lambda'_{20}.\end{aligned}$$

3. Intra-subject variability

$$\begin{aligned} &\mathrm{H}_{0v}\colon \sigma_{\mathrm{WT}}^2/\sigma_{\mathrm{WR}}^2 \geq \lambda_{30} \\ \text{versus}\quad &\mathrm{H}_{av}\colon \sigma_{\mathrm{WT}}^2/\sigma_{\mathrm{WR}}^2 < \lambda_{30}. \end{aligned}$$

The hypothesis for subject-by-formulation interaction can be expressed as

$$\begin{aligned} &\mathrm{H}_{0I}\colon \sigma_{\mathrm{D}}^2/\left(\sigma_{\mathrm{WT}}^2+\sigma_{\mathrm{WR}}^2\right) \geq \lambda_{20}'' \\ \text{versus}\quad &\mathrm{H}_{aI}\colon \sigma_{\mathrm{D}}^2/\left(\sigma_{\mathrm{WT}}^2+\sigma_{\mathrm{WR}}^2\right) < \lambda_{20}''. \end{aligned} \tag{12.3.22}$$

where $\lambda_{20}'' = \lambda_{20}'/(\sigma_{\mathrm{WT}}^2+\sigma_{\mathrm{WR}}^2)$.

In addition, as demonstrated in Chapter 7, the hypothesis for comparing intra-subject variability can also be formulated in terms of difference as follows:

$$\begin{aligned} &\mathrm{H}_{0v}\colon \sigma_{\mathrm{WT}}^2 - \lambda_{30}\sigma_{\mathrm{WR}}^2 \geq 0 \\ \text{versus}\quad &\mathrm{H}_{av}\colon \sigma_{\mathrm{WT}}^2 - \lambda_{30}\sigma_{\mathrm{WT}}^2 < 0. \end{aligned} \tag{12.3.23}$$

Because $T = (\overline{Y}_{\mathrm{T}} - \overline{Y}_{\mathrm{R}})/\sqrt{v(\overline{Y}_{\mathrm{T}} - \overline{Y}_{\mathrm{R}})}$ in Equation 12.2.20 is distributed as a central t-distribution with $N-2$ degrees of freedom, the $100(1-2\alpha)\%$ confidence interval for $\mu_{\mathrm{T}} - \mu_{\mathrm{R}}$ can be constructed as

$$U_a(L_a) = (\overline{Y}_{\mathrm{T}} - \overline{Y}_{\mathrm{R}}) \pm t(\alpha, N-2)\sqrt{v(\overline{Y}_{\mathrm{T}} - \overline{Y}_{\mathrm{R}})}, \tag{12.3.24}$$

where $t(\alpha, N-2)$ is the αth upper quantile of a central t-distribution with $N-2$ degrees of freedom.

For hypothesis of the subject-by-formulation interaction in Equation 11.6.16, the parameter of interest is, in fact, $M_{I5} = \sigma_{\mathrm{D}}^2/(\sigma_{\mathrm{WT}}^2+\sigma_{\mathrm{WR}}^2)$ and the pharmacokinetic responses generated from Design A1 are used to illustrate the procedure. Recall that the four pharmacokinetic responses in 4×1 vector $\boldsymbol{Y}_{ik}$ defined in Equation 12.2.4 are given as

$$\mathbf{Y}_{ik}' = (\mathrm{Y}_{iTk1}, \mathrm{Y}_{iTk2} | \mathrm{Y}_{iRk1}, \mathrm{Y}_{iRk2}), \quad k = 1, 2; \quad i = 1, \ldots, n_k$$

Let two orthogonal contrasts of $\boldsymbol{Y}_{ik}$ be $d_{ik} = \boldsymbol{c}_1\boldsymbol{Y}_{ik}$ in Equation 12.2.10 and $R_{ik} = \boldsymbol{c}_2\boldsymbol{Y}_{ik}$,
where

$$\boldsymbol{c}_1 = (1/2)(1, 1, -1, -1), \tag{12.3.25}$$

and

$$\boldsymbol{c}_2 = (1/2)(1, -1, -1, 1), \quad i = 1, \ldots, n_k, \quad k = 1, 2.$$

It follows that d_{ik} are i.i.d. random variables with variance given as

$$V(d_{ik}) = \sigma_D^2 + (1/2)\left(\sigma_{WT}^2 + \sigma_{WR}^2\right),$$

and R_{ik} are also i.i.d. random variables with variance given as

$$V(R_{ik}) = (1/2)\left(\sigma_{WT}^2 + \sigma_{WR}^2\right).$$

In addition $\{d_{ik}, i = 1, \ldots, n_k, k = 1, 2\}$ and $\{R_{ik}, i = 1, \ldots, n_k, k = 1, 2\}$ are mutually independent. Let

$$MS(S \times F) = v(d_{ik}) = [1/(N-2)]\left[\sum_{k=1}^{2}\sum_{i=1}^{n_k}(d_{ik} - \bar{d}_{\cdot k})^2\right] \quad (12.3.26)$$

and

$$MS(\text{ave}) = [1/(N-2)]\left[\sum_{k=1}^{2}\sum_{i=1}^{n_k}(R_{ik} - \bar{R}_{\cdot k})^2\right]$$

where

$$\bar{d}_{\cdot k} = (1/n_k)\sum_{k=1}^{n_k} d_{ik},$$

and

$$\bar{R}_{\cdot k} = (1/n_k)\sum_{i=1}^{n_k} R_{ik}.$$

It follows that MS (S × F) and MS (ave) are independent and

$$\mathrm{F_{IF}} = \mathrm{MS(S \times F)/MS(ave)} \quad (12.3.27)$$

is distributed as $\{[2\sigma_D^2 + (\sigma_{WT}^2 + \sigma_{WR}^2)]/(\sigma_{WT}^2 + \sigma_{WR}^2)\}F(N-2, N-2)$ where $F(N-2, N-2)$ is a central F distribution with $N-2$ and $N-2$ degrees of freedom. Note that

$$\left[2\sigma_D^2 + \left(\sigma_{WT}^2 + \sigma_{WR}^2\right)\right]/\left(\sigma_{WR}^2 + \sigma_{WR}^2\right) = 2M_{I5} + 1.$$

It follows that the point estimator and $100(1-\alpha)\%$ upper confidence limit for M_{I5} are given, respectively, as

$$\begin{aligned} &m_{I5} = (F_{IF} - 1)/2 \quad \text{and} \\ &U_{IF}\ \{[\mathrm{MS}(S \times F)/\mathrm{MS(ave)}]F(\alpha, N-2, N-2) - 1\}/2, \end{aligned} \quad (12.3.28)$$

where $F(\alpha, N-2, N-2)$ is the αth upper quantile of a central F distribution, with degrees of freedom $N-2$ and $N-2$.

Furthermore, under the normality assumption, the ratio $s^2_{\text{WT, REML}}/s^2_{\text{WR, REML}}$ is distributed as $\sigma^2_{\text{WT}}/\sigma^2_{\text{WR}}$ times a central F distribution with degrees of freedom $N-2$ and $N-2$. It follows that the $100(1-\alpha)\%$ upper confidence limit for $\sigma^2_{\text{WT}}/\sigma^2_{\text{WR}}$ is given as

$$U_v = \left[s^2_{\text{WT, REML}}/s^2_{\text{WR, REML}}\right] F(\alpha,\, N-2,\, N-2), \tag{12.3.29}$$

where $F(\alpha, N-2, N-2)$ is the αth upper quantile of a central F distribution with degrees of freedom $N-2$ and $N-2$.

The Pitman–Morgan two one-sided tests procedure can also be applied to test hypothesis 12.3.23 for the data obtained under Design A1. Define another orthogonal contrast of $\boldsymbol{Y}_{ik}$ as $R'_{ik} = \boldsymbol{c}_3 Y_{ik}$, where $\boldsymbol{c}_3 = (1/2)(1, -1, \lambda_{30}, -\lambda_{30})$. It is easy to verify that

$$V(R'_{ik}) = (1/2)\left(\sigma^2_{\text{WT}} + \lambda_{30}\sigma^2_{\text{WR}}\right),$$

and

$$\text{Cov}(R_{ik},\, R'_{ik}) = (1/2)\left(\sigma^2_{\text{WT}} - \lambda_{30}\sigma^2_{\text{WR}}\right).$$

As a result, the Pitman–Morgan two one-sided tests procedure can be directly applied based on the sample correlation coefficient

$$r_v = \text{SP}(R,\, R')/\sqrt{\text{SS(ave) SS}(R')}, \tag{12.3.30}$$

where

$$\text{SS(ave)} = (N-2)\ \text{MS(ave)},$$

$$\text{SS}(R') = \sum_{k=1}^{2}\sum_{i=1}^{n_k}(R'_{ik} - R'_{.k})^2,$$

$$\text{SP}(R,R') = \sum_{k=1}^{2}\sum_{i=1}^{n_k}\left[(R_{ik} - \overline{R}_{.k})(R'_{ik} - \overline{R}'_{.k})\right],$$

and

$$\overline{R}'_{.k} = (1/n_k)\sum_{k=1}^{n_k} R'_{ik}.$$

The $100(1-\alpha)\%$ upper confidence limit for $\sigma^2_{\text{D}}/[\sigma^2_{\text{WT}} + \sigma^2_{\text{WR}}]$ given in Equation 12.3.28 can be used to assess σ^2_{D} in terms of hypothesis based on M_{15} in Equation 12.3.22. On the other hand, the $100(1-\alpha)\%$ upper confidence limit for σ^2_{D} obtained from the constrained REML method can be used to test hypothesis (2) in Equation 11.6.16 for the subject-by-formulation interaction.

Step 1: Construct the 95% confidence interval (L_a, U_a) for $\mu_T - \mu_R$ according to Equation 12.3.24. If $(L_a, U_a)[\exp(L_a), \exp(U_a)]$ is completely contained within [log0.8, log1.25] [0.8, 1.25], then two formulations are conducted average bioequivalence at the 5% significance level.

Step 2: Construct the 95% upper confidence limits, U_{IF} for M_{I5} according to Equation 12.3.28 or for σ_D^2 by REML method. If it is smaller than the corresponding upper limit (0.2 or 0.3 for M_{I5} or 0.02 or 0.03 for σ_D^2), then the test and reference formulations are bioequivalent in subject-by-formulation at the 5% significance level.

Step 3: Compute the 95% upper confidence limit for $\sigma_{WT}^2/\sigma_{WR}^2$. If as suggested in the 2001 FDA guidance, $\sigma_{WT}^2 = \sigma_{WO}^2 = 0.04$ and $\sigma_{WT}^2 - \sigma_{WR}^2 = 0.02$, then the upper limit for the ratio of the test intra-subject variability to the reference intra-subject variability is 1.5. As a result, the 95% upper confidence limit for $\sigma_{WT}^2/\sigma_{WR}^2$ is smaller than 1.5, then the test and reference formulations are bioequivalent in intra-subject variability. The Pitman–Morgan's two one-sided tests procedure can also be applied in Equation 12.3.30. However, it cannot yield the corresponding 95% upper limit for $\sigma_{WT}^2 - \sigma_{WR}^2$.

Step 4: If the two formulations are bioequivalent in average, the subject-by-formulation interaction and the intra-subject variability as demonstrated at the α significance level in steps 1–3 using the confidence interval (limit) approach, then the test and reference formulations are concluded individual bioequivalent at the α significance level.

Example 12.3.2

Two data sets published in the FDA Web sites (FDA, 1998) are used to illustrate the procedure for the disaggregate criteria. The first data set is the AUC of furosemide employed by Sheiner (1992) to illustrate his proposed method based on M_{I2}. This data set was originally reported by Ekbohm and Melander (1989) and by Grahnén et al. (1980). Table 12.4.1 reproduces the total AUC on the original scale from eight

TABLE 12.4.1: Total AUC of furosemide.

Subject	Sequence	Test 1	Test 2	Reference 1	Reference 2
1	(TRTR)	164.9	162.4	137.3	110.9
2	(TRTR)	268.9	234.9	166.7	209.4
3	(RTRT)	147.2	109.2	184.3	91.2
4	(TRTR)	95.0	108.0	107.8	173.4
5	(RTRT)	175.7	183.7	173.5	146.5
6	(RTRT)	161.0	207.1	194.7	153.7
7	(RTRT)	168.8	241.9	151.3	189.9
8	(TRTR)	62.3	127.7	190.4	189.8

Source: From Ekbohm, G. and Melander, H. *Biometrics*, 45, 1249, 1989.

TABLE 12.4.2: Summary of evaluation of individual bioequivalence of furosemide and ac-5-ASA.

Parameter	Furosemide	ac-5-ASA
μ_T/μ_R		
Estimate[a]	98.1	115.9
90% CI	(81.2, 116.9)	(106.0, 127.3)
σ_{BR}		
Estimate	0.059	0.517
90% CI	(0.000, 0.157)	(0.000, 0634)
σ_{BT}/σ_{BR}		
Estimate	5.487	0.853
90% CI	(0.665, 6.725)	(0.635, 1.058)
σ_{WR}		
Estimate	0.242	0.327
90% CI	(0.108, 0.263)	(0.137, 0.392)
σ_{WT}/σ_{WR}		
Estimate	0.986	0.827
90% CI	(0.543, 1.183)	(0.493, 1.463)
σ_D		
Estimate	0.274	0.076
90% CI	(0.033, 0.373)	(0.008, 0.147)

Source: From Data Sets of Bioequivalence for Individual and Population Bioequivalence, U.S. Food and Drug Administration, 1998.

[a] REML estimates and 90% confidence interval (CI).

subjects under Design A1. The other data set is the AUC data set of *N*-acetyl-5-aminosalicyclic acid (ac-5-ASA) introduced in Table 9.4.3 (Ryde et al., 1991). For this example, the logarithmic transformation of AUC data in Tables 9.4.3 and 12.4.1 is used for evaluation of individual bioequivalence. Table 12.4.2 summarizes the results of these two data sets. For the log-transformed AUC of furosemide, the 90% confidence interval for $\mu_T - \mu_R$ is (81.2, 116.9) and the 95% upper limit for $\sigma^2_{WT}/\sigma^2_{WR}$ by the REML method is $1.40(=1.183^2)$. Both are within their respective equivalence limits (0.8, 1.25) and 1.5. However, the 95% upper confidence limit for σ^2_D is $0.139(=0.373^2)$, which is larger than 0.03. As a result, the two formulations cannot be concluded individual bioequivalence at the 5% significance level according to the disaggregate criteria. For the data set of ac-5-ASA, because the 90% confidence interval for $\mu_T - \mu_R$ is (106.0, 127.3), the two formulations of ac-5-ASA are not individual bioequivalent at the 5% significance level. Note that for ac-5-ASA, the 95% upper confidence limit for $\sigma^2_{WT}/\sigma^2_{WR}$ is $2.14(=1.463^2)$, which is larger than 1.5. However, the 95% upper confidence limit for σ^2_D is $0.0216(=0.147^2)$, which is between 0.02 and 0.03.

12.4 Procedures for Probability-Based Criteria

For the probability-based criteria introduced in Section 12.5, the general formulation of the hypothesis for evaluation of individual bioequivalence is given as

$$\begin{aligned} &\text{H}_0\text{: } P \leq \pi \\ \text{versus } &\text{H}_a\text{: } P > \pi, \end{aligned} \tag{12.4.1}$$

where π is the MINP.

Recall that the individual equivalence ratio given in Equation 11.5.1 is defined in terms of the ratio of the two subject-specific averages, and P_{TIER} is defined as the difference of two subject-specific averages on the log-scale as

$$P_{\text{TIER}} = P\{-r < \mu_{i\text{T}} - \mu_{i\text{R}} < r\},$$

where r is some prespecified constant.

The hypothesis for evaluation based on P_{TIER} is given as

$$\begin{aligned} &\text{H}_0\text{: } P_{\text{TIER}} \leq \pi \\ \text{versus } &\text{H}_a\text{: } P_{\text{TIER}} > \pi. \end{aligned} \tag{12.4.2}$$

When the 75/75 rule is applied, then $-r = \ln(0.75) = -0.2877$ and $\pi = 0.75$.

On the other hand, $P_{\text{d}}(P_r) = P_{\text{TR}} - P_{\text{RR}}(P_{\text{TR}}/P_{\text{RR}})$ is defined in terms of the difference in the observed logarithmic pharmacokinetic responses, for example,

$$P_{\text{TR}} = P\{-r < Y_{i\text{T}} - Y_{i\text{R}} < r\},$$

and

$$P_{\text{RR}} = P\{-r < Y_{i\text{R}} - Y'_{i\text{R}} < r\}.$$

Under the normality assumption, P_{RR} is a constant. The corresponding hypothesis can then be formulated in terms of P_{TR} as

$$\begin{aligned} &\text{H}_0\text{: } P_{\text{TR}} \leq \pi \\ \text{versus } &\text{H}_a\text{: } P_{\text{TR}} > \pi \end{aligned} \tag{12.4.3}$$

P_{TIER} evaluates probability without inclusion of intra-subject variability. As a result, P_{TR} in general is smaller than P_{TIER}. Hypotheses 12.4.2 and 12.4.3 are, therefore, two different hypotheses.

12.4.1 Algorithm for TIER

Anderson and Hauck (1990) consider the following distribution-free procedure based on the binomial distribution for evaluation of individual bioequivalence based on the individual subject ratios (or difference on log-scale) of the pharmacokinetic responses obtained from the standard two-sequence and two-period design.

Step 1: Select the value of r and π.

Step 2: Count the number of subjects whose individual subject difference $Y_{iT} - Y_{iR}$ is within $-r$ and r. Denote this number as X.

Step 3: Find the $100(1-\alpha)\%$ lower confidence limit for P_{TIER}, L_{TIER}, by the following formula:

$$\alpha = \Pr\{X \text{ or more subjects whose } Y_{iT} - Y_{iR} \text{ is within } -r \text{ and } r|\pi = P_{\text{TIER}}\}$$

Step 4: If $L_{\text{TIER}} > \pi$, then the two formulations are concluded individual bioequivalent at the α significance level.

Table 12.4.1 provides the minimal number of subjects required for concluding individual bioequivalence at the 5% significance level and the 95% lower confidence limit L_{TIER} corresponding to 75% of subjects whose differences on the log-scale are within $-r$ and r.

Example 12.4.1

To illustrate the procedure of TIER, we consider the AUC data from two erythromycin formulations given in Table 6.9.1 (Clayton and Leslie, 1981). Columns 7 and 8 of Table 6.9.1 provide the individual ratios of the AUC of the new formulation compared with that of the reference formulation and its logarithmic transformation. We define that a subject is individual bioequivalent if the individual difference in log-AUC is between $\ln(0.7) = -0.3567$ and $\ln(1.4286) = 0.3567$. It can be verified from Table 6.9.1 that only five subjects meet this criterion. The 95% lower confidence limit for P_{TIER} computed is 0.116. If MINP is selected to be 0.75, because $L_{\text{TIER}} < 0.75$, the two formulations cannot be concluded individual bioequivalent. The same conclusion can be reached using Table 12.4.3. The minimal number of subjects required for concluding individual bioequivalence at the 5% significance level is 17 for a sample size of 18 subjects. However, for this data set, only five subjects meet the criteria. Again, the stearate formulation of erythromycin is not individual bioequivalent to the base formulation.

The procedure proposed by Anderson and Hauck (1990) dichotomizes a continuous response into a binary variable. As a result, valuable information is lost during the categorization process. In addition, their procedure is not applicable in the presence of period effect. Furthermore, TIER cannot be extended to assessing individual bioequivalence for the pharmacokinetic responses obtained from the designs other than the standard two-sequence and two-period design. To overcome this deficiency of the procedure for TIER proposed by Anderson and Hauck (1990), under the normality assumption, Liu and Chow (1997b) suggested a two one-sided tests procedure for hypothesis 12.4.3 formulated in terms of P_{TR}. Although the test proposed by Liu and Chow is not expressed as hypothesis 12.4.2 based on P_{TIER},

TABLE 12.4.3: Minimal number of subjects required for concluding individual bioequivalence at the 5% significance level and L_{TIER} corresponding to 75% of subjects whose differences are within $-r$ and r.

Sample Size	0.6667	0.75	0.80	0.9	L_{TIER}
10	10	—	—	—	0.493
11	11	11	—	—	0.530
12	12	12	—	—	0.473
13	12	13	—	—	0.505
14	13	14	14	—	0.534
15	14	15	15	—	0.560
16	15	16	16	—	0.516
17	15	17	17	—	0.539
18	16	17	18	—	0.561
19	17	18	19	—	0.581
20	18	19	20	—	0.544
21	18	20	21	—	0.563
22	19	21	21	—	0.580
23	20	21	22	—	0.596
24	21	22	23	—	0.565
25	21	23	24	—	0.581
26	22	24	25	—	0.595
27	23	25	26	—	0.608
28	24	26	27	—	0.581
29	24	26	28	29	0.594
30	25	27	28	30	0.606
31	26	28	29	31	0.617
32	27	29	30	32	0.594
33	27	30	31	32	0.605
34	28	30	32	34	0.615
35	29	31	33	35	0.625

Source: From Anderson, S. and Hauck, W.W., *J. Pharmacokin. Biopharm.*, 18, 259, 1990.

Hwang and Wang (1997) show that it is also a valid test for hypothesis 12.4.2 under the normality assumption as long as $\pi \geq 0.5$.

As shown in Section 11.7, hypothesis 12.4.3 based on P_{TR} can be reformulated as two one-sided hypotheses in terms of quantiles of a standard normal distribution as

$$\begin{aligned} &\mathrm{H}_{0L}: \theta - z(\omega_0)\sqrt{\sigma_D^2 + \sigma_{WT}^2 + \sigma_{WR}^2} \leq -r \\ \text{versus}\quad &\mathrm{H}_{aL}: \theta - z(\omega_0)\sqrt{\sigma_D^2 + \sigma_{WT}^2 + \sigma_{WR}^2} > -r, \end{aligned} \tag{12.4.4}$$

and

$$\text{H}_{0U}\text{: } \theta + z(\omega_0)\sqrt{\sigma_D^2 + \sigma_{WT}^2 + \sigma_{WR}^2} \geq r$$

$$\text{versus} \quad \text{H}_{aU}\text{: } \theta + z(\omega_0)\sqrt{\sigma_D^2 + \sigma_{WT}^2 + \sigma_{WR}^2} < r,$$

where

$z(\omega_0)$ is the ω_0th quantile of a standard normal random variable
ω_0 is defined in Equation 11.7.5

Under the standard two-sequence and two-period crossover design, it is not possible to obtain separate estimators of σ_D^2, σ_{WT}^2, and σ_{WR}^2 because of identification problem. As a result, it is assumed for the moment that $\sigma_D^2 = 0$ and $\sigma_{WT}^2 = \sigma_{WR}^2$. Under the assumption, T_L and T_U in Equation 4.3.4 for the Schuirmann's two one-sided tests procedure with replacement of θ_L and θ_U, respectively, are also the test statistics for hypothesis 12.4.4. Under normality assumption, T_L and T_U, respectively, follow noncentral t-distribution with $n_1 + n_2 - 2$ degrees of freedom and noncentrality $\{\sqrt{2/[1/n_1) + (1/n_2)]}\}z(\omega_0)$ and $-\{\sqrt{2/[1/n_1) + (1/n_2)]}\}z(\omega_0)$. As a result, individual bioequivalence is concluded at the α significance level if

$$\begin{aligned} T_L &> t(\alpha, \text{NC}, n_1 + n_2 - 2) \quad \text{and} \\ T_U &< -t(\alpha, \text{NC}, n_1 + n_2 - 2), \end{aligned} \tag{12.4.5}$$

where $t(\alpha, \text{NC}, n_1 + n_2 - 2)$ is the αth upper quantile of a noncentral t-distribution with $n_1 + n_2 - 2$ degrees of freedom, and noncentrality parameter $\text{NC} = \{\sqrt{2/[1/n_1) + (1/n_2)]}\}z(\omega_0)$.

Table 12.4.4 gives the critical values for $\pi = 0.67$, 0.75, 0.80, and 0.90 and $n_1 = n_2 = 5$ to 20 by 1. The rejection region for hypothesis 12.4.5 is given as

$$\begin{aligned} R = \{(\overline{Y}_T - \overline{Y}_R, \widehat{\sigma}_d)| &- r + t(\alpha, \text{NC}, n_1 + n_2 - 2)\sqrt{[1/n_1) + (1/n_2)]}\widehat{\sigma}_d \\ &< (\overline{Y}_T - \overline{Y}_R) < r + t(\alpha, \text{NC}, n_1 + n_2 - 2)\sqrt{[1/n_1) + (1/n_2)]}\widehat{\sigma}_d\} \end{aligned} \tag{12.4.6}$$

Figure 12.4.1 presents the rejection for $r = \ln(1.25)$ and $\omega_0 = 12.5\%$ and $n_1 = N_2 = 10$. For comparison, the rejection region of Schuirmann's two one-sided tests procedure for average bioequivalence with the same sample size is also provided in Figure 12.4.1. Because for the same degrees of freedom, $t(\alpha, \text{NC}, n_1 + n_2 - 2) > t(\alpha, 0, n_1 + n_2 - 2)$, as demonstrated in Figure 12.4.1, the rejection for the hypothesis of individual bioequivalence is totally contained within that of average bioequivalence. It follows that conclusion of average bioequivalence generally does not imply individual bioequivalence. On the other hand, conclusion of individual bioequivalence by the two one-sided tests procedure in Equation 12.4.5, however, will guarantee average bioequivalence by Schuirmann's two one-sided tests procedure.

Although the procedure given in Equation 12.4.5 is valid for hypothesis 12.4.2, it is not directly expressed in terms of P_{TIER}. Anderson and Hauck (1990) defined

TABLE 12.4.4: Critical values for two one-sided tests procedure for individual bioequivalence.

	π			
N	**0.67**	**0.75**	**0.80**	**0.90**
5	6.1442	7.0376	7.6884	9.5239
6	6.2424	7.1580	7.8243	9.7011
7	6.3846	7.3295	8.0164	9.9497
8	6.5450	7.5219	8.2316	10.2273
9	6.7217	7.7225	8.4557	10.5160
10	6.8823	7.9252	8.6820	10.8073
11	7.0512	8.1269	8.9070	11.0969
12	7.2182	8.3260	9.1292	11.3826
13	7.3824	8.5219	9.3476	11.6634
14	7.5435	8.7139	9.5619	11.9388
15	7.7015	8.9022	9.7717	12.2086
16	7.8563	9.0865	9.9773	12.4727
17	8.0079	9.2671	10.1786	12.7314
18	8.1564	9.4440	10.3758	13.2330
19	8.3020	9.6173	10.5690	13.2330
20	8.4447	9.7872	10.7585	13.4763

Source: From Liu, J.P. and Chow, S.C., *J. Biopharm. Stat.*, 7, 49, 1997b.

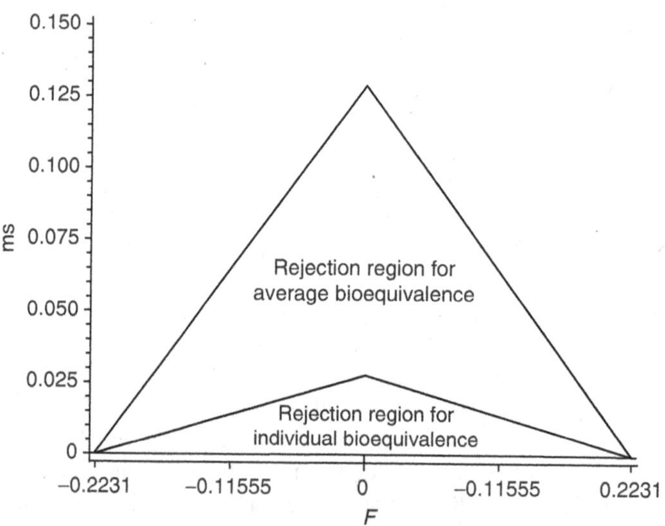

FIGURE 12.4.1: Comparison of rejection region of Schuirmann's two one-sided tests procedure for average bioequivalence and proposed two one-sided tests procedure for individual bioequivalence, $n_1 = n_2 = 10$, and the 0.05 nominal level of significance. Large triangle: Rejection region for average bioequivalence. Small triangle: Rejection region for individual bioequivalence.

the individual equivalence ratio as the ratio of the two subject-specific averages. On the log scale, for the higher-order designs such as Design A1, difference in subject-specific sample means d_{ik} in Equation 12.2.10 is an unbiased estimator for difference in the subject-specific averages. As a result, an estimate for P_{TIER} is given as

$$P_{\text{TIER}} = P\{-r < \overline{Y}_{iTk\cdot} - \overline{Y}_{iRk\cdot} < r\}$$

Consequently, the corresponding two one-sided hypotheses can be expressed as follows:

$$\begin{aligned} &\text{H}_{0\text{L}}:\ \theta - z(\omega_0)\sqrt{\sigma_{\text{D}}^2 + (1/2)\left(\sigma_{\text{WT}}^2 + \sigma_{\text{WR}}^2\right)} \le -r \\ \text{versus}\quad &\text{H}_{\text{aL}}:\ \theta - z(\omega_0)\sqrt{\sigma_{\text{D}}^2 + (1/2)\left(\sigma_{\text{WT}}^2 + \sigma_{\text{WR}}^2\right)} > -r, \end{aligned} \tag{12.4.7}$$

and

$$\begin{aligned} &\text{H}_{0\text{U}}:\ \theta + z(\omega_0)\sqrt{\sigma_{\text{D}}^2 + (1/2)\left(\sigma_{\text{WT}}^2 + \sigma_{\text{WR}}^2\right)} \ge r \\ \text{versus}\quad &\text{H}_{\text{aU}}:\ \theta + z(\omega_0)\sqrt{\sigma_{\text{D}}^2 + (1/2)\left(\sigma_{\text{WT}}^2 + \sigma_{\text{WR}}^2\right)} < r. \end{aligned}$$

It follows that the two one-sided test procedures introduced in the above for evaluation of individual bioequivalence can be directly applied to Design 11.9.1.1 by replacing $\overline{Y}_{\text{T}} - \overline{Y}_{\text{R}}$ and $\widehat{\sigma}_{\text{d}}$ by the corresponding REML estimator of $\mu_{\text{T}} - \mu_{\text{R}}$ and its estimated standard error $\sqrt{v(\overline{Y}_{\text{T}} - \overline{Y}_{\text{R}})}$.

The power function at $\pi_a > \pi$ and $n_1 + n_2 - 2$ is given as

$$\phi(\pi_a) = P\{T_{\text{L}} > t(\alpha, \text{NC}, n_1 + n_2 - 2) \text{ and } T_{\text{U}} < -t(\alpha, \text{NC}, n_1 + n_2 - 2)\} \tag{12.4.8}$$

where

$P\pi_a$ is the probability evaluated by noncentral t-distribution with $(n_1 + n_2 - 2)$ degrees of freedom and noncentrality parameters $\sqrt{2/[(1/n_1) + (1/n_2)]}\ z(\omega_0)$ and $\sqrt{2/[(1/n_1) + (1/n_2)]}\ z(\omega_0)$

$z(\omega_a)$ is the ω_ath upper quantile of a standard normal variable

$\omega_a < \omega_0$ is similarly defined as ω_0

The sample size can be determined by simultaneously evaluating Equation 12.4.7 and

$$P\{T_{\text{L}} > t(\alpha, \text{NC}, n_1 + n_2 - 2)\} = P\{T_{\text{U}} < -t(\alpha, \text{NC}, n_1 + n_2 - 2)\} = \alpha. \tag{12.4.9}$$

Table 12.4.5 provides the total number of subjects required for some selected π and π_a under various designs when the desired power is either 80% or 90%. From Table 12.4.5, one needs a large number of subjects for the desired power to evaluate individual bioequivalence.

TABLE 12.4.5: Total number of subjects ($2n$) required for individual bioequivalence under different designs.

			Design		
Power	$\mathbf{H_0}$	$\mathbf{H_a}$	**2 × 2**	**2 × 3**	**2 × 4**
0.8	0.67	0.90	36	28	16
		0.95	20	16	10
	0.75	0.90	70	54	30
		0.95	30	24	20
0.9	0.67	0.90	46	36	20
		0.95	24	18	10
	0.75	0.90	88	78	38
		0.95	28	28	24

Source: From Liu, J.P. and Chow, S.C., *J. Biopharm. Stat.*, 7, 49, 1997b.

12.4.2 Parametric Algorithm for TIER

Step 1: Determine r and π in hypothesis 12.4.1.

Step 2: Obtain subject-specific sample mean differences as estimators for the subject-specific averages $\mu_{iT} - \mu_{iR}$.

Step 3: Use the subject-specific mean differences as the responses to compute the estimated standard error and T_L and T_U according to Equation 4.3.4.

Step 4: Conclude individual bioequivalence and the α significance level if $T_L > t(\alpha, \text{NC}, n_1 + n_2 - 2)\}$ and $T_U < -t(\alpha, \text{NC}, n_1 + n_2 - 2)$.

Example 12.4.2

We use the log-AUC data from Albert and Smith (1980) to illustrate the above parametric procedure for hypothesis 12.4.1. It is easy to verify that $\overline{Y}_T - \overline{Y}_R = 0.05331$ and $v(\overline{Y}_T - \overline{Y}_R) = 0.07819$. If we choose $-r = \ln(1.25) = 0.2231$, then $T_L = 3.1260$ and $T_U = -1.9202$. It follows that two formulations are average bioequivalent at the 5% significance level because $t(0.05, 18) = 1.7341$.

On the other hand, two formulations can be concluded individual bioequivalent if for at least 75% of the population two formulations are bioequivalent. Then we test whether the upper (or lower) 12.5% quantile of the subject-specific mean differences is not larger (or smaller) than 0.2231 (or −0.2231). The noncentrality parameter corresponding to the 12.5% upper quantile is equal to $\sqrt{2}z(0.125)/\sqrt{10} = 5.1445$. The critical value for the 5% significance level given in Table 12.4.5 is 7.9252. Because $T_L = 3.1260 < 7.9252$ and $T_U = -1.9202 > -7.9252$. Two formulations cannot be concluded individual bioequivalent at the 5% significance level. If the true P_{TIER} is assumed to be 0.90 for the alternative hypothesis 12.4.1 and MINP is set at 0.75 for the null hypothesis 12.4.1, from Table 12.4.6, 30 subjects are required to provide 80% power for the replicated crossover design employed by Albert and

TABLE 12.4.6: Total number of subjects required for individual bioequivalence using tolerance interval approach for $r = \log 1.33 = 0.2877$.

			$\pi = 0.75$		$\pi = 0.80$	
Design	$\mu_T - \mu_R$	**CV**	$\alpha = 0.05$	$\alpha = 0.10$	$\alpha = 0.05$	$\alpha = 0.10$
2 × 2	log0.95	10	18	13	30	21
		12	50	34	210	135
		14	827	158	—	—
		16	—	—	—	—
	0	10	10	7	13	10
		12	17	12	27	19
		14	36	25	100	66
		16	145	94	—	—
		18	—	—	—	—
2 × 4	log0.95	10	7	6	9	7
		12	11	8	14	10
		14	17	12	28	19
		16	32	22	80	53
		18	88	58	—	849
		20	—	—	—	—
	0	10	6	5	7	5
		12	7	6	9	7
		14	10	7	13	9
		16	14	10	20	14
		18	21	15	37	26
		20	37	26	108	71
		22	89	59	—	871
		24	491	310	—	—
		26	—	—	—	—

Source: From Esinhart, J.D. and Chinchilli, V.M., *Int. J. Clin. Pharmacol. Ther.*, 32, 26, 1994b.

Note: — denotes that the required sample size is either greater than 1000 or does not exist.

Smith. For comparison, 20 subjects are needed to achieve the same power for average bioequivalence under the same design.

12.4.3 Algorithm Based on Tolerance Interval

The parametric procedure introduced by Liu and Chow (1997b) is to test, at the 5% risk of type I error, whether P_{TR} is greater than MINP $= \pi$ as stated in hypothesis 12.4.3. On the other hand, Esinhart and Chinchilli (1994a,b) suggest use of a tolerance interval for evaluation based on P_{TR}. A *tolerance interval* is defined as the interval that will contain $100\pi\%$ of the intra-subject differences $Y_{iT} - Y_{iR}$ in the population with probability $100(1-\alpha)\%$. For P_{TR}, MINP in hypothesis 12.4.3 and at the α significance level, the interval $(L_{\text{T}}, U_{\text{T}})$ is said to be a $100(1-\alpha)\%$ tolerance interval of $100\pi\%$ of the distribution of $Y_{i\text{T}} - Y_{i\text{R}}$ if

$$P\{F(U_{\text{T}}) - F(L_{\text{T}}) \geq 100\pi\%\} \geq 100(1-\alpha)\%, \qquad (12.4.10)$$

where $F(\cdot)$ is the distribution function of $Y_{i\text{T}} - Y_{i\text{R}}$.

Under normality assumption, the inequality of Equation 12.4.10 becomes

$$P\{\Phi(U_{\text{T}}) - \Phi(L_{\text{T}}) \geq 100\pi\%\} \geq 100(1-\alpha)\%, \qquad (12.4.10)$$

where $\Phi(\cdot)$ is the cumulative distribution function of a normal distribution with mean $E(Y_{i\text{T}} - Y_{i\text{R}})$ and variance $V(Y_{i\text{T}} - Y_{i\text{R}})$.

Note that $\Phi(U_{\text{T}}) - \Phi(L_{\text{T}}) \geq 100\pi\%$ if and only if $L_{\text{T}} \geq -r$ and $U_{\text{T}} < r$. In addition, the tolerance interval has an interpretation similar to the confidence interval. Suppose that the same bioequivalence studies are repeated independently B times. As a result, B tolerance intervals can be computed. When B becomes larger and larger, at least $100(1-\alpha)\%$ of the B tolerance intervals will cover at least $100\pi\%$ of the distribution of $(Y_{i\text{T}} - Y_{i\text{R}})$. It follows that individual bioequivalence between the test and reference formulations is concluded at the $100(1-\alpha)\%$ level of confidence if the resulting tolerance interval is completely contained within $-r$ and r.

Although there are distribution-free tolerance procedures, they are too conservative to apply to the bioequivalence studies with a usual sample size ranging from 18 to 40 (Esinhart and Chinchilli, 1994a). Hence, only the parametric tolerance interval approach under normality assumption proposed by Esinhart and Chinchilli (1994a,b) is presented here.

Step 1. For each subject, compute the differences in subject-specific sample means between the test and reference formulations.

Step 2. Based on the intra-subject differences, use the estimation procedure described in Section 12.2 to find the least squares estimator for $\mu_{\text{T}} - \mu_{\text{R}}$, $\overline{Y}_{\text{T}} - \overline{Y}_{\text{R}}$, and its standard error denoted by s.

Step 3. Find the root, k_1 by iteratively solving the following equation:

$$\Phi\left(\sqrt{N} + k_1\right) - \Phi\left(\sqrt{N} - k_1\right) = \pi. \qquad (12.4.11)$$

Compute $k_2 = \sqrt{\text{df}/\chi^2(1-\alpha, \text{df})}$, where df is the degrees of freedom associated with s.

Step 4. The upper and lower limits for the $100(1-\alpha)\%$ tolerance interval of $100\pi\%$ of the distribution of $Y_{i\text{T}} - Y_{i\text{R}}$ is given as

$$L_{\text{T}}(U_{\text{T}}) = (\overline{Y}_{\text{T}} - \overline{Y}_{\text{R}}) + cs, \qquad (12.4.12)$$

where $c = k_1k_2$.

Step 5. Two formulations are concluded individual bioequivalent with $(1-\alpha)100\%$ level of confidence if (L_T, U_T) is completely contained within $(-r, r)$.

Given r, $\mu_T - \mu_R$, its standard error, π, and α, Esinhart and Chinchilli (1994b) demonstrate that sample sizes for the $(1-\alpha)100\%$ tolerance interval of $100\pi\%$ of the distribution can be determined by iteratively solving k_1, k_2, and c. Table 12.4.6 provides sample sizes for some selected combinations of r, $\mu_T - \mu_R$, coefficient of variation π, α, and designs. From Table 12.4.6, the required sample sizes increase rapidly after coefficient of variation reaches a moderate size of 16%. When the coefficient of variation goes beyond 24%, the required sample size is either over 1000 or does not even exist.

Example 12.4.3

The log-AUC data of verapamil given in Table 12.3.3 are used to illustrate the tolerance interval approach for evaluation of individual bioequivalence. Recall that a four-sequence and four-period crossover design (TRTR, RTRT, TRRT, RTTR) was employed to compare two formulations of verapamil in 23 subjects. The least-squares estimate for $\mu_T - \mu_R$ is -0.020, and its standard error is 0.051, with 19 degrees of freedom. For $\pi = 0.75$ and $1-\alpha = 0.95$, it can be easily verified that $k_1 = 1.1730$ and $k_2 = \sqrt{19/10.1170} = 1.3704$. It is estimated that 75% of the differences in subject-specific averages at the 95% confidence level lie between -0.1020 and 0.06201 on the log-scale or between 90.3% and 106.4% on the original scale. If r is selected $\ln(1.33) = 0.2877$, then two formulations are indeed individual bioequivalent at the 95% level of confidence.

12.4.4 Algorithm for P_d

As mentioned in Chapter 11, the probability-based criteria can be expressed in terms of either the difference or ratio of P_{TR} and P_{RR}. Under the normality assumption, P_{RR} is a constant. The inference for P_d or P_r reduces to that for P_{TR}. On the other hand, for the nonparametric approach, because the procedures for P_d and P_r are quite similar, here we focus only on the statistical inference for P_d. In addition, except under the strict normality assumption that $\sigma_D^2 = 0$ and $\sigma_{WT}^2 = \sigma_{WR}^2$, analytical results for the inference of P_d are complicated and not yet available, assessment of individual bioequivalence based on P_d has to rely on bootstrap procedures.

Again the bioavailability responses from Design A1 is used for illustration of the procedures proposed by Schall and Luus (1993) and Schall (1995). The stratified bootstrap resampling by sequence will be used. The distribution-free procedure is presented first.

Step 1. Determine r in P_{TR} of Equation 11.5.3 and P_{RR} of Equation 11.5.4 and the equivalence limit. Schall and Luus (1993) selected a value of $r = \log 1.25 = 0.2231$ for their example. On the other hand, Schall (1995) suggested that r should be selected according to the magnitude of the reference intra-subject variability by $r = c\sqrt{2}\sigma_{WR}$. A value of c of 1 is used for the numerical example in Schall (1995).

Step 2. Bootstrap resampling is stratified by sequence. Generate bootstrap samples ($y^*_{iT11}, y^*_{iR11}, y^*_{iT12}, y^*_{iR12}$) by sampling with replacement for n_1 vectors of the four observed pharmacokinetic responses ($y_{iT11}, y_{iR11}, y_{iT12}, y_{iR12}$) in sequence 1. Generate bootstrap samples ($y^*_{iR21}, y^*_{iT21}, y^*_{iR22}, y^*_{iT22}$) by sampling with replacement from n_2 vectors of the four observed pharmacokinetic responses ($y_{iR21}, y_{iT21}, y_{iR22}, y_{iT22}$) in sequence 2.

Step 3. Situation a: r is a prespecified constant.

Use the data set of the bootstrap samples of estimate P_{TR} and P_{RR}, respectively, by the following formulas:

$$p^*_{TR} = (1/2)\sum(1/4n_k)\sum\sum I(|y^*_{iTkl} - y^*_{iRkl'}| < r) \quad \text{and}$$
$$p^*_{RR} = (1/2)\sum(1/n_k)\sum I(|y^*_{iRk1} - y^*_{iRk2}| < r), \tag{12.4.13}$$

where $I(\cdot)$ is an indicator function such that $I(\cdot) = 1$ if $|y^*_{iRk1} - y^*_{iRk2}| < r$; $= 0$ otherwise.

Situation b: $r = c\sqrt{2}\sigma_{WR}$

Use the original data set of estimate $\sqrt{2}\sigma_{WR}$ as

$$\sqrt{2}s_{WR} = \left\{(1/N)\sum\sum(y_{iRk1} - y_{iRk2})^2\right\}^{1/2}.$$

Then estimate P_{TR} and P_{RR}, respectively, as

$$p^*_{TR} = (1/2)\sum(1/4n_k)\sum\sum I\left(|y^*_{iTkl} - y^*_{iRkl'}| < c\sqrt{2}s_{WR}\right) \quad \text{and}$$
$$p^*_{RR} = (1/2)\sum(1/n_k)\sum I\left(|y^*_{iRk1} - y^*_{iRk2}| < c\sqrt{2}s_{WR}\right). \tag{12.4.13}$$

Step 4. Obtain the estimate of P_d as $p^*_d = p^*_{TR} - p^*_{RR}$.

Step 5. Repeat steps 2 and 3 a large number of times, say at least 1000 times.

Step 6. Method a: nonparametric percentile method.

The $100(1-\alpha)\%$ lower confidence limit of P_d is obtained as the $100\alpha\%$ quantile of the B bootstrap value of p^*_d.

Method b: Bias-corrected accelerated method

Let q be the proportion of the bootstrap values of p^*_d smaller than the observed value of p_d computed from the original data set. The $100(1-\alpha)\%$ lower confidence limit of P_d is obtained as

$100\Phi[-z(\alpha)+2z(1-q)]\%$ quantile of the B bootstrap values of p_d^*, where $z(a)$ is the ath upper quantile of a standard normal distribution.

Step 7. Conclude that two formulations are individual bioequivalent at the α significance level if the resulting $100(1-\alpha)\%$ lower confidence limit is larger than the prespecified equivalence limit.

Under the normality assumption, because P_{RR} is a constant, evaluation of individual bioequivalence is performed by the bootstrap procedure based only on P_{TR}, which is given as

$$P_{TR}=\Phi\left\{[\theta+c\sqrt{2}\sigma_{WR}]/\sqrt{\sigma_D^2+\sigma_{WT}^2+\sigma_{WR}^2}\right\} \\ -\Phi\left\{[\theta+c\sqrt{2}\sigma_{WR}]/\sqrt{\sigma_D^2+\sigma_{WT}^2+\sigma_{WR}^2}\right\}, \quad (12.4.14)$$

where $\theta=\mu_T-\mu_R$ and $\Phi(\cdot)$ is the cumulative distribution function of a standard normal distribution.

Schall (1995) suggested use of the analysis of variance with formulation and period effects as fixed effects, and subject and subject-by-formulation interaction as random effects for estimation of θ, σ_{WR}^2, and $\sigma_D^2+\sigma_{WT}^2+\sigma_{WR}^2$. A consistent estimate of P_{TR} can be obtained by substituting their sample estimators of θ, σ_{WR}^2, and $\sigma_D^2+\sigma_{WT}^2+\sigma_{WR}^2$ in Equation 12.4.14. Note that these estimators can also be obtained by the procedures described in Section 12.2. The parametric procedure is given as follows:

Step 1. Determine c in $r=\sqrt{2}\sigma_{WR}$ of P_{TR} of Equation 11.5.3 and the equivalence limit. Compute p_{TR} according to Equation 12.4.14 using the original data set.

Step 2. Bootstrap resampling is stratified by sequence. Generate bootstrap samples $(y_{iT11}^*, y_{iR11}^*, y_{iT12}^*, y_{iR12}^*)$ by sampling with replacement from n_1 vectors of the four observed pharmacokinetic responses $(y_{iT11}, y_{iR11}, y_{iT12}, y_{iR12})$ in sequence 1. Generate bootstrap samples $(y_{iR21}^*, y_{iT21}^*, y_{iR22}^*, y_{iT22}^*)$ by sampling with replacement from n_2 vectors of the four observed pharmacokinetic responses $(y_{iR21}, y_{iT21}, y_{iR22}, y_{iT22})$ in sequence 2.

Step 3. Use the bootstrap data set to compute p_{TR}^* according to Equation 12.4.14.

Step 4. Repeat steps 2 and 3 a large number of times, say 1000 times.

Step 5. Use either nonparametric percentile or bias-corrected accelerated methods described in step 6 for distribution-free procedure to obtain the $100(1-\alpha)\%$ lower confidence limit of P_{TR}.

Step 6. Conclude that two formulations are individual bioequivalent at the α significance level if the resulting $100(1-\alpha)\%$ lower confidence limit is larger than the prespecified MINP.

Example 12.4.4

Schall and Luus (1993) considered the logarithmic transformation of AUC data from a bioequivalence study using a randomized three-period crossover design in which 24 subjects received a reference formulation twice and one of its generic copy once. This product is a combined drug that contains active ingredients: paracetamol and phenylpropanolamine. The value of r was selected either as $\log 1.25=0.2231$ or $\sqrt{2}\sigma_{WR}$. The results are presented in Table 12.4.7. From the original data set in Schall and Luus (1993), the reference intra-subject variability, σ_{WR}, of paracetamol and phenylpropanolamine are 0.0866 and 0.1245, respectively. It follows that r is approximately 0.1247 and 0.1761 for paracetamol and phenylpropanolamine, respectively. The estimated P_{TR} and P_{RR} with $r=0.2231$ are larger than those estimated with $r=\sqrt{2}\sigma_{WR}$. However, the point estimates of P_d by both values are quite close. On the other hand, the 95% lower confidence limits for P_d obtained with $r=\sqrt{2}\sigma_{WR}$ is smaller than those with $r=\log 1.25$.

For the purpose of illustration, we declare the two formulations individual bioequivalent if P_{TR} is not smaller than 20% below P_{RR}. In other words, the equivalence limit based on P_d is selected as −20%. It follows that for active ingredient paracetamol, two formulations can be claimed individual bioequivalent at the 5% significance level by the distribution-free procedure with $r=0.2231$ because an estimated 95% lower confidence limit of −13% is greater than −20%. However if r is chose to be $\sqrt{2}\sigma_{WR}$, then two formulations are not individual

TABLE 12.4.7: Summary of evaluation of individual bioequivalence of paracetamol and phenylpropanolamine based on probability-based criteria.

Method	Parameter	Paracetamol	Phenylpropanolamine
Distribution-free			
$R=\log 1.25$	P_{TR}	0.89	0.74
	P_{RR}	0.91	0.78
	P_d	−0.02	−0.04
	95% lower CL	−0.13	−0.22
$r=\sqrt{2}\sigma_{WR}$	P_{TR}	0.67	0.63
	P_{RR}	0.69	0.65
	P_d	−0.02	−0.02
	95% lower CL	−0.24	−0.30
Parametric			
$r=\sqrt{2}\sigma_{WR}$	P_{TR}	0.60	0.62
	95% lower CL	0.44	0.48

Source: From Schall, R. and Luus, H.G., *Stat. Med.*, 12, 1109, 1993; Schall, R., *Biometrics*, 51, 615, 1995.

bioequivalent. For phenylpropanolamine, two formulations are not individual bioequivalent by either value of r. For the parametric procedure, the point estimates and 95% lower confidence limits for P_{TR} are 60% and 62%, 44% and 48%, respectively, for both active ingredients. Note that the point estimates of P_{TR} are smaller than 75%. As a result, according to 75/75 rule, MINP is selected as 75%, then for both ingredients, the two formulations are not individual bioequivalent. For example, the parametric method seems more conservative than the distribution-free method.

12.5 Generalized *p*–Values for Evaluation of Population Bioequivalence

For most of the aggregate criteria in Table 15.1.1, bootstrap procedures were proposed due to analytic difficulty arising from the presence of the nuisance parameters in these criteria, see Schall and Luus (1993) for M_{I1} and Sheiner (1992) for M_{I2}. In Section 12.3, the statistical procedures for constructing a MLS $100(1-\alpha)\%$ upper confidence limit for the linearized version of M_{I3} were reviewed. However, it is still a large-sample method. As a result, McNally et al. (2003) proposed to apply the technique of generalized p-values for the exact inference of individual bioequivalence based on M_{I3}. The generalized p-value is defined in terms of generalized test variable (GTV) through generalized pivotal quantities (GPQs) proposed by Tsui and Weerahandi (1989), and Weerahandi (1995). We first provide a brief introduction to the GTV and generalized p-values.

Suppose that $\mathbf{X}$ is a random variable whose distribution depends on a vector of unknown parameters $\boldsymbol{\zeta} = (\lambda, \boldsymbol{\upsilon})$, where λ is a scalar parameter of interest and $\boldsymbol{\upsilon}$ is a vector of nuisance parameters. For M_{I3}, $\lambda = M_{I3}$ and $\boldsymbol{\upsilon} = (\theta, \sigma_I^2, \sigma_{WT}^2, \sigma_{WR}^2)'$. Let $\mathbf{x}$ be the observed value of $\mathbf{X}$. A test variable $T(\mathbf{X}; \mathbf{x}, \boldsymbol{\zeta})$ is said to be a generalized test variable if it satisfies the following three properties:

Property A: $T(\mathbf{X}; \mathbf{x}, \boldsymbol{\zeta})$ is free of unknown parameters.

Property B: For fixed $\mathbf{x}$ and $\boldsymbol{\zeta}$, the distribution of $T(\mathbf{X}; \mathbf{x}, \boldsymbol{\zeta})$ does not depend on nuisance parameters, $\boldsymbol{\upsilon}$.

Property C: For fixed $\mathbf{x}$ and $\boldsymbol{\zeta}$, $\Pr\{T(\mathbf{X}; \mathbf{x}, \boldsymbol{\zeta}) \leq t(\lambda\}$ is monotonic in λ.

For hypothesis 12.3.1, the generalized p-value is defined as

$$p = \operatorname*{Sup}_{\lambda \geq \Delta_{I3}} \Pr[\mathrm{T}(\mathbf{X};\, \mathbf{x},\, \xi) \leq \mathrm{t}|\lambda]. \tag{12.4.15}$$

From property C, it can be shown that

$$p = \operatorname*{Sup}_{\lambda \geq \Delta_{I3}} \Pr[\mathrm{T}(\mathrm{X};\, \mathrm{x},\, \xi) \leq \mathrm{t}|\lambda] = \Pr\{\mathrm{T}(\mathrm{X};\, \mathrm{x},\, \zeta) \leq \mathrm{t}|\Delta_{I3}\}. \tag{12.4.16}$$

It follows from Property A and B that the generalized p-value is free of nuisance parameters and hence it can be calculated from the observed PK responses only.

The test formulation is claimed to be individually bioequivalent to the reference formulation at the α significance level if the generalized p-value in Equation 12.4.16 is less than α.

Again, the two-sequence and four-period replicated crossover design in which each subject receives the test and reference formulations twice is used to illustrate the procedures. The method presented below can be directly to other four-period replicated crossover designs with each formulation being administered to each subject twice in each sequence.

For the linearized version of M_{I3}, the parameters are θ, σ_I^2, σ_{WT}^2, and σ_{WR}^2 and their corresponding unbiased estimators are $\widehat{\theta}$, s_I^2, s_{WT}^2, and s_{WR}^2 given in Equation 12.3.11. Define

$$\begin{aligned}&\mathrm{SS_I} = (n_1+n_2-2)s_I^2,\ \mathrm{SS_{WT}} = (n_1+n_2-2)s_{WT}^2, \quad \text{and}\\ &\mathrm{SS_{WR}} = (n_1+n_2-2)s_{WR}^2.\end{aligned} \tag{12.4.17}$$

It can be easily verified that

$$\begin{aligned}Z_\theta &= \frac{\widehat{\theta}-\theta}{\frac{1}{2}\sqrt{\left(\frac{1}{n_1}+\frac{1}{n_2}\right)s_I^2}} = \frac{D-\theta}{\frac{1}{2}\sqrt{\left(\frac{1}{n_1}+\frac{1}{n_2}\right)s_I^2}} \sim N(0,1),\\ U_I &= \frac{\mathrm{SS_I}}{(n_1+n_2-2)\sigma_I^2} \sim \chi^2(n_1+n_2-2),\\ U_{WT} &= \frac{\mathrm{SS_{WT}}}{(n_1+n_2-2)\sigma_{WT}^2} \sim \chi^2(n_1+n_2-2),\end{aligned} \tag{12.4.18}$$

and

$$U_{WR} = \frac{\mathrm{SS_{WR}}}{(n_1+n_2-2)\sigma_{WR}^2} \sim \chi^2(n_1+n_2-2),$$

where $D = \widehat{\theta}$.

In addition, the set of random variables Z_θ, U_I, U_{WT}, and U_{WR} are mutually independent. As mentioned before, for M_{I3}, the parameters of interest are $|\theta|$, σ_I^2, σ_{WT}^2, and σ_{WR}^2. However, McNally et al. (2003) proposed an alternative set of parameters $\boldsymbol{v}^* = (\lambda, \sigma_I^2, \sigma_{WT}^2, \sigma_{WR}^2)$ which has a one-to-one correspondence with $\boldsymbol{v} = (|\theta|, \sigma_I^2, \sigma_{WT}^2, \sigma_{WR}^2)$. For the new parameterization, the parameter of interest is λ, and $(\sigma_I^2, \sigma_{WT}^2, \sigma_{WR}^2)$ is the vector of nuisance parameters. Note that

$$M_{I3} = \lambda = \left(\theta^2 + \sigma_D^2 + \sigma_{WT}^2 - \sigma_{WR}^2\right)/\max\left(\sigma_{WR}^2, \sigma_{WO}^2\right).$$

It follows that

$$\lambda \max\left(\sigma_{WR}^2, \sigma_{WO}^2\right) = \left(\theta^2 + \sigma_D^2 + \sigma_{WT}^2 - \sigma_{WR}^2\right) = \left(\theta^2 + \sigma_I^2 + \frac{1}{2}\sigma_{WT}^2 - \frac{3}{2}\sigma_{WR}^2\right),$$

and

$$\lambda \max\left(\sigma_{\mathrm{WR}}^2, \sigma_{\mathrm{WO}}^2\right) + \tfrac{3}{2}\sigma_{\mathrm{WR}}^2 = \theta^2 + \sigma_{\mathrm{I}}^2 + \tfrac{1}{2}\sigma_{\mathrm{WT}}^2.$$

As a result,

$$\frac{\lambda \max\left(\sigma_{\mathrm{WR}}^2, \sigma_{\mathrm{WO}}^2\right) + \tfrac{3}{2}\sigma_{\mathrm{WR}}^2}{\theta^2 + \sigma_{\mathrm{I}}^2 + \tfrac{1}{2}\sigma_{\mathrm{WT}}^2} = 1, \tag{12.4.19}$$

and the generalized test variable based on M_{13} for evaluation of individual bioequivalence constructed by McNally et al. (2003) is therefore given as

$$\begin{aligned} T(\mathbf{X};\mathbf{x},\boldsymbol{\zeta}) &= \frac{\lambda \max\left(\sigma_{\mathrm{WO}}^2, \dfrac{\mathrm{ss}_{\mathrm{WR}}}{\mathrm{SS}_{\mathrm{WR}}}\sigma_{\mathrm{WR}}^2\right) + 1.5\dfrac{\mathrm{ss}_{\mathrm{WR}}}{\mathrm{SS}_{\mathrm{WR}}}\sigma_{\mathrm{WR}}^2}{\left[d - \dfrac{(D-\theta)}{\sqrt{c^2\sigma_{\mathrm{I}}^2}}\sqrt{\left(c^2\sigma_{\mathrm{I}}^2\dfrac{\mathrm{ss}_{\mathrm{I}}}{\mathrm{SS}_{\mathrm{I}}}\right)}\right]^2 + \dfrac{\mathrm{ss}_{\mathrm{I}}}{\mathrm{SS}_{\mathrm{I}}}\sigma_{\mathrm{I}}^2 + 0.5\dfrac{\mathrm{ss}_{\mathrm{WT}}}{\mathrm{SS}_{\mathrm{WT}}}\sigma_{\mathrm{WT}}^2} \\ &= \frac{\lambda \max\left(\sigma_{\mathrm{WO}}^2, \dfrac{\mathrm{ss}_{\mathrm{WR}}}{U_{\mathrm{WR}}}\right) + 1.5\dfrac{\mathrm{ss}_{\mathrm{WR}}}{U_{\mathrm{WR}}}}{\left[d - Z_\theta\sqrt{\left(c^2\dfrac{\mathrm{ss}_{\mathrm{I}}}{U_{\mathrm{I}}}\right)}\right]^2 + \dfrac{\mathrm{ss}_{\mathrm{I}}}{U_{\mathrm{I}}} + 0.5\dfrac{\mathrm{ss}_{\mathrm{WT}}}{U_{\mathrm{WT}}}}, \end{aligned} \tag{12.4.20}$$

where $c^2 = \dfrac{1}{4}\left(\dfrac{1}{n_1} + \dfrac{1}{n_2}\right)$

In Equation 12.4.18, d, ss_{I}, $\mathrm{ss}_{\mathrm{WT}}$, and $\mathrm{ss}_{\mathrm{WR}}$ are the observed values of random variables D, SS_{I}, $\mathrm{SS}_{\mathrm{WT}}$, and $\mathrm{SS}_{\mathrm{WR}}$ defined in Equation 12.4.18, respectively. Once the observed values of these random variables are obtained, they are considered as known constants. It follows that $\mathrm{T}(\mathbf{X};\mathbf{x},\boldsymbol{\zeta})$ is free of all nuisance parameters. Furthermore, when D, SS_{I}, $\mathrm{SS}_{\mathrm{WT}}$, and $\mathrm{SS}_{\mathrm{WR}}$ are set to equal to their corresponding observed values. $\mathrm{T}(\mathbf{x};\mathbf{x},\boldsymbol{\zeta}) = 1$ and is free of $\boldsymbol{\upsilon}$. Except for λ, all quantities in Equation 12.4.20 are positive. The generalized test variable defined in Equation 12.4.20 is an increasing function of the parameter of interest λ. It follows that $\mathrm{T}(\mathbf{X};\mathbf{x},\boldsymbol{\zeta})$ satisfies Property A to C and it is indeed a generalized test variable. When $\lambda = \Delta_{13}$, the generalized test variable in Equation 12.4.20 becomes

$$T_{\Delta_{13}}(\mathbf{X};\mathbf{x},\boldsymbol{\zeta}) = \frac{\Delta_{13} \max\left(\sigma_{\mathrm{WO}}^2, \dfrac{\mathrm{ss}_{\mathrm{WR}}}{U_{\mathrm{WR}}}\right) + 1.5\dfrac{\mathrm{ss}_{\mathrm{WR}}}{U_{\mathrm{WR}}}}{\left[d - Z_\theta\sqrt{\left(c^2\dfrac{\mathrm{ss}_{\mathrm{I}}}{U_{\mathrm{I}}}\right)}\right]^2 + \dfrac{\mathrm{ss}_{\mathrm{I}}}{U_{\mathrm{I}}} + 0.5\dfrac{\mathrm{ss}_{\mathrm{WT}}}{U_{\mathrm{WT}}}}. \tag{12.4.21}$$

As a result, the generalized p-value based on the generalized test variable for M_{I3} for evaluation of individual bioequivalence is given as

$$\begin{aligned} p\text{-value} &= \Pr[T(X;x,\zeta) < 1 | \lambda = \Delta_{I3}] \\ &= \Pr[T_{\Delta_B}(X;x,\zeta) < 1]. \end{aligned} \tag{12.4.22}$$

For testing hypothesis of individual equivalence, the following Monte-Carlo procedure with the estimation method for determination of the appropriate scale for M_{I3} can be applied to compute the generalized p-value in Equation 12.4.21:

1. Obtain s_{WR}^2 in Equation 12.3.11. If $s_{WR}^2 < \sigma_{WR}^2$, then the constant-scaled criterion of M_{I3} is used. Otherwise, use the reference-scaled criterion.
2. Compute the observed values of D, SS_I, SS_{WT}, and SS_{WR}.
3. Determine the number of simulations, for example, say $M = 10{,}000$. For $1 \leq M \leq 10{,}000$, generate mutually independent chi-square random variables, U_{WT}, and U_{WR} with degrees of freedom $n_1 + n_2 - 2$ and the standard normal deviates Z_θ.
4. Compute the generalized test variable in Equation 12.4.21.
5. Then the generalized p-value is estimated as the proportion that $T_{\Delta_{I3}}(X;x,\zeta) < 1$. In other words,

$$\text{Estimated generalized } p\text{-value} = \frac{1}{M}\sum_{m=1}^{M} I(T_{\Delta_{I3}}(X;x,\zeta) < 1) \tag{12.4.23}$$

McNally et al. (2003) report that the standard error of generalized p-value for a Monte Carlo simulation with a size of 10,000 is approximated 0.2%. If the sample size increases to 100,000, then the standard error can reduce to 0.05%. Hence, we suggest that a sample size of at least 10,000 be required for estimating the generalized p-value for inference of individual bioequivalence based on M_{I3}.

Example 12.5.1

The data set of the AUC of verapamil in a four-sequence and four-period crossover design with 23 normal volunteers is again elected to illustrate the application of generalized p-value to assessing individual bioequivalence. Recall that the point estimators of θ, σ_I^2, σ_{WT}^2, and σ_{WR}^2 are $\hat{\theta} = -0.0196$, $s_I^2 = 0.05924$, $s_{WT}^2 = 0.1271$, and $s_{WR}^2 = 0.0745$, respectively. Hence, the observed values of D, SS_I, SS_{WT}, and SS_{WR} are $d = -0.0196$, $ss_I = 1.4155$, $ss_{WT} = 2.4156$, and $ss_{WR} = 1.1256$, respectively. Because $s_{WR} = 0.2729 > 0.2$, the reference-scaled criterion of M_{I3} is applied with $\Delta_{I3} = 2.4948$. It follows that

$$T_{\Delta_{I3}}(\mathbf{X};\mathbf{x},\zeta) = \frac{2.4948\dfrac{1.4155}{U_{WR}} + 1.5\dfrac{1.4155}{U_{WR}}}{\left[-0.0196 - Z_\theta\sqrt{\left(0.04375\dfrac{1.1256}{U_I}\right)}\right]^2 + \dfrac{1.1256}{U_I} + 0.5\dfrac{2.4156}{U_{WT}}}. \tag{12.4.24}$$

The Monte Carlo procedure described above was applied with a sample of 20,000. For each sample, the standard normal deviates, chi-square random variables U_{WT}, U_{WR}, and U_I were generated to compute the generalized test variable $T(\mathbf{X}; \mathbf{x}, \zeta)$ in Equation 12.4.24. Then the generalized p-value is estimated as the proportion of the generalized test variable being less than 1 which is 0.0186 with a 95% confidence interval (0.0167, 0.0205). Because the generalized p-value is smaller than 0.05, the test formulation of verapamil is individual bioequivalent to the reference formulation at the 5% significance level.

12.6 Discussion

In addition to average, subject-by-formulation interaction and intra-subject variability are required to assess the individual bioequivalence. Total variance is also needed to evaluate the population bioequivalence. However, different criteria are proposed based on different presentations of statistical results or on different combinations of these characteristics. As indicated above, these criteria can be classified into moment-based or probability-based criteria. Furthermore, they can be grouped as aggregate or disaggregate criteria. Various statistical procedures for evaluation of population and individual bioequivalence, therefore, are presented in this chapter. However, currently, there is no comprehensive evaluation of direct comparisons of these criteria and their corresponding statistical procedures.

For the aggregate criterion M_{I3}, the reference- or constant-scaled version is determined by whether the value of estimated σ^2_{WR} from the original data set is greater than $\sigma^2_{W0} = 0.04$. However, s^2_{WR} being greater than 0.04 does not prove that the unknown reference intra-subject variability, σ^2_{WR}, is also greater than 0.04. As a result, the selection of the reference- or constant-scaled version of M_{I3} should be determined by the following hypothesis:

$$\begin{aligned} &H_0\colon\ \sigma^2_{WR} \le \sigma^2_{W0} \\ \text{versus}\quad &H_a\colon\ \sigma^2_{WR} > \sigma^2_{W0}. \end{aligned} \tag{12.4.25}$$

The standard chi-square test based on s^2_{WR} from the original data set can be used to test hypothesis 12.4.25. If the null hypothesis 12.4.25 is rejected at the 5% significance level, then the reference-scaled version of M_{I3} is selected for the all subsequent bootstrap samples. Otherwise, the constant-scaled version is used. The above method is referred to as the test approach by Chow et al. (2003a). The simulation results reported by Chow et al. (2003a) indicated that the test method is conservative when the true intra-subject variability of the reference formulation is less than 0.15. However, the test approach performs better than the estimation method when the reference intra-subject variability is close to 0.2.

For the linearized version of M_{I3}, Chow et al. (2003a) proposed a method for the sample size determination based on the MLS method. The required sample size for the reference-scaled criterion to achieve a $1-\beta$ power is the smallest integer satisfying the following inequality:

TABLE 12.6.1: Size for M_{I3} based on bootstrap procedure.

					Size	
θ	σ^2_{WR}	σ^2_{WT}	σ^2_{D}	M_{I3}	Est.	Test
0.2231	0.01	0.03	0.02	2.25	0.015	0.015
−0.2231	0.01	0.03	0.02	2.25	0.017	0.015
0.2231	0.04	0.06	0.02	2.25	0.039	0.052
−0.2231	0.04	0.06	0.02	2.25	0.026	0.038

Note: Est.: the selection of scale for M_{I3} for bootstrap is determined by the estimate of σ^2_{WR} from the original data set; Test: the selection of scale for M_{I3} for bootstrap is determined by the result of hypothesis testing for Equation 12.4.25 based on the original data set.

$$A + \sqrt{B} + \sqrt{B_\beta}, \tag{12.4.26}$$

where B_β is defined same as B except that α and $1 - \alpha$ are replaced by $1 - \beta$ and β, respectively.

Tables 12.6.1 and 12.6.2 provide the simulation results on the size and power for some selected combinations of θ, σ^2_{WR}, σ^2_{WT}, and σ^2_D based on the bootstrap procedure for M_{I3}, respectively. For the size, the individual bioequivalence limit of 2.25 is used with σ^2_D being set as 0.02. Two thousand bootstrap samples were resampled from each of 1000 randomly simulated samples. From Table 12.6.1, the results also indicate that when the reference intra-subject variability is equal to 0.04, the test method provides a size much closer to the nominal level of 0.05 than the estimation method. However, for both test and estimation methods, with the same value of M_{I3} being 2.25, because of different configurations of the values of θ, σ^2_{WR}, σ^2_{WT}, and σ^2_D, the size ranges from 0.015 to 0.052. The same phenomenon can also be observed from the simulated power presented in Table 12.6.2. From $M_{I3} = 0.5$, the power of the estimation method ranges from 0.718 to 0.936. For the test method, it is from 0.502 to 0.973. In addition, for both procedures, Table 12.6.2 shows that the

TABLE 12.6.2: Power for M_{I3} based on bootstrap procedure.

					Power	
θ	σ^2_{WR}	σ^2_{WT}	σ^2_{D}	M_{I3}	Est.	Test
0	0.08	0.09	0.01	0.25	0.718	0.502
0.005	0.08	0.09	0.05	0.25	0.776	0.552
0.01	0.08	0.09	0	0.5	0.798	0.634
0	0.04	0.05	0.01	0.5	0.799	0.874
0.005	0.04	0.05	0.005	0.5	0.866	0.904
0.01	0.04	0.05	0	0.5	0.936	0.973

Note: Est.: the selection of scale for M_{I3} for bootstrap is determined by the estimate of σ^2_{WR} from the original data set; Test: the selection of scale for M_{I3} for bootstrap is determined by the result of hypothesis testing for Equation 12.4.25 based on the original data set.

powers at $M_{I3} = 0.25$ are less than those at $M_{I3} = 0.50$. Therefore, Tables 12.6.1 and 12.6.2 provide some very disturbing observations. First, at the same value of M_{I3}, the size and power can vary. Secondly, for hypothesis 12.3.1, we would expect that the power function is a deceasing function of M_{I3}. However, the simulation results given in Table 12.6.2 show the contrary. These undesirable properties hinder the implementation of the individual bioequivalence.

Because of the intrigue nature of the aggregate criteria and challenges of statistical inference, there was an explosion of papers in literature between 1992 that Sheiner (1992) presented the concept of individual bioequivalence and 2003 when the U.S. FDA published its guidance on general considerations for bioequivalence. Although the concept of individual bioequivalence is sound, its implementation into regulatory practice was not successful yet. The first reason is the clinical and pharmacokinetic interpretation of the aggregate criteria. It is quite clear about the meaning of the average bioequivalence limit of 0.80 and 1.25 on the original scale. However, nobody knows what an individual bioequivalence limit of 2.4948 actually means and how to interpret it clinically and pharmaceutically on the original scale. Second, due to the masking effects and presence of nuisance parameters, statistical procedures for inference of individual bioequivalence based on aggregate criteria present some serious undesirable and disturbing properties as discussed above. Therefore, after sedimentation over a 10-year period, the U.S. FDA guidance on general considerations for bioequivalence (FDA, 2003), the EMEA guidance on bioequivalence (EMEA, 2001), and the WHO draft guidance on interchangeability multisource drugs (WHO, 2005) still only use the average bioequivalence for regulatory approval of generic or multisource drug products.

Although individual and population bioequivalence are still included in the U.S. FDA guidance on statistical approaches to establishing bioequivalence, due to difficulty experienced by the currently available aggregate criteria, we would recommend that any desirable criteria for evaluation of bioequivalence possess the following properties:

1. Evidence to justify replacement of the current average bioequivalence.
2. Meaningful interpretation of bioequivalence criteria and results on the original scale of pharmacokinetic responses.
3. No masking effect.
4. Availability of unbiased or asymptotically unbiased estimator of the proposed bioequivalence criterion with analytical results on bias.
5. Availability of the analytical results of the statistical properties for the procedures based on the proposed bioequivalence criteria.
6. Meaningful relationship between the power function and parameters in the bioequivalence criteria.
7. Robustness of the procedures.
8. Ability to search for the optimal design based on the procedure.
9. Ability to provide adequate procedures for outlier detection.

Part IV

In Vitro and Alternative Evaluation of Bioequivalence

Chapter 13

Assessment of Bioequivalence for Drugs with Negligible Plasma Levels

13.1 Introduction

In previous chapters, bioequivalence between formulations is evaluated based on pharmacokinetic responses, such as AUC, $C_{\max}$, and $T_{\max}$. These responses are usually determined from the blood or plasma concentration–time curve. For some drug products, however, we may have negligible plasma levels because of their intended routes of administration. These drug products include metered dose inhalers (MDIs), indicated for the relief of bronchospasm in patients with reversible obstructive airway disease; antiulcer agents, such as sucralfate; and topical and vaginal antifungals. Because these products have negligible plasma concentrations, pharmacokinetic responses are no longer adequate for assessment of bioequivalence between drug products. It is thus suggested that some other clinical endpoints be used to assess bioequivalence between drug products.

13.2 Design and Clinical Endpoints

In 1989, the FDA issued guidance for *in vivo* bioequivalence studies of metaproterenol sulfate and albuterol inhalation aerosols (i.e., MDI). In the FDA guidance, it is suggested that a four-sequencer, four-period, double-blind, randomized crossover design be used for comparing drug products with negligible plasma levels. The recommended design evaluates clinical endpoints of two products at two different dose levels. This design is summarized in Table 13.2.1. This design is of particular interest because it consists of two levels of crossover factors: the dose and the product. For the dose, we may classify the four sequences into two strata (e.g., sequences 1 and 2 to stratum 1, and sequences 3 and 4 to stratum 2) and the 4 days into two periods (e.g., days 1 and 2 to period I, and days 3 and 4 to period II). In this case, the design with albuterol MDI can be expressed as follows:

Stratum	Time Block I	Time Block II
1	90 μg	180 μg
2	180 μg	90 μg

The arrangement based on the dose is a standard two-sequence, two-period crossover design. The second level is the product. From the above, it can be seen that each combination of stratum and period (four in total) is also a standard 2 × 2 crossover design, in which the test and reference products are administered at the same dose level.

The advantage of inhalation therapy is that the active ingredient of the drug can be directly delivered to the site of action. In this case, a lower dose can be employed, and the risk of systematic adverse experiences can be minimized. However, as MDI products produce negligible plasma concentrations, the assessment of bioequivalence will have to be based on other meaningful clinical endpoints. Most clinical endpoints recommended by the FDA guidance are derived from the volume of air forced out of lung within 1 second (FEV_1), which is usually measured at 0, 10, 15, 30, 60, 90, 120, 180, 240, 300, and 360 minutes after dosing. For assessment of bioequivalence between MDI products, the FDA guidance requires that the following information obtained from FEV_1 be provided:

1. Onset of therapeutic response
2. Duration of therapeutic response
3. AUC from the onset of the response to hour 3 based on FEV_1–time curve
4. AUC from the onset of the response to the time of termination of the response based on FEV_1–time curve

TABLE 13.2.1: Design for assessment of bioequivalence for MDI products suggested by the FDA 1989 guidance.

Sequence	Day 1	Day 2	Day 3	Day 4
1	A	C	B	D
2	C	A	D	B
3	B	D	A	C
4	D	B	C	A

Formulation	Albuterol	Metaproterenol Sulfate
A	Generic 1 puff	Generic 2 puffs
B	Generic 2 puffs	Generic 3 puffs
C	Reference 1 puff	Reference 2 puffs
D	Reference 2 puffs	Reference 3 puffs
Dose	90 μg/puff	0.65 mg/puff

5. $FEV_{1\,max}$

6. T_{max}

7. FEV_1 at each point

A therapeutic response is defined to be the event such that the postdose FEV_1 measurement exceeds 115% of the baseline value. Onset of the response is the time within 30 minutes postdose when the event of a therapeutic response occurs. Time of onset of the response is calculated by linear interpolation between the first postdose FEV_1 exceeding 115% of the baseline value and the FEV_1 value immediately preceding. The termination of a therapeutic response is defined to be the occurrence of the event of two consecutive FEV_1 measurements falling below 115% of the baseline value before or at hour 6, provided that the event of a therapeutic response has occurred. The time of termination of response is estimated by linear interpolation between the last postdose FEV_1 value exceeding 115% and the first FEV_1 value below 115% after a therapeutic response has occurred. Therefore, the duration of the event of a therapeutic response is the time interval between onset and termination of the response. $FEV_{1\,max}$ and T_{max} can be computed from the FEV_1–time curve in the same way as C_{max} and T_{max} are computed from the plasma concentration–time curve.

13.3 Statistical Considerations

13.3.1 Continuous Endpoint

For each clinical endpoint, there are two major comparisons, which are (1) to assess bioequivalence between two products at each dose, and (2) to differentiate clinical response affected by a twofold difference in dose. In other words, statistical comparisons of interest are

1. Bioequivalence at 90 μg: treatment A versus treatment C

2. Bioequivalence at 180 μg: treatment B versus treatment D

3. Comparison between 90 μg and 180 μg for generic products: treatment A versus treatment B

4. Comparison between 90 μg and 180 μg for reference products: treatment C versus treatment D

For continuous variables such as AUC, under the assumption of normality and compound symmetry, analyses can be performed under model Equation 10.2.1. Table 13.3.1 gives the expected values of sequence-by-period means. The coefficients of linear contrasts of sequence-by-period means for the unbiased ordinary least squares (OLS) estimates of $\theta_{AC} = F_A - F_C$, $\theta_{BD} = F_B - F_D$, $B_A = F_B - F_A$, and $\theta_{DC} = F_D - F_C$ are given in Table 13.3.2 for the situation in which the carryover

TABLE 13.3.1: Expected values of sequence-by-period means for design in Table 13.2.1.

	Period			
Sequence	**I**	**II**	**III**	**IV**
1	$\mu + G_1 + P_1 + F_A$	$\mu + G_1 + P_2 + F_C + C_A$	$\mu + G_1 + P_3 + F_B + C_C$	$\mu + G_1 + P_4 + F_D + C_B$
2	$\mu + G_2 + P_1 + F_C$	$\mu + G_2 + P_2 + F_A + C_C$	$\mu + G_2 + P_3 + F_D + C_A$	$\mu + G_2 + P_4 + F_B + C_D$
3	$\mu + G_3 + P_1 + F_B$	$\mu + G_3 + P_2 + F_D + C_B$	$\mu + G_3 + P_3 + F_A + C_D$	$\mu + G_3 + P_4 + F_C + C_A$
4	$\mu + G_4 + P_1 + F_D$	$\mu + G_4 + P_2 + F_B + C_D$	$\mu + G_4 + P_3 + F_C + C_B$	$\mu + G_4 + P_4 + F_A + C_C$

effect is present. In the absence of carryover effect, the coefficients are listed in Table 13.3.3. From Table 13.3.2, when there are carryover effects, it can be seen that the variance of the unbiased OLS estimates for assessment of bioequivalence between two products is $(33\sigma_e^2)/(20n)$, which is three times as large as that for comparison between two doses of the same product. This is because the design is not a variance-balanced design in presence of the carryover effect. When there are no carryover effects, it can be seen from Table 13.3.3 that all OLS estimates have the same variance $\sigma_e^2/(2n)$, which is the same as the variance of the unbiased OLS estimates obtained from the Williams design with four formulations discussed in Chapter 10. Therefore, unless a sufficient length of washout (FDA guidance requires a washout no less than 24 hours between study days) is provided, the Williams design with four formulations is preferred because it provides a smaller (at least the same) variance of the unbiased OLS estimates with the same number of sequences and periods in the presence of carryover effects.

13.3.2 Binary Endpoint

A patient is considered to be a responder if his or her FEV_1 value exceeds 115% of the baseline value within 30 minutes after dosing. Thus, a therapeutic response is a binary endpoint (i.e., yes or no). Therefore, for a standard two-sequence (RT and TR), two-period crossover design, we only observe one of the following four possible outcomes on each patient: (N, N), (N, Y), (Y, N), and (Y, Y). Note that (N, Y) denotes that the patient does not respond to the drug at period I, but does respond in period II. Table 13.3.4 gives a summary of the response data from a standard 2×2 crossover design in terms of a 2×4 contingency table (observed counts). For example, n_{41} is the number of patients in sequence 1 who responded to the drug in both periods.

The objective of this section is to assess bioequivalence between two products based upon a 90% confidence interval for the ratio of the marginal probability of the response for the test product to that for the reference product after adjustment

TABLE 13.3.2: Coefficients for OLS estimates of pairwise formulation effects for design in Table 13.2.1 (adjusted for carryover effects).

I. Comparisons between Products at the Same Dose

	90 μg $\theta_{AC} = F_A - F_C$					**180 μg** $\theta_{BD} = F_B - F_D$				
	Period					**Period**				
Sequence	**1**	**2**	**3**	**4**	$\Sigma_j C^2_{ajk}$	**1**	**2**	**3**	**4**	$\Sigma_j C^2_{ajk}$
1	26	−8	−17	−1	$1030/(40)^2$	14	−2	−3	−9	$290/(40)^2$
2	−26	8	17	1	$1030/(40)^2$	−14	2	3	9	$290/(40)^2$
3	14	−2	−3	−9	$290/(40)^2$	26	−8	−17	−1	$1030/(40)^2$
4	−14	2	3	9	$290/(40)^2$	−26	8	17	1	$1030/(40)^2$
Variance[a]					$\frac{33}{20n}\sigma^2_e$					$\frac{33}{20n}\sigma^2_e$

II. Comparisons between Doses of the Same Product

	Generic $\theta_{BA} = F_B - F_A$					**Reference** $\theta_{DC} = F_D - F_C$				
	Period					**Period**				
Sequence	**1**	**2**	**3**	**4**	$\Sigma_j C^2_{ajk}$	**1**	**2**	**3**	**4**	$\Sigma_j C^2_{ajk}$
1	−12	−1	14	−1	$342/(40)^2$	0	−7	0	7	$98/(40)^2$
2	0	−7	0	7	$98/(40)^2$	−12	−1	14	−1	$342/(40)^2$
3	12	1	−14	1	$342/(40)^2$	0	7	0	−7	$98/(40)^2$
4	0	7	0	−7	$98/(40)^2$	12	1	−14	1	$342/(40)^2$
Variance[a]					$\frac{11}{20n}\sigma^2_e$					$\frac{11}{20n}\sigma^2_e$

Note: Coefficients are multiplied by 40.

[a] Variance when $n = n_k$ for $1 \le k \le 4$.

TABLE 13.3.3: Coefficients for OLS estimates of pairwise formulation effects for design in Table 13.2.1 (in absence of carryover effects).

I. Comparisons between Products at the Same Dose

	90 µg $\theta_{AC} = F_A - F_C$					180 µg $\theta_{BD} = F_B - F_D$				
	Period					Period				
Sequence	**1**	**2**	**3**	**4**	$\Sigma_j C^2_{ajk}$	**1**	**2**	**3**	**4**	$\Sigma_j C^2_{ajk}$
1	4	−4	0	0	$32/(16)^2$	0	0	4	−4	$32/(16)^2$
2	−4	4	0	0	$32/(16)^2$	0	0	−4	4	$32/(16)^2$
3	0	0	4	−4	$32/(16)^2$	4	−4	0	0	$32/(16)^2$
4	0	0	−4	4	$32/(16)^2$	−4	4	0	0	$32/(16)^2$
Variance[a]					$\frac{1}{2n}\sigma_e^2$					$\frac{1}{2n}\sigma_e^2$

II. Comparisons between Doses at the Same Product

	Generic $\theta_{BA} = F_B - F_A$					Reference $\theta_{DC} = F_D - F_C$				
	Period					Period				
Sequence	**1**	**2**	**3**	**4**	$\Sigma_j C^2_{ajk}$	**1**	**2**	**3**	**4**	$\Sigma_j C^2_{ajk}$
1	−4	0	4	0	$32/(16)^2$	0	−4	0	4	$32/(16)^2$
2	0	−4	0	4	$32/(16)^2$	−4	0	4	0	$32/(16)^2$
3	4	0	−4	0	$32/(16)^2$	0	4	0	−4	$32/(16)^2$
4	0	4	0	−4	$32/(16)^2$	4	0	−4	0	$32/(16)^2$
Variance[a]					$\frac{1}{2n}\sigma_e^2$					$\frac{1}{2n}\sigma_e^2$

Note: Coefficients are multiplied by 16.

[a] Variance when $n = n_k$ for $1 \leq k \leq 4$.

TABLE 13.3.4: Summary of response data for a standard 2 × 2 crossover design (observed counts by response).

	Outcome				
Sequence	**(N, N)**	**(N, Y)**	**(Y, N)**	**(Y, Y)**	**Total**
1 (RT)	n_{11}	n_{21}	n_{31}	n_{41}	$n_{\cdot 1}$
2 (TR)	n_{12}	n_{22}	n_{32}	n_{42}	$n_{\cdot 2}$
Total	$n_{1\cdot}$	$n_{2\cdot}$	$n_{3\cdot}$	$n_{4\cdot}$	$n_{\cdot\cdot}$

Source: From Liu, J.P. and Chow, S.C., *Biom. J.*, 35, 109, 1993.

for period effects. In the following sections, we introduce the following three model-based methods:

1. Weighted least squares (WLS) method (Koch and Edwards, 1988)
2. Log–linear model (Jones and Kenward, 2003)
3. Generalized estimating equations (GEEs) (Liang and Zeger, 1986)

Note that the above three methods are derived based on asymptotic results. To apply these methods, a total sample size of 40 patients, as suggested by the FDA guidance, might be large enough for MDI products. Let P_T and P_R denote the marginal probabilities of a therapeutic response of the test and reference formulations, respectively. Then, it is suggested that the decision rule for assessment of bioequivalence be based on a 90% confidence interval of $\delta = P_T/P_R$. Two products are considered to be bioequivalent if the 90% confidence interval of δ is within the prescribed limits (δ_L, δ_U) (Liu and Chow, 1993).

Similar to continuous data, estimation of direct formulation effect is not valid unless there are no unequal carryover effects (or direct formulation-by-period interaction) (Jones and Kenward, 2003). Therefore, a preliminary test for the presence of unequal carryover effects should be carried out before assessing bioequivalence. This can be done by simply performing the Fisher's exact test (Armitage and Berry, 1987) for association of the following 2 × 2 contingency table (Altham, 1971; Hills and Armitage, 1979; Jones and Kenward, 2003).

n_{11}	n_{41}
n_{12}	n_{42}

13.4 WLS Method

Define $\mathbf{P}_k = (P_{1k}, P_{2k}, P_{3k}, P_{4k})'$ as the 4 × 1 vector of probabilities corresponding to the four possible outcomes in sequence k, where P_{hk}, $h = 1, \ldots, 4$; $k = 1, 2$ are summarized in Table 13.4.1. Let $\mathbf{n}_k = (n_{1k}, n_{2k}, n_{3k}, n_{4k})'$ be the 4 × 1 vector of

TABLE 13.4.1: Summary of response data for a standard 2× 2 crossover design (probabilities by response).

Sequence	Outcome				Total
	(N, N)	(N, Y)	(Y, N)	(Y, Y)	
1 (RT)	P_{11}	P_{21}	P_{31}	P_{41}	1
2 (TR)	P_{12}	P_{22}	P_{32}	P_{42}	1
Total	$P_{1\cdot}$	$P_{2\cdot}$	$P_{3\cdot}$	$P_{4\cdot}$	—

Source: From Liu, J.P. and Chow, S.C., *Biom. J.*, 35, 109, 1993.

observed counts of the four possible outcomes in sequence k, where $k = 1, 2$. Then $\mathbf{n} = (\mathbf{n}_1, \mathbf{n}_2)'$ has a product multinomial distribution with parameter vector $\mathbf{P} = (\mathbf{P}_1, \mathbf{P}_2)'$ and $\mathbf{n}_1$ and $\mathbf{n}_2$ are independent. Let $\mathbf{p} = (\mathbf{p}_1, \mathbf{p}_2)'$ be the 8×1 vector of observed proportions of the four possible outcomes in both sequences, where

$$\mathbf{p}_k = (p_{1k}, p_{2k}, p_{3k}, p_{4k})',$$

$$p_{hk} = \frac{n_{hk}}{n_{\cdot k}},$$

and

$$n_{\cdot k} = \sum_{k=1}^{4} n_{hk}. \tag{13.4.1}$$

Then, $\mathbf{p}$ is an unbiased estimator of $\mathbf{P}$ whose covariance matrix is given by

$$\text{Var}(\mathbf{p}) = \begin{bmatrix} \mathbf{V}_1 & \mathbf{O}_{4\times 4} \\ \mathbf{O}_{4\times 4} & \mathbf{V}_2 \end{bmatrix}, \tag{13.4.2}$$

where

$$\mathbf{V}_k = \frac{1}{n_{\cdot k}}[\mathbf{D}(\mathbf{P}_k) - \mathbf{P}_k\mathbf{P}'_k], \tag{13.4.3}$$

and $\mathbf{D}(\mathbf{P}_k)$ is a 4×4 diagonal matrix with diagonal elements P_{1k}, P_{2k}, P_{3k}, and P_{4k}, where $k = 1.2$.

Let $\mathbf{g} = \mathbf{g}(\mathbf{p})$ be a $t \times 1$ vector of linear function $\mathbf{p}$, which can be expressed as

$$\mathbf{g}(\mathbf{p}) = \mathbf{C}\mathbf{p},$$

where $\mathbf{C}$ is a $t \times 8$ matrix with elements of each row corresponding to the coefficients of linear functions. A consistent estimator of the covariance matrix of $\mathbf{g}$ is then given by

$$V_g = \text{Var}(\mathbf{g}) = \mathbf{C}\,\widehat{\text{Var}}(\mathbf{p})\mathbf{C}', \tag{13.4.4}$$

where

$$\widehat{\text{Var}}(\mathbf{p}) = \begin{bmatrix} \frac{1}{n_{\cdot 1}}[\mathbf{D}(\mathbf{p}_1) - \mathbf{p}_1\mathbf{p}_1'] & \mathbf{O}_{4\times 4} \\ \mathbf{O}_{4\times 4} & \frac{1}{n_{\cdot 2}}[\mathbf{D}(\mathbf{p}_2) - \mathbf{p}_2\mathbf{p}_2'] \end{bmatrix}$$

is a consistent estimator of Var(**p**) in Equation 13.4.2.

If the total sample size is large enough such that **g** has approximately a multivariate normal distribution, then the formulation effect can estimated by fitting a linear model using WLS method. Suppose that we can express the expected value of **g** as a linear model given below

$$\mathbf{E(g)} = \mathbf{Z}\boldsymbol{\beta}, \tag{13.4.5}$$

where

$\mathbf{Z}$ is a $t \times m$ design matrix of full rank with $m \leq t$

$\boldsymbol{\beta}$ is a $m \times 1$ vector of parameters

The WLS estimator of $\boldsymbol{\beta}$ and its consistent estimate of the variance matrix are given by

$$\mathbf{b} = (\mathbf{Z}'\mathbf{V}_g^{-1}\mathbf{Z})^{-1}\mathbf{Z}'\mathbf{V}_g^{-1}\mathbf{g}, \tag{13.4.6}$$

and

$$\mathbf{V}_b = (\mathbf{Z}'\mathbf{V}_g^{-1}\mathbf{Z})^{-1}, \tag{13.4.7}$$

respectively.

The predicted values of **E(g)** are given by

$$\widehat{\mathbf{g}} = \mathbf{Zb}. \tag{13.4.8}$$

Hence, lack of fit of the model 13.4.5 can be evaluated by the Wald statistic, which has the form of residual chi-square with $t - m$ degrees of freedom, that is,

$$\begin{aligned} R_g &= (\mathbf{g} - \mathbf{Zb})'V_g^{-1}(\mathbf{g} - \mathbf{Zb}) \\ &= \mathbf{g}'V_g^{-1}\mathbf{g} - \widehat{\mathbf{g}}'V_g^{-1}\widehat{\mathbf{g}}. \end{aligned} \tag{13.4.9}$$

It should be noted that **g** is not restricted to the linear functions of **p**. However, for estimation of the formulation effect, which is expressed in terms of observed proportions of responses, we consider only linear functions of **p**.

As can be seen from Table 13.4.1, the marginal probability of the occurrence of a therapeutic response for test formulation in sequence 1 is the sum of observing a therapeutic response during period II in sequence 1. Other marginal probabilities by

TABLE 13.4.2: Marginal probabilities of a therapeutic response by sequence and drug product.

Sequence	Marginal Probability: Reference	Marginal Probability: Test
1 (RT)	$P_{1R} = P_{31} + P_{41}$	$P_{1T} = P_{21} + P_{41}$
2 (TR)	$P_{2R} = P_{22} + P_{42}$	$P_{2T} = P_{32} + P_{42}$
Total	$P_R = \frac{1}{2}(P_{1R} + P_{2R})$	$P_T = \frac{1}{2}(P_{1T} + P_{2T})$

Source: From Liu, J.P. and Chow, S.C., *Biom. J.*, 35, 109, 1993.

sequence and formulation can be similarly defined. Table 13.4.2 gives marginal probabilities of a therapeutic response by formulation. In this case, the matrix **C** in Equation 13.4.3 becomes

$$\mathbf{C} = \begin{bmatrix} \mathbf{A} & \mathbf{O}_{2\times 4} \\ \mathbf{O}_{2\times 4} & \mathbf{A} \end{bmatrix}, \tag{13.4.10}$$

where

$$\mathbf{A} = \begin{bmatrix} 0 & 0 & 1 & 1 \\ 0 & 1 & 0 & 1 \end{bmatrix}.$$

Hence, $\mathbf{g} = (p_{1R}, p_{1T}, p_{2T}, p_{2R})'$, where p_{hk} are obtained by replacing P_{hk} in Table 13.4.2 with p_{hk}, $h = 1, 2, 3, 4$, and $k = 1, 2$. Under condition of absence of unequal carryover effects, Koch and Edwards (1988) suggested the following linear model:

$$\mathbf{E}(\mathbf{g}) = \mathbf{E}\begin{bmatrix} p_{1R} \\ p_{1T} \\ p_{2T} \\ p_{2R} \end{bmatrix} = \begin{bmatrix} 1 & 0 & 0 \\ 1 & 1 & 1 \\ 1 & 0 & 1 \\ 1 & 1 & 0 \end{bmatrix} \begin{bmatrix} \beta_1 \\ \beta_2 \\ F \end{bmatrix} = \mathbf{Z}\boldsymbol{\beta}, \tag{13.4.11}$$

where $\boldsymbol{\beta} = (\beta_1, \beta_2, F)'$, β_1 is the probability of a therapeutic response for the reference formulation at period I, β_2 is the period effect, and F is the corresponding formulation effect. Let $\widehat{\boldsymbol{\beta}} = (\widehat{\beta}_1, \widehat{\beta}_2, \widehat{F})'$ be the WLS estimates of $\boldsymbol{\beta}$. Then, the predicted marginal probabilities under model 13.4.11 by sequence and formulation are given by

$$\widehat{\mathbf{g}} = \mathbf{Z}\widehat{\boldsymbol{\beta}} = (\widehat{P}_{1R}, \widehat{P}_{1T}, \widehat{P}_{2T}, \widehat{P}_{2R})'.$$

Hence, the predicted marginal formulation probabilities of a therapeutic response are given by

$$\widehat{\mathbf{P}}_{\mathrm{M}} = \begin{bmatrix} \widehat{P}_{\mathrm{R}} \\ \widehat{P}_{\mathrm{T}} \end{bmatrix} = \begin{bmatrix} \frac{1}{2} & 0 & 0 & \frac{1}{2} \\ 0 & \frac{1}{2} & \frac{1}{2} & 0 \end{bmatrix} \begin{bmatrix} \widehat{P}_{1\mathrm{R}} \\ \widehat{P}_{1\mathrm{T}} \\ \widehat{P}_{2\mathrm{T}} \\ \widehat{P}_{2\mathrm{R}} \end{bmatrix}$$

$$= \mathbf{L}\widehat{g} \tag{13.4.12}$$

Thus, a consistent estimator of the covariance matrix of $\widehat{P}_{\mathrm{M}}$ can be obtained as follows:

$$\widehat{\mathrm{V}}\mathrm{ar}(\widehat{\mathbf{P}}_{\mathrm{M}}) = \begin{bmatrix} V_{\mathrm{RR}} & V_{\mathrm{TR}} \\ V_{\mathrm{TR}} & V_{\mathrm{TT}} \end{bmatrix}$$

$$= \boldsymbol{LZ}(\mathbf{Z}'\mathbf{V}_{\mathrm{g}}^{-1}\mathbf{Z})^{-1}\mathbf{Z}'\boldsymbol{L}'. \tag{13.4.13}$$

A consistent estimate for the bioequivalence measure $\delta = P_{\mathrm{T}}/P_{\mathrm{R}}$ is then given by

$$\widehat{\delta} = \widehat{P}_{\mathrm{T}}/\widehat{P}_{\mathrm{R}}.$$

Hence, based on Fieller's theorem, an approximate $(1 - 2\alpha) \times 100\%$ confidence interval for δ, denoted by $[L, U]$, can be obtained as follows:

$$(L, U) = \frac{-a_2 \pm \left(a_2^2 - 4a_1a_3\right)^{1/2}}{2a_1}, \tag{13.4.14}$$

where

$$a = \widehat{P}_{\mathrm{R}}^2 - z^2(\alpha)V_{\mathrm{RR}},$$

$$a_2 = 2\left[\widehat{P}_{\mathrm{T}}\widehat{P}_{\mathrm{R}} - z^2(\alpha)V_{\mathrm{TR}}\right],$$

$$a_3 = \widehat{P}_{\mathrm{T}}^2 - z^2(\alpha)V_{\mathrm{TT}},$$

and $z(\alpha)$ is the αth upper quantile of a standard normal distribution. Test product is then considered to be bioequivalent to the reference product if (L, U) is within equivalent limits $(\delta_{\mathrm{L}}, \delta_{\mathrm{U}})$.

Example 13.4.1

To illustrate the use of the WLS method, we consider the data from Herson (1991) concerning bioequivalence trials for albuterol MDI indicated for acute bronchospasm. Table 13.4.3 gives response data and time of onset for the responses, which were calculated according to the FDA guidance. For the purpose of illustration, the response data will be used to assess bioequivalence between the test (generic) and the reference products at the dose of 90 μg. For simplicity, we consider the standard 2×2 crossover mode. In other words, sequences 2 and 4 are combined as group 1

TABLE 13.4.3: Response data and time of onset of response.

		Response		Time of Onset (min)	
Group	**Patient**	**Period I**	**Period II**	**Period I**	**Period II**
1 (RT)	1003	Yes	Yes	3.77	3.13
	1004	Yes	No	6.72	30.00[a]
	1006	Yes	Yes	2.69	3.68
	1007	Yes	No	3.74	30.00[a]
	1008	Yes	Yes	6.38	5.84
	1011	Yes	Yes	7.88	5.56
	1014	No	No	30.00[a]	30.00[a]
	1015	Yes	No	9.36	30.00[a]
	1020	Yes	No	6.02	30.00[a]
	1021	Yes	Yes	3.58	8.44
	1022	Yes	Yes	6.26	11.61
	1024	Yes	No	8.75	30.00[a]
	2003	Yes	Yes	6.75	5.51
	2007	Yes	Yes	1.89	3.29
	2015	Yes	Yes	2.85	3.23
	2016	No	No	30.00[a]	30.00[a]
	2018	Yes	Yes	5.39	6.31
	2021	No	Yes	30.00[a]	3.64
2 (TR)	1002	Yes	Yes	4.05	4.88
	1009	Yes	Yes	4.97	7.47
	1010	No	Yes	30.00[a]	13.98
	1012	No	Yes	30.00[a]	4.86
	1013	Yes	Yes	14.35	3.01
	1016	Yes	Yes	8.41	10.20
	1017	Yes	No	9.46	30.00[a]
	1018	Yes	Yes	2.50	1.69
	1025	Yes	No	13.55	30.00[a]
	2004	Yes	Yes	4.70	4.71
	2005	Yes	Yes	4.02	2.38
	2006	Yes	Yes	3.84	3.36
	2009	Yes	Yes	4.91	4.80
	2010	Yes	Yes	12.22	21.55
	2011	Yes	Yes	21.48	2.14
	2012	Yes	Yes	4.58	5.13
	2014	Yes	Yes	0.99	1.79
	2019	Yes	No	6.69	30.00[a]
	2020	No	Yes	30.00[a]	9.27
	2022	No	Yes	30.00[a]	7.09
	2023	No	Yes	30.00[a]	5.56
	2024	Yes	No	8.25	30.00[a]

Source: From Herson, J. Statistical controversies in design and analysis of bioequivalence trials for pharmaceuticals with negligible blood levels: The metered dose inhaler trial. Presented at the 14th Midwest Biopharmaceutical Statistics Workshop, Muncie, IN, 1991.

[a] Censoring observations.

TABLE 13.4.4: Summary of observed counts of a therapeutic response for data given in Table 13.4.3.

	Outcome[a]				
Group	**(N, N)**	**(N, Y)**	**(Y, N)**	**(Y, Y)**	**Total**
1 (RT)	2	1	5	10	18
2 (TR)	0	5	4	13	22
Total	2	6	9	23	40

Source: From Liu, J.P. and Chow, S.C., *Biom. J.*, 35, 109, 1993.

[a] N, nonresponse; Y, response.

and sequences 1 and 3 are combined as group 2, while days 1 and 3 are designated as period I and days 2 and 4 are designated as period II. The observed counts for the response data of the four possible outcomes by group are summarized in Table 13.4.4. The carryover effect can then be evaluated through the association of a 2×2 contingency table, which is constructed from the patients who have the same outcomes during both periods; that is,

2	10	12
0	13	13
2	23	25

The Fisher's exact test gives a two-tailed p-value of 0.220 which indicates no evidence of carryover effects. Therefore, the weighted least squares method can be applied using PROC CATMOD of SAS. Because no patients in group 2 respond in either period, a small constant (10^{-6}) was added to this cell. Table 13.4.5 gives the elements of vector $\mathbf{g}$ that are the observed marginal probabilities of a therapeutic response by group and formulation. The estimates of $\boldsymbol{\beta}$ and their standard errors are given in Table 13.4.6. The results indicate that both period and formulation effects are not significantly different from 0 (p-values >0.15). Note that the chi-square test statistic for lack of fit is 0.58 with a p-value of 0.45. This indicates that model 13.4.11 is adequate for this data set. The predicted marginal probabilities, $\widehat{\mathbf{g}}$ of a therapeutic response by group and drug product and their estimated covariance

TABLE 13.4.5: Summary of observed marginal probabilities of a therapeutic response by group and drug product for data set in Table 13.4.3.

	Marginal Probability	
Group	**Reference**	**Test**
1	0.8333	0.6111
2	0.8182	0.7727
Total	0.8258	0.6919

Source: From Liu, J.P. and Chow, S.C., *Biom. J.*, 35, 109, 1993.

TABLE 13.4.6: Summary of WLS estimates of β for Herson's data.

Parameter	Estimate	SE[a]	Chi-Square	*p*-Value
β_1	0.8740	0.0697	157.02	<0.0001
β_2	−0.0751	0.0909	0.68	0.4086
F	−0.1254	0.0919	1.86	0.1724
Lack of fit			0.58	0.4467

[a] SE, standard error.

matrix are given in Table 13.4.7. The predicted marginal probabilities, $\widehat{\mathbf{g}}$ the predicted marginal formulation probabilities, $\widehat{\mathbf{P}}_M$ can be computed according to Equation 13.4.12, which are given by

$$\widehat{\mathbf{P}}_M = \begin{bmatrix} \widehat{P}_R \\ \widehat{P}_T \end{bmatrix} = \begin{bmatrix} 0.8364 \\ 0.7110 \end{bmatrix}.$$

A consistent estimate of $\text{Var}(\widehat{\mathbf{P}}_M)$ is given by

$$\begin{bmatrix} 0.003442 & -0.000179 \\ -0.000179 & 0.004665 \end{bmatrix}.$$

Hence, a consistent estimate and 90% confidence interval for $\delta = P_T/P_R$ are given by

$$\widehat{\delta} = \frac{0.7110}{0.8364} = 0.8501,$$

and $(L, U) = (0.6984, 1.0344)$, respectively.

As a result, according to the ±20 rule, the test product is not bioequivalent to the reference product with 90% assurance based on the response data.

TABLE 13.4.7: Summary of predicted marginal probabilities by group and drug product.

I. Estimates

	$\widehat{P}_{1R}$	$\widehat{P}_{1T}$	$\widehat{P}_{2T}$	$\widehat{P}_{2R}$
Estimates	0.8740	0.6735	0.7486	0.7989

II. Covariance Matrix

	$\widehat{P}_{1R}$	$\widehat{P}_{1T}$	$\widehat{P}_{2T}$	$\widehat{P}_{2R}$
$\widehat{P}_{1R}$	0.004859	−0.001808	0.001695	0.001356
$\widehat{P}_{1T}$		0.006487	0.002599	0.002079
$\widehat{P}_{2T}$			0.006977	−0.002683
$\widehat{P}_{2R}$				0.006118

13.5 Log–Linear Models

Jones and Kenward (2003) suggested the use of log–linear models for binary response data. In this section, we apply their results to the predicted marginal formulation probabilities to obtain an approximate $(1 - 2\alpha) \times 100\%$ confidence interval for δ for assessing bioequivalence.

For a standard 2×2 crossover design, a pair of binary responses is observed on each subject. Let (X_{i1k}, X_{i2k}) be the observed paired responses on subject i in sequence k. Jones and Kenward (2003) gave a general representation of the probabilities of possible outcomes as follows:

$$\begin{aligned} P_{hk} &= P(X_{i1k} = x_{i1k}, X_{i2k} = x_{i2k}) \\ &= \exp\{\eta_{0k} + \eta_{1k}x_{1lk} + \eta_{2k}x_{i2k} + \eta_{12k}x_{i1k} \cdot x_{i2k}\} \end{aligned} \quad (13.5.1)$$

where η_{0k} is the normalizing term, which was chosen so that the sum of probabilities of the four possible outcomes for sequence k is equal to 1; η_{1k} and η_{2k} are the parameters corresponding to the design, and η_{i2k} is the intra-subject dependence parameter which is included in the model to assess the dependence of the two binary responses observed on the same subject. Note that, under the above model, the possible values for X_{ijk} can be coded either 1 or -1. $X_{ijk} = 1$ indicates that a therapeutic response has occurred. On the other hand, if $X_{ijk} = -1$, then the patient does not respond. The value of η_{12k} depends on the correlation between X_{i1k} and $X_{i2k} \cdot \eta_{12k}$ is positive (negative) if X_{1lk} and X_{i2k} are positively (negatively) correlated. $\eta_{12k} = 0$ indicates that X_{ilk} and X_{i2k} are independent. In this section, we assume that the correlation between two binary responses observed on the same subject is the same from subject to subject in both sequences (i.e., $\eta_{12k} = \eta_{12}$ for all k). Note that the common intra-subject dependence parameter is also known as the average intra-subject dependence parameter.

Let Y_{ijk} be the logit of the probability of a therapeutic response observed during period j on subject i in sequence k; that is,

$$Y_{ijk} = \text{logit}[X_{ijk} = "Y"] = \log\left[\frac{P[X_{ijk} = "Y"}{1 - P[X_{ijk} = "Y"]}\right], \quad (13.5.2)$$

where

$i = 1, 2, \ldots, n_k$
$j = 1, 2$
$k = 1, 2$

Then, according to Jones and Kenward (2003), the explicit representation of the log–linear model for P_{hk} can be constructed by the following steps:

Step 1. Obtain logit probabilities Y_{ijk} as defined in Equation 13.5.2. Under assumption of independence between two binary responses observed on the same subject, the logits of the probabilities of a therapeutic

TABLE 13.5.1: Representation of the logits of the therapeutic response by sequence and period.

	Period	
Sequence	**I**	**II**
1 (RT)	$\mu + P_1 + F_R$	$\mu + P_2 + F_T + C_R$
2 (TR)	$\mu + P_1 + F_T$	$\mu + P_2 + F_R + C_T$

Source: From Liu, J.P. and Chow, S.C., *Biom. J.*, 35, 109, 1993.

response by sequence and period have the same representation as the expected values of the sequence-by-period means for continuous variables under a standard 2 × 2 crossover design. The representation of the logits of probabilities of a therapeutic response by sequence and period are given in Table 13.5.1.

Step 2. Obtain the joint probabilities P_{hk} of four possible outcomes for each sequence under independence by multiplying the probabilities from step 1.

Step 3. Include the intra-subject dependence parameter $\eta = \eta_{12}$ in model 13.5.1. Table 13.5.2 summarizes the resulting model for $\log(P_{hk})$.

In the log–linear model for a standard 2 × 2 crossover design given in Table 13.5.2, P_1, P_2, F_T, F_R, C_T, and C_R are the fixed effects for period, direct formulation, and carryover; μ_1 and μ_2 are normalizing constants; η is the average intra-subejct dependence parameter; and τ has no particular interpretation and other effects are defined as deviations from it.

Let **g(P)** be a 8 × 1 vector with elements of $\log(p_{hk})$. The log–linear model discussed in the above can be expressed as

$$\mathbf{g(P)} = \mathbf{Z\beta}, \tag{13.5.3}$$

where

$$\boldsymbol{\beta} = (\mu_1, \mu_2, \tau, P_2, F_T, C_T, \eta),$$

TABLE 13.5.2: Log–linear model for a standard 2 × 2 crossover design.

		Period II	
Sequence	**Period I**	**No**	**Yes**
1	No	$\mu_1 + \eta$	$\mu_1 + \tau + P_2 + F_T + C_R - \eta$
	Yes	$\mu_1 + \tau + P_1 + F_R - \eta$	$\mu_1 + 2\tau + C_R + \eta$
2	No	$\mu_2 + \eta$	$\mu_2 + \tau + P_2 + F_R + C_T - \eta$
	Yes	$\mu_2 + \tau + P_1 + F_T - \eta$	$\mu_2 + 2\tau + C_T + \eta$

and

$$\mathbf{Z} = \begin{bmatrix} 1 & 0 & 0 & 0 & 0 & 0 & 1 \\ 1 & 0 & 1 & 1 & 1 & -1 & -1 \\ 1 & 0 & 1 & -1 & -1 & 0 & -1 \\ 1 & 0 & 2 & 0 & 0 & -1 & 1 \\ 0 & 1 & 0 & 0 & 0 & 0 & 1 \\ 0 & 1 & 1 & 1 & -1 & 1 & -1 \\ 0 & 1 & 1 & -1 & 1 & 0 & -1 \\ 0 & 1 & 2 & 0 & 0 & 1 & 1 \end{bmatrix}.$$

Note that the estimation of direct formulation effect is valid only in the absence of carryover effects (Jones and Kenward, 2003). Therefore, the column corresponding to C_T in the design matrix $\mathbf{Z}$ can be omitted when there is no evidence of carryover effects. The carryover effect can be examined by Fisher's exact test as described in the Section 13.4.

Agresti (2002) pointed out that the correct likelihood ratio test, maximum likelihood estimation of the parameters, and consistent estimates of their covariance matrix can be obtained if the observed counts n_{hk} are independent Poisson variables with no constraints on μ_1 and μ_2. From this result, the statistical package, GLIM (Generalized Linear Interactive Modeling) (Numerical Algorithm Group, 2008) can be directly applied by specifying log link function and Poisson errors.

Similar to the WLS method, the predicted values of $\mathbf{g(P)}$ is obtained as follows:

$$\widehat{\mathbf{g}}(\mathbf{P}) = \mathbf{Zb},$$

where $\mathbf{b}$ is the maximum likelihood estimator of $\boldsymbol{\beta}$.

Hence, the maximum likelihood estimator of $\mathbf{P}$ is given by

$$\widehat{P}_{hk} = \exp(\widehat{g}_{hk}), \quad h = 1, 2, 3, 4, \quad k = 1, 2. \tag{13.5.4}$$

Let $\widehat{\mathbf{P}} = (\widehat{P}_{11}, \widehat{P}_{21}, \ldots, \widehat{P}_{42})'$. Then a consistent estimator of the covariance matrix of $\mathbf{P}$ is given by

$$\widehat{\mathrm{Var}}(\widehat{\mathbf{P}}) = \mathrm{Diag}(\widehat{P}_{hk})\,\widehat{\mathrm{Var}}(\widehat{g})\,\mathrm{Diag}(\widehat{P}_{hk}), \tag{13.5.5}$$

where $\mathrm{Diag}(\widehat{\mathbf{P}}_{hk})$ is an 8×8 diagonal matrix with diagonal elements $\widehat{P}_{hk}$, and $\widehat{\mathrm{Var}}(\widehat{\mathbf{g}})$, is a consistent estimator of $\mathrm{Var}(\widehat{\mathbf{g}})$ which is given by

$$\widehat{\mathrm{Var}}(\widehat{\mathbf{g}}) = \mathbf{Z}\,\widehat{\mathrm{Var}}(\mathbf{b})Z',$$

where $\widehat{\mathrm{Var}}(\mathbf{b})$ is a consistent estimator of $\mathrm{Var}(\mathbf{b})$.

The predicted marginal formulation probabilities $\widehat{\mathbf{P}}_{\mathrm{M}}$ can then be obtained as

$$\widehat{\mathbf{P}}_{\mathrm{M}} = (\widehat{P}_{\mathrm{R}}, \widehat{P}_{\mathrm{T}})' = \mathbf{LC}\widehat{P} \tag{13.5.6}$$

where **L** and **C** are defined in Equations 13.4.12 and 13.4.10, respectively.

A consistent estimator of the covariance matrix of $\widehat{\mathbf{P}}_{\mathrm{M}}$ is then given by

$$\begin{aligned}\widehat{\mathrm{V}}\mathrm{ar}(\widehat{\mathbf{P}}_{\mathrm{M}}) &= \begin{bmatrix} V_{\mathrm{RR}} & V_{\mathrm{TR}} \\ V_{\mathrm{TR}} & V_{\mathrm{TT}} \end{bmatrix} \\ &= \mathbf{LC}\,\widehat{\mathrm{V}}\mathrm{ar}(\widehat{\mathbf{P}})\mathbf{C}'\mathbf{L}'\end{aligned} \tag{13.5.7}$$

Therefore, in a similar manner, the maximum likelihood estimator and an approximate $(1 - 2\alpha) \times 100\%$ confidence interval for δ can be obtained.

13.6 Generalized Estimating Equations

When the total sample size is large, as an alternative, the technique of GEEs by Liang and Zeger (1986) may be useful for estimation of period and direct formulation effects in the absence of carryover effects. However, this method treats X_{i1k} and X_{i2k} as they were independent although X_{i1k} and X_{i2k} are not independent. The logistic regression uses the representation of the logits of a therapeutic response specified in Table 13.5.1 with the deletion of the carryover effects C_{R} and C_{T}. Define

$$\mathbf{X}_{ik} = (X_{1lk}, X_{i2k})'$$

and

$$\mathbf{Z}_{ik} = (\mathbf{z}'_{i1k}, \mathbf{z}_{i2k})'$$

where $\mathbf{z}_{ijk}$ is the row of the design matrix **Z** corresponding to the jth period of subject i in sequence k, $i = 1, \ldots, n_k$; $k = 1, 2$. Note that, for the representation of the logits with the carryover effects deleted, $\mathbf{Z}_{ik}$ is a 2×3 matrix. Let $\widehat{\boldsymbol{\Sigma}}(\mathbf{b})$ be a "naive" estimator of the covariance matrix of the estimator **b** obtained under the assumption that X_{ilk} and X_{i2k} are independent. Then, a consistent estimator of the covariance matrix of **b** regardless of the true underlying correlation structure between the two binary responses observed on the same subject is given by Zeger and Liang (1986) as

$$\widehat{\mathrm{V}}\mathrm{ar}(\mathbf{b}) = \widehat{\boldsymbol{\Sigma}}(\mathbf{b})\mathbf{S}_{\mathrm{R}}\widehat{\boldsymbol{\Sigma}}(\mathbf{b}), \tag{13.6.1}$$

where

$$\mathbf{S}_{\mathrm{R}} = \sum_{k=1}^{2} \sum_{i=1}^{n_k} \mathbf{Z}'_{ik}[\mathbf{x}_{ik} - \widehat{\mathbf{P}}_{ik}]\,[\mathbf{x}_{ik} - \widehat{\mathbf{P}}_{ik}]'\mathbf{Z}_{ik}, \tag{13.6.2}$$

$$\begin{aligned} \widehat{P}_{ik} &= (\widehat{P}_{i1k}, \widehat{P}_{i2k})', \\ \widehat{P}_{ijk} &= \widehat{P}(X_{ijk} = "\,Y") = [1 + \exp(-\mathbf{Z}'_{ijk}\mathbf{b})]^{-1}, \end{aligned} \tag{13.6.3}$$

where
$i = 1, 2, \ldots, n_k$
$j = 1, 2$
$k = 1, 2$

$\widehat{\mathrm{V}}\mathrm{ar}(\mathbf{b})$ is not only a consistent estimator, but is also a robust estimator of the covariance matrix of **b** in the sense that it is still a consistent estimator even though the correlation between X_{i1k} and X_{i2k} is misspecified. $\widehat{\mathrm{V}}\mathrm{ar}(\mathbf{b})$ is referred to as an "information sandwich." Note that there are only four possible values for vector $\mathbf{z}_{ijk}$ if the carryover effects are excluded from the model. Therefore, only four possible predicted probabilities $\widehat{\mathbf{P}}_{ijk}$ in Equation 13.6.3 can be obtained. These four probabilities are actually the predicted marginal probabilities by sequence and formulation, i.e., $\widehat{P}_{1\mathrm{R}}$, $\widehat{P}_{1\mathrm{T}}$, $\widehat{P}_{2\mathrm{T}}$ and $\widehat{P}_{2\mathrm{R}}$. As a result, a consistent estimator of the marginal formulation probabilities P_{M} and a robust consistent estimator of its covariance matrix are given by, respectively,

$$\widehat{\mathbf{P}}_{\mathrm{M}} = L(\widehat{P}_{1\mathrm{R}}, \widehat{P}_{1\mathrm{T}}, \widehat{P}_{2\mathrm{T}}, \widehat{P}_{2\mathrm{R}})', \tag{13.6.4}$$

and

$$\widehat{\mathrm{V}}\mathrm{ar}(\widehat{\mathbf{P}}_{\mathrm{M}}) = \mathbf{L}\mathbf{L}_{\mathrm{T}}\mathbf{Z}\,\widehat{\mathrm{V}}\mathrm{ar}(\mathbf{b})\mathbf{Z}'\mathbf{L}_{\mathrm{T}}\mathbf{L}', \tag{13.6.5}$$

where
L is defined as Equation 13.4.12
$\mathbf{L}_{\mathrm{T}}$ is a 4×4 diagonal matrix with diagonal elements $-\widehat{P}_{fk}(1 - \widehat{P}_{fk})$, $f = \mathrm{R}, \mathrm{T}$, $k = 1, 2$

and

$$\mathbf{Z} = \begin{bmatrix} 1 & -1 & -1 \\ 1 & 1 & 1 \\ 1 & -1 & 1 \\ 1 & 1 & -1 \end{bmatrix}.$$

Hence, similarly, based on the GEEs, a consistent estimate and an approximate $(1 - 2\alpha) \times 100\%$ confidence interval can be obtained.

TABLE 13.6.1: Summary of test results of carryover effects.

Estimate	Log–Linear	GEEs[a]
$C = C_T - C_R$	0.6760	0.3332
SE[b]	1.1090	1.0185
p-value	0.5422	0.7435

Source: From Liu, J.P. and Chow, S.C., *Biom. J.*, 35, 109, 1993.
[a] GEEs, generalized estimating equations.
[b] SE, standard error.

Example 13.6.1

Again, we use the response data given in Table 13.4.3 to illustrate the log–linear model and the GEEs method. Table 13.6.1 summarizes the results of carryover effects in the presence of other effects for a log–linear model and the generalized estimation equations method. Because both methods indicate that there is no evidence of unequal carryover effects (p-values >0.50), the same models were fitted without carryover effects. The results for both methods are summarized in Table 13.6.2. The deviance for a log–linear model with scale parameter 1 is 3.822 which yields a p-value of 0.15. Therefore, the log–linear model without carryover effects is an adequate model for this data set. The predicted marginal probabilities by group and drug product are given in Table 13.6.3 for both methods. Note that both methods yield identical estimates for the parameters. This is probably due to the following reasons: (1) the log–linear model in Table 13.5.2 is actually derived from the model for logits in Table 13.5.1 (Agresti, 2002; Chapter 6); (2) the magnitude of the estimated average intra-subject dependence is too small to have any influence on prediction. However, the estimated variances of the predicted marginal probability obtained by the generalized estimating equations method are much smaller than those by the log–linear model.

TABLE 13.6.2: Summary of results from log–linear model and GEEs method.

	Log–Linear Model			GEEs Method		
Parameter	Estimate	SE	p-Value	Estimate	SE	p-Value
Intercept	0.1306	0.5670	0.8178	1.2153	0.4992	0.0149
μ	−0.2680	0.3306	0.4176			
τ	1.2210	0.63681	0.0009			
$P_2 - P_1$	−0.5020	0.5464	0.3582	−0.5038	0.5938	0.3962
$F_T - F_R$	−0.7586	0.5600	0.1755	−0.7616	0.5738	0.1845
η	~0.0055	0.2318	0.9810			

Source: From Liu, J.P. and Chow, S.C., *Biom. J.*, 35, 109, 1993.

TABLE 13.6.3: Summary of predicted marginal probabilities by group and drug product.

Method		$\widehat{P}_{1R}$	$\widehat{P}_{1T}$	$\widehat{P}_{2T}$	$\widehat{P}_{2R}$
Log–linear	Estimates	0.8639	0.6417	0.7477	0.7932
	$\widehat{P}_{1R}$	0.09920	0.06815	−0.00379	−0.00414
	$\widehat{P}_{1T}$		0.06277	−0.00229	−0.00256
	$\widehat{P}_{2T}$			0.02727	0.01990
	$\widehat{P}_{2R}$				0.02871
GEEs	Estimate	0.8639	0.6417	0.7477	0.7932
	$\widehat{P}_{1R}$	0.00586	0.00159	0.00546	0.00456
	$\widehat{P}_{1T}$		0.02408	0.01086	0.00996
	$\widehat{P}_{2T}$			0.01416	0.00305
	$\widehat{P}_{2R}$				0.01082

Source: From Liu, J.P. and Chow, S.C., *Biom. J.*, 35, 109, 1993.

To compare the three methods discussed in Sections 13.4, 13.5, and 13.6, the predicted marginal formulation probabilities, consistent estimates of δ and 90% confidence interval for δ for each method are summarized in Table 13.6.4. According to the ± 20 rule, the three methods reach the same conclusion of bioinequivalence. However, among these methods, the weighted least squares method gives the narrowest confidence interval, whereas the log–linear model yields a much wider confidence interval when compared with the other two methods.

TABLE 13.6.4: Summary of predicted marginal formulation probabilities by method.

Method		$\widehat{P}_R$	$\widehat{P}_T$	$\widehat{\delta} = \widehat{P}_T/\widehat{P}_R$	90% CI
WLS	Estimate	0.8364	0.7110	85.01%	(69.84%, 103.44%)
	$\widehat{P}_R$	0.003422	−0.000179		
	$\widehat{P}_T$		0.004665		
Log–linear	Estimate	0.8285	0.6947	83.85%	(61.31%, 104.22%)
	$\widehat{P}_R$	0.02990	0.02043		
	$\widehat{P}_T$		0.02136		
GEEs	Estimate	0.8285	0.6947	83.85%	(67.79%, 106.23%)
	$\widehat{P}_R$	0.006449	0.005015		
	$\widehat{P}_T$		0.014990		

Source: From Liu, J.P. and Chow, S.C., *Biom. J.*, 35, 109, 1993.

13.7 Analysis of Time to Onset of a Therapeutic Response

As defined in Section 13.2, a therapeutic response is the event that the FEV_1 measurement evaluated within 30 minutes after dosing exceeds 115% of its baseline value. If a patient has the same outcomes of a therapeutic response to both test and reference products (i.e., either his or her FEV_1 measurements for both test and reference products exceeds [or do not exceed] 115% of their baseline values within 30 minutes after administration), the time to onset of the response for one product may be longer than that of the other product. Therefore, although the test and reference products may be bioequivalent relative to occurrence of a therapeutic response, they may not be bioequivalent on the time to onset of the response. Hence, time to onset of a therapeutic response is another clinical endpoint, which can be derived from FEV_1–time curve, to characterize the profile of bioequivalence of MDI products.

For the analysis of time to the onset of a therapeutic response, several methods for paired times are available, for example, the paired Prentice–Wilcoxon statistic by O'Brien and Fleming (1987) and the parametric models proposed by Huster et al. (1989). However, these methods are either for test of equality or derived under a particular form of distribution. None of these methods takes into account the structure of crossover design. Holt and Prentice (1974) and Kalbfleisch and Prentice (1980), however, modified the proportional hazards model for paired failure times that can be extended to estimate the direct formulation effect and its asymptotic confidence interval under the structure of a standard 2×2 crossover design with the assumption of no carryover effects (also see France et al. 1991). This method is essentially a sign test, which can be derived from a binary logistic model. Hence, bioequivalence for the time to onset of a therapeutic response between two products can be assessed using the $100\,(1 - 2\alpha)\%$ asymptotic confidence interval for hazard ratio of the test product to the reference product.

Let $\mathbf{X}_{ik} = (X_{iRk}, X_{iTk})'$ where X_{ifk} is the time to onset of a therapeutic response (defined as response time), censored or uncensored, of product f for subject i in the sequence k. Also, let $\mathbf{z}_{ik} = (\mathbf{z}'_{iRk}, \mathbf{z}'_{iTk})'$ be the corresponding covariate matrices, $i = 1, \ldots, n_k$; $k = 1, 2$. Then, under a proportional hazards model, the hazard function for product f of subject i in sequence k can be expressed as

$$\lambda_{ifk}(x) = \lambda_{0ik}(x)\exp(\mathbf{z}'_{ifk}\boldsymbol{\beta}), \tag{13.7.1}$$

where

$\lambda_{0ik}(x)$ is an underlying baseline hazard function assumed to be unknown, but different from subject to subject

$\boldsymbol{\beta} = (P, F)$, in which $P = P_2 - P_1$ and $F = F_T - F_R$ are the period and formulation effects, respectively

If the time to occurrence is continuous, Kalbfleisch and Prentice (1980) showed that a partial likelihood (or conditional likelihood) with the form of a binary logistic likelihood can be constructed as the product (over all subjects) of the conditional probability of the ranks of the bivariate response times given the smallest response time of subject i in sequence k, $i = 1, 2, \ldots, n_k$, $k = 1, 2$. This partial likelihood is formed based on subjects whose smallest response time is not censored. As we rank the response times within each subject, not across all subjects, there are only two possible ranks for each subject. Without loss of generality, we choose 0 and 1 for the two possible values as follows:

$$y_{ik} = \begin{cases} 0 & \text{if } x_{i\mathrm{R}k} > x_{i\mathrm{T}k} \\ 1 & \text{if } x_{i\mathrm{R}k} < x_{i\mathrm{T}k}, \end{cases} \tag{13.7.2}$$

where

x_{ifk} are the observed response time
$i = 1, 2, \ldots, n_k$
$f = \mathrm{R}, \mathrm{T}$
$k = 1.2$

Let $\mathbf{v}_{ik} = \mathbf{z}_{i\mathrm{T}k} - \mathbf{z}_{i\mathrm{R}k}$, $i = 1, 2, \ldots, n_k$; $k = 1, 2$. Then the inference on $\boldsymbol{\beta}$ can be obtained by fitting a binary logistic regression with dependent variable y_{ik} and vector of explanatory covariates $\mathbf{v}_{ik}$. Because the elements of $\boldsymbol{\beta}$ are expressed in terms of the period and formulation effects and $P_1 + P_2 = 0$ and $F_\mathrm{T} + F_\mathrm{R} = 0$, there are only two possible values of $\mathbf{v}_{ik}$, which are given in Table 13.7.1. Let $\widehat{P}$ and $\widehat{F}$ be the resulting estimators of period and formulation effects obtained from fitting the logistic regression, and S_P^2 and S_F^2 be the corresponding estimated asymptotic variances obtained from the inverse of the observed information matrix. Then an approximate $(1 - 2\alpha) \times 100\%$ confidence interval of the hazard ratio of the test product to the reference product, denoted by (L, U), is given by

$$(L, U) = \exp[\widehat{F} \pm z(\alpha) S_\mathrm{F}] \tag{13.7.3}$$

Two products are considered to be bioequivalent on time to onset of a therapeutic response at the α level of significance if (L, U) is within the prespecified equivalent limits $(\delta_\mathrm{L}, \delta_\mathrm{U})$.

TABLE 13.7.1: Values of $\mathbf{z}'_{ifk}$ and $\mathbf{v}'_{ik}$ for proportional hazards model (in absence of carryover effects).

	Formulation		
Sequence	$z'_{i\mathrm{R}k}$	$z'_{i\mathrm{R}k}$	v'_{ik}
1 (RT)	(−1/2, −1/2)	(1/2, 1/2)	(1,1)
2 (TR)	(1/2, −1/2)	(−1/2, 1/2)	(−1,1)

Source: From Liu, J.P. and Chow, S.C., *Biom. J.*, 35, 109, 1993.

It can be easily verified that

$$\widehat{F} = \frac{1}{2}(\widehat{\beta}_1 + \widehat{\beta}_2),$$
$$\widehat{P} = \frac{1}{2}(\widehat{\beta}_1 - \widehat{\beta}_2),$$

and

$$\widehat{S_F^2} = \widehat{S_P^2} = \frac{1}{4}\left(S_1^2 + S_2^2\right), \tag{13.7.4}$$

where

$\widehat{\beta}_k$ is the estimator of the intercept of the logistic regression with dependent variable y_{ik} and intercept term as the only explanatory covariate for sequence k

S_k^2 is the corresponding estimator for the asymptotic variance, $k = 1, 2$

Kalbfleisch and Prentice (1980) pointed out that the omission of the subjects whose smallest response times are censored will not introduce systematic bias for estimation of period and formulation effects. However, too many subjects with smallest censored response times will certainly have an impact on the efficiency of these estimates.

Example 13.7.1

The time to onset of a therapeutic response for Herson's data set, listed in Table 13.4.3, is used to illustrate the method suggested in this section. Because a therapeutic response is defined within 30 minutes after dosing, the response time is censored at 30 minutes after administration. Patients 1014 and 2016 of group 1 are not included in the logistic regression from the analysis because both response times of the two patients are censored. The results using the logistic regression are summarized in Table 13.7.2. An estimate of the hazard ratio of the test product to the reference

TABLE 13.7.2: Summary of results of response time.

	Number of Patients Whose		**Formulation**	
Group	$X_{iRk} > X_{iTk}$	$X_{iRk} < X_{iTk}$	**Effect (SE)**	**90% CI**
1	5	11	−0.789 (0.539)	(−1.676, 0.099)
2	11	11	0.000 (0.426)	(−0.701, 0.701)
Period effect			−0.394 (0.344)	(−0.960, 0.171)
Formulation effect			−0.394 (0.344)	(−0.960, 0.171)
Hazard ratio[a]			67.42%	(38.30%, 118.69%)

Source: From Liu, J.P. and Chow, S.C., *Biom. J.*, 35, 109, 1993.

[a] Hazard ratio of the test product to the reference product.

product is 67.42% with the corresponding 90% confidence interval being (38.30%, 118.69%). As a result, according to the ±20 rule, the test product is not bioequivalent to the reference product based on the time to onset of therapeutic response.

13.8 Discussion

For the WLS method, because there is an empty cell in the 2×4 contingency table constructed for the data from Table 13.4.3, a small constant (correction factor) was added to the cell to fit the linear model. Agresti (2002) pointed out that different small constants may have a strong influence on the results of the WLS methods. To investigate this, a sensitivity analysis was performed to study the influence of adding constants of four different sizes on the estimates and 90% confidence interval of δ. The results are summarized in Table 13.8.1. It seems that, at least for the data considered here, the WLS method yields rather robust estimates and 90% confidence interval for δ. However, the WLS method may not be useful if there are continuous covariates, such as baseline FEV_1.

For the log–linear model and the GEEs method, both methods are maximum likelihood procedures, which depend only on the marginal totals, not on individual cell counts. Therefore, both methods are robust to zero cell counts. However, sometimes they can be computationally intensive. Although we may consider the more complex crossover design by the method described in Jones and Kenward (2003) for binary response data, the GEEs method seems more appealing. For example, for the design in Table 13.2.1, as recommended by the FDA, we can obtain consistent estimates of various effects simply by fitting a logistic regression with the model specified in Table 13.3.1 as if all binary responses were independent. A consistent estimate of the covariance matrix of various effects can also be obtained by the same procedure as described in Section 13.6. Examples of application of GEEs to crossover designs can be found in Diggle et al. (1994). All computations can be performed using PROC LOGISTIC, PROC IML, or PROC GENMOD of SAS.

Jung and Su (1995) proposed a nonparametric procedure of the ratio of median failure times for correlated censored data. They also used for data in Table 13.9 as an example to illustrate their procedure. The median time to onset of the therapeutic

TABLE 13.8.1: Sensitivity analysis of WLS for data given Table in 13.4.3.

Correction Constant	$\hat{\delta}$ (%)	90% Confidence Interval
1×10^{-6}	85.01	(69.84%, 103.44%)
1×10^{-4}	85.01	(69.84%, 103.44%)
1×10^{-2}	85.00	(69.83%, 103.43%)
0.5	84.56	(69.36%, 103.03%)

response is estimated as 6.02 and 8.25 minutes for reference and test products, respectively. As a result, the ratio of the median times to onset of the therapeutic response of test to reference products is estimated as 1.37 with the corresponding 95% confidence interval of 0.82 and 2.38. Therefore, at the 2.5% significance level and an equivalence limit of ±20%, the products cannot be concluded bioequivalent in the time to onset of the therapeutic response. However, their method fails to take into account the structure of crossover designs. Feingold and Gillespie (1996) suggest alternative methods to analyze censored data obtained under crossover designs. However, their interval estimation is not consistent with their hypothesis testing procedure, although their estimation procedure omits undefined data that may produce biased estimates.

In this chapter, we focused on the assessment of bioequivalence between MDI products using response data and time to onset of a therapeutic response as primary clinical endpoints. However, the FDA guidance suggests that seven clinical endpoints be analyzed. This raises a question of whether one, or some of them, or all of these endpoints should be used for determination of sample size at the planning stage of trials of this kind. In addition, the methods discussed in this chapter depend on the asymptotic results. Therefore, further research on the calculation of the corresponding power is needed if binary response data is the primary endpoint.

For other drugs, such as topical antifungals or antiulcer agents, Huque and Dubey (1990) suggested a three-arm parallel placebo-controlled, randomized design, which consists of the test and reference products and a placebo group. Bioequivalence is assessed only after superiority of both the test and reference products over the placebo is established. Huque and Dubey (1990) also discussed issues of interim analysis, choice of equivalence limits, multicenter studies, and assessment of bioequivalence under a generalized mixed-effects model for binary responses.

This chapter considers clinical endpoints for evaluation of bioequivalence between the test and reference formulation. However, clinical endpoints must be measured and collected from clinical trials in targeted patient population. This type of equivalence trials is referred to as the clinical equivalence trials with clinical endpoints whose variability is much higher than that of pharmacokinetic responses such as AUC from normal health volunteers. Consequently, the sample size required will be much higher for the clinical equivalence trials than the traditional bioequivalence trials. Furthermore, the cost of the clinical equivalence trial will be much higher and duration will much longer than the traditional bioequivalence trials. On the other hand, much of variability observed in the clinical endpoints is mainly due to the variation caused by different use of MDI by patients and may not be due to the variation of the product itself. As a result, clinical endpoints may not be sensitive to detect potential differences between the test and reference formulations. From a perspective of regulatory agencies, approval of the generic product of MDI is based on the evidence of equivalence between the generic and innovative product of MDI. Therefore, the U.S. FDA in 2003 issued the draft guidance on *Bioavailability and Bioequivalence Studies for Nasal Aerosols and Nasal Sprays for Local Action* (FDA, 2003c). In this guidance, for solution formulations of locally acting nasal drug products, bioequivalence can be established using the *in vitro* methods. The concept and statistical procedures for evaluation of *in vitro* bioequivalence are introduced and discussed in Chapter 14.

Chapter 14

In Vitro *Bioequivalence Testing*

14.1 Introduction

As indicated earlier, bioequivalence testing is considered as a surrogate for clinical evaluation of the therapeutic equivalence of drug products based on the *Fundamental Bioequivalence Assumption* that when two drug products (e.g., a brand-name drug and its generic copy) are equivalent in bioavailability, they will reach the same therapeutic effect. Although bioavailability for *in vivo* bioequivalence studies is usually assessed through the measures of the rate and extent to which the drug product is absorbed into the bloodstream of human subjects, for some locally acting drug products such as nasal aerosols (e.g., metered-dose inhalers) and nasal sprays (e.g., metered-dose spray pumps) that are not intended to be absorbed into the bloodstream, bioavailability may be assessed by measurements intended to reflect the rate and extent to which the active ingredient or active moiety becomes available at the site of action. For those local delivery drug products, the FDA indicates that bioequivalence may be assessed, with suitable justification, by *in vitro* bioequivalence studies alone (see, e.g., Part 21 Codes of Federal Regulations Section 320.24). In practice, although it is recognized that *in vitro* methods are less variable, easier to control, and more likely to detect differences between products if they exist, the clinical relevance of the *in vitro* tests or the magnitude of the differences in the tests are not clearly established until a draft guidance on bioavailability and bioequivalence studies for nasal aerosols and nasal sprays for local action (FDA, 1999c) and a draft guidance on nasal spray and inhalation solution, suspension and spray drug product (FDA, 1999d) were issued by the FDA. The 1999 FDA draft guidance on bioavailability and bioequivalence was subsequently revised and issued in 2003 (FDA, 2003c,d). The 2003 FDA draft guidance indicates that *in vitro* bioequivalence can be established through seven *in vitro* tests. These *in vitro* tests include tests for (1) single actuation content through container life, (2) droplet size distribution by laser diffraction, (3) drug in small particles/droplets, or particle/droplet size distribution by cascade impactor, (4) drug particle size distribution by microscopy, (5) spray pattern, (6) plume geometry, and (7) priming and re-priming (see Table 14.1.1). For bioequivalence assessment of the seven *in vitro* tests, the FDA classifies statistical methods as either the nonprofile analysis or the profile analysis.

TABLE 14.1.1: Required *in vitro* tests for assessment of bioequivalence.

Test	Description
1	Single actuation content through container life
2	Droplet size distribution by laser diffraction
3	Drug in small particles/droplets or particle/droplet size distribution by cascade impactor
4	Drug particle size distribution by microscopy
5	Spray pattern
6	Plume geometry
7	Priming and re-priming

Section 14.2 provides a review of the design and the seven *in vitro* tests recommended by the FDA. Regulatory requirements and statistical methods as suggested in the 1999 FDA draft guidances are given in Sections 14.3 and 14.4, respectively. An example is given in Section 14.5 to illustrate the use of the statistical methods. Formulas and procedures for sample size calculation based on the suggested statistical methods are derived in Section 14.6. Recent development regarding profile analysis and nonprofile analysis are discussed in the last section of this chapter.

14.2 Study Design and Data Collection

For the assessment of *in vitro* bioequivalence, the FDA requires that seven *in vitro* testing of single actuation content uniformity through container life, droplet/particle size distribution, spray pattern, plume geometry, and priming/re-priming be done to demonstrate comparable delivery characteristics between two drug products. In this section, a brief description of the recommended study design and each of the seven *in vitro* tests are given.

14.2.1 Study Design

According to the FDA, three lots/sublots from each product are required to be tested for *in vitro* emitted dose uniformity, droplet size distribution, spray pattern, plume geometry, priming/re-priming, and tail-off profile. For each *in vitro* test, ten samples are randomly drawn from each lot. Samples are randomized for *in vitro* tests. The analysts will not have access to the randomization codes. An automated actuation station with a fixed setting (actuation force, dose time, return time, and hold time) is usually used for the *in vitro* tests.

14.2.2 Emitted Dose Uniformity, Priming/Re-Priming, and Tail-Off Profile

Following the FDA's recommendations, the priming, emitted dose uniformity, priming/re-priming, and tail-off tests maybe tested in the following setting. Three individual lots of test product and reference product are evaluated. For each lot, ten samples are then tested for pump priming, unit spray content through life, and tail-off studies. Then, additional samples for each lot are evaluated for the prime hold study (re-prime study).

For each sample unit, spray samples are collected for sprays 1–8 and analyzed in order to determine the minimum number of actuations required before the pump delivers the labeled dose of drug (sprays 1–8). To characterize emitted dose uniformity at the beginning of unit life, spray 9 is collected. Sprays 10–15 are wasted by the automatic actuation station. Spray 16 is collected in the middle of unit life. Sprays 17–20 are wasted. Sprays 21–23 are collected at the end of the unit life. Additional sprays after spray 23 are collected and analyzed to determine the tail-off profile.

Ten additional samples are drawn randomly from each lot of drug product for the pump prime hold study. For each unit, the first 12 sprays (sprays 1–12) are wasted. Sprays 13 and 14 are collected as fully primed sprays. The unit is then stored undisturbed for 24 hours. Within each lot, five samples are placed in the upright position, while the other five samples are placed in a side position. After that, sprays 15–17 are collected. The unit is then stored undisturbed in its former position for another 24 hours. After that, the doses emitted by sprays 18–20 are collected. All spray samples are weighted in order to obtain re-priming characteristics.

14.2.3 Spray Pattern

A spray pattern produced by a nasal spray pump evaluates in part the integrity and the performance of the orifice and pump mechanism in delivering a dose to its intended site of deposition. Measurements can be made on the diameter of the horizontal intersection of the spray plume at different distances from the actuator tip. Spray patterns are usually measured at three distances (e.g., 1, 2, and 4 cm) at both the beginning (sprays 8–10) and the end (sprays 17–19) of unit life. As a result, a total of six spray patterns are collected from each sample unit. For each spray pattern image, the diameters (the longest and shortest diameters denoted by D_{max} and D_{min}, respectively) and the ovality (which is defined by the ratio of the longest to the shortest diameters) are measured.

14.2.4 Droplet Size Distribution

For a test of droplet size distribution, methods of laser diffraction and cascade impaction are commonly used. These methods are briefly described below.

Laser diffraction: For a test of droplet size distribution using laser diffraction particle analyzer, each sample unit is first primed by actuating the pump eight times using an automatic actuation station. Droplet size distribution is then determined at three distances (e.g., 3, 5, and 7 cm) from the laser beam and at the beginning, the middle, and the end of unit life. At each distance, three measurements of delay times (plume, formation, start of dissipation, and intermediate measurements) and overall evaluation are used to characterize the droplet size. As a result, a total of 36 measurements are recorded for each sample unit.

Cascade impaction: When the spray pump is actuated in the nasal cavity, a fine mist of droplets is generated. Droplets that are greater than nine in diameter are considered nonrespirable and are therefore useful for nasal deposition. As recommended in the 1999 FDA draft guidance (FDA, 1999c), the data should be reported as follows:

Group 1: Adaptor (expansion chamber, i.e., 5 L flask), rubber gasket, throat, and Stage 0.

Group 2: Stage 1.

Group 3: Stage 2 to filter.

Each sample unit is first primed by actuating the pump seven times using an automatic actuation station. Droplet size distribution is then determined at the beginning and the end of the life of the sample. Thus, a total of six groups of results are reported for each spray unit.

14.2.5 Plume Geometry

Plume geometry is performed on the nasal spray plume that is allowed to develop into an unconstrained space that far exceeds the volume of nasal cavity. It represents a frozen moment in spray plume development that is viewed from two axes perpendicular to the axis of plume development. The samples should be actuated vertically. Prime the pump with 10 actuations until a steady fine mist is produced from the pump. A fast–speed video camera is placed in front of the sample bottle and starts recording. Repeat the test by rotating the actuator 90° to the previous actuator placement so that two side views are at 90° to each other (two perpendicular planes) and, relative to the axis of the plume of the spray, are captured when actuated into space. Spray plumes are characterized at three stages: early upon formation, as the plume starts to dissipate, and at some intermediate time. Longest vertical distance (LVD), widest horizontal distance (WHD), and plume angle (ANG) are recorded and analyzed.

14.3 Bioequivalence Limit

Similar to the assessment of individual bioequivalence and population bioequivalence, the 1999 FDA draft guidance recommends the following criterion for bioequivalence limit be used (FDA, 1999c):

$$\frac{(\text{average BE limit in natural log scale})^2 + \text{variance terms offset}}{\text{scaling variance}}.$$

As it can be seen, in order to obtain the bioequivalence (BE) limit, there are three quantities that need to be specified. They are (1) average BE limit, (2) variance terms offset, and (3) scaling variance, respectively. The FDA guidances indicate that the final specification of those parameters should be based on the results of the on-going simulation study. However, the following values are recommended in the 1999 FDA draft guidance.

Due to the small variability of *in vitro* measurements, at the present time, the FDA recommends that the ratio of geometric means should fall within 0.90 and 1.11 (FDA, 1999c). As a result, a value of 0.90 is recommended as the average BE limit for *in vitro* data. The objective of variance terms offset is to allow some difference among the total variances that may be inconsequential. As a result of the low variability of *in vitro* measurements, the FDA recommends that a value of 0 should be taken based on the guidance of population and individual bioequivalence. In practice, however, a value of 0.01 may be accepted by the FDA for variance terms offset depending upon the nature of the drug products under investigation. The purpose of scaling variance is to adjust the BE criterion depending upon the reference product variance. When the reference variance is greater than the scaling variances, the limit is widened. On the other hand, the limit is narrowed when reference variance is less than scaling variance. The FDA indicates that the choice of the scaling variance should be at least 0.1. As a result, the specification of 0.90 for the average BE limit, 0.0 for the variance offset, and 0.10 for scaling standard deviation gives the following BE limit:

$$\theta_{\mathrm{BE}} = \frac{(\log 0.9)^2 + 0}{(0.1)^2} = 1.11. \tag{14.3.1}$$

More specifically, let y_{T}, y_{R}, and y'_{R} be independent *in vitro* bioavailabilities, where y_{T} is from the test product and y_{R} and y'_{R} are from the reference product. The two products are said to be *in vitro* bioequivalent if $\theta < \theta_{\mathrm{BE}}$, where

$$\theta = \frac{E(y_{\mathrm{R}} - y_{\mathrm{T}})^2 - E(y_{\mathrm{R}} - y'_{\mathrm{R}})^2}{\max\left\{\sigma_0^2,\, E(y_{\mathrm{R}} - y'_{\mathrm{R}})^2/2\right\}}. \tag{14.3.2}$$

θ_{BE} is a prespecified equivalence limit, and σ_0^2 is a prespecified constant. Values of σ_0^2 and θ_{BE} can be found in the 1999 FDA draft guidance (FDA, 1999c). According to the FDA draft guidances, *in vitro* bioequivalence can be claimed if the hypothesis that $\theta \geq \theta_{\mathrm{BE}}$ is rejected at the 5% level of significance, provided that the ratio of geometric means between the two drug products is within 0.90 and 1.11.

14.4 Statistical Methods

For assessment of bioequivalence for the seven *in vitro* tests, in addition to the so-called noncomparative analysis, the FDA classifies statistical methods as either nonprofile analysis or profile analysis (see also Wang et al., 2000; Chow et al., 2003), which are briefly described below.

14.4.1 Noncomparative Analysis

For each *in vitro* test, the FDA requires that a noncomparative analysis be performed. Noncomparative analysis refers to the statistical summarization of the bioavailability data by descriptive statistics. As a result, means, standard deviations, and coefficients of variation (CVs) in percentage of the seven *in vitro* tests should be documented. More specifically, the overall sample means for a given formulation should be averaged over all samples (e.g., bottles/canisters), life stages (except for priming and re-priming evaluations), and lots or batches. In addition to the overall means, means at each life stage for each batch averaged over all bottles/canisters and for each life stage averaged over all lots (or batches) should be presented. For profile data, means, standard deviations, and percent CVs should be reported for each stage. The between-lot (or between-batch), within-lot (or within-batch) between-sample (e.g., bottle or canister), and within-sample (e.g., bottle or canister) between-life stage variability should be evaluated through appropriate statistical models.

14.4.2 Nonprofile Analysis

The FDA classifies statistical methods for assessment of the seven *in vitro* bioequivalence tests for nasal aerosols and sprays as either the nonprofile analysis or the profile analysis. In this chapter we focus on the nonprofile analysis, which applies to tests for dose or spray content uniformity through container life, droplet size distribution, spray pattern, and priming and re-priming. For nonprofile analysis, commonly used criterion for assessment of *in vitro* bioequivalence is given in Equation 14.3.1.

Suppose that m_{T} and m_{R} canisters from respectively the test and the reference products are randomly selected for *in vitro* bioequivalence testing and one observation from each canister is obtained. The data can be described by the following model:

$$y_{jk} = \mu_k + \varepsilon_{jk}, \quad j = 1, \ldots, m_k, \tag{14.4.1}$$

where

$k = \mathrm{T}$ for the test product
$k = \mathrm{R}$ for the reference product
μ_{T} and μ_{R} are fixed product effects
ε_{jk}'s are independent random measurement errors distributed as $N(0, \sigma_k^2)$, $k = \mathrm{T}, \mathrm{R}$

Under model 14.4.1, the parameter θ in Equation 14.3.2 becomes

$$\theta = \frac{(\mu_{\mathrm{T}} - \mu_{\mathrm{R}})^2 + \sigma_{\mathrm{T}}^2 - \sigma_{\mathrm{R}}^2}{\max\{\sigma_0^2, \sigma_{\mathrm{R}}^2\}}, \tag{14.4.2}$$

and $\theta < \theta_{\mathrm{BE}}$ if and only if $\zeta < 0$, where

$$\zeta = (\mu_{\mathrm{T}} - \mu_{\mathrm{R}})^2 + \sigma_{\mathrm{T}}^2 - \sigma_{\mathrm{R}}^2 - \theta_{\mathrm{BE}} \max\{\sigma_0^2, \sigma_{\mathrm{R}}^2\}. \tag{14.4.3}$$

as indicated in the 1999 FDA draft guidance (FDA, 1999c), the above linearized criteria can be expressed as

$$\zeta_1 = (\mu_T - \mu_R)^2 + \sigma_T^2 - \sigma_R^2 - \theta_{BE}\,\sigma_R^2 \quad \text{for } \sigma_R > \sigma_0$$

and (14.4.4)

$$\zeta_2 = (\mu_T - \mu_R)^2 + \sigma_T^2 - \sigma_R^2 - \theta_{BE}\,\sigma_0^2 \quad \text{for } \sigma_R < \sigma_0$$

To test bioequivalence at level 5%, it suffices to construct a 95% upper confidence bound for ζ. Under model 14.4.1, the best unbiased estimator of $\delta = \mu_T - \mu_R$ is

$$\hat{\delta} = \bar{y}_T - \bar{y}_R \sim N\left(0, \frac{\sigma_T^2}{m_T} + \frac{\sigma_R^2}{m_R}\right),$$

where $\bar{y}_k$ is the average of y_{jk} over j for a fixed k. The best unbiased estimator of σ_k^2 is

$$s_k^2 = \frac{1}{m_k - 1}\sum_{j=1}^{m_k}(y_{jk} - \bar{y}_k)^2 \sim \frac{\sigma_k^2\,\chi_{m_k-1}^2}{m_k - 1},$$

where $k = \mathrm{T}$, R, and χ_t^2 denotes the central chi-square distribution with t degrees of freedom. Using the method in Hyslop et al. (2000) for individual bioequivalence testing, an approximate 95% upper confidence bound for ζ in Equation 14.4.3 is

$$\tilde{\zeta}_U = \hat{\delta}^2 + s_T^2 - s_R^2 - \theta_{BE}\max\{\sigma_0^2, s_R^2\} + \sqrt{U},$$

where U is the sum of the following three quantities:

$$\left[\left(|\hat{\delta}| + z_{0.95}\sqrt{\frac{s_T^2}{m_T} + \frac{s_R^2}{m_R}}\right)^2 - \hat{\delta}^2\right]^2,$$

$$s_T^4\left(\frac{m_T - 1}{\chi_{0.05;\,m_{T-1}}^2} - 1\right)^2,$$

and

$$(1 + c\theta_{BE})^2 s_R^4\left(\frac{m_R - 1}{\chi_{0.95;\,m_{R-1}}^2} - 1\right)^2.$$

$c = 1$ if $s_R^2 \geq \sigma_0^2$, $c = 0$ if $s_R^2 < \sigma_0^2$, z_a is the ath quantile of the standard normal distribution, and $\chi_{t;a}^2$ is the ath quantile of the central chi-square distribution with t degrees of freedom. *In vitro* bioequivalence can be claimed if $\tilde{\zeta}_U < 0$. This procedure is recommended by the FDA guidances.

Note that for the calculation of the 95% upper confidence bounds for the linearized criteria given in Equation 14.4.4, FDA uses the following notations (FDA, 1999c):

$$\hat{\zeta}_1 = (\mathrm{E}_0 + \mathrm{E}_1 + \mathrm{E}_{2\mathrm{rs}}) + (\mathrm{U}_0 + \mathrm{U}_1 + \mathrm{U}_{2\mathrm{rs}})^{\frac{1}{2}}$$

and

$$\hat{\zeta}_2 = (\mathrm{E}_0 + \mathrm{E}_1 + \mathrm{E}_{2\mathrm{cs}} - \theta_{\mathrm{BE}}\sigma_0^2) + (\mathrm{U}_0 + \mathrm{U}_1 + \mathrm{U}_{2\mathrm{cs}})^{\frac{1}{2}}, \tag{14.4.5}$$

where $\hat{\zeta}_1$ and $\hat{\zeta}_2$ are $\hat{\zeta}_\mathrm{U}$ according to the linearized criteria given in Equation 14.4.4, and

$$\begin{aligned} \mathrm{E}_0 &= \hat{\delta}^2, \\ \mathrm{E}_1 &= s_\mathrm{T}^2, \\ \mathrm{E}_{2\mathrm{rs}} &= -(1 + \theta_{\mathrm{BE}})s_\mathrm{R}^2/m_\mathrm{R}, \\ \mathrm{E}_{2\mathrm{cs}} &= -s_\mathrm{R}^2, \end{aligned}$$

and

$$\mathrm{H}_0 = \max\{\mathrm{LCL}^2, \mathrm{UCL}^2\},$$

where (LCL, UCL) are the confidence internal for δ, and

$$\mathrm{H}_1 = \frac{(m_\mathrm{T} - 1)\mathrm{E}_1}{\chi^2_{0.05;\, m_\mathrm{T}-1}},$$

$$\mathrm{H}_{2\mathrm{rs}} = \frac{(m_\mathrm{R} - 1)\mathrm{E}_{2\mathrm{rs}}}{\chi^2_{0.95;\, m_\mathrm{R}-1}},$$

$$\mathrm{H}_{2\mathrm{cs}} = \frac{(m_\mathrm{R} - 1)\mathrm{E}_{2\mathrm{cs}}}{\chi^2_{0.95;\, m_\mathrm{R}-1}},$$

and $\mathrm{U}_i = (\mathrm{H}_i - \mathrm{E}_i)^2$ for $i = 0$, 1, 2rs, and 2cs.

As indicated in the 1999 FDA draft guidance, the FDA requires that m_k be at least 30. However, $m_k = 30$ may not be enough to achieve a desired power of the bioequivalence test in some situations (see, e.g., the simulation results in Section 14.6). Increasing m_k can certainly increase the power, but in some situations, obtaining replicates from each canister may be more practical, and cost effective.

14.4.3 Profile Analysis

As indicated in the 1999 FDA draft guidance (FDA, 1999c), profile analysis using a confidence interval approach should be applied to cascade impactor or multistage liquid impringer (MSLI) for particle size distribution. Equivalence may be assessed based on chi-square differences. The idea is to compare the profile difference between test product and reference product samples to the profile variation between reference product samples. More specifically, let y_{ijk} denote the observation from the jth subject's ith stage of the kth treatment. Given a sample (j_0) from test product and two samples (j_1, j_2) from reference products and assuming that there are a total of S stages, the profile distance between test and reference is given by

$$d_{\mathrm{TR}} = \sum_{i=1}^{S} \frac{\left[y_{ij_0\mathrm{T}} - \frac{1}{2}(y_{ij_1\mathrm{R}} + y_{ij_2\mathrm{R}})\right]^2}{\left[y_{ij_0\mathrm{T}} + \frac{1}{2}(y_{ij_1\mathrm{R}} + y_{ij_2\mathrm{R}})\right]}$$

Similarly, the profile variability within reference is defined as

$$d_{\mathrm{RR}} = \sum_{i=1}^{S} \frac{(y_{ij_1\mathrm{R}} - y_{ij_2\mathrm{R}})^2}{\frac{1}{2}(y_{ij_1\mathrm{R}} + y_{ij_2\mathrm{R}})}$$

For a given triplet sample of (Test, Reference 1, Reference 2), the ratio of d_{TR} and d_{RR}, i.e.,

$$rd = \frac{d_{\mathrm{TR}}}{d_{\mathrm{RR}}}$$

can then be used as a bioequivalence measure for the triplet samples between the two drug products. For a selected sample, the 95% upper confidence bound of $E(rd) = E(d_{\mathrm{TR}}/d_{\mathrm{RR}})$ is then used as a bioequivalence measure for the determination of bioequivalence. In other words, if the 95% upper confidence bound is less than the bioequivalence limit, then we claim that the two products are bioequivalent. The 1999 FDA draft guidance recommends a bootstrap procedure to construct the 95% upper bound for $E(rd)$ (FDA, 1999c). The procedure is described below.

Assume that the samples are obtained in a two-stage sampling manner. In other words, for each treatment (test or reference), three lots are randomly sampled. Within each lot, 10 samples (e.g., bottles or canisters) are sampled. The following is quoted from the 1999 FDA draft guidance regarding the bootstrap procedure to establish profile bioequivalence (FDA, 1999c).

For an experiment consisting of three lots each of test and reference products, and with 10 canisters per lot, the lots can be matched into six different combinations of triplets with two different reference lots in each triplet. The 10 canisters of a test lot can be paired with the 10 canisters of each of the two reference lots in $(10 \text{ factorial})^2 = (3{,}628{,}800)^2$ combinations in each of the lot triplets. Hence a random sample of the N canisters pairing of the six Test–Reference 1–Reference 2 lot triplets is needed. rd is estimated by the sample mean of the rd's calculated for the triplets in 10 selected samples of N. Note that the FDA recommends that $N = 500$ be considered.

14.5 Example

A pharmaceutical company is interested in conducting an *in vitro* study to characterize the *in vitro* performance of one of their products of butorphanol tartrate nasal solution relative to that of Stadol NS (reference listed drug) in terms of the droplet size distribution based on the FDA guidance entitled *Guidance for Industry on Bioavailability and Bioequivalence Studies for Nasal Spray for Local Action* (FDA, 1999c, 2003c). For illustration purpose, we will only focus on the assessment of bioequivalence in droplet size distribution.

14.5.1 Study Design

To demonstrate comparable delivery characteristics between the test product of butorphanol and the reference product of Stadol NS, three lots/sublots from each product was tested for *in vitro* droplet size distribution. A list of the lots to be tested is given in Table 14.5.1.

For the droplet size distribution test, as suggested by the FDA draft guidances, 10 samples were randomly drawn from each lot. The analysts did not have access to the randomization codes. The droplet size distribution was tested using the laser diffraction particle analyzer. Droplet size distribution was determined at three distances, 3, 5, and 7 cm from the laser beam, and at the beginning, the middle, and the end of unit life. At each distance, the measurements at the middle portion (stable portion) of the plume were used to characterize the droplet size. At each distance, each sample was actuated three times. As a result, a total of 27 measurements were performed for each sample unit.

14.5.2 Statistical Methods

For the *in vitro* bioavailability (BA) and the BE studies, as indicated in the FDA draft guidances for nasal aerosols and nasal sprays products, descriptive statistics, nonprofile analysis, and profile analysis of collected *in vitro* data are usually considered for the assessment of the comparability between two drug products. In what

TABLE 14.5.1: List of lots for the *in vitro* study.

Product	Lot Number
Test product of butorphanol	TP0001
	TP0002
	TP0003
Reference product of Stadol NS	RP0001
	RP0002
	RP0003

follows, descriptive statistics and nonprofile analysis for assessment of equivalence between droplet size distributions are briefly outlined.

14.5.2.1 Descriptive Statistics

For each factor considered in the study, mean, standard deviation, and the relative standard deviation (RSD) or the CV be obtained to document the accuracy of the collected *in vitro* data, according to the acceptance criteria as specified in the FDA draft guidances (FDA, 1999c, 2003c).

14.5.2.2 Nonprofile Analysis

As indicated in the FDA draft guidances for nasal aerosols and nasal sprays products, nonprofile analysis using a confidence interval approach applies to the dose or spray content uniformity through unit life, droplet size distribution, spray pattern, and priming and re-priming. The method consists of (1) a criterion that allows the comparison, (2) a confidence interval for the criterion, and (3) a bioequivalence limit for the criterion, which is briefly described below.

Criterion for Comparison: As indicated earlier in this chapter, the *in vitro* population bioequivalence criterion and the bioequivalence limit are given below:

$$\frac{(\mu_{\mathrm{T}} - \mu_{\mathrm{R}})^2 + \left(\sigma_{\mathrm{T}}^2 - \sigma_{\mathrm{R}}^2\right)}{\sigma_{\mathrm{R}}^2} \leq \theta$$

where

μ_{T}, σ_{T} and μ_{R}, σ_{R} are the means and standard deviation for the test product and the reference product, respectively

θ is the bioequivalence limit

As discussed earlier, based on this criterion, a typical approach is to construct a 95% confidence interval for the criterion and compare the upper 95% confidence bound with the bioequivalence limit. We conclude that the two products are bioequivalent if the 95% upper confidence bound for the criterion is less than the bioequivalence limit and the ratio of the geometric means falls within 90% and 111%.

Note that as indicated in the FDA draft guidances for nasal aerosol and nasal spray products, the upper limit may be interpreted by the population distance ratio (PDR). The PDR is the ratio of the test–reference distance (in the log scale) to the reference–reference distance. The population bioequivalence criterion, denoted by PBC, is related to the PDR by

$$\mathrm{PDR} = \left(1 + \frac{\mathrm{PBC}}{2}\right)^{1/2}.$$

Thus, we may substitute the bioequivalence limit for PBC to express the upper limit in the PDR scale. The specification of 0.90 for the average limit, 0 for the variance offset, and 0.10 for the scaling standard deviation corresponds to an upper limit of

PDR of 1.25. As a result, we may solve the above equation for PBC, which is given by PBC = 1.125. The FDA draft guidances indicate that *in vitro* bioequivalence is concluded if the 95% upper confidence bound is less than or equal to 1.125 and the ratio of geometric means falls within the limits of 90% and 111%.

Determining a 95% Upper Confidence Bound: For construction of a 95% upper confidence bound for the criterion, the FDA draft guidances suggest that the method proposed by Hyslop et al. (2000) in conjunction with the procedures proposed by Lee and Fineberg (1991) and Hsu et al. (1994) be used. The idea of the method by Hyslop et al. (2000) is to linearize the bioequivalence criterion as follows:

$$\eta = (\mu_T - \mu_R)^2 + \sigma_T^2 - (1 + \theta)\,\sigma_R^2 \leq 0.$$

Then apply the method of BLUE (best linear unbiased estimate) and the moment-based estimators for the variance components. Note that a detailed description of the method can be found in Appendix B of the 1999 FDA guidance. On the basis of the linearized criterion, the FDA suggests constructing a 95% confidence interval for and then compares the upper 95% confidence bound of with zero. We conclude that the two products are bioequivalent if the 95% upper confidence bound for is less than zero and the ratio of the geometric means falls within 90% and 111%.

14.5.2.3 Results

The spray droplet size distribution of test product and reference product was evaluated and compared using the nonaerodynamic method of laser diffraction analyzer. Modern laser diffraction instrumentation provided plots of obscuration (optical concentration) or percent transmission (%T), which is denoted by Dx, where x is the percent of transmission. Thus, the droplet size distribution (D_{10}, D_{50}, D_{90}) over the entire life of a single spray can be obtained. The droplet size distribution data D_{50} and SPAN, which is defined as $(D_{90}\text{–}D_{10})/D_{50}$, by life stage and by distance, are given in Tables 14.5.2 and 14.5.3, respectively. Tables 14.5.4 and 14.5.5 provide descriptive statistics for D_{50} and SPAN, respectively. The overall means and standard deviations of D_{50} and SPAN by distance are given in Table 14.5.6. The ratio of raw means and the ratio of geometric means between the test product and the reference product for D_{50} and SPAN by distance and by life stage are summarized in Table 14.5.7. As it can be seen from the above table that for D_{50} and SPAN, the ratios of raw means and geometric means fell within the limits of 90% and 111% as required by the 1999 FDA draft guidances (FDA, 1999c,d).

Estimates of the between-lot variation, between-sample within lot variation, and between-life stage within sample variation were obtained using the method of restricted maximum likelihood estimation (REML), as suggested by the FDA draft guidance. The results for D_{50} and SPAN based on the raw data and the log-transformed data are summarized in Tables 14.5.8 through 14.5.11, respectively. Tables 14.5.12 and 14.5.13 summarize the results of bioequivalence assessment based on D_{50} and SPAN by distance, according to the test procedure as outlined in the FDA draft guidance, respectively. The results from D_{50} and SPAN support bioequivalence

TABLE 14.5.2: Data listing for particle sizing by laser diffraction—D_{50}.

				Bottle/Can #									
Distance (cm)	**Product**	**Lot #**	**Life Stage**	**1**	**2**	**3**	**4**	**5**	**6**	**7**	**8**	**9**	**10**
3	Test	TP0001	Beg	66.90	52.10	64.97	64.13	84.01	55.63	57.32	64.89	50.89	49.00
			Mid	68.63	50.92	61.89	61.29	86.39	58.84	58.27	57.13	51.63	49.60
			End	73.45	50.35	63.50	62.06	86.92	64.67	57.41	56.61	55.84	53.20
		TP0002	Beg	52.17	53.03	61.76	61.04	55.12	64.58	59.46	58.60	97.94	66.17
			Mid	50.78	48.81	57.59	65.97	52.63	56.01	52.62	52.73	99.90	63.54
			End	48.97	51.72	60.17	67.76	52.30	56.07	53.76	52.97	91.84	62.21
		TP0003	Beg	61.13	56.70	57.60	60.97	67.30	52.82	69.54	44.15	64.32	73.43
			Mid	58.63	59.53	54.94	63.03	64.46	51.90	52.63	45.48	57.95	66.17
			End	55.67	58.13	52.48	59.12	62.68	50.90	53.25	44.66	58.67	59.81
	Reference	RP0001	Beg	56.99	67.71	75.09	62.88	61.23	84.28	60.95	60.66	62.09	58.10
			Mid	53.63	66.70	71.19	61.61	58.87	84.06	57.01	67.09	61.79	71.65
			End	66.45	66.44	72.04	58.60	57.28	79.19	56.76	66.87	54.35	68.67
		RP0002	Beg	66.21	58.86	50.62	53.45	63.72	58.13	38.13	59.23	63.94	59.75
			Mid	63.55	62.84	56.38	48.06	55.60	51.79	38.78	56.75	58.61	57.90
			End	62.06	60.71	57.07	47.61	55.30	52.95	41.36	54.88	57.02	56.18
		RP0003	Beg	43.62	71.08	49.60	56.47	57.59	53.82	54.42	45.12	55.90	72.81
			Mid	54.25	60.53	46.36	56.32	56.96	50.94	52.44	44.91	56.03	67.32
			End	42.21	62.44	46.91	52.38	56.80	51.61	52.48	45.61	55.33	69.43
5	Test	TP0001	Beg	51.12	47.05	52.27	52.12	66.50	48.07	52.30	49.52	45.81	40.86
			Mid	57.99	45.61	53.56	51.72	59.21	50.72	50.42	50.03	46.82	43.91
			End	66.22	46.41	55.79	54.73	63.18	51.37	51.36	52.95	49.22	49.37
		TP0002	Beg	47.19	44.58	52.08	55.72	46.56	46.62	48.64	46.80	89.22	54.06
			Mid	46.01	48.81	52.85	58.33	46.10	50.68	46.18	46.60	95.82	54.12
			End	47.04	47.13	54.09	59.80	47.97	51.10	48.83	45.99	85.87	58.23
		TP0003	Beg	49.36	49.99	45.58	55.45	53.20	42.81	49.89	40.95	52.62	54.71
			Mid	50.42	54.73	48.53	52.80	57.43	47.00	49.78	41.93	51.96	58.49
			End	52.86	53.96	48.49	52.32	55.70	47.34	49.82	48.58	52.66	54.64

(*continued*)

TABLE 14.5.2 (continued): Data listing for particle sizing by laser diffraction—D_{50}.

				Bottle/Can #									
Distance (cm)	**Product**	**Lot #**	**Life Stage**	**1**	**2**	**3**	**4**	**5**	**6**	**7**	**8**	**9**	**10**
	Reference	RP0001	Beg	48.50	58.73	61.76	52.51	52.86	71.53	52.44	56.34	47.65	54.43
			Mid	50.66	60.15	64.95	52.78	51.79	69.02	52.03	58.77	54.89	59.22
			End	52.30	58.91	68.79	52.16	54.76	73.02	51.39	58.61	50.26	58.49
		RP0002	Beg	55.86	51.26	45.52	48.42	53.36	48.29	40.70	47.55	48.51	47.23
			Mid	55.12	51.21	51.91	46.71	48.06	47.44	39.66	50.69	49.81	54.22
			End	54.80	51.00	48.09	46.63	52.30	49.59	40.83	51.52	49.81	52.40
		RP0003	Beg	43.44	56.03	43.63	51.59	50.18	47.11	49.81	42.51	50.93	62.19
			Mid	46.66	52.43	45.77	52.27	53.46	48.53	47.49	43.31	51.17	61.48
			End	44.26	54.19	45.53	50.04	50.59	49.14	46.66	43.71	51.89	62.90
7	Test	TP0001	Beg	49.17	48.62	50.16	50.70	56.39	49.30	51.65	51.04	48.26	44.89
			Mid	67.92	48.27	54.18	51.06	55.78	52.30	53.00	51.11	49.23	46.58
			End	62.11	48.64	57.51	51.80	58.89	51.12	52.72	53.79	51.65	51.41
		TP0002	Beg	46.37	46.30	51.98	58.44	46.82	49.58	48.40	46.95	75.46	53.90
			Mid	49.63	49.94	54.57	61.07	47.33	51.40	47.66	48.99	80.29	54.16
			End	49.00	50.85	52.85	60.77	49.59	52.25	49.85	49.19	81.40	61.72
		TP0003	Beg	51.30	51.46	48.47	59.15	51.75	47.18	51.70	43.30	52.23	58.83
			Mid	50.34	53.52	50.17	56.37	55.16	48.77	54.23	45.56	50.08	56.38
			End	54.48	56.25	51.04	56.58	57.80	48.20	51.40	44.71	51.20	55.70
	Reference	RP0001	Beg	51.31	54.52	58.44	48.73	49.97	67.06	54.86	56.10	53.85	55.14
			Mid	52.76	57.56	65.59	50.28	53.00	69.52	50.04	61.80	52.19	60.12
			End	54.14	65.58	66.03	48.88	53.27	62.15	51.11	60.53	52.00	60.03
		RP0002	Beg	55.87	48.01	47.80	46.51	50.20	49.32	43.26	48.65	58.25	51.71
			Mid	54.97	54.89	53.75	51.47	49.69	50.90	44.42	50.74	52.53	54.23
			End	56.23	51.53	50.05	47.88	52.33	53.70	43.76	51.62	52.36	52.13
		RP0003	Beg	46.49	56.15	46.37	52.36	49.53	48.17	49.13	47.45	51.71	61.11
			Mid	46.52	55.11	49.33	49.43	52.29	51.05	48.35	47.40	54.06	60.15
			End	46.93	54.49	45.90	52.58	51.06	51.18	48.18	44.34	50.98	58.96

TABLE 14.5.3: Data listing for particle sizing by laser diffraction—SPAN.

				Bottle/Can #									
Distance (cm)	**Product**	**Lot #**	**Life Stage**	**1**	**2**	**3**	**4**	**5**	**6**	**7**	**8**	**9**	**10**
3	Test	TP0001	Beg	1.86	1.94	1.93	1.76	2.22	1.91	1.88	1.84	1.81	1.92
			Mid	1.75	1.82	1.87	1.79	2.22	1.81	1.88	1.82	1.89	1.90
			End	1.75	1.85	1.86	1.75	2.23	1.79	1.90	1.88	1.80	1.86
		TP0002	Beg	1.79	1.87	1.92	1.99	1.99	2.08	1.74	1.92	1.64	1.88
			Mid	1.80	1.83	1.90	1.79	1.84	1.87	1.73	1.82	1.61	1.83
			End	1.76	1.80	1.87	1.79	1.82	1.83	1.74	1.81	1.65	1.80
		TP0003	Beg	2.07	2.10	2.06	2.09	1.95	2.00	1.95	1.79	2.04	2.02
			Mid	1.82	1.92	2.00	1.92	1.94	1.89	1.90	1.86	1.98	1.89
			End	1.81	1.92	1.98	2.02	1.81	1.91	1.92	1.89	1.93	1.84
	Reference	RP0001	Beg	1.94	1.94	1.88	1.91	1.95	1.85	1.86	2.05	1.90	2.08
			Mid	1.85	1.85	1.87	1.90	1.97	1.81	1.80	1.98	1.84	1.96
			End	1.83	1.83	1.85	1.93	1.93	1.85	1.89	1.92	2.02	1.93
		RP0002	Beg	1.89	2.22	2.32	1.87	2.21	2.35	1.87	1.88	1.86	2.01
			Mid	1.86	2.08	2.26	1.87	2.04	2.15	1.78	1.88	1.86	1.96
			End	1.78	2.13	2.13	1.87	2.04	2.16	1.82	1.82	1.88	1.81
		RP0003	Beg	2.04	1.94	1.95	1.98	2.03	1.88	1.96	1.91	1.93	1.94
			Mid	2.04	1.92	1.91	1.95	1.85	1.92	1.91	1.87	1.90	1.92
			End	1.92	1.84	1.83	1.99	1.91	1.91	1.93	1.84	1.87	1.85
5	Test	TP0001	Beg	1.92	1.72	1.88	1.84	2.46	1.83	1.91	1.80	1.67	1.58
			Mid	1.85	1.67	1.90	1.88	2.45	1.79	1.85	1.75	1.65	1.64
			End	1.73	1.61	1.90	1.74	2.36	1.76	1.86	1.78	1.66	1.69
		TP0002	Beg	1.87	1.60	1.90	1.76	1.77	1.87	1.82	1.73	1.71	1.95
			Mid	1.63	1.68	1.87	1.79	1.76	1.80	1.79	1.68	1.63	1.90
			End	1.70	1.65	1.85	1.68	1.75	1.74	1.71	1.66	1.64	1.84
		TP0003	Beg	1.87	1.92	1.88	1.71	1.92	1.66	1.84	1.35	1.97	1.96
			Mid	1.79	1.88	1.81	1.88	1.88	1.76	1.80	1.41	1.89	1.95
			End	1.76	1.89	1.75	1.87	1.83	1.76	1.86	1.59	1.91	1.85

(*continued*)

TABLE 14.5.3 (continued): Data listing for particle sizing by laser diffraction—SPAN.

Distance (cm)	Product	Lot #	Life Stage	Bottle/Can #									
				1	2	3	4	5	6	7	8	9	10
	Reference	RP0001	Beg	1.72	1.97	2.01	2.17	1.92	1.94	1.85	2.07	1.89	2.11
			Mid	1.81	1.95	1.87	1.98	1.88	1.97	1.71	1.88	1.78	2.09
			End	1.90	1.96	1.82	1.99	1.84	1.95	1.75	1.93	1.87	2.07
		RP0002	Beg	1.83	1.94	2.16	1.82	2.29	1.98	1.49	1.87	1.94	2.03
			Mid	1.83	1.93	2.03	1.81	1.85	2.02	1.51	1.80	1.74	1.80
			End	1.76	2.00	1.97	1.69	1.78	2.01	1.49	1.84	1.74	1.71
		RP0003	Beg	1.67	1.93	1.66	1.84	1.96	1.88	1.91	1.66	1.91	1.98
			Mid	1.78	1.83	1.71	1.79	1.85	1.78	1.90	1.70	1.90	1.90
			End	1.58	1.87	1.64	1.78	1.80	1.79	1.77	1.66	1.88	1.89
7	Test	TP0001	Beg	1.60	1.34	1.40	1.58	2.28	1.42	1.51	1.37	1.29	1.20
			Mid	1.78	1.30	1.66	1.56	1.97	1.51	1.43	1.36	1.33	1.35
			End	1.66	1.33	1.58	1.54	2.04	1.49	1.63	1.51	1.37	1.41
		TP0002	Beg	1.38	1.34	1.74	1.46	1.47	1.49	1.48	1.46	1.81	1.76
			Mid	1.36	1.43	1.67	1.48	1.42	1.51	1.51	1.37	1.76	1.73
			End	1.40	1.48	1.58	1.52	1.47	1.48	1.59	1.40	1.77	1.78
		TP0003	Beg	1.59	1.71	1.60	1.50	1.66	1.33	1.70	1.24	1.76	1.70
			Mid	1.52	1.66	1.48	1.57	1.70	1.42	1.60	1.15	1.64	1.62
			End	1.60	1.63	1.45	1.55	1.60	1.44	1.56	1.17	1.63	1.60
	Reference	RP0001	Beg	1.54	1.71	1.88	1.79	1.59	1.94	1.47	1.72	1.53	1.77
			Mid	1.57	1.83	1.94	1.74	1.64	1.85	1.51	1.69	1.67	1.77
			End	1.43	1.80	1.75	1.72	1.58	1.91	1.55	1.75	1.50	1.89
		RP0002	Beg	1.67	1.65	1.44	1.53	1.44	1.99	1.33	1.56	1.55	1.52
			Mid	1.75	1.65	1.75	1.52	1.50	1.61	1.27	1.52	1.41	1.64
			End	1.68	1.65	1.68	1.53	1.57	1.72	1.30	1.55	1.47	1.55
		RP0003	Beg	1.23	1.59	1.37	1.55	1.72	1.52	1.55	1.26	1.73	1.87
			Mid	1.29	1.65	1.36	1.57	1.62	1.45	1.51	1.29	1.64	1.79
			End	1.30	1.66	1.39	1.48	1.63	1.54	1.51	1.35	1.65	1.79

TABLE 14.5.4: Summary statistics of laser diffraction—D_{50} (micrometer).

		Test Product					Reference Product					Ratio of
Laser Diffraction–D_{50}		N	**Mean**	**G. Mean**[a]	**SD**	**CV (%)**	N	**Mean**	**G. Mean**[a]	**SD**	**CV (%)**	**G. Mean**[a] **(%)**
Overall		270	55.06	54.40	9.380	17.03	270	54.44	53.93	7.640	14.03	100.9
For each distance												
	3.0 cm	90	60.05	59.27	10.50	17.48	90	58.44	57.76	8.98	15.36	102.6
	5.0 cm	90	52.26	51.70	8.66	16.58	90	52.08	51.70	6.51	12.49	100.0
	7.0 cm	90	52.88	52.54	6.54	12.37	90	52.80	52.54	5.39	10.21	100.0
For each life stage												
Beginning	3.0 cm	30	61.59	60.81	10.52	17.08	30	59.42	58.68	9.41	15.83	103.6
	5.0 cm	30	51.06	50.47	8.82	17.27	30	51.36	50.99	6.49	12.64	99.0
	7.0 cm	30	51.33	51.03	6.00	11.69	30	51.93	51.70	5.11	9.83	98.7
Middle	3.0 cm	30	59.33	58.51	10.99	18.52	30	58.33	57.68	8.94	15.32	101.5
	5.0 cm	30	52.29	51.67	9.41	17.99	30	52.39	52.04	6.26	11.94	99.3
	7.0 cm	30	53.17	52.81	6.84	12.86	30	53.47	53.21	5.51	10.30	99.2
End	3.0 cm	30	59.24	58.51	10.15	17.13	30	57.57	56.92	8.78	15.25	102.8
	5.0 cm	30	53.43	52.98	7.82	14.64	30	52.49	52.08	6.92	13.18	101.7
	7.0 cm	30	54.15	53.81	6.66	12.29	30	53.00	52.72	5.61	10.58	102.1
For each lot and life stage												
		LOT# TP0001					Lot# RP0001					
Beginning	3.0 cm	10	60.98	60.24	10.40	17.05	10	65.00	64.54	8.53	13.13	93.3
	5.0 cm	10	50.56	50.20	6.66	13.17	10	55.67	55.30	7.02	12.62	90.8
	7.0 cm	10	50.02	49.94	2.93	5.86	10	55.00	54.79	5.15	9.36	91.1
Middle	3.0 cm	10	60.46	59.69	10.79	17.84	10	65.36	64.85	8.85	13.53	92.1
	5.0 cm	10	51.00	50.78	4.96	9.73	10	57.43	57.14	6.13	10.67	88.9
	7.0 cm	10	52.94	52.67	5.94	11.22	10	57.29	56.94	6.78	11.83	92.5
End	3.0 cm	10	62.40	61.63	10.86	17.40	10	64.67	64.24	7.84	12.12	95.9
	5.0 cm	10	54.06	53.75	6.27	11.60	10	57.87	57.45	7.63	13.19	93.6
	7.0 cm	10	53.96	53.82	4.19	7.76	10	57.37	57.07	6.23	10.86	94.3

(*continued*)

TABLE 14.5.4 (continued): Summary statistics of laser diffraction—D_{50} (micrometer).

Laser Diffraction–D_{50}		Test Product					Reference Product					Ratio of
		N	Mean	G. Mean[a]	SD	CV (%)	N	Mean	G. Mean[a]	SD	CV (%)	G. Mean[a] (%)
		Lot# TP0002					Lot# RP0002					
Beginning	3.0 cm	10	62.99	61.99	13.12	20.83	10	57.20	56.59	8.20	14.33	109.5
	5.0 cm	10	53.15	52.03	13.19	24.81	10	48.67	48.51	4.18	8.59	107.3
	7.0 cm	10	52.42	51.83	9.00	17.17	10	49.96	49.79	4.40	8.81	104.1
Middle	3.0 cm	10	60.06	58.74	15.03	25.03	10	55.03	54.54	7.33	13.31	107.7
	5.0 cm	10	54.55	53.17	15.08	27.64	10	49.48	49.29	4.41	8.91	107.9
	7.0 cm	10	54.50	53.82	9.95	18.26	10	51.76	51.67	3.18	6.14	104.2
End	3.0 cm	10	59.78	58.78	12.61	21.10	10	54.51	54.18	6.10	11.19	108.5
	5.0 cm	10	54.61	53.65	12.00	21.97	10	49.70	49.55	3.88	7.82	108.3
	7.0 cm	10	55.75	55.05	10.14	18.18	10	51.16	51.05	3.38	6.61	107.8
		Lot# TP0003					Lot# RP0003					
Beginning	3.0 cm	10	60.80	60.22	8.56	14.07	10	56.04	55.33	9.618	17.16	108.8
	5.0 cm	10	49.46	49.23	4.94	9.99	10	49.74	49.42	6.108	12.28	99.6
	7.0 cm	10	51.54	51.34	4.81	9.33	10	50.85	50.66	4.701	9.25	101.3
Middle	3.0 cm	10	57.47	57.14	6.38	11.09	10	54.61	54.25	6.562	12.02	105.3
	5.0 cm	10	51.31	51.09	4.95	9.65	10	50.26	50.03	5.140	10.23	102.1
	7.0 cm	10	52.06	51.94	3.61	6.93	10	51.37	51.22	4.158	8.09	101.4
End	3.0 cm	10	55.54	55.30	5.30	9.55	10	53.52	52.99	8.076	15.09	104.4
	5.0 cm	10	51.64	51.56	2.89	5.59	10	49.89	49.62	5.698	11.42	103.9
	7.0 cm	10	52.74	52.58	4.17	7.91	10	50.46	50.29	4.347	8.61	104.5

[a] G. Mean, geometric mean.

TABLE 14.5.5: Summary statistics of laser diffraction—SPAN.

Laser Diffraction—SPAN		Test Product					Reference Product					Ratio of
		N	Mean	G. Mean[a]	SD	CV (%)	*N*	Mean	G. Mean[a]	SD	CV (%)	G. Mean[a] (%)
Overall		270	1.74	1.73	0.215	12.34	270	1.80	1.79	0.206	11.43	96.6
For each distance												
	3.0 cm	90	1.88	1.88	0.115	6.13	90	1.94	1.94	0.116	5.99	97.1
	5.0 cm	90	1.80	1.79	0.164	9.09	90	1.86	1.86	0.144	7.75	96.7
	7.0 cm	90	1.54	1.53	0.182	11.85	90	1.60	1.59	0.171	10.71	96.0
For each life stage												
Beginning	3.0 cm	30	1.93	1.93	0.125	6.49	30	1.98	1.98	0.134	6.76	97.6
	5.0 cm	30	1.82	1.81	0.181	9.94	30	1.91	1.91	0.167	8.70	95.2
	7.0 cm	30	1.54	1.53	0.217	14.12	30	1.60	1.59	0.189	11.78	96.0
Middle	3.0 cm	30	1.86	1.86	0.102	5.47	30	1.93	1.92	0.105	5.43	96.8
	5.0 cm	30	1.80	1.79	0.168	9.33	30	1.85	1.84	0.116	6.30	97.3
	7.0 cm	30	1.53	1.52	0.172	11.28	30	1.60	1.59	0.170	10.65	95.5
End	3.0 cm	30	1.85	1.85	0.104	5.64	30	1.91	1.91	0.099	5.18	96.9
	5.0 cm	30	1.78	1.77	0.142	7.98	30	1.82	1.82	0.135	7.39	97.5
	7.0 cm	30	1.54	1.53	0.157	10.19	30	1.60	1.59	0.159	9.97	96.6
For each lot and life stage												
		Lot# TP0001					Lot# RP0001					
Beginning	3.0 cm	10	1.91	1.90	0.124	6.50	10	1.94	1.93	0.076	3.94	98.4
	5.0 cm	10	1.86	1.85	0.237	12.73	10	1.97	1.96	0.132	6.74	94.3
	7.0 cm	10	1.50	1.48	0.301	20.11	10	1.69	1.69	0.157	9.28	87.5
Middle	3.0 cm	10	1.88	1.87	0.130	6.95	10	1.88	1.88	0.066	3.52	99.4
	5.0 cm	10	1.84	1.83	0.234	12.70	10	1.89	1.89	0.110	5.83	96.9
	7.0 cm	10	1.53	1.51	0.221	14.47	10	1.72	1.72	0.132	7.67	88.1

(*continued*)

TABLE 14.5.5 (continued): Summary statistics of laser diffraction—SPAN.

Laser Diffraction—SPAN		Test Product					Reference Product					Ratio of
		N	Mean	G. Mean[a]	SD	CV (%)	*N*	Mean	G. Mean[a]	SD	CV (%)	G. Mean[a] (%)
End	3.0 cm	10	1.87	1.86	0.138	7.39	10	1.90	1.90	0.060	3.16	98.2
	5.0 cm	10	1.81	1.80	0.212	11.72	10	1.91	1.91	0.092	4.84	94.4
	7.0 cm	10	1.56	1.55	0.201	12.94	10	1.69	1.68	0.165	9.75	91.9
		Lot# TP0002					**Lot# RP0002**					
Beginning	3.0 cm	10	1.88	1.88	0.130	6.92	10	2.05	2.04	0.204	9.96	92.1
	5.0 cm	10	1.80	1.80	0.104	5.81	10	1.94	1.92	0.215	11.09	93.3
	7.0 cm	10	1.54	1.53	0.167	10.84	10	1.57	1.56	0.179	11.42	98.2
Middle	3.0 cm	10	1.80	1.80	0.081	4.52	10	1.97	1.97	0.153	7.77	91.4
	5.0 cm	10	1.75	1.75	0.095	5.42	10	1.83	1.83	0.149	8.12	95.9
	7.0 cm	10	1.52	1.52	0.146	9.58	10	1.56	1.56	0.150	9.60	97.6
End	3.0 cm	10	1.79	1.79	0.060	3.36	10	1.94	1.94	0.153	7.86	92.1
	5.0 cm	10	1.72	1.72	0.074	4.31	10	1.80	1.79	0.162	9.01	96.0
	7.0 cm	10	1.55	1.54	0.136	8.77	10	1.57	1.57	0.124	7.90	98.5
		Lot# TP0003					**Lot# RP0003**					
Beginning	3.0 cm	10	2.01	2.00	0.093	4.61	10	1.96	1.96	0.050	2.54	102.5
	5.0 cm	10	1.81	1.80	0.190	10.52	10	1.84	1.84	0.128	6.95	97.9
	7.0 cm	10	1.58	1.57	0.173	10.96	10	1.54	1.53	0.207	13.42	102.9
Middle	3.0 cm	10	1.91	1.91	0.053	2.79	10	1.92	1.92	0.051	2.65	99.6
	5.0 cm	10	1.81	1.80	0.150	8.33	10	1.81	1.81	0.075	4.13	99.2
	7.0 cm	10	1.54	1.53	0.160	10.44	10	1.52	1.51	0.168	11.05	101.3
End	3.0 cm	10	1.90	1.90	0.069	3.61	10	1.89	1.89	0.052	2.73	100.7
	5.0 cm	10	1.81	1.80	0.095	5.26	10	1.77	1.76	0.107	6.05	102.4
	7.0 cm	10	1.52	1.52	0.141	9.28	10	1.53	1.52	0.155	10.14	99.6

[a] G. Mean, geometric mean.

TABLE 14.5.6: Overall means and standard deviations of D_{50} and SPAN by distance.

Test product	3 cm	60.05 ± 10.50	1.88 ± 0.12
	5 cm	52.26 ± 8.66	1.80 ± 0.16
	7 cm	52.88 ± 6.54	1.54 ± 0.18
Reference product	3 cm	58.44 ± 8.98	1.94 ± 0.12
	5 cm	52.08 ± 6.51	1.86 ± 0.14
	7 cm	52.80 ± 5.39	1.60 ± 0.17

TABLE 14.5.7: Ratio of raw means and ratio of geometric means for D_{50} and SPAN by distance and by life stage.

Test/Reference	Distance (cm)	Life Stage	D_{50} (%)	SPAN (%)
Ratio of raw means	3	Beginning	103.6	97.6
		Middle	101.7	96.8
		End	102.9	97.0
	5	Beginning	99.4	95.2
		Middle	99.8	97.5
		End	101.8	97.5
	7	Beginning	98.8	96.2
		Middle	99.4	95.5
		End	102.2	96.6
Ratio of geometric means	3	Beginning	103.6	97.6
		Middle	101.5	96.8
		End	102.8	96.9
	5	Beginning	99.0	95.2
		Middle	99.3	97.3
		End	101.7	97.5
	7	Beginning	98.7	96.0
		Middle	99.2	95.5
		End	102.1	96.6

TABLE 14.5.8: Summary of standard variations of laser diffraction based on raw data—D_{50} (micrometer).

Parameter: Laser Diffraction—D_{50} **Variation**	**Test Product**	**Reference Product**	**Total**
Between-lot	0.0000 (0.0000)	16.0548 (4.0068)	5.5223 (2.3500)
Between-sample within-lot	66.9224 (8.1806)	30.8621 (5.5554)	48.8923 (6.9923)
Between-life stage within-sample	26.4055 (5.1386)	17.6877 (4.2057)	22.0465 (4.6954)
Total	93.3277 (9.6606)	64.6047 (8.0377)	76.4611 (8.7442)

Note: Variance components were estimated by REML. The numbers in parentheses are the corresponding standard deviations.

TABLE 14.5.9: Summary of standard variations of laser diffraction based on raw data—SPAN.

Variation	Test Product	Reference Product	Total
Between-lot	0.0000 (0.0000)	0.0010 (0.0309)	0.0001 (0.0093)
Between-sample within-lot	0.0132 (0.1149)	0.0072 (0.0851)	0.0102 (0.1011)
Between-life stage within-sample	0.0338 (0.1839)	0.0346 (0.1860)	0.0342 (0.1850)
Total	0.0470 (0.2169)	0.0428 (0.2069)	0.0445 (0.2110)

Note: Variance components were estimated by REML. The numbers in parentheses are the corresponding standard deviations.

TABLE 14.5.10: Summary of standard variation of laser diffarction based on log scale—D_{50} (log of μm).

Variation	Test Product	Reference Product	Total
Between-lot	0.0000 (0.0000)	0.0050 (0.0710)	0.0018 (0.0427)
Between-sample within-lot	0.0168 (0.1296)	0.0100 (0.0998)	0.0134 (0.1157)
Between-life stage within-sample	0.0072 (0.0851)	0.0053 (0.0727)	0.0063 (0.0791)
Total	0.0240 (0.1550)	0.0203 (0.1424)	0.0215 (0.1465)

Note: Variance components were estimated by REML. The numbers in parentheses are the corresponding standard deviations.

TABLE 14.5.11: Summary of standard variation of laser diffraction based on log scale—SPAN.

Variation	Test Product	Reference Product	Total
Between-lot	0.0000 (0.0000)	0.0004 (0.0191)	0.0000 (0.0057)
Between-sample within-lot	0.0041 (0.0638)	0.0024 (0.0491)	0.0032 (0.0569)
Between-life stage within-sample	0.0124 (0.1113)	0.0116 (0.1079)	0.0120 (0.1096)
Total	0.0405 (0.2012)	0.0347 (0.1862)	0.0367 (0.1917)

Note: Variance components were estimated by REML. The numbers in parentheses are the corresponding standard deviations.

TABLE 14.5.12: *In vitro* bioequivalence assessment of D_{50}.

I. Height = 3 cm
Population BE criterion:[a] −0.034344
Estimated linearized criteria:[b] −0.043366

Parameter Estimate i	E_i	H_i	U_i
0	0.000670	0.005159	0.000000
1	0.024883	0.032449	0.000057
2rs	−0.050828	−0.040383	0.000109
2cs	−0.023919	−0.019004	0.000024

II. Height = 5 cm
Population BE criterion: −0.032992
Estimated linearized criteria: −0.039696

Parameter Estimate i	E_i	H_i	U_i
0	0.000000	0.001487	0.000000
1	0.019767	0.025777	0.000036
2rs	−0.030735	−0.024418	0.000040
2cs	−0.014463	−0.011491	0.000009

III. Height = 7 cm
Population BE criterion:[a] −0.038074
Estimated linearized criteria:[b] −0.042340

Parameter Estimate i	E_i	H_i	U_i
0	0.000000	0.000965	0.000000
1	0.012393	0.016160	0.000014
2rs	−0.020682	−0.016432	0.000018
2cs	−0.009733	−0.007733	0.000004

[a] Population BE criterion: 95% upper bound of η
[b] Estimated linearized criteria: point estimate of η

TABLE 14.5.13: *In vitro* bioequivalence assessment of SPAN.

I. Height = 3 cm
Population BE criterion:[a] −0.042505
Estimated linearized criteria:[b] −0.043805

Parameter Estimate i	E_i	H_i	U_i
0	0.000871	0.002195	0.000000
1	0.003640	0.004747	0.000001
2rs	−0.007045	−0.005597	0.000002
2cs	−0.003315	−0.002634	0.000000

II. Height = 5 cm
Population BE criterion:[a] −0.039696
Estimated linearized criteria:[b] −0.042348

(*continued*)

TABLE 14.5.13 (continued): *In vitro* bioequivalence assessment of SPAN.

Parameter Estimate i	E_i	H_i	U_i
0	0.001151	0.003409	0.000001
1	0.007663	0.009994	0.000005
2rs	−0.013096	−0.010405	0.000007
2cs	−0.006163	−0.004896	0.000002

III. Height = 7 cm
Population BE criterion:[a] −0.037067
Estimated linearized criteria:[b] −0.041787

Parameter Estimate i	E_i	H_i	U_i
0	0.001656	0.005424	0.000000
1	0.013330	0.017382	0.000016
2rs	−0.025016	−0.019875	0.000026
2cs	−0.011772	−0.009353	0.000006

[a] Population BE criterion: 95% upper bound of η
[b] Estimated linearized criteria: point estimate of η

between the test product and the reference product. The upper 95% confidence bounds for η for D_{50} and SPAN by distance are summarized in Table 14.5.14.

14.5.2.4 Conclusion

On the basis of the analyses of test results of the droplet size distribution, no significant differences between the test product and the reference product were detected. In addition, the assessment of *in vitro* population bioequivalence, according to the bioequivalence criterion suggested in the above mentioned FDA guidance, supports equivalence in the delivery characteristics between the test product and the reference listed drug.

14.6 Sample Size Determination

In view of the fact that the FDA requires $m_k \geq 30$ and that $m_k = 30$ and $n_k = 1$ may not produce a test with sufficient power, Chow et al. (2003) proposed a procedure for determining sample sizes as follows.

TABLE 14.5.14: The upper 95% confidence bounds for η by distance for D_{50} and SPAN.

Distance (cm)	D_{50}	SPAN
3	−0.034344	−0.042505
5	−0.032992	−0.039696
7	−0.038074	−0.037067

As a typical approach, Chow et al. (2003a) choose $m = m_T = m_R$ and $n = n_T = n_R$ so that the power of the bioequivalence test reaches a given level β (say 80%) when the unknown parameter vector $\psi = (\delta, \sigma^2_{BT}, \sigma^2_{BR}, \sigma^2_{WT}, \sigma^2_{WR})$ is set at some initial guessing value $\tilde{\psi}$ for which the value of ζ (denoted by $\tilde{\zeta}$) is negative. Let U be given in the definition of $\widehat{\zeta}_U$ and U_β be the same as U but with 5% and 95% replaced by $1-\beta$ and β, respectively. Since

$$P\left(\widehat{\zeta}_U < \zeta + \sqrt{U} + \sqrt{U_\beta}\right) \approx \beta,$$

the power of the bioequivalence test, $P(\widehat{\zeta}_{\tilde{U}} < 0)$, is approximately larger than β if $\zeta + \sqrt{U} + \sqrt{U_\beta} \leq 0$. Let $\tilde{U}$ and $\tilde{U}_\beta$ be U and U_β, respectively, with $(\widehat{\delta}, s^2_{BT}, s^2_{BR}, s^2_{WT}, s^2_{WR})$ replaced by $\tilde{\psi}$. Then, the sample sizes $m = m_T = m_R$ and $n = n_T = n_R$ that produce a test with power approximately β should satisfy

$$\tilde{\zeta} + \sqrt{\tilde{U}} + \sqrt{\tilde{U}_\beta} \leq 0. \tag{14.6.1}$$

From the results described in Section 14.4, having a large m and a small n is an advantage when mn, the total number of observations for one treatment, is fixed. Thus, we propose the following procedure:

Step 1. Set $m = 30$ and $n = 1$. If Equation 14.6.1 holds, stop and the required sample sizes are $m = 30$ and $n = 1$; otherwise, go to Step 2.

Step 2. Let $n = 1$ and find a smallest integer m_* such that Equation 14.6.1 holds. If $m_* \leq m_+$ (the largest possible number of canisters in a given problem), stop and the required sample sizes are $m = m_+$ and $n = 1$; otherwise, go to Step 3.

Step 3. Let $m = m_+$ and find a smallest integer n_* such that Equation 14.6.1 holds. The required sample sizes are $m = m_+$ and $n = n_*$.

If in practice it is much easier and inexpensive to obtain more replicates than to sample more canisters, then Steps 2–3 in the previous procedure can be replaced by

Step 2′. Let $m = 30$ and find a smallest integer n such that Equation 14.6.1 holds. The required sample sizes are $m = 30$ and $n = n_*$.

Since selecting sample sizes according to Equation 14.6.1 only produces a test with approximate power β, we conduct a simulation study to examine the actual power corresponding to the selected sample sizes according to Steps 1–3 (or Steps 1 and 2′). That is, for a given combination of parameter values in Table 14.6.1, we select sample sizes m_* and n_* according to Steps 1–3 or Steps 1 and 2′ with $\beta = 80\%$; and then compute the actual power p corresponding to the selected m_* and n_* by 10,000 simulations. Note that m_+ is set to be ∞ in the simulation so that Step 3 is not needed. The results in Table 14.6.1 show that the selected sample sizes produce a test with power $\geq 75\%$ except for two cases where the power is about 73%.

TABLE 14.6.1: Selected sample sizes m_* and n_* and the actual power p when $\theta_{BE} = 1.125$ and $\sigma_0 = 0.2$ (10,000 simulations).

					Step 1	Step 2		Step 2′	
σ_{BT}	σ_{BR}	σ_{WT}	σ_{WR}	δ	p	m_*, n_*	p	m_*, n_*	p
0	0	0.25	0.25	0.05300	0.4893	55,1	0.7658	30,2	0.7886
					0.5389	47,1	0.7546	30,2	0.8358
		0.25	0.50	0.4108	0.6391	45,1	0.7973	30,2	0.8872
				0.2739	0.9138	—	—	—	—
		0.50	0.50	0.10610	0.4957	55,1	0.7643	30,2	0.7875
					0.5362	47,1	0.7526	30,2	0.8312
0.25	0.25	0.25	0.25	0.07500	0.4909	55,1	0.7774	30,3	0.7657
					0.5348	47,1	0.7533	30,2	0.7323
		0.25	0.50	0.4405	0.5434	57,1	0.7895	30,3	0.8489
				0.2937	0.8370	—	—	—	—
		0.50	0.50	0.11860	0.4893	55,1	0.7683	30,2	0.7515
					0.5332	47,1	0.7535	30,2	0.8091
0.50	0.25	0.25	0.50	0.11860	0.4903	55,1	0.7660	30,4	0.7586
					0.5337	47,1	0.7482	30,3	0.7778
0.25	0.50	0.25	0.25	0.2937	0.8357	—	—	—	—
		0.50	0.25	0.11860	0.5016	55,1	0.7717	30,4	0.7764
					0.5334	47,1	0.7484	30,3	0.7942
		0.25	0.50	0.5809	0.6416	45,1	0.7882	30,2	0.7884
				0.3873	0.9184	—	—	—	—
		0.50	0.50	0.3464	0.6766	38,1	0.7741	30,2	0.8661
				0.1732	0.8470	—	—	—	—
0.50	0.50	0.25	0.50	0.3464	0.6829	38,1	0.7842	30,2	0.8045
				0.1732	0.8450	—	—	—	—
		0.50	0.50	0.15000	0.4969	55,1	0.7612	30,3	0.7629
					0.5406	47,1	0.7534	30,2	0.7270

Note: In Step 1, $m_* = 30$, $n_* = 1$.

14.6.1 Numerical Example

We consider an *in vitro* bioequivalence study between two nasal spray products (a test and a reference). According to FDA's draft guidances, the sponsor has to demonstrate similar drug delivery characteristics to the nasal cavity between the test and the reference products. This example contains data from one of the characteristics. There are 30 sampled canisters from each treatment and two replicates are obtained within each canister. A total of $2 \times 30 \times 2 = 120$ data are listed in Table 14.6.2.

Using the formulas in Section 14.4, we obtain the following statistics and conclusion:

TABLE 14.6.2: Data listing for bioequivalence testing of nasal spray products.

Test Product		Reference Product	
Replicate 1	**Replicate 2**	**Replicate 1**	**Replicate 2**
0.561666	1.125871	−0.039464	−0.432529
0.798124	1.430523	0.307254	0.267646
0.436184	−0.222413	0.253502	−0.119584
−0.024528	0.393267	−0.648004	−1.177679
−0.090290	−0.627502	0.301081	−0.494485
−0.272998	−0.153278	−0.616031	−0.191127
0.218929	−0.727645	−0.308066	0.234591
−0540058	−0.053589	0.365324	−0.522845
−0.764153	0.368896	−0.151981	−0.391525
0.806935	1.073829	−0.313767	0.146926
0.285985	−0.079857	0.570084	−0.689592
−0.202443	−0.131901	−0.770030	−0.251785
0.443907	−0.043639	0.015629	0.458543
−0.164041	−0.688999	−0.468089	−0.501593
−1.065702	0.403384	0.167847	−0.268849
−0.320509	−0.584669	0.551757	0.733643
0.390335	−0.033335	0.069074	0.181878
−0.547364	0.351125	−0.006792	0.042096
0.113892	0.321204	−1563092	−0.869159
−0.201228	0.978660	−0.221517	−0.407714
0.416043	−0.643256	−0.624500	0.594661
−0.462978	0.780152	0.171163	1.107604
0.523478	−0.851068	0.386695	−0.810703
0.179169	0.040342	−1.273343	−0.050407
0.486552	0.564771	0.463084	0.172705
1.122766	0.070407	0.214514	0.385597
0.748173	0.236006	−0.208575	−0.301824
1.440898	0.262185	0.628295	−0.131757
−0.327088	0.314147	−0.562163	−1.000834
0.719226	0.428375	−0.794484	0.050426

$$\widehat{\delta} = -0.268069,$$
$$s_{\mathrm{BT}}^2 = 0.197011,\ s_{\mathrm{BR}}^2 = 0.185969,$$
$$s_{\mathrm{WT}}^2 = 0.182724,\ s_{\mathrm{WR}}^2 = 0.287895,$$
$$s_{\mathrm{T}}^2 = s_{\mathrm{BT}}^2 + \tfrac{1}{2}s_{\mathrm{WT}}^2 = 0.29889,$$
$$s_{\mathrm{R}}^2 = s_{\mathrm{BR}}^2 + \tfrac{1}{2}s_{\mathrm{WR}}^2 = 0.329916,$$
$$\widehat{\zeta}_{\mathrm{U}} = -0.091582 < 0.$$

Thus, we conclude bioequivalence.

It is of interest to know what happens if we do not have replicates, i.e., from each canister we only have one observation. For this purpose, we delete the second observation in each canister from Table 14.6.2 and apply the formulas in the FDA draft guidances (see Section 14.4). The results are given as follows:

$$\begin{aligned}\widehat{\delta} &= -0.252149,\\ s_{\mathrm{T}}^2 &= 0.307987,\\ s_{\mathrm{R}}^2 &= 0.331149,\\ U &= 0.120758,\end{aligned}$$

and

$$\tilde{\zeta}_{\mathrm{U}} = 0.015377 < 0.$$

Thus, we conclude bioinequivalence.

In this example, estimates of parameters (δ and variances) based on data without replication are very similar to those based on data with replication. But the values of U, which determines the upper confidence bound for ζ, are very different in two cases. This indicates that in this example, the design of 30 canisters for each treatment without replication does not provide enough power in claiming bioequivalence when the two products are in fact bioequivalence.

14.7 Discussion

14.7.1 Nonprofile Analysis

Suppose that there are n_k replicates from each canister for product k. Let y_{ijk} be the ith replicate in the jth canister under product k. Let b_{jk} be the between-canister variation and e_{ijk} be the within-canister measurement error. Then

$$y_{ijk} = \mu_k + b_{jk} + e_{ijk}, \quad i = 1, \ldots, n_k, \quad j = 1, \ldots, m_k, \tag{14.7.1}$$

where b_{jk}'s and e_{ijk}'s are independent, $b_{jk} \sim N(0, \sigma_{\mathrm{B}k}^2)$ and $e_{ijk} \sim N(0, \sigma_{\mathrm{W}k}^2)$. Under model Equation 14.7.1, the total variances σ_{T}^2 and σ_{R}^2 are equal to $\sigma_{\mathrm{BT}}^2 + \sigma_{\mathrm{WT}}^2$ and $\sigma_{\mathrm{BR}}^2 + \sigma_{\mathrm{WR}}^2$, respectively, i.e., the sums of between-canister and within-canister variances. The parameter θ in Equation 14.3.2 is still given by Equation 14.4.2 and $\theta < \theta_{\mathrm{BE}}$ if and only if $\zeta < 0$, where ζ is given in Equation 14.4.3. Under model 14.7.1, the best unbiased estimator of $\delta = \mu_{\mathrm{T}} - \mu_{\mathrm{R}}$ is

$$\widehat{\delta} = \bar{y}_{\mathrm{T}} - \bar{y}_{\mathrm{R}} \sim N\left(0, \frac{\sigma_{\mathrm{BT}}^2}{m_{\mathrm{T}}} + \frac{\sigma_{\mathrm{BR}}^2}{m_{\mathrm{R}}} + \frac{\sigma_{\mathrm{WT}}^2}{m_{\mathrm{T}} n_{\mathrm{T}}} + \frac{\sigma_{\mathrm{WR}}^2}{m_{\mathrm{R}} n_{\mathrm{R}}}\right),$$

where $\bar{y}_k$ is the average of y_{ijk} over i and j for a fixed k.

To construct a confidence bound for ζ in Equation 14.4.3 using the approach in Hyslop et al. (2000), it suffices to find independent, unbiased, and chi-square distributed estimators of σ_{T}^2 and σ_{R}^2 that are independent of $\hat{\delta}$. These estimators, however, are not available when $n_k > 1$. Note that

$$\sigma_k^2 = \sigma_{\mathrm{B}k}^2 + n_k^{-1}\sigma_{\mathrm{W}k}^2 + \left(1 - n_k^{-1}\right)\sigma_{\mathrm{W}k}^2, \quad k = \mathrm{T}, \mathrm{R},$$

$\sigma_{\mathrm{B}k}^2 + n_k^{-1}\,\sigma_{\mathrm{W}k}^2$ can be estimated by

$$s_{\mathrm{B}k}^2 = \frac{1}{m_k - 1}\sum_{j=1}^{m_k}\left(\bar{y}_{jk} - \bar{y}_k\right)^2 \sim \frac{\left(\sigma_{\mathrm{B}k}^2 + n_k^{-1}\sigma_{\mathrm{W}k}^2\right)\chi_{m_k-1}^2}{m_k - 1},$$

where $\bar{y}_{jk}$ is the average of y_{ijk} over i; $\sigma_{\mathrm{W}k}^2$ can be estimated by

$$s_{\mathrm{W}k}^2 = \frac{1}{m_k(n_k - 1)}\sum_{j=1}^{m_k}\sum_{i=1}^{n_k}\left(y_{ijk} - \bar{y}_{jk}\right)^2 \sim \frac{\sigma_{\mathrm{W}k}^2\chi_{m_k(n_k-1)}^2}{m_k(n_k - 1)},$$

and $\hat{\delta}$, $s_{\mathrm{B}k}^2$, $s_{\mathrm{W}k}^2$, $k = \mathrm{T}, \mathrm{R}$, are independent. Thus, applying the approach in Hyslop et al. (2000), we obtain the following approximate 95% upper confidence bound for ζ as follows:

$$\begin{aligned}\hat{\zeta}_{\mathrm{U}} = {} & \hat{\delta}^2 + s_{\mathrm{BT}}^2 + \left(1 - n_{\mathrm{T}}^{-1}\right)s_{\mathrm{WT}}^2 - s_{\mathrm{BR}}^2 - \left(1 - n_{\mathrm{R}}^{-1}\right)s_{\mathrm{WR}}^2 \\ & - \theta_{\mathrm{BE}}\max\left\{\sigma_0^2, s_{\mathrm{BR}}^2 + \left(1 - n_{\mathrm{R}}^{-1}\right)s_{\mathrm{WR}}^2\right\} + \sqrt{U},\end{aligned}$$

where U is the sum of the following five quantities:

$$\left[\left(|\hat{\delta}| + z_{0.95}\sqrt{\frac{s_{\mathrm{BT}}^2}{m_{\mathrm{T}}} + \frac{s_{\mathrm{BR}}^2}{m_{\mathrm{R}}}}\right)^2 - \hat{\delta}^2\right],$$

$$s_{\mathrm{BT}}^4\left(\frac{m_{\mathrm{T}} - 1}{\chi_{0.05;\,m_{\mathrm{T}}-1}^2} - 1\right)^2,$$

$$\left(1 - n_{\mathrm{T}}^{-1}\right)s_{\mathrm{WT}}^4\left(\frac{m_{\mathrm{T}}(n_{\mathrm{T}} - 1)}{\chi_{0.05;\,m_{\mathrm{T}}(n_{\mathrm{T}}-1)}^2} - 1\right)^2,$$

$$(1 + \theta_{\mathrm{BE}})^2 s_{\mathrm{BR}}^4\left(\frac{(m_{\mathrm{R}} - 1)}{\chi_{0.05;\,m_{\mathrm{R}}-1}^2} - 1\right)^2,$$

and

$$(1 + c\theta_{\text{BE}})^2 \left(1 - n_{\text{R}}^{-1}\right) s_{\text{WR}}^4 \left(\frac{m_{\text{R}}(n_{\text{R}} - 1)}{\chi^2_{0.95;\, m\text{R}}(n_{\text{R}} - 1)} - 1 \right)^2,$$

and $c = 1$ if $s_{\text{BR}}^2 + (1 - n_{\text{R}}^{-1})s_{\text{BR}}^2 \geq \sigma_0^2$ and $c = 0$ if $s_{\text{BR}}^2 + (1 - n_{\text{R}}^{-1})s_{\text{WR}}^2 < \sigma_0^2$. *In vitro* bioequivalence can be claimed if $\hat{\zeta}_{\text{U}} < 0$. If the difference between models 14.4.1 and 14.7.1 is ignored and the confidence bound $\hat{\zeta}_{\text{U}}$ with m_k replaced by $m_k n_k$ (instead of $\hat{\zeta}_{\text{U}}$) is used, then the asymptotic size of the test procedure is not 5%.

Simulation Results: We consider a simulation study to examine the finite sample performance (type I error probability and power) of the *in vitro* bioequivalence test described in Section 14.4. For each combination of variance parameters shown in Table 14.7.1, data are generated according to model 14.7.1. When the type I probability is considered, the value of $\delta = \mu_{\text{T}} - \mu_{\text{R}}$ is chosen so that $\zeta = 0$ (i.e., two products are not bioequivalent). When the power is considered, values of δ are selected so that $\zeta < 0$. The values of θ_{BE} and σ_0 are chosen to be 1.125 and 0.2, respectively, according to the FDA draft guidances. We consider the case where $m_{\text{T}} = m_{\text{R}} = m$ and $n_{\text{T}} = n_{\text{R}} = n$ and $(m, n) = (60, 1)$ (50, 1) (40, 1) (30, 1) (30, 2), and (30, 3). The reason to consider these combinations of sample sizes is that $(m, n) =$ (30, 1) is the minimum sample size required by the FDA draft guidances. If $m = 30$ is not enough, then we may increase either m (to 40, 50, or 60) or n (to 2 or 3).

TABLE 14.7.1: Type I error probabilities of bioequivalence test when $\theta_{\text{BE}} = 1.125$ and $\sigma_0 = 0.2$ (10,000 simulations).

				Sample Size (m, n)					
σ_{BT}	σ_{BR}	σ_{WT}	σ_{WR}	**(60, 1)**	**(50, 1)**	**(40, 1)**	**(30, 1)**	**(30, 2)**	**(30, 3)**
0	0	0.25	0.25	0.0431	0.0427	0.0388	0.0381	0.0390	0.0471
		0.25	0.50	0.0479	0.0421	0.0433	0.0411	0.0503	0.0517
		0.50	0.50	0.0431	0.0408	0.0410	0.0382	0.0431	0.0470
0.25	0.25	0.25	0.25	0.0391	0.0430	0.0395	0.0373	0.0433	0.0423
		0.25	0.50	0.0444	0.0439	0.0449	0.0444	0.0451	0.0493
		0.50	0.50	0.0414	0.0423	0.0455	0.0424	0.0429	0.0454
0.50	0.25	0.25	0.50	0.0414	0.0412	0.0412	0.0402	0.0415	0.0436
		0.50	0.50	0.0389	0.0361	0.0408	0.0353	0.0353	0.0404
0.25	0.50	0.25	0.25	0.0434	0.0396	0.0428	0.0437	0.0401	0.0454
		0.50	0.25	0.0439	0.0442	0.0419	0.0396	0.0405	0.0391
		0.25	0.50	0.0431	0.0444	0.0446	0.0395	0.0460	0.448
		0.50	0.50	0.0406	0.0431	0.0406	0.0379	0.0385	0.0420
0.50	0.50	0.25	0.25	0.0416	0.0430	0.0418	0.0369	0.0380	0.0392
		0.50	0.25	0.0398	0.0404	0.0360	0.0365	0.0350	0.0341
		0.25	0.50	0.0452	0.0453	0.0400	0.0391	0.0463	0.0439
		0.50	0.50	0.0468	0.0473	0.0401	0.0432	0.0425	0.0411

The simulation results for the type I error probability based on 10,000 runs are given in Table 14.7.1. The type I error probability ranges from 3.41% to 5.17% It is under the nominal level 5% in all but two cases and are generally close to 5%. The following are some observations:

1. Except for the cases where $\sigma_{\mathrm{T}}^2 > \sigma_{\mathrm{R}}^2$ (the total variability of the test product is larger than that of the reference product), a reasonable power (say 80%) can be reached by either increasing the total number of observations or decreasing the value of ζ. For cases where $\sigma_{\mathrm{T}}^2 > \sigma_{\mathrm{R}}^2$ in the simulation, the chance of claiming bioequivalence is small when the two products are in fact bioequivalent.

2. The sample sizes $m = 30$ and $n = 1$ do not lead to a satisfactory power unless $\sigma_{\mathrm{T}}^2 > \sigma_{\mathrm{R}}^2$.

3. When the between-canister variances are nonzero, having more canisters is preferred than having more replicates within each canister (if the power of the bioequivalence test is the only concern). In all cases, the choice of $m = 60$ and $n = 1$ is better than the choice of $m = 60$ and $n = 2$ although the total number of observations are the same. The choice of $m = 60$ and $n = 1$ is even better than the choice of $m = 30$ and $n = 3$ in 11 out of 13 cases, although the latter has a larger total number of observations. In fact, the choice of $m = 30$ and $n = 3$ is even worse than the choice of $m = 50$ and $n = 1$ in some cases.

4. When $\sigma_{\mathrm{BT}}^2 = \sigma_{\mathrm{BR}}^2 = 0$ (i.e., there is no canister-to-canister variation), the data sets for the cases of $(m, n) = (60, 1)$ and $(m, n) = (30, 2)$ are the same, but the test procedures are different, since, in the case of $(m, n) = (30, 2)$, we do not assume that one knows that $\sigma_{\mathrm{BT}}^2 = \sigma_{\mathrm{BR}}^2 = 0$. However, the results show that the two procedures have almost the same power.

14.7.2 Profile Analysis

The bootstrap procedure described in Section 14.4 has received much attention and criticisms since it was introduced by the FDA. Major criticisms are described below.

First, the statistical properties of this procedure are unknown. It includes two aspects. One is that the statistical model, which should be used to describe the profile data, is not clearly defined in the FDA draft guidances. In addition, even under an appropriate statistical model, the statistical properties of the bootstrap procedure are still unknown. More specifically, it is not clear whether the bootstrap sample means a consistent estimator for *E*(*rd*). As a result, the 95% percentile of the bootstrap samples may not be an appropriate 95% upper bound for *E*(*rd*). These questions are not addressed in the FDA draft guidances.

Second, no criteria are given regarding the passage or failure of the bioequivalence study. This is the issue that confuses most researchers/scientists in practice. After the conduct of a valid trial and an appropriate statistical analysis following the FDA draft guidance, the sponsor still cannot tell if its product has passed or failed the bioequivalence test. This is a direct consequence of our first point (i.e., the statistical properties of the recommended bootstrap procedure are unknown).

Third, the simulation study using different random number generation schemes may produce contradictory results. It is possible for a good product to fail the bioequivalence test simply because of bad luck. It is also possible for a bad product to pass the bioequivalence test with an "appropriate" choice of random number generation scheme. As a result, researchers/scientists tend to rely more on the descriptive statistics of the two products in order to assess their bioequivalence instead of the bootstrap procedure. The proposed bootstrap procedure recommended by the FDA is not as reliable as it should be.

As a result, further research of profile analysis becomes a problem of interest in practice. More specifically, the questions of interest include (1) What statistical model should be used to describe the profile data? (2) Is $E(rd)$ defined by the FDA a good parameter for characterizing the bioequivalence between test and reference products? (Can we define the test-to-reference distance and reference-to-reference variability differently?) (3) What bioequivalence limit should we use to evaluate the *in vitro* bioequivalence between two products based on appropriate model, parameter, and bioequivalence criterion?

14.7.3 Multiple Strengths

As indicated in the 2003 FDA draft guidance, a small number of nasal sprays for local action are available in two strengths (lower and higher strength) such as ipratropium bromide nasal spray and beclomethasone dipropionate nasal spray. Lower strengths of a product would achieve the lower dose per actuation using a lower concentration formulation, without changing the actuator and metering valve or pump used in the higher strength product. The FDA recommends that the bioavailability of lower or higher strength solution formulation nasal sprays be used on conduct of all applicable *in vitro* tests described earlier in this chapter. Table 14.7.2 lists *in vitro* tests recommended by the FDA to document bioequivalence of the lower strength of the test product to the low-strength of the reference product provided bioequivalence of the high-strength product has been documented. It should be noted that for establishment of bioequivalence, the FDA recommends that the same protocols and acceptance criteria be used for both low-strength and high-strength products.

Chapter 15

In Vitro *Dissolution Profiles Comparison*

15.1 Introduction

In vivo bioequivalence studies are surrogate trials for assessing equivalence between a test and a reference formulations based on the rate and extent of drug absorption in humans without actually performing clinical trials to establish similar effectiveness and safety. The *Fundamental Bioequivalence Assumption* implies that bioequivalent formulations are therapeutically equivalent and can be used interchangeably. After a drug is approved for commercial marketing, there may be some changes in chemistry, manufacturing, and controls for drug production. Therefore, scientifically, the test formulation manufactured after the changes must show formulation quality and performance similar to that of the currently accepted reference formulation before it can be approved for commercial use. On the other hand, drug absorption depends on the dissolved state of drug product, and dissolution testing provides a rapid *in vitro* assessment of the rate and extent of drug release. Leeson (1995), therefore, suggested that *in vitro* dissolution testing be used as a surrogate for *in vivo* bioequivalence studies to assess equivalence between the test and reference formulations for postapproval changes.

On November 30, 1995, the FDA issued the guidance *Immediate Release Solid Oral Dosage Forms*; *Scale-up and Postapproval Changes*: *Chemistry, Manufacturing, and Controls*; *In Vitro Dissolution Testing*; *In Vivo Bioequivalence Documentation.* This guidance is known as the scale-up and post-approval change (SUPAC) guidance. SUPAC provides recommendations to sponsors of new drug applications (NDAs), abbreviated new drug applications (ANDAs), and abbreviated antibiotic drug applications (AADAs), which intend, during the postapproval period to change (1) the components or compositions, (2) the site of manufacture, (3) the scale-up or scale-down of manufacture, or (4) the manufacturing (process and equipment) of an immediate-release oral formulation. For each type of change, the SUPAC also defines (1) levels of changes; (2) recommended chemistry, manufacturing, and controls test for each level of change; (3) *in vitro* dissolution or *in vivo* bioequivalence tests for each level of change; and (4) documentation that should support the change. Table 15.1.1 provides a summary of required *in vitro* dissolution and *in vivo* bioequivalence tests for different levels and types of changes specified in the SUPAC. Except for bioequivalence study for level 3 changes in components, composition, and process, most other changes require only

TABLE 15.1.1: Summary of *in vitro* dissolution and *in vivo* bioequivalence tests required in the SUPAC.

Type	Level	Dissolution	Bioequivalence
Components and composition	1	None beyond application/ compendial requirement	None
	2	HP and HS: case A LP and HS: case B HP and LS: case C	None
	3	Case B	Full BE study
Site	1	None beyond application/ compendial requirement	None
	2	None beyond application/ compendial requirement	None
	3	Case B	None
Batch size	1	None beyond application/ compendial requirement	None
	2	Case B	None
Manufacturing equipment	1	None beyond application/ compendial requirement	None
	2	Case C	
Process	1	None beyond application/ compendial requirement	None
	2	Case B	None
	3	Case B	BE study

Note: HP, high permeability; LP, low permeability; HS, high solubility; LS, low solubility.

dissolution tests, which should be conducted on at least 12 individual dosage units. On the other hand, as indicated in the FDA guidances (FDA, 1997b, 2003e) and the WHO draft guideline (WHO, 2005a,b), for immediate-release products with multiple strengths, the *in vivo* bioequivalence study may be conducted only at the highest dose. Under some conditions, *in vivo* bioequivalence studies on one or more lower doses can be waived based on dissolution tests. According to the biopharmaceutics classification system (BCS), based on aqueous solubility and intestinal permeability, an active pharmaceutical ingredient can be classified into the following four classes (Amidon et al., 1995):

Class I: High solubility, high permeability

Class II: Low solubility, high permeability

Class III: High solubility, low permeability

Class IV: Low solubility, low permeability

In addition, for consideration of biowaiver, the WHO guidelines on multisource drug products classified the drug products according to their dissolving rate. A generic drug product is classified as a very rapidly dissolving if at least 85% of the labeled amount of the drug substance dissolves within 15 minutes using a basket apparatus at 100 rpm or a paddle apparatus at 75 rpm in a volume of less than 900 mL in each of the following media: (1) pH 1.2 HCl solution, (2) a pH 4.5 acetate buffer, and (3) a pH 6.8 phosphate buffer. On the other hand, no less than 85% of the labeled amount of the drug substance for a rapidly dissolving generic drug product dissolves in 30 minutes using a basket apparatus at 100 rpm or a paddle apparatus at 75 rpm in a volume of less than 900 mL in each of the following media: (1) pH 1.2 HCl solution, (2) pH 4.5 acetate buffer, and (3) pH 6.8 phosphate buffer. The U.S. FDA guidance on *Waiver of In Vivo Bioavailability and Bioequivalence Studies for Immediate-Release Solid Oral Dosage Forms Based on a Biopharmaceutics Classification System* (FDA, 2000) recommends the biowaiver only for the drug substance that is highly soluble and highly permeable (Class I). On the other hand, under some conditions, the WHO guidance (2005a) also considers the biowaiver for the highly soluble and low permeable drug substances (Class III). Although the U.S. FDA and WHO may have different criteria for biowaiver of *in vivo* bioequivalence studies, similarity in dissolution profiles between the generic and reference drug product at different strengths must be established via *in vitro* dissolution testing to approve the generic drug products.

In Section 15.2, *in vitro* dissolution testing is briefly described. In addition, concepts and criteria for assessment of similarity of dissolution profiles are provided. In general, the FDA guidance (FDA, 1997b) classified the criteria into model-independent and model-dependent approaches. The FDA guidance refers the model-dependence to as the differential shapes among dissolution profiles rather than the distributional assumption of the responses. Some comments are given regards the advantages and drawbacks of various criteria based on the two approaches. In Section 15.3, statistical procedures are introduced to evaluate the similarity of dissolution profiles between the generic and reference drug products. These include similarity and difference factors suggested in the FDA guidance (FDA, 1997b). In Section 15.4, the procedures based on the multivariate confidence region are surveyed. These include the procedure suggested in the FDA guidance (FDA, 1997b) and those by Eaton, Muirhead, and Steeno (2003) and Saranadasa and Krishnamoorthy (2005). Final remarks and discussion are given in Section 15.5.

15.2 Criterion for Assessment of Similarity between Dissolution Profiles

A typical dissolution test instrument usually consists of six vessels for agitated medium. Each vessel is of the size of one liter. The dissolution testing procedure, as recommended by the FDA guidance (FDA, 1995, 1997b), puts 12 dosage units (tablets or capsules) into agitated medium. Then a basket or a paddle is handed down to excite the medium. The 1997 FDA guidance (FDA, 1997b) suggests that a dissolution testing be performed at a 15 minutes interval to generate a dissolution profile under the basket method at 50/100 rpm or a paddle method at 50/75 rpm. With respect to the characteristics of the drug products, at different prespecified time points, samples are taken and analyzed by some validated assays using certain techniques such as chromatography or UV spectroscopy. In general, the sampling time points are every 15 minutes for the first hour and every hour afterwards.

The variable of interest is the cumulative percentage of dosage unit dissolved in the medium at a particular time point. Let Y_{hti} as the cumulative percentage dissolved for dosage unit i at sampling time point t for formulation h, where $i=1,\ldots, I$, $t=1,\ldots, n$, $h=\text{T, R}$, and T and R denote the test and reference formulation, respectively. Therefore, the dissolution profile of dosage unit i for formulation h is represented by the vector of cumulative dissolution rates over n time points

$$\mathbf{Y}_{hi} = (Y_{h1i}, \ldots, Y_{hni})', \tag{15.2.1}$$

with corresponding population mean vector

$$\boldsymbol{\mu}_h = (\mu_{h1}, \ldots, \mu_{hn})', \tag{15.2.2}$$

where

$$\begin{aligned} \mu_{ht} &= E(Y_{hti}) \\ i &= 1,\ldots, I \\ t &= 1,\ldots, n \\ h &= \text{T, R} \end{aligned}$$

Because Y_{hti} is the cumulative percentage dissolved at time point t, it follows that

$$Y_{h1i} \leq Y_{h2i} \leq \cdots \leq Y_{hni} \quad \text{and} \quad \mu_{h1} \leq \mu_{h2} \leq \cdots \leq \mu_{hn}.$$

The objective for evaluation of similarity of dissolution profiles between the test and reference formulation is to assess the closeness between two mean dissolution vectors $\boldsymbol{\mu}_\text{T}$ and $\boldsymbol{\mu}_\text{C}$.

The approaches recommended by the FDA guidance (FDA, 1995, 1997) can be classified into two categories. The first is the model-independent approach which does not require the knowledge of the shape of the dissolution profile and to fit a model that can adequately describe the dissolution profile. On the other hand, the model-dependent methods must select the most appropriate model to fit the dissolution profiles for the test and reference formulations. However, similarity of dissolution profiles must consider (1) the overall profile similarity and (2) similarity at each sampling time point. In order to achieve these two objectives, based on Moore and Flanner (1996), both the SUPAC guidance (FDA, 1995) and guidance on dissolution testing (FDA, 1997b) suggest the similarity and difference factor for assessment of similarity. The similarity factor is then defined as the logarithmic reciprocal square root transformation of 1 plus the mean-squared (the average sum of squares) difference in mean cumulative percentage dissolved between the test and reference formulations over all sampling time points. That is,

$$f_2 = 50 \log\left\{\left[1 + \frac{Q}{n}\right]^{-0.5} \cdot 100\right\}, \tag{15.2.3}$$

where

$$Q = \sum_{t=1}^{n} (\mu_{Rt} - \mu_{Tt})^2, \tag{15.2.4}$$

and log denotes the logarithm based on 10.

On the other hand, the difference factor is the sum of the absolute difference in mean cumulative percentage dissolved between the test and reference formulations divided by the sum of the mean cumulative dissolved of the reference formulation.

$$f_1 = \frac{\sum_{t=1}^{n} |\mu_{Ri} - \mu_{Ti}|}{\sum_{t=1}^{n} \mu_{Ri}}. \tag{15.2.5}$$

The guidance on dissolution testing (FDA, 1997) made the following recommendations on the design, sampling time points, and precision of the measurements:

1. Dissolution measurements of the test and reference formulations should be obtained under the exactly the same considerations. The sampling time points should be the same (e.g., 15, 30, 45, 60 minutes) for both formulations.

2. For both formulations, only one measurement after 85% cumulative dissolution is reached.

3. Because the sample mean dissolution is used to estimate μ_{ht}, the percent coefficient of variation should be less than 20% at the earlier points up to 15 minutes and 10% at other sampling time points.

It should be noted that the definitions of f_1 and f_2 provided by Moore and Flanner (1996) and in the SUPAC and guidance on dissolution testing are not clear whether they are defined based on the population means or the sample averages. However, following the traditional statistical inference with ability for evaluation of error probability, we define both f_1 and f_2 based on the population mean dissolution rates. It follows that f_1 and f_2 are population parameters for assessment of similarity of dissolution profiles between the test and reference formulations.

If there is no difference in mean cumulative percentages at all time points, the value of f_2 is 100. On the other hand, theoretically, Q could be 100,000 and, hence, the corresponding f_2 is 0. The range of the similarity factor, therefore, is between 0 and 100. With respect to f_1, if the mean cumulative percentages dissolved for the test formulation are equal to that for the reference formulation at all time points, then f_1 is 0. However, although it is quite impossible to occur in practice, when the mean cumulative percentages dissolved of the test formulation are zero at all time points, then f_1 is 100. Although the range of both of f_1 and f_2 is from 0 to 100, the direction in assessment of similarity is completely opposite. A value of 100 for f_2 is completely similar while it is completely dissimilar for f_1. On the other hand, a value of 0 for f_2 is completely dissimilar while it is completely similar for f_1. The guidance on dissolution testing (FDA, 1997) suggests that two dissolution profiles are similar if the difference factor f_1 is less than 15. This implies that similarity of the dissolution profiles between the test and reference formulations can be claimed if the absolute mean difference in cumulative percentage between the test and reference formulations is no less than 15% of the total mean cumulative dissolution rate of the reference formulation.

For f_2, both SUPAC and the FDA guidance on dissolution testing recommend that the dissolution profile of the test formulation is similar to that of the reference formulation if f_2 is greater than 50. Shah et al. (1998) show that if the mean difference in cumulative percentage is 10 for all sampling time point, then Q/n is 100. It follows that

$$\begin{aligned} f_2 &= 50 \cdot \log[(\sqrt{101}) \cdot 100] \\ &= 50 \cdot \log(9.95037) \\ &= 49.89 \\ &\approx 50. \end{aligned}$$

Therefore, f_2 is greater than 50 if the difference in mean cumulative percentage is less than 10% at all time points. Since all SUPAC related guidance issued by the FDA and the draft guidance on bioequivalence by the WHO adopted f_2 as the criterion for evaluation of dissolution profiles between the test and reference formulations. In what follows, we focus on f_2 and its inference. First of all, we notice that f_2 is location invariant.

Q is the sum of squares of mean differences in cumulative percentage dissolved. It remains unchanged if the mean cumulative percentage dissolved of both formulations shifting by the same amount (Liu et al., 1997). Because f_2 is a continuous function of Q, f_2 also remains unchanged. The data sets provided by Tsong (1995) and Chow and Ki (1997) can be used to illustrate this concept. The cumulative percentage dissolved of both test and reference formulations is subtracted by amounts of 0, 15, 28, 35, 47, 55, and 65, respectively, at sampling time points 1, 2, 3, 4, 6, 8, and 10 hours. Table 15.2.1 displays the averages and variances by formulation and time point for the original data and transformed data with location change. Figures 15.2.1 and 15.2.2 give the average dissolution profiles of two formulations, in percentage label claimed for the test and reference formulations, respectively. For the original data, $Q=48.85$ with the corresponding $f_2=72.45$. Since f_2 is between 50 and 100, we claim that the two profiles are similar. From Table 15.2.1, the average of cumulative percentage dissolved for the transformed

TABLE 15.2.1: Summary statistics for the dissolution data.

Formulation	Time Points (in Hours)	Original		Location Change	
		Average	Variance	Average	Variance
Reference	1	45.08	10.27	45.08	10.27
	2	54.00	11.64	39.00	11.64
	3	62.50	11.00	34.50	11.00
	4	67.08	14.08	32.08	14.08
	6	74.75	15.48	27.75	15.48
	8	80.25	17.66	25.25	17.66
	10	85.33	20.24	20.33	20.24
Test	1	36.50	1.91	36.50	1.91
	2	50.08	5.17	35.08	5.17
	3	62.17	2.15	34.17	2.15
	4	68.75	4.75	33.75	4.75
	6	79.33	6.42	32.33	6.42
	8	86.42	13.90	31.42	13.90
	10	92.00	5.82	27.00	5.82
		$Q=48.85$	$f_2=77.45$	$q=48.85$	$f_2=77.45$

Source: From Tsong, Y., Statistical assessment of mean differences between two dissolution data sets. Presented at the 1995 Drug Information Association Dissolution Workshop, Rockville, Maryland, 1995.

data decreases as time increases. The values of Q and f_2, however, remain unchanged as 48.85 and 72.45, respectively.

Even though, in practice, it is impossible for average cumulative percentage dissolved to be a decreasing function of sampling time points, according to the criterion based on f_2, for the transformed data with the location changes, the test formulation is claimed similar to the reference because of the same value of f_2. This

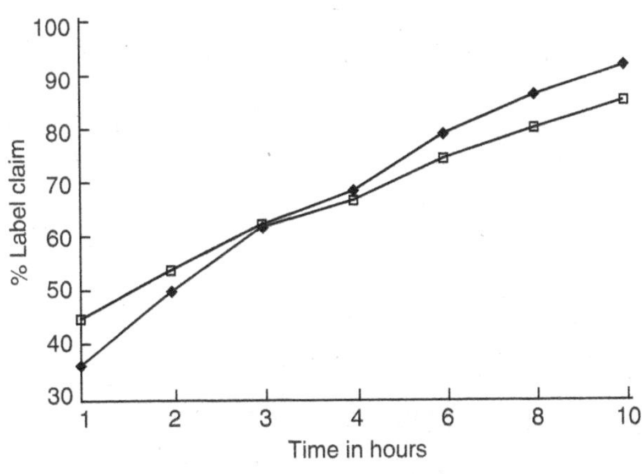

FIGURE 15.2.1: Mean percentage label claim by time in hours.

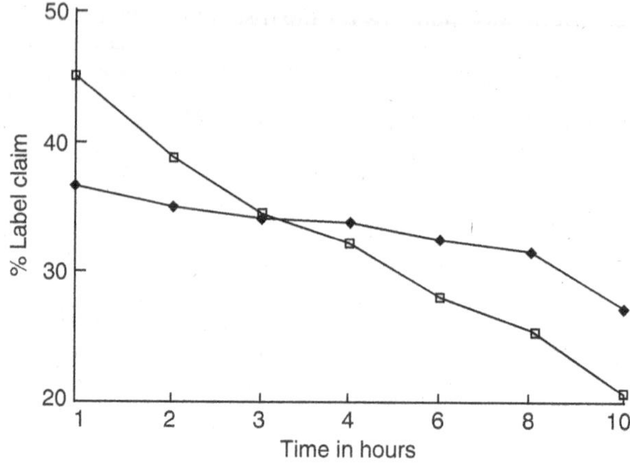

FIGURE 15.2.2: Mean percentage label claim by time in hours for transformed data.

example illustrates a serious deficiency in the use of the similarity factor in assessment of similarity between dissolution profiles. The similarity factor is not only insensitive to the shape of the curves, but also it cannot take into account the information of unequal spacing between sampling time points. In addition, the SUPAC guidance requires that dissolution testing for cases B and C must be performed until the time point when the asymptote is reached. It is impossible for f_2 to differentiate a dissolution profile with the asymptote reached from that without achieving asymptote. On the other hand, the USP/NF also specifies in the individual monographs the minimum amount of cumulative percentage of active ingredient dissolved achieved at certain sampling time points. For example, the SUPAC requests that dissolution testing for case C drug products must be performed at 15, 30, 45, 60, and 120 minutes until either 90% of the drug from the drug product is dissolved, or an asymptote is reached. Therefore, it does not matter whether the asymptote is reached or the amount of cumulative percentage dissolved reaches 90%, two dissolution profiles will be declared similar as long as f_2 is between 50 and 100.

When the within-batch coefficient of variation exceeds 15%, the U.S. FDA guidance on dissolution testing recommends the use of a multivariate model-independent procedure. The steps suggested by the FDA guidance are given in the following:

1. To use the multivariate statistical distance (MSD) based on the interbatch differences from reference formulation (standard approved) to establish the similarity limits.

2. To obtain the estimate of MSD between the test and reference formulations.

3. To obtain a 90% confidence interval of true MSD between the test and reference formulations.

4. If the upper limit of the 90% confidence interval is less than or equal to the similarity limit determined in (1), then the dissolution profile of the test formulation is declared to be similar to that of the reference formulation.

The FDA guidance on dissolution testing suggests that the model-dependent approaches for assessment of similarity of dissolution profiles include the following steps:

1. Determine the most appropriate statistical model for the dissolution profiles for the test and reference formulations. The FDA guidance also recommends a model with no more than three parameters such as linear, quadratic, logistic, probit or Weibull models.
2. Fit the data for the profile generated for each unit to the most appropriate model.
3. Based on variation of the estimates of the parameters of the fitted model for test units, obtain a similarity region from the reference formulation.
4. Calculate the MSD for the model parameters between the test and reference formulations.
5. Obtain the 90% confidence region for the true difference between the test and reference formulations.
6. If the 90% confidence region is within the limits of the similarity region, the test formulation is claimed to have a dissolution profile to the reference formulation.

In all SUPAC guidances and the WHO draft guideline on multisource drug products, similarity factor f_2 is selected to evaluate the similarity of dissolution profiles between the test and reference formulations. Therefore, we focus on the statistical inference of f_2 although we review the statistical properties of f_1 and procedures based on model-independent multivariate confidence region (Eaton et al., 2003; Saranadasa and Krishnamoorthy, 2005).

15.3 Inference for Similarity Factors

The upper limit of the possible range of f_2 is 100, which is the same as the upper limit for f_2 specified in the SUPAC. As a result, one has to consider only the lower limit of f_2 for assessment of similarity between dissolution profiles. In other words, the dissolution profile of the test formulation is claimed to be similar to that of the reference if f_2 is greater than a number less than 100, say 50, as suggested in the SUPAC guidance. In contrast with the criterion for average bioequivalence, which can be formulated as an interval hypothesis for the ratio of average bioavailabilities between 0.8 and 1.25, implementation of the similarity factor f_2 is, in fact, a one-sided problem for assessment of similarity between two dissolution profiles. As a result, the hypothesis for evaluation of similarity of dissolution profiles between the test and reference formulations based on similarity factor is formulated as the following one-sided hypothesis:

$$\begin{aligned} &\text{H}_0\text{: } f_2 \leq \theta_0 \\ \text{versus } &\text{H}_\text{a}\text{: } f_2 > \theta_0, \end{aligned} \tag{15.3.1}$$

where θ_0 is set as 50 by the FDA and WHO guidelines.

One of the natural estimators of f_2 is to replace the population mean dissolution rates by their corresponding sample means calculated from at least 12 dosage units at each time point. Let

$$\overline{Y}_{ht\cdot} = \frac{1}{I}\sum_{i=1}^{I} Y_{hti}.$$

Then an estimator of f_2 is given as

$$\begin{aligned} \widehat{f_2} &= 50 \log[(1 + W/n)^{-1/2} \cdot 100] \\ &= 100 - 25 \log(1 + W/n), \end{aligned} \tag{15.3.2}$$

where

$$W = \sum_{t=1}^{n} (\overline{Y}_{\text{R}t\cdot} - \overline{Y}_{\text{T}t\cdot})^2.$$

Following Ma et al. (2000), assume that $\mathbf{Y}_{hi}$ follows an $n \times 1$ multivariate normal distribution with mean vector $\boldsymbol{\mu}_h$ and covariance matrix $\boldsymbol{\Sigma}_h$, $h = \text{T, R}$. Define $\mathbf{D}$ as the vector of the differences in sample mean vector of cumulative dissolution rates, i.e., $\mathbf{D} = \overline{\mathbf{Y}}_\text{R} - \overline{\mathbf{Y}}_\text{T}$, where $\overline{\mathbf{Y}}_h = (\overline{Y}_{h1\cdot}, \ldots, \overline{Y}_{hn\cdot})$. It follows that D is distributed as a $t \times 1$ multivariate normal distribution with mean vector $\boldsymbol{\mu}_\text{D}$ and covariance matrix $\boldsymbol{\Sigma}_\text{D}$, where $\boldsymbol{\mu}_\text{D} = \boldsymbol{\mu}_\text{R} - \boldsymbol{\mu}_\text{T}$, and $\boldsymbol{\Sigma}_\text{D} = (\boldsymbol{\Sigma}_\text{R} + \boldsymbol{\Sigma}_\text{T})/I$. Since $W = \mathbf{D}'\mathbf{D}$, it follows that

$$\begin{aligned} E(W) &= \boldsymbol{\mu}_\text{D}'\boldsymbol{\mu}_\text{D} + tr(\boldsymbol{\Sigma}_\text{D}) \\ &= \boldsymbol{\mu}_\text{D}'\boldsymbol{\mu}_\text{D} + \sigma_\text{D}^2 \\ &= Q + \sigma_\text{D}^2 \end{aligned} \tag{15.3.3}$$

where

$\sigma_\text{D}^2 = \frac{1}{I}\sum_{t=1}^{n}(\sigma_{\text{R}t}^2 + \sigma_{\text{T}t}^2)$

σ_{ht}^2 is the tth diagonal element of $\boldsymbol{\Sigma}_h$, $t = 1, \ldots, n$; $h = \text{T, R}$

The result of $E(W)$ in Equation 15.3.3 holds even without normality assumption. Although $\widehat{f_2}$ is a continuous function of W, as shown in Ma et al. (1999), its probability density distribution is very complicated even under the normality assumption. However, the expected value of $\widehat{f_2}$ can be approximated by the Taylor's series expansion about $E(W)$

$$
\begin{aligned}
E(\widehat{f_2}) &\approx 100 - 25\log[1 + E(W)/n] \\
&= 100 - 25\log[1 + Q/n + \sigma_D^2] \\
&\leq 100 - 25\log[1 + Q/n] \\
&= f_2.
\end{aligned}
$$

Therefore, $\widehat{f_2}$ is conservative in evaluation of dissolution similarity (Shah et al., 1998). However, because $\widehat{f_2}$ converges in probability to f_2 as I goes large, then $\widehat{f_2}$ is asymptotically unbiased when the number of dosage units at each time points becomes large. Because the distribution of $\widehat{f_2}$ is very complicated, both Ma et al. (2000) and Shah et al. (1998) recommend the use of nonparametric bootstrap method to evaluate its sampling distribution for hypothesis 15.3.1. The procedures of non-parametric bootstrap method for evaluation of the similarity of dissolution profiles are outlined below:

1. Based on the dosage units, generate bootstrap samples $\mathbf{y}_{hi}^* = (y_{h1i}^*, \ldots, Y_{hni}^*)'$ by sampling with replacement from I n-variate vectors of the observed cumulative percentage dissolved $\mathbf{Y}_{hi} = (\mathrm{Y}_{h1i}, \ldots, \mathrm{Y}_{hni})'$. Sampling unit is the dosage unit. In addition, sampling should be carried out independently for the samples of dosages units and separately from the test and reference formulations.

2. Compute $\widehat{f_2^*}$ based on the bootstrap samples using formula 15.3.2.

3. Repeat steps 1 and 2 a large number of times, say 5,000.

4. Use the $\alpha 100\%$ percentile of the sampling distribution of $\widehat{f_2^*}$ as the $(1-\alpha)$ 100% lower confidence limit of f_2.

5. Conclude that the dissolution profile of the test formulation is similar to the reference formulation at the α significance level if the $(1-\alpha)100\%$ lower confidence limit of f_2 is greater than 50.

Ma et al. (2000) report the results of a simulation study about the bias of $\widehat{f_2}$, and size and power of the bootstrap procedure for evaluation of similarity of dissolution profiles based on hypothesis 15.3.1.

The random samples of the simulation were generated under the following assumptions: (1) $\mu_{Rt} - \mu_{Tt} = \delta$, for $t = 1, \ldots, n$, and (2) $\mathbf{\Sigma}_T = \mathbf{\Sigma}_R = \sigma_S^2 \mathbf{J}_n + \sigma_e^2 \mathbf{I}_n$ where σ_S^2 is the between-unit variance, σ_e^2 is the within-unit variance, $\mathbf{J}_n$ is a $n \times n$ matrix of 1, and $\mathbf{I}_n$ is the $n \times n$ identity matrix. Table 15.3.1 provides the empirical bias of $\widehat{f_2}$ when the total variation is 27.6312 which represents a coefficient of variation about 6.6% at the mean cumulative dissolution rate of 80%. From Table 15.3.1, the f_2 is severely underestimated by $\widehat{f_2}$ when δ is zero. The magnitude of underestimation ranges from 10% to 24%. However, as δ increases, magnitude of bias decreases and bias becomes positive. In addition, the absolute magnitude of bias is a monotonically decreasing function of the number of dosage units. From the results of simulation, it demonstrates that $\widehat{f_2}$ severely underestimates f_2 when δ is zero and f_2 is 100 for the dissolution

TABLE 15.3.1: Empirical bias of $\widehat{f_2}$.

		$\delta=0$			$\delta=6$		
N	I	$a=0.2$	$a=0.5$	$a=0.8$	$a=0.2$	$a=0.5$	$a=0.8$
3	6	−22.25	−21.64	−20.31	−0.44	0.48	1.59
	12	−16.42	−15.85	−14.79	−0.18	0.35	1.04
	18	−13.35	−12.98	−12.19	−0.04	0.24	0.71
	24	−11.41	−11.00	−10.15	0.01	0.20	0.44
5	6	−23/47	−22.47	−20.77	−1.02	0.15	1.29
	12	−17.20	−16.55	−15.26	−0.47	0.10	0.73
	18	−13.97	−13.83	−12.29	−0.31	0.15	0.64
	24	−111.90	−11.38	−10.43	−0.24	0.08	0.49
7	6	−23.87	−22.90	−20.88	−1.21	−0.07	1.36
	12	−17.55	−16.79	−15.40	−0.59	0.17	0.80
	18	−14.34	−13.59	−12.45	−0.39	0.08	0.57
	24	−12.11	−11.66	−10.61	0.23	0.05	0.43

Source: Reproduced from Ma, M.C., Wang, B.B.C, Liu, J.P., and Tsong, Y., *J. Biopharm. Stat.*, 10, 229, 2000.

Note: $a=\sigma_S^2/(\sigma_S^2+\sigma_e^2)$ and $\sigma_S^2+\sigma_e^2=27.6312$; N, the number of sampling time points and I, the number of dosage units.

profiles of the test and reference formulations being the same. To overcome this drawback, Shah et al. (1998) suggest the following estimator of f_2:

$$\begin{aligned}\widetilde{f_2} &= 50\log[(1+W^*/n)^{-1/2}\cdot 100]\\ &= 100-25\log(1+W^*/n), \end{aligned} \tag{15.3.4}$$

where

$$W^* = W - \sum_{t=1}^{n}\left(S_{Rt}^2+S_{Tt}^2\right)/I.$$

and S_{ht}^2 is the sample estimator of σ_{ht}^2.

However, its performance in reduction of bias and in testing hypothesis 15.3.1 was not thoroughly investigated.

Table 15.3.2 presented the empirical size reported by Ma et al. (2000) in testing hypothesis 15.3.1 based on the bootstrap procedures based on $\widehat{f_2}$. The total variances considered in the simulation are 7.5, 64, and 128 which represent about CV of 3.4%, 10%, and 14% at the mean cumulative percent dissolved of 80%. As mentioned before, a CV of 14% is allowed for dissolution at early time points, e.g., 15 minutes. On the other hand, as specified in the FDA guidance in dissolution testing, a CV of 10% is allowed for the time points after 15 minutes while in a typical dissolution experiment a CV of 3.4% for cumulative percent dissolved is commonly observed. In general the size of the bootstrap procedures based on $\widehat{f_2}$ is a decreasing function of total variation. In addition, the size approaches to the nominal level of 5%

TABLE 15.3.2: Empirical size of $\widehat{f_2}$.

		$a = \sigma_S^2/(\sigma_S^2 + \sigma_e^2)$		
Total Variance	***I***	**0.2**	**0.5**	**0.8**
7.5	6	5.4	6.3	7.8
	12	4.6	5.0	4.9
	18	4.2	4.8	5.1
	24	4.1	4.5	4.1
64	6	3.0	4.5	6.9
	12	2.7	5.5	5.3
	18	3.3	3.9	5.3
	24	3.2	4.6	5.3
128	6	0.4	1.3	3.2
	12	1.9	3.3	4.9
	18	2.0	4.2	4.9
	24	2.6	3.8	4.7

as the dosage units increases. Furthermore, the empirical size increases as the between-unit variation increases. However, the bootstrap procedure based on $\widehat{f_2}$ is quite conservative as demonstrated by the most of the empirical sizes being less than the nominal level of 5% when total variation is large. But when the proportion of the between-unit variation reaches 80% and the number of dosage units is 6, the size becomes inflated above the nominal level of 5%. Figure 15.3.1 provides an empirical power curve when the CV is 10% at the 80% mean cumulative percent dissolved and

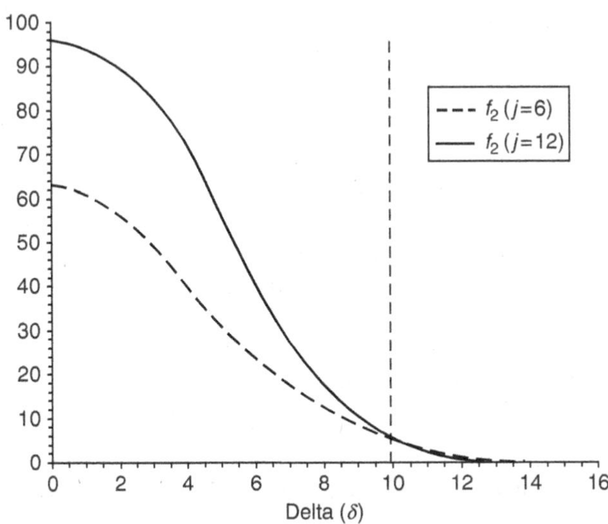

FIGURE 15.3.1: Empirical power curve of f_2 for total variation = 64, I = 12, n = 4.

the number of dosage units is 6 or 12. From Figure 15.3.1, the power is an increasing power of the number of dosage units and is a decreasing function of δ. This figure also indicates that the power is only about 64% at $\delta=0$ when the CV is 10%. However, when the number of dosage units is 12 the power at $\delta=0$ can reach to 95%. This concurs that the number of dosage units should be at least 12 suggested by the FDA guidance.

With respect to the difference factor f_1, its maximum likelihood estimator can be obtained by substituting the population means by their corresponding sample means. It follows that

$$\widehat{f_1} = \frac{\sum_{t=1}^{n} |\overline{Y}_{Rt\cdot} - \overline{Y}_{Tt\cdot}|}{\sum_{t=1}^{n} \overline{Y}_{Rt\cdot}}. \tag{15.3.5}$$

Although $\widehat{f_1}$ is a consistent estimator of f_1, it is not unbiased and the unbiased estimator of f_1 does not exist. In addition, the distribution of $\widehat{f_1}$ is very complicated and intractable. As a result, the U.S. FDA guidance and the WHO draft guideline select f_2 as the criterion for assessment of similarity for dissolution profiles between the test and reference formulations.

15.4 Approaches Based on Multivariate Confidence Regions

Hypotheses 15.3.1 for assessing similarity of dissolution profiles between the test and reference formulations can be expressed in terms of the average Euclidean distance of the population mean differences in cumulative percent dissolved as follows:

$$\begin{aligned} &\text{H}_0\text{: } \boldsymbol{\mu}_D'\boldsymbol{\mu}_D/n \geq 100 \\ \text{versus } &\text{H}_a\text{: } \boldsymbol{\mu}_D'\boldsymbol{\mu}_D/n < 100. \end{aligned} \tag{15.4.1}$$

In addition, if $|\mu_{Tt} - \mu_{Rt}| < 10$, for all $t = 1, \ldots, n$, then the alternative hypothesis 15.4.1 is true. As a result, the similarity of dissolution profile can be constructed on the rectangular neighborhood by the following hypothesis:

$$\begin{aligned} &\text{H}_0\text{: } |\mu_{Tt} - \mu_{Rt}| \geq 10 \quad \text{for at least one } t, \\ \text{versus } &\text{H}_a\text{: } |\mu_{Tt} - \mu_{Rt}| < 10 \quad \text{for all } t. \end{aligned} \tag{15.4.2}$$

Hypothesis 15.4.2 can be further decomposed into the following n subhypothesis:

$$\begin{aligned} &\text{H}_{0i}\text{: } |\mu_{Tt} - \mu_{Rt}| \geq 10, \\ \text{versus } &\text{H}_{ai}\text{: } |\mu_{Tt} - \mu_{Rt}| < 10, \; t = 1, \ldots, n. \end{aligned} \tag{15.4.3}$$

Note that hypothesis 15.4.2 implies hypothesis 15.4.1. However, the reverse is not true. The reason is that the hypothesis 15.4.1 is based on an aggregate criterion while n disaggregate criteria were employed in hypothesis 15.4.2. As a result, several testing procedures for hypothesis 15.4.2 were proposed based on the multivariate confidence region (Tsong et al., 1996; Eaton et al., 2003, and Saranadasa and Krishnamoorthy, 2005).

Let $\mathbf{S}_T$ and $\mathbf{S}_R$ be the sample covariance matrices for the test and reference formulations, respectively. Under the assumption of homogeneity of covariance matrix, an unbiased estimator of the common population covariance matrix Σ is

$$\begin{aligned}\mathbf{S}_P &= \frac{(I-1)\mathbf{S}_T + (I-1)\mathbf{S}_R}{(2I-2)} \\ &= \frac{\mathbf{S}_T + \mathbf{S}_R}{2}.\end{aligned}$$

It follows that $\mathbf{D}$ is distributed as a $t \times 1$ multivariate normal distribution with mean vector $\boldsymbol{\mu}_D$ and covariance matrix Σ/I and $2(I-1)\mathbf{S}_P$ follows a Wishart distribution with parameter $2\boldsymbol{\Sigma}/I$ and degrees of freedom $2(I-1)$.

As pointed out by Eaton et al. (2003), Wang et al. (1999) show that the intersection–union test and likelihood ratio test will give the same two one-sided tests procedures. Reject H_0 in Equation 15.4.2 if the $100(1-\alpha)\%$ for $\mu_{Tt} - \mu_{Rt}$ given as

$$(\overline{Y}_{Tt} - \overline{Y}_{Rt}) \pm t(\alpha,\ 2(I-1))2s_{tt}/I \tag{15.4.4}$$

is totally contained within $(-10, 10)$, where s_{tt} is the $(t \cdot t)$ diagonal element of $\mathbf{S}_P$, for all $t = 1, \ldots, n$.

On the other hand, the $100(1-\alpha)\%$ confidence region for $\boldsymbol{\mu}_D$ is given as

$$\begin{aligned}c(\overline{\mathbf{D}},\ \mathbf{S}_P) = \Bigg\{ &\boldsymbol{\mu}_D : (\overline{\mathbf{D}} - \boldsymbol{\mu}_D)'\mathbf{S}_P^{-1}(\overline{\mathbf{D}} - \boldsymbol{\mu}_D) \\ &\le \frac{[2(I-1)n]}{[2(I-1)-n+1]} F(\alpha,\ n,\ 2(I-1)-n+1) \Bigg\}.\end{aligned} \tag{15.4.5}$$

The two one-sided tests procedure constructed from the $100(1-\alpha)\%$ confidence region for $\boldsymbol{\mu}_D$ rejects in Equation 15.4.2 if $(\overline{Y}_{Tt} - \overline{Y}_{Rt}) \pm c2s_{tt}/I$ is totally contained within $(-10, 10)$, where

$$c^2 = \frac{[2(I-1)n]}{[2(I-1)-n+1]} F(\alpha,\ n,\ 2(I-1)-n+1).$$

Both procedures given in Equations 15.4.4 and 15.4.5 focus on the disaggregate criteria of rectangular neighborhood. Therefore, these two procedures are extremely conservative if the number of sampling time point becomes large.

To overcome the conservatism of the hypothesis based on disaggregate criteria, Saranadasa and Krishnamoorthy (2005) proposed a testing method under the assumption that the mean difference of cumulative percent dissolved is the same for all sampling time point. In other words, they assume that $\boldsymbol{\mu}_D = \delta \mathbf{1}_n$, where $\mathbf{1}_n$ is an $n \times 1$ vector of 1. As a result, the hypothesis for evaluation of similarity of dissolution profiles between the test and reference formulations can be expressed in terms of δ as follows:

$$\begin{aligned} &\mathrm{H_0}\text{: } \delta \geq 10 \text{ or } \delta \leq -10 \\ \text{versus } &\mathrm{H_a}\text{: } -10 < \delta < 10. \end{aligned} \tag{15.4.6}$$

The estimated generalized least squares estimator of δ is then given as

$$\widehat{\delta} = \frac{\mathbf{1}'_n \mathbf{S}_\mathrm{P}^{-1} \mathbf{D}}{\mathbf{1}'_n \mathbf{S}_\mathrm{P}^{-1} \mathbf{1}_n}. \tag{15.4.7}$$

Saranadasa and Krishnamoorthy (2005) apply the transformation suggested by Halperin (1961) to obtain the distribution of $\widehat{\delta}$. Define $\mathbf{A}$ as a $n \times n$ matrix

$$\mathbf{A} = \begin{pmatrix} 1 & \mathbf{0}' \\ \mathbf{1}_{n-1} & -\mathbf{I}_{(n-1)\times(n-1)} \end{pmatrix}.$$

The transformation of $\mathbf{D}$ can be expressed as

$$\mathbf{AD} = \begin{pmatrix} \overline{d} \\ \overline{\mathbf{X}} \end{pmatrix}, \tag{15.4.8}$$

where $\overline{d} = \mathrm{D}_i$; $\overline{x}_1 = \mathrm{D}_1 - \mathrm{D}_2, \ldots, \overline{x}_{n-1} = \mathrm{D}_{n-1} - \mathrm{D}_n$.

Express

$$\mathbf{A} = \begin{pmatrix} a_{11} & \mathbf{0}' \\ \mathbf{a}_{21} & \mathbf{A}_{22} \end{pmatrix} \quad \text{and} \quad 2(I-1)\mathbf{S}_\mathrm{P} = \begin{pmatrix} v_{11} & \mathbf{v}_{12} \\ \mathbf{v}_{21} & \mathbf{V}_{22} \end{pmatrix}.$$

Note that a_{11} and v_{11} are scalar and

$$2(I-1)\mathbf{A}\mathbf{S}_\mathrm{P}\mathbf{A}' = \begin{pmatrix} w_{dd} & \mathbf{w}_{dX} \\ \mathbf{w}_{Xd} & \mathbf{W}_{XX} \end{pmatrix},$$

where

$$\begin{aligned} w_{dd} &= v_{11}, \\ \mathbf{w}_{dX} &= a_{11} v_{11} \mathbf{a}'_{21} + a_{11} \mathbf{v}_{12} \mathbf{A}_{22}, \\ \mathbf{w}_{Xd} &= \mathbf{a}_{21} v_{11} a_{11} + \mathbf{A}_{22} \mathbf{v}_{21} a_{11}, \\ \mathbf{W}_{XX} &= \mathbf{a}_{21} v_{11} \mathbf{a}'_{21} + \mathbf{A}_{22} \mathbf{v}_{21} \mathbf{a}'_{21} + \mathbf{a}_{21} \mathbf{v}_{21} \mathbf{A}_{22} + \mathbf{A}_{22} \mathbf{V}_{22} \mathbf{A}'_{22}. \end{aligned}$$

It can be shown that conditionally $\widehat{\delta}$ is distributed as a normal distribution with mean δ and variance

$$2\sigma_{dd\cdot x}(1 + G)/I,$$

where $G = I\overline{\mathbf{X}}'\mathbf{W}_{XX}^{-1}\overline{\mathbf{X}}/2$.

An estimator of $\sigma_{dd\cdot x}$ is given as

$$\widehat{\sigma}_{yy\cdot x} = \frac{w_{dd} - \mathbf{w}_{dX}\mathbf{W}_{XX}^{-1}\mathbf{w}_{Xd}}{2(I-1) - n - 1}, \tag{15.4.9}$$

which is independent of G.

Saranadasa and Krishnamoorthy (2005) show that conditional given G, the following statistic

$$T = \frac{(\widehat{\delta} - \delta)}{\sqrt{2\widehat{\sigma}_{dd\cdot x}(1 + G)/I}} \tag{15.4.10}$$

is distributed as a central t-distribution with $2(I-1) - n - 1$ degrees of freedom.

Denote $\text{SE} = \sqrt{2\widehat{\sigma}_{dd\cdot X}(1 + G)/I}$ and $t = t(\alpha, 2(I-1) - n - 1)$. A $100(1 - 2\alpha)\%$ confidence interval for δ is given as $\widehat{\delta} \pm t(SE)$. It follows that the null hypothesis 15.4.6 is rejected and the dissolution profile of the test formulation is similar to that of the reference formulation at the α significance level if the $100(1 - 2\alpha)\%$ confidence interval for δ is completely contained within -10, 10. This procedure is in fact based on an aggregate criterion because it assumes that the mean differences in cumulative percentage dissolved are the same for all time points. However, this assumption needs to be verified before its application. The impact of violation of a constant mean difference on the size and power of the testing procedure requires further investigation.

The method proposed by Tsong et al. (1996) is another approach to assessing similarity of dissolution profiles based on the model-independent multivariate confidence region procedures recommended in the 1997 FDA guidance on dissolution testing. Define the MSD as the Mahalanobis distance. Let δ be the maximum allowable similarity limit at sampling time t based on interbatch difference in dissolution from the reference formulation, for $t = 1, \ldots, n$. Then the tolerance limit for global similarity based on δ is the Mahalanobis distance based on $\delta\mathbf{1}_n$ and the pooled sample covariance matrix $\mathbf{S}_\text{P}$

$$\text{TL} = \delta^2\mathbf{1}'\mathbf{S}_\text{P}^{-1}\mathbf{1}. \tag{15.4.11}$$

Let MSD_M be the maximum value of the Mahalanobis distance based on $\boldsymbol{\mu}_\text{D}$ and $\mathbf{S}_\text{P}$ computed over the $100(1 - \alpha)\%$ confidence region for $\boldsymbol{\mu}_\text{D}$

$$\text{MSD}_\text{M} = \sup_{\mu_\text{D} \in C(\overline{D},\, S_\text{P})} \boldsymbol{\mu}_\text{D}'\mathbf{S}_\text{P}^{-1}\boldsymbol{\mu}_\text{D}. \tag{15.4.12}$$

The decision is to declare the similarity of dissolution profiles between the test and reference formulations at the α significance level if $\text{MSD}_\text{M} < \text{TL}$.

Eaton et al. (2003) pointed out that one of the drawbacks for this procedure is that both the tolerance limit for global similarity TL and the maximum Mahalanobis distance MSD_M involve both the unknown parameters and statistics calculated from the data. As a result, the criterion for evaluation of dissolution similarity is not defined on parameters. In addition, the performance in decision making with regards to the type I and type II errors for this procedure has not been investigated and reported in the literature yet.

15.5 Example

We consider the dataset first given in Shah et al. (1998) which was used again in Ma et al. (2000). This dataset consists of the cumulative percentages dissolved at 30, 60, 90, and 180 minutes for one prechange batch (reference batch) and five postchange batches (test batches). The number of dosage units for all six batches is 12. The individual cumulative percentages of dissolution at each sampling time point can be found in Shah et al. (1998) and Ma et al. (2000). Table 15.5.1 provides the average cumulative percentages and their corresponding standard deviations. Shah, et al. also presented the estimated covariance and correlation matrices for each batch. They reported that the correlations among sampling time points fluctuate from a negative correlation of −0.54 to a positive correlation of 0.93. Therefore, there is no clear pattern of correlation among different sampling time point and different

TABLE 15.5.1: Average cumulative percentage dissolved of prechange and five postchange batches.

		Time Points (Minutes)			
Batches	**Statistics**	**30**	**60**	**90**	**180**
Prechange	Mean	34.92	59.50	79.27	95.08
(Reference)	S.D.	2.4	2.8	3.0	2.7
Postchange 1	Mean	40.34	67.15	87.01	97.73
(Test 1)	S.D.	4.3	6.6	5.0	1.6
Postchange 2	Mean	49.33	65.33	86.75	102.83
(Test 2)	S.D.	3.0	5.1	3.7	1.9
Postchange 3	Mean	25.80	50.64	67.00	88.60
(Test 3)	S.D.	2.5	2.4	2.7	2.7
Postchange 4	Mean	15.08	59.50	79.27	95.08
(Test 4)	S.D.	2.3	2.8	3.0	2.7
Postchange 5	Mean	43.39	77.96	86.33	98.58
(Test 5)	S.D.	1.5	1.7	2.9	2.1

Source: Reproduced from Shah, V.P., Tsong, Y., Sathe, P., and Liu, J.P., *Pharm. Res.*,1998; Ma, M.C., Wang, B.B.C, Liu, J.P., and Tsong, Y., *J. Biopharm. Stat.*, 10, 229, 2000.

Note: S.D. = Standard deviation.

batches. Most of the differences in the average cumulative percentages dissolved are less than 10% except for that at 30 minutes test batch 2, at 90 minutes of test batch 3, at 30 minutes of test batch 4, and at 60 minutes of test batch 5 with average differences more than 15%, 12%, 19%, and 17%, respectively.

Because the average cumulative percentages of dissolution of test batch 4 are the same as those of reference batch at all sampling time points except for 30 minutes at which a difference of 19.84% is observed, we use the data from test batch 4 and reference batch to illustrate the procedure for assessment of dissolution similarity based on the similarity factor f_2 recommended by the U.S. FDA and the WHO guidelines. Since the mean difference is 19.84%, $W = 19.84^2 = 393.6256$ and

$$\begin{aligned}\widehat{f_2} &= 100 - 25\log(1 + 393.6256)\\ &= 100 - (25)(49.9354)\\ &= 100 - 49.9354\\ &= 50.0646.\end{aligned}$$

According to the U.S. FDA guidance on dissolution testing, SUPAC, and the general considerations of bioequivalence, the dissolution profile of test batch 4 can be claimed similar to that of reference batch because $\widehat{f_2} = 50.0646 > 50$. However, this approach fails to take the sampling distribution of $\widehat{f_2}$ into account and no statement of probability of type I error can be made. In addition, the type I error rate of this approach can be as high as 50%. Therefore, we apply the bootstrap procedure described above. To obtain a precise inference, the number of bootstrap samples for this dataset is 10,000. The sampling distribution of $\widehat{f_2}$ obtained by the bootstrap procedure is a little skewed to the right. The bootstrap mean and median are 49.99 and 49.97. In addition, the 5% percentile of the bootstrap sampling distribution is 48.39 which is less than 50. Consequently, based on the bootstrap procedure, the dissolution profile of test batch 4 cannot be claimed to be similar to that of reference batch at the 5% significance level.

Table 15.5.2 provides the individual results for evaluation of similarity of dissolution profiles between each of five postchange batches and the prechange batch. As shown in Table 15.5.2, the bootstrap means are quite close to the observed $\widehat{f_2}$

TABLE 15.5.2: Results of comparisons of dissolution profiles.

Comparisons	Observed f_2	Bootstrap Mean	5% Percentile	Conclusion on Similarity
T1 versus R	60.035	60.425	53.219	Yes
T2 versus R	51.082	51.022	48.275	No
T3 versus R	51.184	51.194	48.372	No
T4 versus R	50.066	49.993	48.392	No
T5 versus R	48.052	48.022	46.022	No

Source: From Ma, M.C., Wang, B.B.C, Liu, J.P., and Tsong, Y., *J. Biopharm. Stat.*, 10, 229, 2000.
Note: T = test (Postchange batch); R = reference (Prechange batch). The number of bootstrap samples = 10,000.

although in general the bootstrap means are smaller than the observed $\widehat{f}_2$. In addition, only the 5% percentile of the bootstrap sampling distribution of test batch 1 is greater than 50. It follows that at the 5% significance level and a value of f_2 of 50, only the dissolution profile of test batch 1 can be claimed to be similar to that of reference batch. As mentioned before, except for test batch 1, all test batches have the difference in average cumulative dissolved from those of reference batch exceeding 10% at a least one sampling time points. This illustrates that f_2 is very sensitive to a large average difference at a single time point. It also demonstrates that the dissolution profiles between the test and reference formulations with a mean difference greater than 10% at more than one time point cannot be claimed to be similar. This is another reason why 50 is chosen to be allowable lower limit for similarity factor f_2.

15.6 Discussion

For generic drug products and the postapproval changes for the innovative products as well as changes of formulations during the clinical development, comparing *in vitro* dissolution profiles is the first and a must step for establishment of bioequivalence. In this chapter, we review the concept, criteria, and inference for evaluation of similarity of dissolution profiles. The fundamental criteria for evaluation of similarity of dissolution profiles between the test and reference formulations are the sum of squares of differences in mean cumulative percentages dissolved divided by the number of sampling time points which is Q/n. However, to have a criterion with a possible range from 0 to 100, the FDA guidance recommends an artificial logarithmic reciprocal square root transformation of Q/n is performed. This transformation results in an unnecessary complication of the sampling distribution for the maximum likelihood estimator of f_2 (Ma et al., 1999). In addition, a value of f_2 greater than 50 is equivalent to that Q/n is less than 100. This implies that hypothesis in Equation 15.3.1 formulated under f_2 is the same as hypothesis in Equation 15.4.1 expressed in terms of Q/n.

On the other hand, it is not very clear that f_2 given in the U.S. FDA guidance on dissolution testing, and WHO draft guidance on multisource drug products is defined in terms of population means or sample averages. In addition, these guidances recommend that the dissolution profiles of two formulations can be claimed similar if f_2 is greater than 50. Consequently, many pharmaceutical companies claim that the dissolution profile of the test formulation is similar to that of the reference formulation if the observed $\widehat{f}_2$ is greater than 50. Furthermore, most of health authorities accept this practice of claim of similarity using f_2 by pharmaceutical companies despite the warning of uncontrollable inflation of type I error by Liu et al. (1997) and Eaton et al. (2003). For a proper appraisal of the type I error rate, we believe and strongly recommend that assessment of similarity of dissolution profiles follow the concept of evaluation of bioequivalence and perform in the context of hypothesis testing using the confidence interval.

Hypothesis in Equation 15.4.2 is formulated in terms of mean difference at individual time points. Therefore, it is defined by the disaggregate criteria. As a result, any procedure for testing hypothesis 15.4.2 will be very conservative. On the other hand, all other hypotheses in this chapter are defined in terms of aggregate criteria such as f_2 or Q/n. Current procedures based on these aggregate criteria are maximum likelihood methods and their performance in terms of estimation and hypothesis testing in finite sample has not been thoroughly investigated. Therefore, comprehensive empirical investigation and comparisons of the statistical procedures described in Sections 15.3 and 15.4 should be conducted as soon as possible. On the other hand, the estimation of aggregate criteria involves nuisance parameters. The generalized pivotal quantities may shed light on handling the nuisance parameters. The research on application of generalized pivotal quantities to the exact inference for these aggregate criteria in evaluation of dissolution similarity is urgently needed.

Part V

Other Bioequivalence Studies

Chapter 16

Meta-Analysis for Bioequivalence Review

16.1 Introduction

When a brand-name drug is going off patent, the innovator drug company will usually develop a new formulation to extend its exclusivity in the marketplace. At the same time, generic drug companies may file an ANDA submission to the U.S. FDA for approval of generic copies of the brand-name drug. No generic copy of the brand-name drug can be made without regulatory approval confirming that they work as well as the brand-name drug based on bioequivalence testing. When a generic drug is claimed bioequivalent to the brand-name drug, it is assumed that they will reach the equivalent therapeutic effect, or that they are therapeutically equivalent. As indicated earlier, this statement is true only under the *Fundamental Bioequivalence Assumption.* Under the current FDA regulations, a patient may switch from the brand-name drug to its generic copies provided the generic copies have been shown to be bioequivalent to the brand-name drug. Although a generic drug is all right to substitute for any other generic or innovator drug product, the FDA, however, does not indicate that a patient may switch from a generic drug to another for all drug products, even though both of the generic drugs have been shown to be bioequivalent to the brand-name drug. Therefore, an interesting question for the physicians and the patients is whether the brand-name drug and its generic copies can be used interchangeably, especially when different generic copies of the same innovator drug product are available and competition among generic copies is fierce.

Basically, drug interchangeability can be classified as a drug prescribability and drug switchability (Chow and Liu, 1995a). Drug prescribability is usually referred to as the physician's choice for prescribing an appropriate drug for his or her patients between the brand-name drug and its generic copies. The underlying assumption of drug prescribability is that the brand-name drug and its generic copies can be used interchangeably in terms of their efficacy and safety. To ensure drug prescribability, it is suggested that, in addition to average bioequivalence, population bioequivalence, which accounts for both average and variability of bioavailability, be established. On the other hand, drug switchability is referred to as the switch of a drug (e.g., a brand-name drug or its generic copies) to an alternative drug (e.g., a generic copy) within the same subject for whom the concentration of the drug has been titrated to a steady, efficacious, and safe level. To ensure drug switchability, it is recommended that individual bioequivalence be considered. The concept of individual bioequivalence is to ensure bioequivalence within individual subjects according to some criteria. The issues of drug prescribability and switchability have been discussed in chapters 11 and 12.

Recently, as more generic drugs become available, the quality, safety, and efficacy of generic drugs have become a public concern because it is very likely that a patient may switch from one generic drug to another. This situation is particularly true in developing countries where only cheaper generic copies are available. There is a tremendous debate on the quality, safety, and efficacy of generic drugs because they are not identical in terms of inactive ingredients that are binded and bulked, coated and colored, and may vary from one version to another. The current FDA guidance and many regulatory agencies around the world require only that evidence of equivalence in average bioavailabilities between the brand-name drug and its generic copies be provided. Bioequivalence between generic copies of the brand-name drug is not required. Therefore, whether the brand-name drug and its generic copies can be used interchangeably has become a safety concern. To address this issue, Chow and Liu (1997) proposed the performance of a meta-analysis based on average bioequivalence for bioequivalence review. The idea of a meta-analysis is to provide an overview of bioequivalence among generic drugs based on data from independent bioequivalence trials (or submissions). The purpose is to assess not only bioequivalence among generic drugs of the same brand-name drug, but also to provide a tool to monitor the performance of the approved generic copies of the same brand-name drug. In Chow and Liu's approach, a rather restricted, yet strong assumption of inter-subject and intra-subject variances is made, which limits its practical use. To overcome this problem, Chow and Shao (1999) propose an alternative method for meta-analysis that relaxes the assumption. The proposed alternative meta-analysis increases statistical power when the inter-subject variability is not too large.

In Section 16.2, the method of meta-analysis for bioequivalence trials proposed by Chow and Liu (1997) is outlined. A numerical example is given to illustrate Chow and Liu's method in Section 16.3. In Section 16.4, an alternative method for meta-analysis proposed by Chow and Shao (1999) is discussed. A brief discussion is given in Section 16.5.

16.2 Meta-Analysis for Average Bioequivalence

16.2.1 Statistical Model

Let Y_{ijk} be the pharmacokinetic response of interest. Then, model 4.1.1 is useful in describing Y_{ijk} which is given as

$$Y_{ijk} = \mu + S_{ik} + F_{(j,k)} + P_j + e_{ijk}, \qquad (16.2.1)$$

where

μ is the overall mean

S_{ik} is the random effect of the ith subject in the kth sequence, where $i = 1, \ldots, n_k$ and $k = 1, 2$

P_j is the fixed effect of the jth period, where $j = 1, 2$ and $\sum_{j=1}^{2} P_j = 0$

$F_{(j,k)}$ is the direct fixed effect of the drug in the kth sequence that is administered at the jth period, and $\Sigma_{j,k} F_{(j,k)} = 0$

e_{ijk} is the within-subject random error in observing Y_{ijk}

The primary assumptions of the above statistical model are that (1) S_{ik} are i.i.d. with mean 0 and variance σ_S^2, and e_{ijk} are independently distributed with mean 0 and variance σ_e^2 and (2) S_{ik} and e_{ijk} are mutually independent. Under model 16.2.1, for each pharmacokinetic parameter, a 90% confidence interval for μ_T/μ_R can be constructed to assess average bioequivalence, where $\mu_T = \mu + F_T$ and $\mu_R = \mu + F_R$ are the true means for the test product and the reference product, respectively. Average bioequivalence is claimed if the constructed 90% confidence interval is within (80%, 125%), provided that log-transformed data are used for analysis.

16.2.2 Chow and Liu's Method for Meta-Analysis

Suppose there are H different bioequivalence trials. Each bioequivalence trial compares a generic drug with the same brand-name drug. To combine these H studies, Chow and Liu (1997) proposed to perform a meta-analysis for a systemic overview of bioequivalence among the H generic copies of the same brand-name drug. The method of meta-analysis proposed by Chow and Liu (1997) is described in the following. To perform a meta-analysis by combining the H independent studies, we make the following assumptions:

1. Same standard two-sequence, two-period crossover design was conducted with n_{h1} and n_{h2} subjects at sequences 1 and 2, respectively, where $h = 1, \ldots, H$.

2. Same statistical model 16.2.1 for the two-sequence, two-period crossover design was used for assessing bioequivalence based on the log-transformed data.

3. Inter-subject variabilities are the same for all studies (i.e., $\sigma_{Sh}^2 = \sigma_S^2$ for all h).

4. Intra-subject variabilities are the same for all studies (i.e., $\sigma_{eh}^2 = \sigma_e^2$ for all h).

Let μ_{Rh} and μ_{Th} be the true means for the reference product and the hth test product, respectively. Denote by $\overline{Y}_{Rh}$ and $\overline{Y}_{Th}$ the least squares means for the reference product and the test product from the hth bioequivalence study. Then, assuming that $\mu_{Rh} = \mu_R$ for all h, we have

$$\begin{pmatrix} \overline{Y}_{Rh} \\ \overline{Y}_{Th} \end{pmatrix} \sim N\left(\begin{pmatrix} \mu_R \\ \mu_{Th} \end{pmatrix}, \frac{1}{4}\left(\frac{1}{n_{h1}} + \frac{1}{n_{h2}}\right) \begin{bmatrix} \sigma_e^2 + \sigma_S^2 & \sigma_S^2 \\ \sigma_S^2 & \sigma_e^2 + \sigma_S^2 \end{bmatrix} \right),$$

where $h = 1, \ldots, H$. Also, let $\overline{Y} = (\overline{Y}_{R1}, \overline{Y}_{T1}, \ldots, \overline{Y}_{Rh}, \overline{Y}_{Th})'$. Then, $\overline{Y}$ follows a multivariate normal distribution with mean μ and variance–covariance matrix $\boldsymbol{\Sigma}$, where $\boldsymbol{\mu} = (\mu_R, \mu_{T1}, \ldots, \mu_R, \mu_{TH})'$ and

$$\boldsymbol{\Sigma} = C \otimes \left(\sigma_e^2 \mathbf{I}_2 + \sigma_S^2 \mathbf{J}_2\right),$$

where

$$C = \begin{bmatrix} c_1 & & \\ & \ddots & \\ & & c_H \end{bmatrix}, \quad c_h = \frac{1}{4}\left(\frac{1}{n_{h1}} + \frac{1}{n_{h2}}\right),$$

and

$$\mathbf{I}_2 = \begin{bmatrix} 1 & 0 \\ 0 & 1 \end{bmatrix}, \quad \mathbf{J}_2 = \begin{bmatrix} 1 & 1 \\ 1 & 1 \end{bmatrix}.$$

To combine the data from the H studies, we first test for the homogeneity of the reference products among the H studies. For a given study h, the variance of the least squares mean of the reference product is given by

$$\begin{aligned} \operatorname{Var}(\overline{Y}_{Rh}) &= \frac{1}{4}\left(\frac{1}{n_{h1}} + \frac{1}{n_{h2}}\right)\left(\sigma_e^2 + \sigma_S^2\right) \\ &= c_h\left(\sigma_e^2 + \sigma_S^2\right). \end{aligned}$$

Therefore, if we let $\overline{Y}_R = (\overline{Y}_{R1}, \ldots, \overline{Y}_{RH})'$, then $\overline{Y}_R$ follows a distribution with mean μ_R and variance V_R, where

$$\mu_R = (\mu_R, \ldots, \mu_R)' \quad \text{and} \quad V_R = \left(\sigma_e^2 + \sigma_S^2\right)C.$$

Hence, a combined estimate of μ_R can be obtained as the weighted mean of $\overline{Y}_{R1}, \ldots, \overline{Y}_{RH}$ with the corresponding weight being the inverse of its variance. That is,

$$\begin{aligned} \widehat{\mu}_R &= \sum_{h=1}^{H}\left(\frac{\dfrac{1}{c_h(\sigma_e^2 + \sigma_S^2)}\overline{Y}_{Rh}}{\sum_{h=1}^{H}\dfrac{1}{c_h(\sigma_e^2 + \sigma_S^2)}}\right) \\ &= \sum_{h=1}^{H}\left(\frac{\dfrac{1}{c_h}\overline{Y}_{Rh}}{\sum_{h=1}^{H}\dfrac{1}{c_h}}\right) \\ &= \sum_{h=1}^{H}\left(\frac{\omega_h \overline{Y}_{Rh}}{H\overline{\omega}}\right), \end{aligned} \tag{16.2.2}$$

where

$$\omega_h = \frac{1}{c_h} \quad \text{and} \quad \overline{\omega} = \frac{1}{H}\sum_{h=1}^{H} \omega_h.$$

It can be seen from Equation 16.2.2 that the weights are independent of the unknown variance $\sigma_e^2 + \sigma_S^2$, which depends only on the sample sizes of the H studies. Therefore, we may consider the following statistic to test the null hypothesis of homogeneity of the reference products among the studies:

$$\chi_R^2 = \sum_{h=1}^{H} \frac{1}{c_h}(\overline{Y}_{Rh} - \widehat{\mu}_R)^2$$

It can be verified that χ_R^2 follows a chi-square distribution with (H – 1) degrees of freedom. Hence, we would reject the null hypothesis of homogeneity at the α level of significance if

$$\chi_R^2 > \chi^2(\alpha, \mathrm{H} - 1),$$

where $\chi^2(\alpha, \mathrm{H} - 1)$, is the αth upper quantile of a chi-square distribution with (H – 1) degrees of freedom. Note that an estimate of the variance of $\widehat{\mu}_R$ is given by

$$\widehat{\mathrm{V}}\mathrm{ar}(\widehat{\mu}_R) = \frac{1}{2\sum_{h=1}^{H}\left(\frac{1}{c_h}\right)}\left(\widehat{\sigma}_e^2 + \widehat{\sigma}_S^2\right).$$

Estimates for the inter-subject variance and intra-subject variance can also be obtained, respectively, as follows:

$$\widehat{\sigma}_S^2 = \frac{\sum_{h=1}^{H}(n_{h1} + n_{h2} - 2)\mathrm{MSR}_h}{\sum_{h=1}^{H}(n_{h1} + n_{h2} - 2)},$$

and

$$\widehat{\sigma}_e^2 = \frac{\sum_{h=1}^{H}(n_{h1} + n_{h2} - 2)\mathrm{MSE}_h}{\sum_{h=1}^{H}(n_{h1} + n_{h2} - 2)},$$

where MSR_h and MSE_h are mean squares due to subject and mean squared error obtained from the analysis of variance table of the hth study.

If we fail to reject the null hypothesis of homogeneity, a combined estimate of drug effect and its corresponding confidence intervals can be obtained. Let

$$\widehat{d}_h = \overline{Y}_{Th} - \overline{Y}_{Rh}, \quad h = 1, \ldots, H,$$

be the difference of the least squares means between the test product and the reference product of the hth study. If we assume that μ_{Th}, $h=1,\ldots,H$, are the same for all studies (i.e., $\mu_{Th}=\mu_T$, for all h), a combined estimate for $\mu_T-\mu_R$ is the weighted means of d_h, i.e.,

$$\bar{d}=\sum_{h=1}^{H}\left(\frac{\frac{1}{c_h}d_h}{\sum_{h=1}^{H}\frac{1}{c_h}}\right),$$

and its variance is given as

$$\mathrm{Var}(\bar{d})=\frac{\sigma_e^2}{\sum_{h=1}^{H}\frac{1}{c_h}}.$$

Therefore, a $(1-2\alpha)\times 100\%$ confidence interval, denoted by (L, U), can be obtained as follows:

$$(L,\ U)=\bar{d}\pm t\left(\alpha,\ \sum_{h=1}^{H}(n_{h1}+n_{h2}-2)\right)\sqrt{\widehat{\mathrm{Var}}(\bar{d})}$$

where

$t[\alpha, \sum_{h=1}^{H}(n_{h1}+n_{h2}-2)]$ is the upper αth quantile of a t distribution with $\sum_{h=1}^{H}(n_{h1}+n_{h2}-2)$ degrees of freedom

$\widehat{\mathrm{Var}}(\bar{d})$ is an estimate of $\mathrm{Var}(d)$ which is given by

$$\widehat{\mathrm{Var}}(\bar{d})=\frac{\hat{\sigma}_e^2}{\sum_{h=1}^{H}\frac{1}{c_h}}.$$

Similarly, we can assess bioequivalence between two test products from two studies, say studies h and h'. Let $D_{hh'}=\mu_{Th}-\mu_{Th'}$ for $h\neq h'$. An intuitive estimate of $D_{hh'}$ is given by

$$\widehat{D}_{hh'}=(\bar{Y}_{Th}-\bar{Y}_{Rh})-(\bar{Y}_{Th'}-\bar{Y}_{Rh'}).$$

It can be verified that the expected value and variance of $D_{hh'}$ are given by

$$\begin{aligned}E(\widehat{D}_{hh'})&=(\mu_{Th}-\mu_R)-(\mu_{Th'}-\mu_R)\\&=\mu_{Th}-\mu_{Th'},\end{aligned}$$

and

$$\mathrm{Var}(\widehat{D}_{hh'})=\frac{1}{2}\left[\left(\frac{1}{n_{h1}}+\frac{1}{n_{h2}}\right)+\left(\frac{1}{n_{h'1}}+\frac{1}{n_{h'2}}\right)\right]\sigma_e^2.$$

Therefore, $\widehat{D}_{hh'}$ is an unbiased estimator of $D_{hh'}$. As a result, a $(1-2\alpha)\times 100\%$ confidence interval for $\mu_{Th}-\mu_{Th'}$ can be obtained as follows:

$$\widehat{D}_{hh'} \pm t\left(\alpha, \sum_{h=1}^{H}(n_{h1}+n_{h2}-2)\right)\sqrt{\widehat{\text{V}}\text{ar}(\widehat{D}_{hh'})}$$

where

$$\widehat{\text{V}}\text{ar}(\widehat{D}_{hh'}) = \frac{1}{2}\left[\left(\frac{1}{n_{h1}}+\frac{1}{n_{h2}}\right)+\left(\frac{1}{n_{h'1}}+\frac{1}{n_{h'2}}\right)\right]\widehat{\sigma}_{\text{e}}^2$$

Note that we recommended that $\widehat{\sigma}_{\text{e}}^2$ be used because it was obtained based on data from all studies, rather than studies h and h' alone. For any given two generic copies of the same brand-name drug, the above confidence interval can be applied to assess whether they are bioequivalent to each other and, hence, to determine whether they can be used interchangeably.

Example 16.2.1

To illustrate the proposed meta-analysis methodology for bioequivalence review, consider a numerical example that consists of three data sets of hypothetical log-transformed AUC. Suppose these three data sets are collected from three independent bioequivalence trials. In each trial, standard two-sequence, two-period crossover experiment was conducted with 24 healthy male subjects (i.e., $n_{h1}=n_{h2}=12$ for all h) to assess bioequivalence between a test product and the same reference product. The log-transformed AUC data for the three studies are listed in Table 16.2.1. Model 16.2.1 was employed to perform statistical analysis for each data set. The results are summarized in Table 16.2.2. It can be verified from Table 16.2.2 that the test statistic for homogeneity of the reference products among the three studies (i.e., χ_{R}^2) is given by

$$\chi_{\text{R}}^2 = 0.0000528$$

which is less than $\chi^2(0.05, 2) = 5.99$. Thus, we fail to reject the null hypothesis of homogeneity at the 5% level of significance. Therefore, we can combine the data to perform a meta-analysis.

From the combined data, a combined estimate of the reference mean is 4.6676. If we assume that the test means, $\mu_{\text{T}h}$, $h=1, 2, 3$ are the same for all h (i.e., $\mu_{\text{T}h}=\mu_{\text{T}}$), then an estimate for $\mu_{\text{T}}-\mu_{\text{R}}$ and its corresponding 90% confidence interval based on the combined data are given by

$$\bar{d} = 0.01252,$$

and

$$(L, U) = (0.00865, 0.01638) \text{ or } (100.9\%, 101.7\%).$$

The combined 90% confidence interval for $\mu_{\text{T}}=\mu_{\text{R}}$ supports the conclusion of bioequivalence between the test products and the reference product. However, an

TABLE 16.2.1: AUC and log(AUC) for studies 1–3.

Subject	Sequence	Period	Drug	AUC	Log(AUC)
Study 1					
1	1	1	Reference	115	4.74493
1	1	2	Test	88	4.47734
2	1	1	Reference	101	4.61512
2	1	2	Test	85	4.44265
3	1	1	Reference	99	4.59512
3	1	2	Test	86	4.45435
4	1	1	Reference	99	4.59512
4	1	2	Test	86	4.45435
5	1	1	Reference	100	4.60517
5	1	2	Test	85	4.44265
6	1	1	Reference	120	4.78749
6	1	2	Test	102	4.62497
7	1	1	Reference	110	4.70048
7	1	2	Test	93	4.53260
8	1	1	Reference	111	4.70953
8	1	2	Test	94	4.54329
9	1	1	Reference	114	4.73620
9	1	2	Test	95	4.55388
10	1	1	Reference	120	4.78749
10	1	2	Test	100	4.60517
11	1	1	Reference	120	4.78749
11	1	2	Test	101	4.61512
12	1	1	Reference	103	4.63473
12	1	2	Test	88	4.47734
13	2	1	Test	89	4.48864
13	2	2	Reference	102	4.62497
14	2	1	Test	90	4.49981
14	2	2	Reference	108	4.68213
15	2	1	Test	89	4.48864
15	2	2	Reference	104	4.64439
16	2	1	Test	88	4.47734
16	2	2	Reference	104	4.64439
17	2	1	Test	85	4.44265
17	2	2	Reference	101	4.61512
18	2	1	Test	86	4.45435
18	2	2	Reference	102	4.62497
19	2	1	Test	95	4.55388
19	2	2	Reference	114	4.73620
20	2	1	Test	91	4.51086
20	2	2	Reference	109	4.69135
21	2	1	Test	84	4.43082
21	2	2	Reference	100	4.60517

TABLE 16.2.1 (continued): AUC and log(AUC) for studies 1–3.

Subject	Sequence	Period	Drug	AUC	Log(AUC)
22	2	1	Test	84	4.43082
22	2	2	Reference	99	4.59512
23	2	1	Test	85	4.44265
23	2	2	Reference	101	4.61512
24	2	1	Test	84	4.43082
24	2	2	Reference	101	4.61512
Study 2					
1	1	1	Reference	115.2	4.74667
1	1	2	Test	108.0	4.68213
2	1	1	Reference	101.2	4.61710
2	1	2	Test	105.0	4.65396
3	1	1	Reference	99.2	4.59714
3	1	2	Test	106.0	4.66344
4	1	1	Reference	99.2	4.59714
4	1	2	Test	106.0	4.66344
5	1	1	Reference	100.2	4.60717
5	1	2	Test	105.0	4.65396
6	1	1	Reference	120.2	4.78916
6	1	2	Test	122.0	4.80402
7	1	1	Reference	110.2	4.70230
7	1	2	Test	113.0	4.72739
8	1	1	Reference	111.2	4.71133
8	1	2	Test	114.0	4.73620
9	1	1	Reference	114.2	4.73795
9	1	2	Test	115.0	4.74493
10	1	1	Reference	120.2	4.78916
10	1	2	Test	120.0	4.78749
11	1	1	Reference	120.2	4.78916
11	1	2	Test	121.0	4.79579
12	1	1	Reference	103.2	4.63667
12	1	2	Test	108.0	4.68213
13	2	1	Test	109.0	4.69135
13	2	2	Reference	102.2	4.62693
14	2	1	Test	110.0	4.70048
14	2	2	Reference	108.2	4.68398
15	2	1	Test	109.0	4.69135
15	2	2	Reference	104.2	4.64631
16	2	1	Test	108.0	4.68213
16	2	2	Reference	104.2	4.64631
17	2	1	Test	105.0	4.65396
17	2	2	Reference	101.2	4.61710

(*continued*)

TABLE 16.2.1 (continued): AUC and log(AUC) for studies 1–3

Subject	Sequence	Period	Drug	AUC	Log(AUC)
18	2	1	Test	106.0	4.66344
18	2	2	Reference	102.2	4.62693
19	2	1	Test	115.0	4.74493
19	2	2	Reference	114.2	4.73795
20	2	1	Test	111.0	4.70953
20	2	2	Reference	109.2	4.69318
21	2	1	Test	104.0	4.64439
21	2	2	Reference	100.2	4.60717
22	2	1	Test	104.0	4.64439
22	2	2	Reference	99.2	4.59714
23	2	1	Test	105.0	4.65396
23	2	2	Reference	101.2	4.61710
24	2	1	Test	104.0	4.65539
24	2	2	Reference	101.2	4.61710
Study 3					
1	1	1	Reference	115.185	4.74654
1	1	2	Test	126.000	4.83628
2	1	1	Reference	101.185	4.61695
2	1	2	Test	123.000	4.81218
3	1	1	Reference	99.185	4.59699
3	1	2	Test	124.000	4.82028
4	1	1	Reference	99.185	4.59699
4	1	2	Test	124.000	4.82028
5	1	1	Reference	100.185	4.60702
5	1	2	Test	123.000	4.81218
6	1	1	Reference	120.185	4.78903
6	1	2	Test	140.000	4.94164
7	1	1	Reference	110.185	4.70216
7	1	2	Test	131.000	4.87520
8	1	1	Reference	111.185	4.71120
8	1	2	Test	132.000	4.88280
9	1	1	Reference	114.185	4.73782
9	1	2	Test	133.000	4.89035
10	1	1	Reference	120.185	4.78903
10	1	2	Test	138.000	4.92725
11	1	1	Reference	120.185	4.78903
11	1	2	Test	139.000	4.93447
12	1	1	Reference	103.185	4.63652
12	1	2	Test	126.000	4.83628
13	2	1	Test	127.000	4.84419
13	2	2	Reference	102.185	4.62678

TABLE 16.2.1 (continued): AUC and log(AUC) for studies 1–3.

Subject	Sequence	Period	Drug	AUC	Log(AUC)
14	2	1	Test	128.000	4.85203
14	2	2	Reference	108.185	4.68384
15	2	1	Test	127.000	4.84419
15	2	2	Reference	104.185	4.64617
16	2	1	Test	126.000	4.83628
16	2	2	Reference	104.185	4.65617
17	2	1	Test	123.000	4.81218
17	2	2	Reference	101.185	4.61695
18	2	1	Test	124.000	4.82028
18	2	2	Reference	102.185	4.62678
19	2	1	Test	133.000	4.89035
19	2	2	Reference	114.185	4.73782
20	2	1	Test	129.000	4.85981
20	2	2	Reference	109.185	4.69304
21	2	1	Test	122.000	4.80402
21	2	2	Reference	100.185	4.60702
22	2	1	Test	122.000	4.80402
22	2	2	Reference	99.185	4.59699
23	2	1	Test	123.000	4.81218
23	2	2	Reference	101.185	4.61695
24	2	1	Test	122.000	4.80402
24	2	2	Reference	101.185	4.61695

unbiased estimate of the difference in means between test product 1 and test product 3 is given by

$$\widehat{D}_{13} = -0.35233.$$

Moreover, the 90% confidence interval for $\mu_{T1} = \mu_{T3}$ is (−0.366, −0.339) or (69.4%, 71.3%), which is below the bioequivalence limits of (80%, 125%). The

TABLE 16.2.2: Statistical results of the three studies.

	Study 1	Study 2	Study 3
Reference mean	4.66637	4.66826	4.66811
Test mean	4.49479	4.69663	4.84877
MSE	0.00031	0.00038	0.00047
Difference	−0.17158	0.02838	0.18075
Lower CI limit[a]	−0.18035	0.01877	0.17001
Upper CI limit[a]	−0.16282	0.03799	0.19150
90% CI (in %)[b]	(83.5%, 85.0%)	(101.9%, 103.9%)	(118.5%, 121.1%)

[a] In log scale.

[b] In original scale.

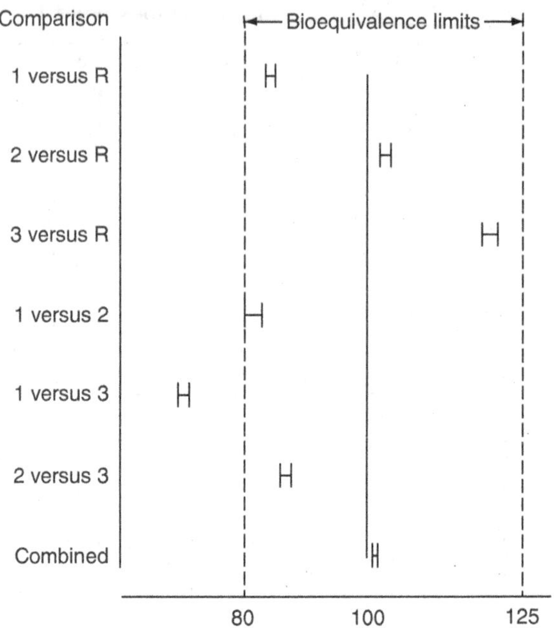

FIGURE 16.2.1: Meta-analysis of bioequivalence studies.

result indicates that test product 1 is not bioequivalent to test product 3. Figure 16.2.1 summarizes the comparison between each of the three test products and the reference product and the comparison among the three test products.

16.3 Alternative Method for Meta-Analysis

16.3.1 No-meta Method for Bioequivalence

To introduce an alternative method for the meta-analysis proposed by Chow and Shao (1999), we first consider the following presentation of the statistical model for a standard two-sequence, two-period crossover experiment. Let Y_{ijk} be the original or the log-transformation of the pharmacokinetic response of interest (e.g., the area under the blood or plasma concentration–time curve [AUC] or the maximum concentration [$C_{\max}$]) of the ith subject in the jth period and the kth sequence of the trial. The following statistical model is assumed:

$$Y_{ijk} = \mu + F_l + P_j + Q_k + S_{ikl} + e_{ijk}, \tag{16.3.1}$$

where

μ is the overall mean

P_j is the fixed effect of the jth period ($j=1$, 2, and $P_1+P_2=0$)

Q_k is the fixed effect of the kth sequence ($k=1$, 2, and $Q_1+Q_2=0$)

F_l is the fixed effect of the lth drug formulation (when $j=k$, $l=T$, test formulation; when $j \neq k$, $l=R$, the reference formulation; $F_{\mathrm{T}}+F_{\mathrm{R}}=0$)

S_{ikl} is the random effect of the ith subject in the kth sequence under drug formulation l

$\mathbf{S}_{ik}=(\mathrm{S}_{ik\mathrm{T}},\ \mathrm{S}_{ik\mathrm{R}})$, $i=1,\ldots,n_k$, $d=1$, 2, are i.i.d. bivariate normal random vectors with mean 0 and an unknown covariance matrix

$$\begin{pmatrix} \sigma_{\mathrm{BT}}^2 & \rho\sigma_{\mathrm{BT}}\sigma_{\mathrm{BR}} \\ \rho\sigma_{\mathrm{BT}}\sigma_{\mathrm{BR}} & \sigma_{\mathrm{BR}}^2 \end{pmatrix}$$

e_{ijk}'s are independent random errors distributed as $N(0, \sigma_{Wl}^2)$, and S_{ik}'s and e_{ijk}'s are independent.

Note that σ_{BT}^2 and σ_{BR}^2 are inter-subject variances and σ_{WT}^2 and σ_{WR}^2 are intra-subject variances, and that $\sigma_{\mathrm{TT}}^2=\sigma_{\mathrm{BT}}^2+\sigma_{\mathrm{WT}}^2$ and $\sigma_{\mathrm{TR}}^2=\sigma_{\mathrm{BR}}^2+\sigma_{\mathrm{WR}}^2$ are called total variances for the test and reference formulations, respectively.

The average bioequivalence index is $\delta=F_{\mathrm{T}}-F_{\mathrm{R}}$. Let $\bar{y}_{jk}$ be the sample average of the observations in the jth period and the kth sequence. Under the assumed statistical model,

$$\overline{Y}_{11}-\overline{Y}_{12} \sim N\left(\delta+P_1-P_2,\ \frac{\tau^2}{n_1}\right),$$

and

$$\overline{Y}_{21}-\overline{Y}_{22} \sim N\left(-\delta+P_1-P_2,\ \frac{\tau^2}{n_2}\right),$$

where $\tau^2=\sigma_{\mathrm{BT}}^2+\sigma_{\mathrm{BR}}^2-2\rho\sigma_{\mathrm{BT}}\sigma_{\mathrm{BR}}+\sigma_{\mathrm{WT}}^2+\sigma_{\mathrm{WR}}^2=\sigma_{\mathrm{TT}}^2+\sigma_{\mathrm{TR}}^2-2\rho\sigma_{\mathrm{BT}}\sigma_{\mathrm{BR}}$. Consequently,

$$\widehat{\delta}=\frac{1}{2}(\overline{Y}_{11}-\overline{Y}_{12}-\overline{Y}_{21}+\overline{Y}_{22}) \sim N\left[\delta,\ \frac{\tau^2}{4}\left(\frac{1}{n_1}+\frac{1}{n_2}\right)\right].$$

A $(1-2\alpha)\times 100\%$ confidence interval for δ is given by

$$\widehat{\delta} \pm t(\alpha,\ n_1+n_2-2)\frac{\widehat{\tau}}{2}\sqrt{\frac{1}{n_1}+\frac{1}{n_2}}, \tag{16.3.2}$$

where $t(\alpha,\ m)$ is the upper αth quantile of the t distribution with m degrees of freedom,

$$\widehat{\tau}^2 = \frac{(n_1 - 1)s_{D1}^2 + (n_2 - 1)s_{D2}^2}{n_1 + n_2 - 2}, \tag{16.3.3}$$

and s_{Dk}^2 is the sample variance based on the differences $\{Y_{i1k} - Y_{i2k}, i = 1, \ldots, n_k\}$, $k = 1, 2$.

16.3.2 Meta-Analysis for Bioequivalence between Test and Reference Drugs

Suppose that there are H independent bioequivalence studies. Each bioequivalence study compares a generic drug (test formulation) and the same brand-name drug (reference formulation). We assume that data from the brand-name drug in different studies are from the same population. However, data from generic drugs may have different populations. An additional subscript h is added to the responses so that Y_{ijkh} is the observation as defined in Section 16.3.1, but is from the hth bioequivalence study. We shall similarly define F_{lh}, P_{jh}, Q_{kh}, δ_h, S_{iklh}, e_{ijklh}, $\delta_{\mathrm{BT}h}^2$, $\sigma_{\mathrm{BR}h}^2$, $\sigma_{\mathrm{WT}h}^2$, $\sigma_{\mathrm{WR}h}^2$, $\sigma_{\mathrm{TT}h}^2$, $\sigma_{\mathrm{TR}h}^2$, ρ_h, τ_h^2, $\overline{Y}_{jkh}$, and n_{kh}. The assumption that data from the brand-name drug are from the same population is the same as

$$F_{\mathrm{RH}} = F_{\mathrm{R}}, \quad \sigma_{\mathrm{BR}h}^2 = \sigma_{\mathrm{BR}}^2, \quad \sigma_{\mathrm{WR}h}^2 = \sigma_{\mathrm{WR}}^2 \quad \text{for all } h. \tag{16.3.4}$$

Because there are more data for the reference formulation (under the above assumption), it is possible to perform a meta-analysis and obtain a more powerful statistical procedure than that described in Section 16.2, especially when H is large. Under the above assumption and based on data from the H studies, the best unbiased estimator of $\mu_{\mathrm{R}} = \mu + F_{\mathrm{R}}$ is

$$\widehat{\mu}_{\mathrm{R}} = \sum_{h=1}^{H} a_h \overline{Y}_{\mathrm{R}h},$$

where $\overline{Y}_{\mathrm{R}h} = (\overline{Y}_{21h} + \overline{Y}_{12h})/2$ and

$$a_h = \frac{1}{c_h} \Big/ \sum_{h=1}^{H} \frac{1}{c_h}, \quad c_h = \frac{1}{4}\left(\frac{1}{n_{1h}} + \frac{1}{n_{2h}}\right). \tag{16.3.5}$$

Let $\overline{Y}_{\mathrm{T}h} = (\overline{Y}_{11h} + \overline{Y}_{22h})/2$. Then using all H data sets $\delta_h = F_{\mathrm{T}h} - F_{\mathrm{R}}$ is

$$\widetilde{\delta}_h = \overline{Y}_{\mathrm{T}h} - \widehat{\mu}_{\mathrm{R}}, \tag{16.3.6}$$

whereas δ_h using data in study h, is estimated by

$$\widehat{\delta}_h = \overline{Y}_{\mathrm{T}h} - \overline{y}_{\mathrm{R}h}. \tag{16.3.7}$$

However, neither $\widetilde{\delta}_h$ nor $\widehat{\delta}_h$ is always better than the other. The variance of $\widetilde{\delta}_h$ is

$$\begin{aligned}
\mathrm{Var}(\widetilde{\delta}_h) &= \mathrm{Var}(\overline{Y}_{\mathrm{T}h}) + \sum_{h=1}^{H} a_h^2 V(\overline{Y}_{\mathrm{R}h}) - 2a_h \mathrm{Cov}(\overline{Y}_{\mathrm{T}h}, \overline{Y}_{\mathrm{R}h}) \\
&= c_h \sigma_{\mathrm{TT}h}^2 + \sigma_{\mathrm{TR}}^2 \sum_{h=1}^{H} a_h^2 c_h - 2a_h c_h \rho_h \sigma_{\mathrm{BT}h} \sigma_{\mathrm{BR}} \\
&= c_h \sigma_{\mathrm{TT}h}^2 + C_H \sigma_{\mathrm{TR}}^2 - 2C_H \rho_h \sigma_{\mathrm{BT}h} \sigma_{\mathrm{BR}} \\
&= (c_h - C_h)\sigma_{\mathrm{TT}h}^2 + C_H \tau_h^2,
\end{aligned}$$

whereas the variance of $\widehat{\delta}_h$ is

$$\mathrm{Var}(\widehat{\delta}_h) = c_h \tau_h^2,$$

where ${\tau_h}^2 = {\sigma_{\mathrm{TT}h}}^2 + {\sigma_{\mathrm{TR}}}^2 - 2\rho_h \sigma_{\mathrm{BT}h} \sigma_{\mathrm{BR}}$ and

$$C_H = \left(\sum_{h=1}^{H} \frac{1}{c_h} \right)^{-1}.$$

Consequently,

$$\begin{aligned}
\mathrm{Var}(\widehat{\delta}_h) - \mathrm{Var}(\widetilde{\delta}_h) &= (c_h - C_H)\left(\tau_h^2 - \sigma_{\mathrm{TT}h}^2\right) \\
&= (c_h - C_H)\left(\sigma_{\mathrm{TR}}^2 - 2\rho_h \sigma_{\mathrm{BT}h} \sigma_{\mathrm{BR}}\right),
\end{aligned}$$

that is, combining data sets leads to a more efficient estimator of δ_h if, and only if, the total variance of the reference formulation is larger than two times that of the covariance between the two observations from the same subject. In the extreme case, where $\rho_h = 1$ and $\sigma_{\mathrm{BT}h} = \sigma_{\mathrm{BR}}$, combining data sets is better, if and only if, the intra-subject variance σ_{WR}^2 is larger than the inter-subject variance σ_{BR}^2, under the reference formulation. Intuitively, a large between-subject variance results in a large variability among different data sets and, thus, reduces the efficiency in meta-analysis.

We will now describe how to construct a 90% confidence interval for δ_h using $\widetilde{\delta}_h$, rather than $\widehat{\delta}_h$, for both balanced and unbalanced cases.

Balanced Case: Assume that sample sizes are the same for all studies (i.e., $n_{kh} = n_k$ for all h). Then a_h's in Equation 16.3.5 are all equal to H^{-1}. Let

$$Z_{i1h} = Y_{i11h} - \frac{1}{H} \sum_{h=1}^{H} Y_{i21h} \quad i = 1, \ldots, n_1,$$

$$Z_{i2h} = Y_{i22h} - \frac{1}{H} \sum_{h=1}^{H} Y_{i21h} \quad i = 1, \ldots, n_2,$$

and $\bar{Z}_{kh}$ be the average of $\{Z_{ikh}, \mathrm{i} = 1, \ldots, n_k\}$, $k = 1, 2$. Then

$$\widetilde{\delta}_h = \frac{\overline{Z}_{1h} + \overline{Z}_{2h}}{2}.$$

Let s^2_{zkh} be the sample variance based on $\{Z_{ikh}, i = 1, \ldots, n_k\}$ and

$$\widehat{\omega}^2_h = \frac{(n_1 - 1)s^2_{z1h} + (n_2 - 1)s^2_{z2h}}{n_1 + n_2 - 2}.$$

Then a $(1 - 2\alpha) \times 100\%$ confidence interval for δ_h is given by

$$\widetilde{\delta}_h \pm t(\alpha, n_1 + n_2 - 2)\frac{\widehat{\omega}_h}{2}\sqrt{\frac{1}{n_1} + \frac{1}{n_2}}. \tag{16.3.8}$$

The above confidence interval is more efficient (shorter) than the confidence interval obtained from the study h if

$$\text{Var}(\widehat{\delta}_h) > \text{Var}(\widetilde{\delta}_h).$$

Unbalanced Case: If some sample sizes from different studies are different, then it is difficult to obtain an exact confidence interval for δ_h. We derive an approximate confidence interval for δ_h in the case where C_H is negligible (i.e., $\sum_{h=1}^{H} \frac{1}{c_h}$ is large). Let n_0 be the smallest sample size over all sequences and studies. Then

$$\sum_{h=1}^{H} \frac{1}{c_h} \geq 2n_0 H.$$

Note that if $n_0 = 10$ and $H = 3$, $\sum_{h=1}^{H} \frac{1}{c_h} \geq 60$. If C_H is negligible, then the variance of $\widetilde{\delta}_h$ is approximately $c_h \sigma^2_{\text{TT}h}$ and the distribution of $\widetilde{\delta}_h / (\sqrt{c_h}\widehat{\sigma}_{\text{TT}h})$ is approximately the t distribution with $n_{1h} + n_{2h} - 2$ degrees of freedom, where

$$\widehat{\sigma}^2_{\text{TT}h} = \frac{(n_{1h} - 1)s^2_{11h} + (n_{2h} - 1)s^2_{22h}}{n_{1h} + n_{2h} - 2}, \tag{16.3.9}$$

and s^2_{jkh} is the sample variance based on the data in the jth period, kth sequence, and hth study. An approximately $(1 - 2\alpha) \times 100\%$ confidence interval for δ_h is then given by

$$\widetilde{\delta}_h \pm t(\alpha, n_{1h} + n_{2h} - 2)\frac{\widehat{\sigma}_{\text{TT}h}}{2}\sqrt{\frac{1}{n_{1h}} + \frac{1}{n_{2h}}}.$$

16.3.3 Bioequivalence among Generic Copies

To assess two test drugs (generic copies), say h and h', we consider the parameter $\delta_{hh'} = F_{\text{T}h} - F_{\text{T}h'}$. Because $F_{\text{T}h} - F_{\text{T}h'} = \delta_h - \delta_{h'}$, both $\widehat{\delta}_h - \widehat{\delta}_{h'}$ and $\widetilde{\delta}_h - \widetilde{\delta}_{h'}$ are unbiased estimators of $\delta_{hh'}$. Note that

$$\widetilde{\delta}_h - \widetilde{\delta}_{h'} = \overline{y}_{\text{T}h} - \overline{y}_{\text{T}h'},$$

where $\bar{y}_{Th} = (\bar{y}_{11h} + \bar{y}_{22h})/2$. These two estimators of $\delta_{hh'}$ are normally distributed with variances, respectively,

$$\mathrm{Var}(\widehat{\delta}_h - \widehat{\delta}_{h'}) = c_h \tau_h^2 + c_{h'} \tau_{h'}^2,$$

and

$$\mathrm{Var}(\widetilde{\delta}_h - \widetilde{\delta}_{h'}) = c_h \sigma_{\mathrm{TT}h}^2 + c_{h'} \sigma_{\mathrm{TT}h'}^2.$$

Because $\sigma_{\mathrm{TT}h}^2$ and $\sigma_{\mathrm{TT}h'}^2$ (τ_h^2 and $\tau_{h'}^2$) are generally different, it is difficult to derive a good exact confidence interval for $\delta_{hh'}$ (this is called Behrens–Fisher problem). When n_{kh}'s are large, we can use the following approximate confidence interval:

$$\widetilde{\delta}_h - \widetilde{\delta}_{h'} \pm z(\alpha)\sqrt{c_h \widehat{\sigma}_{\mathrm{TT}h}^2 + c_{h'} \widehat{\sigma}_{\mathrm{TT}h'}^2},$$

or

$$\widehat{\delta}_h - \widehat{\delta}_{h'} \pm z(\alpha)\sqrt{c_h \widehat{\tau}_h^2 + c_{h'} \widehat{\tau}_{h'}^2},$$

where $z(\alpha)$ is the upper αth quantile of the standard normal distribution, $\sigma_{\mathrm{TT}h}^2$ is given by Equation 16.3.9,

$$\widehat{\tau}_h^2 = \frac{(n_{1h} - 1)s_{D1h}^2 + (n_{2h} - 1)s_{D2h}^2}{n_{1h} + n_{2h} - 2},$$

and s_{Dkh}^2 is given by Equation 16.3.3, but based on the data in study h.

When n_{kh}'s are small, the following exact method can be applied. Consider first the case where $n_{kh} = n_{kh'}$, $k = 1, 2$. Thus, $c_h = c_{h'}$. Define

$$d_{i1hh'} = Y_{i11h} - Y_{i11h'}, \quad i = 1, \ldots, n_{1h}, \tag{16.3.10}$$

$$d_{i2hh'} = Y_{i22h} - Y_{i22h'}, \quad i = 1, \ldots, n_{2h}. \tag{16.3.11}$$

Let $s_{khh'}^2$ be the sample variance based on $\{d_{ikhh'}, i = 1, \ldots, n_{kh}\}$, $k = 1, 2$, and

$$s_{hh'}^2 = \frac{(n_{1h} - 1)s_{1hh'}^2 + (n_{2h} - 1)s_{2hh'}^2}{n_{1h} + n_{2h} - 2}.$$

Then an exact $(1 - 2\alpha) \times 100\%$ confidence interval for $\delta_{hh'}$ is

$$\widetilde{\delta}_h - \widetilde{\delta}_{h'} \pm t(\alpha, n_{1h} + n_{2h} - 2)\sqrt{2c_h s_{hh'}^2}. \tag{16.3.12}$$

Similarly, if we replace $\widetilde{\delta}_h - \widetilde{\delta}_{h'}$ in Equation 16.3.12 by $\widehat{\delta}_h - \widehat{\delta}_{h'}$, $d_{i1hh'}$ in Equation 16.3.10 by

$$(Y_{i11h} - Y_{i12h}) - (Y_{i11h'} - Y_{i12h'}), \quad i = 1, \ldots, n_{1h}, \tag{16.3.13}$$

and $d_{i2hh'}$ in Equation 16.3.11 by

$$(Y_{i22h} - Y_{i21h}) - (Y_{i22h'} - Y_{i21h'}), \quad i = 1, \ldots, n_{2h}, \tag{16.3.14}$$

then Equation 16.3.12 still provides an exact $(1 - 2\alpha) \times 100\%$ confidence interval for $\delta_{hh'}$.

When $n_{kh} \neq n_{kh'}$ for some k, we can still use the interval given by Equation 16.3.12 by changing n_{1h} in Equation 16.3.10 (or in Equation 16.3.13) to $\min(n_{1h}, n_{1h'})$ and changing n_{2h} in Equation 16.3.11 (or in Equation 16.3.14) to $\min(n_{2h}, n_{2h'})$. This interval is exact, but conservative.

When there are more than three generic copies ($H > 2$), we may use simultaneous confidence intervals for $\delta_{hh'}$, $h \neq h'$, to assess bioequivalence among all H generic copies. The simplest way to obtain simultaneous confidence intervals is to apply Bonferroni's method, that is, to use the individual confidence interval for $\delta_{hh'}$ proposed in this section and adjust the confidence coefficient from $(1 - 2\alpha) \times 100\%$ to $\left(1 - \frac{\alpha}{H-1}\right) \times 100\%$.

Example 16.3.1

To illustrate the proposed alternative meta-analysis methodology for bioequivalence review, consider an example consisting of three data sets of hypothetical log-transformed AUC. It is assumed that these three data sets were collected from three independent bioequivalence trials. In each trial, the standard two-sequence, two-period crossover design was conducted with 24 healthy subjects to assess bioequivalence between a test product and the same brand-name drug product. The log-transformed AUC data for the three studies are listed in Table 16.3.1.

First, we calculate 90% confidence intervals for δ_h (effect of test h vs. reference), using the proposed meta-analysis (balanced case) and nonmeta method for each study h. The results are listed in Table 16.3.2. In all cases, intervals from meta-analysis are shorter.

Next, we compute 90% confidence intervals for $\delta_{hh'}$ (effect of test h vs. test h'), using the meta-analysis and nonmeta methods (the exact methods). The results are also listed in Table 16.3.2. Again, all intervals from meta-analysis are shorter. Because the bioequivalence limits are $\delta_L = -0.2231$ and $\delta_U = 0.2231$, none of the test drugs can be claimed to be bioequivalent to each other from the nonmeta analysis. The conclusion from meta-analysis is different. Test drugs 1 and 3, and test drugs 2 and 3 can be claimed to be bioequivalent to each other, which indicates that meta-analysis in this example is more efficient (has a better power). However, test drugs 1 and 2 can still not be claimed to be bioequivalent, based on the available results from three studies.

In general it seems to be a good idea to compute confidence intervals using both meta and nonmeta methods and to compare the results.

TABLE 16.3.1: Data from 2 × 2 crossover and three studies.

	Study 1		Study 2		Study 3	
	Period 1	**Period 2**	**Period 1**	**Period 2**	**Period 1**	**Period 2**
Sequence 1	4.7715	4.6025	4.6974	4.4814	4.9622	4.7198
	4.6557	4.5414	4.6818	4.9480	4.7994	4.7665
	4.6107	4.5170	4.5329	4.4697	4.6686	4.5408
	4.5566	4.7277	4.9905	4.5137	4.6045	4.7574
	4.6165	4.6979	4.7481	4.7476	4.6134	4.3737
	4.6446	4.7441	4.7420	4.6282	4.7692	4.5999
	4.5156	4.4945	4.5469	4.6518	4.5495	4.9195
	4.7461	4.8767	4.9154	4.3600	4.9369	4.6509
	4.5275	4.8566	4.7344	4.8155	4.8391	4.5823
	4.5848	4.6482	4.6322	4.6847	4.7146	4.4432
	4.4630	4.6441	4.6611	4.5936	4.6918	4.8072
	4.6954	4.7787	4.9243	4.7327	4.6751	4.5374
Sequence 2	4.6645	4.6104	4.4902	4.6058	4.6001	4.6721
	4.7719	4.5316	4.7208	4.7824	4.4820	4.6282
	4.6804	4.9791	4.8940	4.9102	4.6419	4.7608
	4.9572	4.4743	4.6753	4.9106	4.8766	4.4202
	4.4570	4.7782	4.6354	4.8466	4.7865	4.6704
	4.8333	4.7906	4.6973	4.8401	4.4985	5.0941
	4.8327	4.6732	4.6558	4.6844	4.7723	4.5420
	4.6009	4.4802	4.6164	4.8815	4.6581	4.4687
	4.7402	4.7901	4.6977	4.8506	4.7311	4.4645
	4.4748	4.7378	4.5732	4.9825	4.7698	4.8313
	4.8065	4.4383	4.6282	4.8060	4.5879	4.5909
	4.4772	4.3670	4.8046	4.9338	4.3235	4.8580

TABLE 16.3.2: 90% Confidence intervals.

	Meta-Analysis	**No-meta**
Test 1 versus reference	(−0.0892, 0.0217)[a]	(−0.1291, 0.0152)[a]
Test 2 versus reference	(0.0760, 0.1734)[a]	(0.0656, 0.1949)[a]
Test 3 versus reference	(−0.0296, 0.1109)[a]	(−0.0342, 0.0949)[a]
Test 1 versus test 2	(−0.2468, −0.0701)	(−0.3366, −0.0379)
Test 1 versus test 3	(−0.1605, 0.0117)[a]	(−0.2160, 0.0305)
Test 2 versus test 3	(−0.0110, 0.1790)[a]	(−0.0818, 0.2258)

[a] Cases for which bioequivalence can be claimed.

16.4 Efficiency of Meta-Analysis

As indicated earlier, we have

$$\begin{aligned}\text{Var}(\widehat{\delta}_h) - \text{Var}(\widetilde{\delta}_h) &= (c_h - C_H)\left(\tau_h^2 - \sigma_{\text{TT}h}^2\right) \\ &= (c_h - C_H)\left(\sigma_{\text{TR}}^2 - 2\rho_h\sigma_{\text{BT}h}\sigma_{\text{BR}}\right).\end{aligned}$$

As a result, combining independent bioequivalence trials will lead to a more efficient estimator of δ_h if, and only if, the total variance of the reference formulation is larger than two times that of the covariance between the two observations from the same subject. In the extreme case, in which $\rho_j = 1$ and $\sigma_{\text{BT}h} = \sigma_{\text{BR}}$, combining independent bioequivalence trials is better if, and only if, the intra-subject variance σ_{WR}^2 is larger than the inter-subject variance σ_{BR}^2, under the reference formulation. Intuitively, a large between-subject variance results in a large variability among different data sets and thus reduces the efficiency in meta-analysis.

Chow and Shao (1999) proposed a simple testing hypothesis procedure that can be used to test

$$\begin{aligned} &\text{H}_0\colon \text{Var}(\widehat{\delta}_h) \le \text{Var}(\widetilde{\delta}_h) \\ \text{versus } &\text{H}_a\colon \text{Var}(\widehat{\delta}_h) > \text{Var}(\widetilde{\delta}_h)\end{aligned} \tag{16.4.1}$$

to determine whether $\widetilde{\delta}_h$ is more efficient than $\widetilde{\delta}_h$, in determining whether a meta-analysis should be performed. Note that the above hypotheses are equivalent to the following hypotheses:

$$\begin{aligned} &\text{H}_0\colon \tau_h^2 \le \sigma_{\text{TT}h}^2 \\ \text{versus } &\text{H}_a\colon \tau_h^2 > \sigma_{\text{TT}h}^2.\end{aligned}$$

Let h be fixed. Consider first the case of $n_{1h} = n_{2h} = n_h$. Define $X_{i1h} = Y_{i11h} - Y_{i12h} + Y_{i21h} - Y_{i22h}$ and $X_{i2h} = Y_{i11h} + Y_{i22h}$. Then X_{i1h}'s and X_{i2h}'s are independent. Let s_{xjh}^2 be the sample variance based on X_{ijh}, $i = 1, \ldots, n_h$, $j = 1, 2$. Then $(n_h - 1)\, s_{x1h}^2/(2\tau_n^2)$ and $(n_h - 1)s_{x2h}^2/2\sigma_{\text{TT}h}^2$ are independently distributed as the chi-square distribution with degrees of freedom $n_h - 1$, and $F_h = s_{xlh}^2/s_{x2h}^2$ has the F distribution with degrees of freedom $n_h - 1$ and $n_h - 1$ under the hypothesis $\tau_h^2 = \sigma_{\text{TT}h}^2$. Thus, an exact size α-test rejects H_0 when F_h is larger than the upper α quantile of the F distribution with degrees of freedom $n_h - 1$ and $n_h - 1$.

When $n_{1h} \neq n_{2h}$, a simple method is to take $n_h = \min(n_{1h}, n_{2h})$ and perform the previously proposed test.

Example 16.4.1

To illustrate the proposed test for the efficiency of a meta-analysis for bioequivalence review, consider Example 16.3.1, which consists of three data sets of hypothetical log-transformed AUC. It is assumed that these three data sets were collected from three independent bioequivalence trials. In each trial, a standard two-sequence, two-period crossover design was conducted with 24 healthy subjects to assess bioequivalence between a test product and the same brand-name drug product. The log-transformed AUC data for the three studies are listed in Table 16.3.1.

The F_h ratios in this example are given by $F_1 = 1.918$, $F_2 = 1.190$, and $F_3 = 1.915$. This indicates that the method based on meta-analysis should be more efficient, but the difference may not be very significant.

16.5 Discussion

Under the current FDA regulation, an ANDA submission for bioequivalence approval is on the first-come-first-serve basis. At each approval process, it is to compare one generic copy to the innovator drug product alone. Thus, meta-analysis may not be practical for regulatory decision before approval. However, it does provide a useful tool to evaluate postapproval bioequivalence among generic copies of the same brand-name drug. On the other hand, people may change jobs, and hence the health insurance plan may also be changed accordingly. Different health insurance plans may provide different generic copies of the same innovator drug product. Even within the same health plan, generic copies may vary due to the cost and other considerations. When the number of important innovator drug products going off patent increases and the market share of the generic copies grows, bioequivalence among generic copies of the same brand-name drug becomes a very important public health issue. We urge the regulatory agencies to conduct the meta-analysis of bioequivalence review for some important categories of drug products. If the results indicate that the approved generic copies are not bioequivalent to one another, the health authorities should at least issue a warning to prohibit the substitution of these generic copies because of safety consideration.

For clinical trials, Dubey recommends that treatment-by-study interaction be examined to avoid uncombinable studies (Dubey, 1988). In this chapter, we combined independent bioequivalence trials based on the fact that they reached the same conclusion of bioequivalence compared with the same reference product. Example 16.2.1, however, reveals that there is a significant treatment-by-study interaction. It is then of interest to study bioequivalence among the test products in the existence of treatment-by-study interaction. This needs further investigation.

In this chapter, we introduce meta-analysis methods, assuming that the effect owing to the study is a fixed effect. When there are many generic copies of the same brand-name drug, we may consider a random effect model, similar to that proposed by DerSimonian and Laird (1986) and modify the meta-analysis procedures as described in this chapter.

Chapter 17

Population Pharmacokinetics

17.1 Introduction

For a given drug product, it is of interest to study how the drug moves through the body and the processes of movement such as absorption (A), distribution (D), metabolism (M), and excretion (E) after drug administration. This leads to the study of pharmacokinetics (PK). The key concept of a PK study is to study *what the body does to the drug*, which is usually characterized by ADME of a drug product after administration. In practice, however, we cannot measure concentrations at the site of action directly. Instead, we can measure concentrations in blood, plasma, or serum that reflects ADME at the site of action. The site of action is defined as the site at which the drug will have its effect. Concentrations have valuable information regarding ADME that allows manipulation of concentrations in early drug development so that the concentrations will remain within therapeutic window (or index) for safety and efficacy. Note that the establishment of bioequivalence described in previous chapters is to show that the primary PK parameters such as AUC and $C_{\max}$, which reflect the extent and rate of absorption of the test product are not too high to avoid toxicity (safety) at one-side and are not too low to produce response (efficacy) for the other side as compared to those of the reference product.

Population pharmacokinetics (population PK) is the study of the sources and correlates of variability in drug concentrations among individuals who are the target patient population receiving clinically relevant doses of a drug of interest (Aarons, 1991). Thus, population PK is to study the relationship between dose and concentration for both individuals and the population of individuals. The study of individual PK parameters has become very popular because it is a representative sample of a population of such individuals. Individual PK parameters are usually estimated by fitting a PK model. The analysis of PK responses has emerged as a useful approach to ascertaining the nature of drug disposition in patient populations. Although such an analysis permits the evaluation of associations between patient characteristics and variation in drug disposition, it usually involves a nonlinear mixed effects model, which presents certain statistical and PK modeling difficulties. Such an analysis is usually performed after a considerably large database of concentrations, doses, and patient characteristics is established. For estimation of population PK parameters, a traditional approach is to employ a so-called standard two-stage (STS) method. At the first stage, we estimate individual parameters. Then, we treat the estimates as samples to obtain a confidence interval for the population parameters. This method, however, does not account for the variability of the estimates obtained from the first stage. To avoid individual estimates, Sheiner et al. (1972, 1977) proposed an alternative first-order (FO) method for estimation of the mean and variance of the population parameters by minimizing an extended least squares criterion. This method, which uses a nonlinear mixed effect model, is available in the software NONMEM (Beal and Sheiner, 1980). Several other methods, including parametric and nonparametric, have been developed. These methods include the use of the EM algorithm (Dempster et al., 1977) and the Bayesian approach (Racine-Poon, 1985). In addition, Prevost, in an unpublished report, proposed an iterative two-stage method (ITS) that uses a linearization of the model around the estimated parameters, under the assumption of a normal distribution of parameters (Steimer et al., 1984). The ITS method has been investigated by Lindstrom and Bates (1990) under different approximations. For nonparametric methods, Mallet (1986) developed a method based upon maximum likelihood of the whole set of individual measurements. Schumitzky (1990) also proposed a nonparametric algorithm to estimate the distribution using an EM estimation approach. For a one-compartment model, these methods are available on the software NPEM (Jellife et al., 1990). For application of a recent development in linear and nonlinear mixed effects model to population PK, see Davidian and Giltinan (1995), Vonesh and Chinchilli (1997), and Davidian (2003).

As one of the primary objectives of a population PK study is to estimate accurately and precisely the kinetic parameters in a population and the population parameters quantify the mean kinetics in the population, the inter-individual kinetic variability, and the intra-individual variability of measured kinetic responses, it is suggested that a valid and efficient design should be used in order to produce accurate and reliable estimates of population parameters. For this purpose, some design factors such as the number of subjects, the number of concentrations measured in each individual, and the sampling times of the biologic fluid (e.g., blood) in which the drug concentration is determined are necessarily considered for achieving the desired degree of accuracy and precision of the estimates of the population parameters. These design factors can be controlled to a certain extent by conducting a prospective population kinetic study. The most widely accepted theoretical approach of determining optimal sampling times for PK studies is probably based on the Fisher information matrix. A commonly used criterion for determining optimal sampling times is to maximize the determinant of the Fisher information matrix (or equivalently minimize the inverse of the determinant), which is known as the D-optimality criterion. Following the concept of D-optimality, two approaches are commonly considered in designing a population PK study. These two approaches are the population Fisher information matrix (PFIM) approach (Wang and Endrenyi, 1992) and the informative block randomized (IBR) approach (Ette et al., 1994).

The remaining of this chapter is organized as follows. In Section 17.2, regulatory requirements for the use of population PK in pharmaceutical development are given. Approaches for population PK modeling are described in Section 17.3.

Approaches to the design of population PK studies are discussed in Section 17.4. An example is given in Section 17.5 to illustrate statistical methods described in this chapter. Section 17.6 provides some concluding remarks including study protocol, concerns/challenges of the population approach in population PK, the relationship between PK and pharmacodynamics (PD), the use of computer simulation, and software application.

17.2 Regulatory Requirements

In 1999, the FDA issued guidance on population PK (FDA, 1999b). In this guidance, the FDA provides some recommendations on design and analysis of a population PK study. Also, included in this guidance are data handling such as missing data and outliers, PK model development and validation. These requirements are briefly summarized below.

17.2.1 Population PK Analysis

As indicated in the 1999 FDA guidance on population PK, the population model defines at least two levels of hierarchy. At the first level, PK observations in an individual such as concentrations are viewed as arising from an individual probability model, whose mean is given by a PK model quantified by individual-specific parameters. At the second level, the individual parameters are regarded as random variables. Since the focus of a population PK study is on population of individual PK parameters, the FDA suggests the two commonly used methods, namely the two-stage approach and the nonlinear mixed effects modeling approach should be considered in population PK analysis. As pointed out by the FDA, although the traditional two-stage approach (when applicable) can yield adequate estimates of population characteristics, it may not be applicable in sparse data situations because individual parameters may not be estimable. The STS approach and the nonlinear mixed effects modeling approach are discussed in detail in Section 17.3.

17.2.2 Study Design

At the planning of a population PK study, it is suggested that certain preliminary PK information and the drug's major elimination pathways in humans should be available. In addition, a sensitive and specific assay capable of measuring the drug and all metabolites of clinical relevance should be available. When designing a population PK study, FDA suggests that some design considerations such as sampling times, number of samples per subject, and number of subjects be considered for an accurate and reliable assessment of population characteristics. Optimizing the sampling design is of particular importance when severe limitations exist on the number of subjects or samples per subject (e.g., in pediatric patients or the elderly). FDA recommends some informative designs proposed in the literature (e.g., Hashimoto and Sheiner, 1991; Johnson et al., 1996; Sun et al., 1996) be used to ensure that there are enough patients not only for an accurate and precise estimation of the population parameters, but also for detection of any subgroup differences with a desired power.

17.2.3 Population PK Model Development/Validation

For development of population PK model, the FDA suggests that the objectives and hypotheses be stated clearly. It is recommended that all assumptions inherent in the population analysis be explicitly expressed. The criteria and rationale for model building procedures dealing with confounding, covariate, and parameter redundancy should be stated clearly. The steps taken for model building should be outlined clearly to permit the reproducibility of the analysis. For a developed population PK model, the FDA recommends that the reliability of the analysis results be examined through diagnostic plots, including predicted versus observed concentration, predicted concentration superimposed on the data, and posterior estimates of parameters versus covariate values. Whenever possible, evaluation for robustness using sensitivity analysis should be conducted.

For validation of a population PK model, since there is no consensus on an appropriate statistical approach for validation of population PK models, the FDA suggests focusing on the predictive performance aspect of validation either through an external or an internal validation. External validation is the application of the developed model to a new data set (validation data set) from another study, while internal validation refers to the use of data splitting (e.g., cross-validation) and resampling techniques (e.g., bootstrapping). The predictive performance aspect of validation is defined as the evaluation of the predictability of the model developed using a learning or index data set when applied to a validation data set not used for model building and parameter estimation.

Note that the FDA indicated that not all population PK models need to be validated. The population PK analysis results will be incorporated in the drug label. Model validation is encouraged and model validation procedures should be an integral part of the protocol. If population PK models are developed to explain variability with no dosage adjustment recommendation envisaged and to provide descriptive information for labeling, models can be tested for stability only.

17.2.4 Missing Data and Outlier

In population PK studies, missing values commonly occur at either PK response or covariates. Missing data is a potential source of bias. Excluding all subjects with any missing data will decrease the sample size. Thus, in certain situations, it may be better to impute missing values rather than to delete those subjects with missing values from analysis. As indicated in the 1999 FDA guidance (FDA, 1999b), although many methods for imputation are available in the literature, the performance of imputation techniques in this context is not well studied. Thus, the FDA suggests that imputation procedure should be described and a detailed explanation of how such imputations was done and the underlying assumptions made should be provided.

For outliers, either outlying individuals (inter-subject variability) or outlying data points (intra-subject variability), the FDA requires that the reasons for declaring an outlying data point should be statistically convincing and if possible be prespecified in the study protocol.

17.2.5 Timing for Application

The use of the population PK approach can help increase understanding of the quantitative relationship among drug input patterns, patient characteristics, and drug disposition. It is helpful in situation when the investigator wishes to identify factors that affect drug behavior, or explain variability in a target population. The population PK approach is especially helpful in certain adaptive study designs such as dose finding studies in early stage of drug development.

As indicated in the 1999 FDA guidance (FDA, 1999b), the FDA advises that in certain circumstances such as (1) when the population for which the drug is intended is quite heterogeneous and (2) when the target concentration window is believed to be relatively narrow, the population PK approach is most likely to add value when a reasonable a priori expectation exists that inter-subject kinetic variation may warrant altered dosing for some subgroups in the target population. The FDA also pointed out that the population PK approach is most likely used in phase I and late phase IIb of clinical development for estimation of population parameters of a response surface model where information is gathered on how the drug will be used in subsequent stages of drug development (see also Sheiner, 1997). However, the FDA also noted that in phase I and much of phase IIb studies where patients are usually sampled extensively, complex methods of data analysis may not be needed.

The population PK approach can also be used in early phase IIa and III of drug development to gain information on drug safety (efficacy) and to gather additional information on drug PK in special populations. The population PK approach can also be useful in phase IV studies such as postmarketing surveillance or labeling change.

17.3 Population PK Modeling

As indicated earlier, the movement of a drug administered to a patient is studied via some population characteristics that describe absorption, distribution, metabolism, and elimination (ADME) of the drug. These population characteristics are measured by some PK parameters such as the fraction of each dose which is absorbed when the drug is given by the oral route (absorption), volume of distribution of the drug with respect to its concentration (distribution), and the clearance of the drug with respect to its concentration in plasma (elimination). In practice, it is of interest to learn about the variation of PK parameters in a target patient population. This leads to the study of population PK modeling. In what follows, several approaches for estimation of population characteristics of PK parameters are described.

17.3.1 Traditional Two-Stage Method

The traditional approach for estimation of population characteristics of PK parameters consists of two stages, which is described below. At the first stage, for each of a number of patients, enough dosages are administered and enough plasma concentrations are drawn to allow the PK parameters to be estimated for each individual. Estimates of these PK parameters are often obtained based on a *deterministic* PK model (e.g., a one-compartment model or a multiple-compartment model). Then, at the second stage, based on estimates of the PK parameters obtained from each individual, an analysis of covariance model is considered to avoid effects due to possible confounding and interaction among covariates (e.g., demographics or patient characteristics) and to study the treatment effects (e.g., dosage and route of administration) and between-individual variation.

As pointed out by Sheiner et al. (1997), there are obvious obstacles to this traditional approach including the ethical issue and cost. From statistical point of view, the traditional approach suffers the following disadvantages. First, the use of estimates based on a deterministic model from each individual does not take into consideration of the variability of each individual (i.e., intra-individual variability). Second, sparse or haphazard sampling of each subject may not provide accurate and reliable estimates of the PK parameters for each subject. To overcome this problem, the frequency of sampling for blood drawn is necessary, which leads to the ethical concern as pointed out by Sheiner et al. (1997). Third, the traditional approach may not be useful in describing population characteristics when there are a lot of demographic, physiological, and behavioral characteristics recorded for each subject such as weight, age, renal function, race, ethnicity, disease status, and so on which are often of interest to the investigator.

17.3.2 Nonlinear Mixed Effects Modeling Approach

As an alternative to the traditional two-stage method, the FDA suggests the use of nonlinear mixed effects modeling approach. The approach of nonlinear mixed effects modeling is a nonlinear regression model that accounts for both fixed and random effects. It provides an estimation of population characteristics that define the population distribution of the PK and pharmacodynamic (PD) parameters.

In the 1970s, Sheiner et al. (1972, 1977) laid the foundations of population PK modeling. They showed how, with data collected as part of routine patient cares, such modeling can estimate the average values of PK parameters and the inter-individual variances of those parameters in a patient population. With such sparsely sampled data from patients, their methodology produced estimates that were similar to published values derived with traditional methods.

17.3.2.1 First-Order Method

Let y_{ij} be the jth (plasma or serum) concentration obtained from the ith subject, where $j = 1, \ldots, n_i$ and $i = 1, \ldots, m$ and $N = \sum_{i=1}^{m} n_i$ is the total number of observations. Also, let x_{ij} be conditions of jth measurement (e.g., times, doses) from the ith subject. As discussed earlier, our focus is not on population mean concentration, but on population of individual PK parameters. This leads to the use of nonlinear mixed effects model. Following the concept of two-stage approach, for the first stage, we consider the so-called intra-subject PK model. Consider the following model:

$$y_{ij} = f(x_{ij}, \beta_i) \cdot e_{ij}, \tag{17.3.1}$$

where

$$E(y_{ij}|\beta_i) = f(x_{ij}, \beta_i),$$
$$\text{Var}(y_{ij}|\beta_i) = v\left[f(x_{ij}, \beta_i), \xi\right],$$

in which f dictated by compartment model, superposition of past doses, β_i is a $p \times 1$ vector of PK parameters, as an example

$$\beta_i = (F_i, Cl_i, V_{di})' \tag{17.3.2}$$

as considered in Sheiner et al. (1977). For the second stage, we consider the inter-subject population model as follows:

$$\beta_i = d(a_i, \beta, b_i),$$

where a_i is the subject characteristic (covariate) of the ith subject and b_i is a $k \times 1$ vector of random effects which follows a k-variate distribution with mean 0 and variance–covariance matrices D. As a result, the two-stage hierarchy leads to the following intra-subject PK model (Stage 1):

$$\begin{aligned} y_i &= f_i(\beta_i) \cdot e_i \\ &= f_i(\beta_i) \cdot R_i^{1/2}(\beta_i, \xi) \cdot \varepsilon_i, \end{aligned} \tag{17.3.3}$$

where

$$E(y_i|b_i) = f_i(\beta_i),$$
$$\text{Var}(y_i|b_i) = R_i(\beta_i, \xi).$$

Note that

$$P_{y|b}(y_i|x_{i1}, \ldots, x_{in_i}, a_i, \beta, b_i, \xi) = P_{y|b}(y_i|\beta, b_i, \xi).$$

For the inter-subject population model (Stage 2), we have

$$\beta_i = d(a_i, \beta, b_i),$$

where

$$b_i \sim H = N_k(0, D).$$

Under this two-stage hierarchical model, the objectives are to (1) determine d (i.e., the relationship between PK and covariates), (2) estimate β (i.e., the relationship between PK and covariates), (3) estimate H (i.e., the variation in population), and (4) estimate β_i (i.e., characterize individuals and consequently optimize or individualized dosing). For achieving these objectives, we consider maximizing the following likelihood function for obtaining the maximum likelihood estimates:

$$\begin{aligned} l(\beta, \xi, H) &= \prod_{i=1}^{m} l_i(\beta, \xi, H) \\ &= \prod_{i=1}^{m} P_{y|b}(y_i|\beta, b_i, \xi) dH(b_i). \end{aligned} \tag{17.3.4}$$

Due the complexity of the likelihood function (i.e., nonlinear in b_i), there exists no closed forms for the maximum likelihood estimates if it is not intractable. Beal and Sheiner (1982) considered first-order approximation about $b_i = 0$ assuming that $P_{y|b}$ is normal and $H = N_k(0, D)$. In other words, they considered

$$\begin{aligned} y_i &= f_i[d(a_i, \beta, b_i)] + R_i^{1/2}[d(a_i, \beta, b_i), \xi] \cdot \varepsilon_i \\ &\approx f[d(a_i, \beta_i, 0)]_i + Z_i(\beta, 0) b_i + R_i^{1/2}[d(a_i, \beta, 0)] \cdot \varepsilon_i. \end{aligned} \tag{17.3.5}$$

Then, approximate l_i by the n_i-variate normal with

$$E(y_i) \approx f_i[d(a_i, \beta, 0)],$$

and

$$\text{Var}(y_i) \approx R_i\{d(a_i, \beta, 0)\} + Z_i(\beta, 0)\, DZ_i'(\beta, 0).$$

This was implemented in the FORTRAN program in NONMEM (it was referred to as the FO method).

17.3.2.2 Example

As an example, consider the specific case of digoxin as described in Sheiner et al. (1977). Suppose the population characteristics describing absorption, distribution, and elimination of the drug are of particular interest to the investigator. For absorption, the PK parameter considered is F_{oral}, which is the fraction of each dose that is absorbed when the drug is given by oral route. For distribution, the volume of distribution, denoted by V_d, of the drug with respect to its concentration in plasma is examined. For elimination, the clearance of the drug (Cl) with respect to its concentration in plasma is assessed. Suppose we wish to model the kinetics of a drug using the one-compartment open model. Without loss of generality, we only consider the single-dose case. Let C_{ij} be the ith measured plasma concentration in the jth individual at time t_{ij}. Thus, the one-compartment open model leads to

$$C_{ij} = \left(\frac{F_j \cdot D_j}{V_{dj}}\right) \exp(-\text{Cl}_j / V_{dt} \cdot t_{ij}), \tag{17.3.6}$$

where

F_j is the fraction of drug absorbed by the jth individual when receiving a dose by the chosen route

D_j is the dose received by the jth individual

V_{dj} is the volume of distribution for the drug in the jth individual

Cl_j is the drug clearance for the jth individual, and t_{ij} is the time of drawing the ith sample in the jth individual ($t_{ij} = 0$ at the time of administration of the dose D_j)

Note that although there are three unknown parameters: F_j, V_{dj}, and Cl_j, only two constants, F_j/V_{dj} and Cl_j/V_{dj} could be estimated for any individual from one single study. Now, suppose that drug clearance can be described by the following relation:

$$\text{Cl}_j = A + B \cdot \text{Cl}_j^{\text{Cr}}, \tag{17.3.7}$$

where Cl_j^{Cr} is the creatinine clearance for the jth individual, a quantity that can be directly measured or can be estimated from other data such as serum creatinine value, A and B are some fixed constants which relate drug clearance to creatinine clearance. Further, suppose that the volume of distribution depends on renal function and has the following relationship:

$$V_{dj} = D + E \cdot \text{Cl}_j^{\text{Cr}}, \tag{17.3.8}$$

where D and E are some fixed constants, which must be estimated from data. As it can be seen that models 17.3.1 through 17.3.3 are deterministic. To have an accurate and reliable assessment of population characteristics, we should take into consideration the variabilities associated with each deterministic model. This leads to

$$\begin{aligned} C_{ij} &= \left(\frac{F_j \cdot D_j}{V_{dj}}\right) \exp(-\text{Cl}_j / V_{dj} \cdot t_{ij}) \cdot \varepsilon_{ij}, \\ \text{Cl}_j &= A + B \cdot \text{Cl}_j^{\text{Cr}} + \eta_j^{\text{Cr}}, \\ V_{dj} &= D + E \cdot \text{Cl}_j^{\text{Cr}} + \eta_j^{V}, \end{aligned} \tag{17.3.9}$$

where ε_{ij}, η_j^{Cr}, and η_j^V follow normal distribution with mean 0 and variances σ_ε^2, σ_{Cl}^2, and σ_V^2, respectively. Sheiner et al. (1977) suggested linearizing model 17.3.4 first and then considering an approximation based on the first-term Taylor series expansion. After some algebra, model 17.3.4 becomes

$$C_{ij} = M_{ij}\left[1 + \left(\frac{\mathrm{Cl}_j}{V_{dj}^2} t_{ij} - \frac{1}{V_{dj}}\right)\eta_j^V - \frac{t_{ij}}{V_{dj}}\eta_j^{\mathrm{Cr}}\right] + \left(\alpha^2 M_{ij}^2 + 1\right)^{1/2}\varepsilon_{ij}, \qquad (17.3.10)$$

where

$$M_{ij} = \left(\frac{F \cdot D_j}{V_{dj}}\right)\exp(-\mathrm{Cl}_j/V_{dj} \cdot t_{ij}),$$

and F is the assumed constant bioavailability. Thus, we have

$$\begin{aligned}\mathrm{Var}(C_{ij}) = {} & M_{ij}^2\left(\frac{\mathrm{Cl}_j}{V_{dj}^2} t_{ij} - \frac{1}{V_{dj}}\right)^2 \sigma_V^2 + M_{ij}^2\left(\frac{t_{ij}}{V_{dj}}\right)^2 \sigma_{\mathrm{Cl}}^2 \\ & -2\left(\frac{\mathrm{Cl}_j}{V_{dj}^2} t_{ij} - \frac{1}{V_{dj}}\right)\left(\frac{t_{ij}}{V_{dj}}\right) M_{ij}^2 \sigma_{V,\mathrm{Cl}}^2 + \left(\alpha^2 M_{ij}^2 + 1\right)\sigma_\varepsilon^2,\end{aligned}$$

where $\sigma_{V,\mathrm{Cl}}^2$ is the population covariance between Cl_j and V_{dj}.

17.3.2.3 Other Approximations

The first order approximation is obviously biased and there is a room for improvement. A better approximation based on Laplace's approximation has been proposed in the literature (Bates and Lindstrom, 1990; Wolfinger, 1993; and Vonesh, 1996).

Assume that H is $N_k(0, D)$, $p_{y\,|\,b}$ is normal with $R_i(\xi)$. Then, we have

$$l_i = (2\pi)^{-(n_i+k)/2}\int |D|^{-1/2}\exp[-q(y_i, b_i)/2]db_i,$$

where

$$q(y_i, b_i) = [y_i - f_i(\beta_i)']R_i^{-1}(\xi)[y_i - f_i(\beta_i)] + b_i' D^{-1} b_{i.}.$$

Thus, we can solve $q'(y_i, b_i) = 0$ for $\hat{b}_i$. It can be verified that for large n_i

$$l_i \approx (2\pi)^{-n_i/2}|D|^{-1/2}\left|q''(y_i, \widehat{b}_i)/2\right|^{-1/2}\exp[-q(y_i, \widehat{b}_i)/2].$$

Thus, $l_i \approx n_i$-variate normal with

$$E(y_i) \approx f_i\left\{d(a_i, \beta, \widehat{b}_i)\right\} - Z_i\left\{\beta, \widehat{b}_i\right\}\widehat{b}_i,$$

and

$$\text{Var}(y_i) \approx Z_i\left\{\beta, \widehat{b}_i\right\} D Z_i'\left\{\beta, \widehat{b}_i\right\} + R_i(\xi).$$

As indicated by Davidian (2003), this approximation works remarkably well for sparse (i.e., small n_i) population PK data as long as intra-subject variation is small. This approximation has been implemented in many software packages. For example, nlme of S-plus, %nlinmix of SAS, and NONMEM.

Note that Mallet (1986) proposed the use of completely nonparametric approach for estimation of H. On the other hand, Davidian and Gallant (1993) assumed H has a nice density and estimate H along with other model components.

17.3.2.4 Bayesian Approach

Wakefield (1996) and Müller and Rosner (1997) proposed a three-stage hierarchy Bayesian approach by the following stages. For the first stage (Stage 1), consider

$$\begin{aligned} y_i &= f_i(\beta_i) \cdot e_i \\ &= f_i(\beta_i) \cdot R_i^{1/2}(\beta_i, \xi) \cdot \varepsilon_i, \end{aligned}$$

where

$$\begin{aligned} E(y_i|b_i) &= f_i(\beta_i), \\ \text{Var}(y_i|b_i) &= R_i(\beta_i, \xi), \end{aligned}$$

and

$$P_{y|b}(y_i|x_{i1}, \ldots, x_{in_i}, a_i, \beta, b_i, \xi) = P_{y|b}(y_i|\beta, b_i, \xi).$$

At the second stage (Stage 2), consider

$$\beta_i = d(a_i, \beta, b_i),$$

where

$$b_i \sim P_b|D(b_i|D) \text{ of } b_i \sim H.$$

At the third stage (Stage 3), assume the following hyperprior:

$$(\beta, \xi, D) \sim p_{\beta,\xi,D}(\beta, \xi, D).$$

Note that this approach has been implemented in PKBugs, which a WinBUGS interface with built-in PK models.

17.4 Design of Population PK

As discussed in Section 17.3, the analysis of population PK parameters usually involves a nonlinear mixed effects model, the estimates of inter-subject (or inter-individual), intra-subject (or intra-individual) variability, and measurement error are extremely important. A relatively large inter-subject variability may indicate that more patients are needed to have sound statistical inference for the parameters. On the other hand, if the intra-subject variability is much larger than the inter-subject variability, more plasma samples may be needed to characterize the plasma concentration–time curve. An appropriate nonlinear mixed effects model should be able to account for these variations. For a PK model, it is of interest to estimate the population parameters and the difference in parameters between groups such as treatment group, sex, age, and race. The estimation of population parameters can be obtained based on plasma concentrations over time. Statistical inference for the difference in parameters between groups may be considered for assessing bioequivalence based on a preselected decision rule. The interpretation of these parameters, however, is important in evaluation of drug performances within and between groups.

When planning a population PK study, the design factors such as the number of subjects, the number of concentrations measured in each individual, and the sampling times of the biologic fluid (e.g., blood) in which the drug concentration is determined are necessarily considered for achieving optimal accuracy and precision of the estimates of the population parameters. In practice, the most widely accepted theoretical approach of determining optimal sampling times for PK studies is based on the Fisher information matrix. A commonly used criterion for determining optimal sampling times is to maximize the determinant of the Fisher information matrix (or equivalently minimize the inverse of the determinant), i.e., the D-optimality criterion. In other words, the design factors should be selected in order to reach D-optimality.

Sheiner and Beal (1983) and Al-Banna et al. (1990) studied the effect of these design factors in terms of the bias and precision of population kinetic parameters estimated obtained by the first-order method via computer simulation. Hashimoto and Sheiner (1991), on the other hand, explored the design of experiments in PK/PD investigations. Wang and Endrenyi (1992) considered a large sample approach for evaluation of the variances of parameter estimates for a population PK study. Their method was referred to as PFIM approach. Sun et al. (1996) proposed using an informative block (profile) randomized (IBR) approach to investigate the effect of sample times recording error (both systematic and random) on the estimates of the population PK parameters. When designing a population PK study, the FDA encourages that these informative designs be considered. Such designs should include enough patients in important subgroups to ensure accurate and precise parameter estimation and the detection of any subgroup differences. In what follows, the PFIM design and IBR design of population PK studies are described.

17.4.1 Population Fisher's Information Matrix Approach

Wang and Endrenyi (1992) proposed a large sample approach to evaluate the approximate asymptotic variances (or coefficients of variation) of the maximum likelihood estimators. The information is used to facilitate the selection of favorable experimental designs that lead to the precise estimation of population kinetic parameters by the first-order method. Wang and Endrenyi (1992) noted that the first-order method is identical to the maximum likelihood approach (applied to the first-order model) under the assumption of normally distributed errors. Thus estimated variances might be normally distributed after suitable transformation.

Let β and $\hat{\beta}$ denote, respectively, a vector of k parameters and the corresponding vector of the maximum likelihood estimators. Let V represent the variance–covariance matrix of $\hat{\beta}$. Thus, the diagonal elements of V are the variances and the off-diagonal elements are the pairwise covariances of the elements of $\hat{\beta}$ Further, let J denote the inverse of V, i.e., $J = V^{-1}$, where each element of J, j_{rs} is given by

$$j_{rs} = E\left(\frac{\partial_l}{\partial\beta_r}\cdot\frac{\partial_l}{\partial\beta_r}\right) = -E\left(\frac{\partial^2 l}{\partial\beta_r\partial\beta_s}\right), \quad r = 1,\ldots,k; \quad s = 1,\ldots,k \qquad (17.4.1)$$

where

l is the log-likelihood function
E is the expectation of the random variable in the equation
J is the Fisher's information matrix

Wang and Endrenyi (1992) proposed to estimate the information matrix J from the data using the following approximation:

$$j_{rs} \approx \left(\frac{\partial_l}{\partial\beta_r}\cdot\frac{\partial_l}{\partial\beta_r}\right) \approx -\left(\frac{\partial^2 l}{\partial\beta_r\partial\beta_s}\right), \quad r = 1,\ldots,k; \quad s = 1,\ldots,k. \qquad (17.4.2)$$

In practice, it is very tedious, if not impossible, to calculate the expected variances based on Equation 17.4.1, even for a simple kinetic model and a simple design. On the other hand, the computation of the observed variances by Equation 17.4.2 is quite feasible with the use of computers. The observed variances obtained from Equation 17.4.2 approach their true values as the sample size (i.e., the number of individuals) in the sample becomes larger.

It should be noted that in the context of population PK, the population kinetic parameters constitute β, the kinetic responses (e.g., drug concentrations) form the observations, and the dose and sampling times are examples of independent variables. Statistically, the set of kinetic responses from a given individual is regarded as a single observation in the multivariate sense. Moreover, the observations from different individuals are assumed to be independent. Thus, the sample size in a population kinetic study is the number of subjects.

The large sample approach, which is referred to as PFIM approach, in conjunction with computer simulation is applied to facilitate the design of experiments that aim at the estimation of population PK parameters. PFIM approach proposed by Wang and Endrenyi (1992) is a numerical procedure that evaluates the efficiency of the different sampling designs, from which the most favorable one is selected. In addition, Wang and Endrenyi (1992) indicated that due to its efficiency and effectiveness in assessing the variability of parameter estimates, the PFIM approach can serve as a tool for studying the relationship between experimental design and the precision of population parameter estimates. After selecting a suitable design for a prospective population PK study, the biases of the parameter estimates may be evaluated and the variability of the estimates confirmed by applying the simulation method for that design. If the calculated biases turn out to be substantial, the estimates obtained following data collection and analysis can be adjusted accordingly.

17.4.2 IBR Approach

Ette et al. (1994) proposed a method that combines the efficiency of D-optimality criteria and the robustness afforded by random sampling. This method was referred to as the IBR design. Based on the D-optimality criteria, Ette et al. (1994) considered three alternative sampling procedures with respect to the average PK parameter estimates. These sampling schemes include (1) the informative sampling scheme, (2) the randomized sampling scheme, and (3) the IBR sampling scheme, which are described below.

In the informative sampling scheme, each subject has an identical sampling scheme with sampling times specified according to the D-optimality criteria with all of the samples constrained to be within a specified sampling interval. In the randomized sampling scheme, samples are chosen at random from within the sampling intervals, while in the IBR sampling scheme, the sampling interval is divided into contiguous intervals and equal numbers of samples are chosen at random from each interval.

Ette et al. (1994) compared the efficiency of these informative sampling schemes with that of a conventional sampling scheme, in which sampling times are approximately equal-spaced on a log-scale. The population PK parameter estimates obtained with the conventional sampling scheme are found to be inferior to those obtained from the informative, randomized, and IBR schemes. The performances of the three sampling schemes are similar in terms of the accuracy and precision of population PK parameter estimates. Sun et al. (1996) investigated the effect of sample times recording error (both systematic and random) on the estimation of population PK parameters under an IBR design for a drug with two compartment PKs for both single-dose and multiple-dose administrations. The PK profile was divided into three blocks and each subject was sampled across the blocks providing two samples per block. Sun et al. (1996) observed that negative systematic error in the recording of sample times resulted in efficient estimation of volume terms, whereas positive systematic error favored the efficient estimation of the clearance terms. These errors resulted in sufficient samples being located in critical regions for the estimation of volume terms (negative systematic error) and clearance terms (positive systematic error). Sun et al. (1996) concluded that the efficiency in the estimation of clearance was not severely compromised for moderate sampling time recording errors.

Roy and Ette (2005) compared the PFIM D-optimal and IBR designs and indicated that the IBR design is preferred for pragmatic reasons. Pragmatism would detect the use of designs that are easy to implement without loss of efficiency and clinical trial simulations should be used to choose the appropriate design to meet study objectives.

17.4.3 Remarks

As indicated in the 1999 FDA guidance for *Population Pharmacokinetics* (FDA, 1999b), three broad approaches (with increasing information content) exist for obtaining information about PK variability. These approaches include (1) single-trough sampling design, (2) multiple-trough sampling design, and (3) full population PK sampling design. For the single-trough sampling design, a single blood sample is obtained from each patient at, or close to, the trough of the drug concentrations, shortly before the next dose, and a frequency distribution of plasma or serum levels in the sample of patients is calculated. The FDA pointed out that this approach will give a fairly accurate picture of the variability in trough concentrations in the target population under the assumptions that (1) the sample size is large, (2) the assay and sampling errors are small, and (3) the dosing regimen and sampling times are identical for all patients. In practice, however, these assumptions are usually not met. Thus, the use of the single-trough sampling design is not encouraged except in situations where it is absolutely necessary.

For the multiple-trough sampling design, two or more blood samples are obtained near the trough of steady-state concentrations from most or all patients. In addition to relating blood concentration to patient characteristics, it is possible to separate inter-individual and residual variabilities. A multiple-trough sampling design requires fewer subjects than that of the single-trough sampling design. In addition, the relationship of trough levels to patient characteristics can be evaluated with greater precision.

The full population PK sampling design is referred to a sampling design that blood samples are drawn from subjects at various times (typically one to six time points) following drug administration. The full population PK sampling design is also known as the experimental population PK design or full PK screen. The objective of the full population PK sampling design is to obtain, where feasible, multiple drug levels per patient at different times to describe the population PK profile. This design permits an estimation of PK parameters of the drug in the study population and an explanation of variability using the nonlinear mixed effects modeling approach. As indicated in the 1999 FDA guidance, the full population PK sampling design should be planned to explore the relationship between the PK of a drug and demographic and pathophysiological features of the target population (with its subgroups) for which the drug is being developed.

17.5 Example

To illustrate statistical methods described in the previous sections, consider the theophylline data from Pinheiro and Bates (1995). Serum concentrations of the drug theophylline were collected in 12 subjects over a 25 hours period after oral administration of the drug. The concentration data are given in Table 17.5.1. Pinheiro and Bates (1995) considered the following first-order compartment model:

$$C_{it} = \frac{Dk_{ei}k_{ai}}{\mathrm{Cl}_i(k_{ai} - k_{ei})}[e^{-k_{ei}t} - e^{-k_{ai}t}] + e_{it},$$

where

C_{it} is the observed concentration of the ith subject at time t
D is the dose of theophylline, k_{ei} is the elimination rate constant for subject i
k_{ai} is the absorption rate constant for subject i
Cl_i is the clearance for subject i
e_{it} are normal errors

To allow for random variability between subjects, Pinheiro and Bates (1995) further assumed that

$$\mathrm{Cl}_i = e^{\beta_1 + b_{i1}},$$
$$k_{ai} = e^{\beta_2 + b_{i2}},$$
$$k_{ei} = e^{\beta_3},$$

where

β's denotes fixed-effect parameters
b's denote random-effect parameters with an unknown covariance matrix

Under the above setting, the PROC NLMIXED procedure of SAS as given in Table 17.5.2. In Table 17.5.2, PARMS statement specifies starting values for the three β's and the four variance–covariance parameters. The clearance and rate constants are defined using SAS programming statements, and the conditional model for the data is defined to be normal with mean PRED and variance S2. The two random effects are B1 and B2, and their joint distribution is defined in the RANDOM statement. Note that brackets are used to define their mean vector (two zeros) and the lower triangle of their variance–covariance matrix (a general 2×2 matrix). A summary of the above PROC NLMIXED is given in Table 17.5.3, where specification lists the

TABLE 17.5.1: Theophylline concentration data in 12 subjects.

Subjects	Time	Concentration	Dose	Weight	Subjects	Time	Concentration	Dose	Weight	Subjects	Time	Concentration	Dose	Weight
1	0.00	0.74	4.02	79.6	5	0.00	0.00	5.86	54.6	9	0.00	0.00	3.10	86.4
1	0.25	2.84	4.02	79.6	5	0.30	2.02	5.86	54.6	9	0.30	7.37	3.10	86.4
1	0.57	6.57	4.02	79.6	5	0.52	5.63	5.86	54.6	9	0.63	9.03	3.10	86.4
1	1.12	10.50	4.02	79.6	5	1.00	11.40	5.86	54.6	9	1.05	7.14	3.10	86.4
1	2.02	9.66	4.02	79.6	5	2.02	9.33	5.86	54.6	9	2.02	6.33	3.10	86.4
1	3.82	8.58	4.02	79.6	5	3.50	8.74	5.86	54.6	9	3.53	5.66	3.10	86.4
1	5.10	8.36	4.02	79.6	5	5.02	7.56	5.86	54.6	9	5.02	5.67	3.10	86.4
1	7.03	7.47	4.02	79.6	5	7.02	7.09	5.86	54.6	9	7.17	4.24	3.10	86.4
1	9.05	6.89	4.02	79.6	5	9.10	5.90	5.86	54.6	9	8.80	4.11	3.10	86.4
1	12.12	5.94	4.02	79.6	5	12.00	4.37	5.86	54.6	9	11.60	3.16	3.10	86.4
1	24.37	3.28	4.02	79.6	5	24.35	1.57	5.86	54.6	9	24.43	1.12	3.10	86.4
2	0.00	0.00	4.40	72.4	6	0.00	0.00	4.00	80.0	10	0.00	0.24	5.50	58.2
2	0.27	1.72	4.40	72.4	6	0.27	1.29	4.00	80.0	10	0.37	2.89	5.50	58.2
2	0.52	7.91	4.40	72.4	6	0.58	3.08	4.00	80.0	10	0.77	5.22	5.50	58.2
2	1.00	8.31	4.40	72.4	6	1.15	6.44	4.00	80.0	10	1.02	6.41	5.50	58.2
2	1.92	8.33	4.40	72.4	6	2.03	6.32	4.00	80.0	10	2.05	7.83	5.50	58.2
2	3.50	6.85	4.40	72.4	6	3.57	5.53	4.00	80.0	10	3.55	10.21	5.50	58.2
2	5.02	6.08	4.40	72.4	6	5.00	4.94	4.00	80.0	10	5.05	9.18	5.50	58.2
2	7.03	5.40	4.40	72.4	6	7.00	4.02	4.00	80.0	10	7.08	8.02	5.50	58.2
2	9.00	4.55	4.40	72.4	6	9.22	3.46	4.00	80.0	10	9.38	7.14	5.50	58.2
2	12.00	3.01	4.40	72.4	6	12.10	2.78	4.00	80.0	10	12.10	5.68	5.50	58.2
2	24.30	0.90	4.40	72.4	6	23.85	0.92	4.00	80.0	10	23.70	2.42	5.50	58.2
3	0.00	0.00	4.53	70.5	7	0.00	0.15	4.95	64.6	11	0.00	0.00	4.92	65.0
3	0.27	4.40	4.53	70.5	7	0.25	0.85	4.95	64.6	11	0.25	4.86	4.92	65.0

(*continued*)

TABLE 17.5.1 (continued): Theophylline concentration data in 12 subjects.

Subjects	Time	Concentration	Dose	Weight	Subjects	Time	Concentration	Dose	Weight	Subjects	Time	Concentration	Dose	Weight
3	0.58	6.90	4.53	70.5	7	0.50	2.35	4.95	64.6	11	0.50	7.24	4.92	65.0
3	1.02	8.20	4.53	70.5	7	1.02	5.02	4.95	64.6	11	0.98	8.00	4.92	65.0
3	2.02	7.80	4.53	70.5	7	2.02	6.58	4.95	64.6	11	1.98	6.81	4.92	65.0
3	3.62	7.50	4.53	70.5	7	3.48	7.09	4.95	64.6	11	3.60	5.87	4.92	65.0
3	5.08	6.20	4.53	70.5	7	5.00	6.66	4.95	64.6	11	5.02	5.22	4.92	65.0
3	7.07	5.30	4.53	70.5	7	6.98	5.25	4.95	64.6	11	7.03	4.45	4.92	65.0
3	9.00	4.90	4.53	70.5	7	9.00	4.39	4.95	64.6	11	9.03	3.62	4.92	65.0
3	12.15	3.70	4.53	70.5	7	12.05	3.53	4.95	64.6	11	12.12	2.69	4.92	65.0
3	24.17	1.05	4.53	70.5	7	24.22	1.15	4.95	64.6	11	24.08	0.86	4.92	65.0
4	0.00	0.00	4.40	72.7	8	0.00	0.00	4.53	70.5	12	0.00	0.00	5.30	60.5
4	0.35	1.89	4.40	72.7	8	0.25	3.05	4.53	70.5	12	0.25	1.25	5.30	60.5
4	0.60	4.60	4.40	72.7	8	0.52	3.05	4.53	70.5	12	0.50	3.96	5.30	60.5
4	1.07	8.60	4.40	72.7	8	0.98	7.31	4.53	70.5	12	1.00	7.82	5.30	60.5
4	2.13	8.38	4.40	72.7	8	2.02	7.56	4.53	70.5	12	2.00	9.72	5.30	60.5
4	3.50	7.54	4.40	72.7	8	3.53	6.59	4.53	70.5	12	3.52	9.75	5.30	60.5
4	5.02	6.88	4.40	72.7	8	5.05	5.88	4.53	70.5	12	5.07	8.57	5.30	60.5
4	7.02	5.78	4.40	72.7	8	7.15	4.73	4.53	70.5	12	7.07	6.59	5.30	60.5
4	9.02	5.33	4.40	72.7	8	9.07	4.57	4.53	70.5	12	9.03	6.11	5.30	60.5
4	11.98	4.19	4.40	72.7	8	12.10	3.00	4.53	70.5	12	12.05	4.57	5.30	60.5
4	24.65	1.15	4.40	72.7	8	24.12	1.25	4.53	70.5	12	24.15	1.17	5.30	60.5

TABLE 17.5.2: PROC NLMIXED procedure of SAS.

```
proc nlmixed data = theoph;
  parms beta1 = −3.22 beta2 = 0.47 beta3 = −2.45
  s2b1 = 0.03 cb12 = 0 s2b2 = 0.4 s2 = 0.5;
  cl = exp(beta1 + b1);
  ka = exp(beta2 + b2);
  ke = exp(beta3);
  pred = dose*ke*ka*(exp(-ke*time)-exp(-ka*time))/cl/
  (ka-ke);
  model conc ~ normal(pred,s2);
  random b1 b2 ~ normal([0,0],[s2b1,cb12,s2b2])
  subject = subject;
run;
```

setup of the model and dimensions indicates that there are 132 observations, 12 subjects, and 7 parameters.

PROC NLMIXED of SAS selects 5 quadrate points for each random effect, which produces a total grid of 25 points over which quadrate is performed. The PROC NLMIXED of SAS begins with a set of initial values (Table 17.5.4) and then provides iteration history (Table 17.5.5). Table 17.5.5 indicates that 10 iterations are required for the dual quasi-Newton algorithm to achieve convergence. The fitting information

TABLE 17.5.3: Summary of PROC NLMIXED of SAS.

NLMIXED Procedure	
Specifications	
Data set	WORK.THEOPH
Dependent variable	Conc
Distribution for dependent variable	Normal
Random effects	b1 b2
Distribution for random effects	Normal
Subject variable	Subject
Optimization technique	Dual quasi-Newton
Integration method	Adaptive Gaussian Quadrature
Dimensions	
Observations used	132
Observations not used	0
Total observations	132
Subjects	12
Maximum observations per subject	11
Parameter	7
Quadrature points	5

TABLE 17.5.4: Starting values of PROC NLMIXED of SAS.

Parameters							
beta1	beta2	beta3	s2b1	cb12	s2b2	s2	NegLogLike
−3.22	0.47	−2.45	0.03	0	0.4	0.5	177.789945

are summarized in Table 17.5.6, which lists the final optimized values of the log-likelihood function and two information criteria in two different forms. Table 17.5.7 contains the maximum likelihood estimates of the parameters. Both S2B1 and S2B2 are marginally significant, indicating between-subject variability in the clearances and absorption rate constants, respectively. Note that there does not appear to be a significant covariance between them, as seen by the estimate of CB12. The estimates of β_1, β_2, and β_3 are close to the adaptive quadrature estimates listed in Table 3 of Pinheiro and Bates (1995). However, Pinheiro and Bates (1995) used a Cholesky-root parameterization for the random-effect variance matrix and a logarithmic parameterization for the residual variance. The PROC NLMIXED of SAS, on the other hand, uses the parameterization as given in Table 17.5.8, which yields similar results.

17.6 Discussion

17.6.1 Study Protocol

A population PK study is either considered as an add-on to a clinical trial or a stand-alone study. It should be noted that the objectives of the add-on population PK study should not compromise the objectives of the primary clinical study. In practice,

TABLE 17.5.5: History of iterations.

Iteration History					
Iter	**Calls**	**NegLogLike**	**Diffraction**	**MaxGrad**	**Slope**
1	5	177.776248	0.013697	2.873367	−63.0744
2	8	177.7643	0.011948	1.698144	−4.75239
3	10	177.757264	0.007036	1.297439	−1.97311
4	12	177.755688	0.001576	1.441408	−0.49772
5	14	177.7467	0.008988	1.132279	−0.8223
6	17	177.746401	0.000299	0.831293	−0.00244
7	19	177.746318	0.000083	0.724198	−0.00789
8	21	177.74574	0.000578	0.180018	−0.00583
9	23	177.745736	3.88E-6	0.017958	−8.25E-6
10	25	177.745736	3.222E-8	0.000143	−6.51E-8

Note: GCONV convergence criterion satisfied.

TABLE 17.5.6: Fitting information.

Fit Statistics	
−2 Log likelihood	355.5
AIC (smaller is better)	369.5
BIC (smaller is better)	372.9
Log likelihood	−177.7
AIC (smaller is better)	−184.7
BIC (smaller is better)	−186.4

a stand-alone population PK study is more comprehensive. As indicated in the 1999 FDA guidance on population PK, a study design protocol should include (1) a clear statement of the objectives of the population PK analysis, (2) sampling design, (3) data collection procedures, (4) data checking procedures, (5) procedures for handling missing data, (6) specific PK parameters to be estimated, (7) covariates to be estimated, (8) model assumptions and model selection criteria, (9) sensitivity analysis and validation procedure (if planned), and (10) special user-friendly case report forms for PK evaluation.

17.6.2 Concerns and Challenges

In population modeling, statistical methods for assessment of means and variances of PK parameters for a patient population are well established based on sparse data collected under conditions of routine patient care. However, Nedelman (2005) indicated that there are the following potential concerns: (1) unobserved confounding variables may bias the statistical inferences, (2) conditions under which data are collected may lead to inaccuracies of reporting or recording, (3) correlations among important predictor variables may reduce statistical efficiency, and (4) costs cannot be controlled by principles of study design. To overcome these problems, Nedelman (2005) proposed a method for diagnosing the possible presence of confounding. In addition, Nedelman (2005) also proposed a model to capture the influences of data inaccuracies.

In practice, there are many issues/challenges when implementing a population PK as an add-on to clinical trial. These issues/challenges include, but are not limited to (1) the maintenance of blinding (2) data management or data merging in multicenter trials, (3) modifying inclusion/exclusion criteria without compromising primary objectives of the clinical trial, (4) complexity of PK procedures, and (5) monitoring PK aspects of study such as dosing history, demographics, sampling times, and sample processing and handling.

17.6.3 PK/PD

As indicated earlier, the key concept of a PK study is to study what the body does to the drug, while the key concept of a PD study is to study what the drug does to the

TABLE 17.5.7: Summary of parameter estimates.

Parameter Estimates

Parameter	Estimate	Standard Error	Degrees of Freedom	*t* Value	Pr > |*t*|	Alpha	Lower	Upper	Gradient
beta1	−3.2268	0.05950	10	−54.23	<.0001	0.05	−3.3594	−3.0942	−0.00009
beta2	0.4806	0.1989	10	2.42	0.0363	0.05	0.03745	0.9238	3.645E − 7
beta3	−2.4592	0.05126	10	−47.97	<.0001	0.05	−2.5734	−2.3449	0.000039
s2b1	0.02803	0.01221	10	2.30	0.0445	0.05	0.000833	0.05523	−0.00014
cb12	−0.00127	0.03404	10	−0.04	0.9710	0.05	−0.07712	0.07458	−0.00007
s2b2	0.4331	0.2005	10	2.16	0.0560	0.05	−0.01353	0.8798	−6.98E − 6
s2	0.5016	0.06837	10	7.34	<.0001	0.05	0.3493	0.6540	6.133E − 6

TABLE 17.5.8: Alternative parameterization in SAS.

```
proc nlmixed data = theoph;
   parms 111 = -1.5 12 = 0 113 = -0.1 beta1 = -3 beta2 = 0.5
   beta3 = -2.5
   ls2 = -0.7;
   s2 = exp(ls2);
   11 = exp(111)
   13 = exp(113);
   s2b1 = 11*11*s2;
   cb12 = 12*11*s2;
   s2b2 = (12*12 + 13*13)*s2;
   cl = exp(beta1 + b1);
   ka = exp(beta2 + b2);
   ke = exp(beta3);
   pred = dose*ke*ka*(exp(-ke*time)-exp(-ka*time)) /cl/ (ka-ke);
   model conc ~ normal (pred, s2);
   random b1 b2 ~ normal ([0, 0], [s2b1, cb12, s2b2]) subject = subject;
run;
```

body. Figure 17.6.1 illustrates the relationship between PK and PD and among dose, concentration and response. As a result, a PK/PD study is to study the relationship between dose and response, which provides insight information regarding (1) how best to choose doses at which to evaluate a drug, (2) how best to use a drug in a population, and (3) how best to use a drug to treat individual patients or subpopulations of patients. As it can be seen from Figure 17.6.1 that PK is to study the relationship between dose and concentration.

PK is only part of the full story. Population PK/PD study collects PK/PD data on same subjects. Suppose PD responses y_{ij}^* at times t_{ij}^*. Consider the plasma concentration C_{ij} taken at t_{ij}^*. Then, the intra-subject PD model could be described as follows:

$$y_{ij}^* = g(C_{ij}, a_i) + e_{ij}^*.$$

As a result, the intra-subject joint PK/PD model can be described as follows:

$$y_{ij} = f(x_{ij}, \beta_i) + e_{ij}, y_{ij}^* = g[f(x_{ij}^*, \beta_i)a_i] + e_{iju}^*,$$

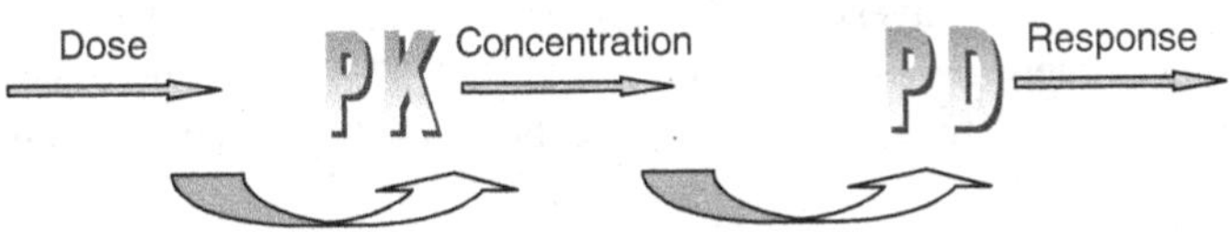

FIGURE 17.6.1: The relationship between PK and PD.

where

$$\beta_i = d(a_i, \beta, b_i), a_i = d^*(a_i, a, b_i^*),$$

and

$$(\beta_i', a_i') \sim H.$$

17.6.4 Computer Simulation

Due the complexity of a population PK study, it is suggested that a trial simulation be conducted to evaluate the performance of various designs for population PK studies for design selection. Trial simulation is a process that uses computers to mimic the conduct of a population PK study by creating virtual patients and extrapolating (or predicting) PK responses for each virtual patient based on pre-specified PK models. In practice, trial simulation of often considered to predict potential PK responses under different assumptions and various design scenarios at the planning stage of a population PK study for better planning (i.e., for achieving optimal accuracy and precision for estimation of population characteristics of the target patient population under study) of the actual study.

17.6.5 Software Application

For population PK studies, many software packages are available. Most of them were developed based on maximum likelihood approach. To name a few, these software packages include (1) NONMEN (Beal and Sheiner, 1982), which was the first software package developed for population PK/PD analyses, (2) NLME (Pinheiro and Bates, 2000), which is a generic function of S-Plus (Insightful, Seattle, Washington), (3) NLINMIX (Wolfinger, 1993) and PROC NLMIXED, which are a macro and a generic function of SAS (SAS Institute, Cary, North Carolina), and (4) WinNonlin or WinNonlinMix (Pharsight, Mountain View, California). These approaches also allow the evaluation of the influence of individual covariates on the parameters through the addition of fixed-effect parameters, or the incorporation of interoccasions variability, which quantifies the variability of the parameters of one individual during different occasions of sampling through the addition of random effects with variances to be estimated (Karlson and Sheiner, 1993). Softwares for analysis based on other approaches are also available. For example, NPLM (Mallet, 1986) is developed for nonparametric maximum likelihood approach. On the other hand, SAS macros for Bayesian EM algorithm (Racine-Poon and Smith, 1990) are also available. Edler (1998) provided a list of PK/PD software packages that were available up to 1998. This list included 72 software packages. This list, however, has not yet been updated.

Chapter 18

Other Pharmacokinetic Studies

18.1 Introduction

In addition to the assessment of bioequivalence (BE) in average bioavailability (BA) in terms of the pharmacokinetic (PK) responses, such as AUC and $C_{\max}$, it is also important to study the behaviors of those PK responses that may provide useful information for evaluation of drug efficacy and safety. For this purpose, some studies related to BA, such as drug interaction studies, dose proportionality studies, steady-state analyses, food-effect BA and fed BE studies, are often conducted to study the behavior of the plasma concentrations in terms of AUC and other PK responses.

In practice, it is not uncommon that more than one drug may be given to a patient at the same time. Therefore, it is important to examine the relative BA of the study drug when it is co-administered with food or other medications. For this purpose, a drug-to-drug interaction study is usually conducted to study the effect of other medications on the study drug and the effect of the study drug on other drugs. On the other hand, a food-effect BA study is usually conducted to assess the potential influence of the food on the rate and extent of absorption of the study drug when it is administrated right after a meal. A study of this kind can certainly provide valuable information on the efficacy or safety of the study drug which should be provided in the drug interactions, warnings and precautions, clinical pharmacology, and dosage and administration sections of the drug label.

When a new compound is discovered, it is important to determine an appropriate dose so that the drug can reach its maximum therapeutic effect with minimum toxicity. If there is a linear relation between AUC and dose, then an optimal dose level can be obtained to reach a desired blood AUC for therapeutic effect. Therefore, it is of interest to determine whether there exists a linear relationship between the PK measures of systemic exposure and the dose level through a dose proportionality (or linearity) study.

The objective of a steady-state analysis is to determine whether the plasma concentrations of the active ingredients of the study drug can reach and maintain at an almost constant level after multiple dosing. This analysis provides useful information for evaluation of drug safety.

In the following sections (Sections 18.2 through 18.5), more details on drug-to-drug interaction studies, dose proportionality studies, steady-state analyses, and food-effect BA, and fed BE studies are provided. A brief discussion is given in Section 18.6.

18.2 Drug Interaction Studies

In the pharmaceutical industry, when a new drug product is developed, it is often of interest to investigate the effect of concurrent usage of the drug with other medications on PK characteristics and therapeutic effects of both the new drug product and the other co-administered medications. As the population of most countries in the world is aging, the proportion of the patients treated by more than one drug is also increasing. For example, some asthma patients may also require medications for their hypertension; cancer or AIDS patients often need antibiotics to treat opportunistic infections. Therefore, can an asthma patient with treatment of a β-agonist also receive a β-blocker for his or her hypertension? On the other hand, because of the recent advance on biotechnology and genomics, knowledge of the mechanisms of drug-to-drug interactions at molecular level with their impact on the safety and efficacy of the patients becomes available. This information about the safety and efficacy obtained by the new technology should be provided in the appropriate section of the label of the approved drug product. As a result, recently, the U.S. FDA issued a draft guidance on *Drug Interaction Studies—Study Design, Data Analysis, and Implications for Dosing and Labeling* (FDA, 2006e).

18.2.1 Possible Mechanisms of Drug-to-Drug Interactions

There might be many different causes for drug-to-drug interactions, which may have an impact on the safety and efficacy of the study drug when it is co-administrated with other medications. One of the most important reasons for drug-to-drug interaction is metabolic routes of elimination through the cytochrome P450 family (CYP) of enzymes, which can be inhibited, activated, or induced by co-administered drug treatment. For co-administration of a new study drug and other medications, drug-to-drug interactions often occur due to the following reasons. First, the metabolism of the study drug can be significantly inhibited or induced by the co-administered medications. Second, the study drug itself can also inhibit or induce the metabolisms of the co-administered medications. As a result, these inhibition or induction can tremendously increase or decrease the blood concentrations of the study drug or the concomitant medications which ultimately alter the safety and efficacy profile of both the study drug and the concomitant medications. Another possible mechanism for drug-to-drug interactions is the transporter-based interactions which have been increasingly recognized. Examples are the interaction between digoxin and quinidine, fexofenadine and ketoxonazole or erythromycin, penicillin and probenecid. These interactions involve the protein-displacement or enzyme inhibition partially due to the inhibition of transport protein such as P-glycoprotein (P-gp) or organic anion transporter (OAT).

Consequently, the 2006 FDA draft guidance recommends that with proper *in vitro* probes and a careful selection of interaction drugs, the potential for drug-to-drug interaction can be investigated early in the development stage. These early studies can provide important information about dose, concentration, response relationships in the general population, specific populations, and individuals. The 2006 FDA draft guidance reflects FDA's current view on the requirements for documentation of the metabolism of the study drug and its interactions with other medications as a part of adequate assessment of its safety and effectiveness. Although the 2006 FDA draft guidance provides detailed description about the *in vitro* studies, we will focus on the design and data analysis of *in vivo* drug-to-drug interaction studies with PK endpoints as the primary endpoints.

18.2.2 General Considerations of *In Vivo* Drug Interaction Studies

Following the 2006 FDA draft guidance, the substrate (S) is defined as the drug studied to be determined whether its exposure is changed by another drug. On the other hand, an interacting drug (I) is the one that may change the exposure of other drugs. A new drug product can be either a substrate or an interacting drug. For the same reason, the approved drugs can also act as substrates or interacting drugs. As mentioned early, the new study drug may alter the metabolism of CYP450 enzymes, and hence change the concentrations of the approved drugs. In this situation, the new study drug is the interacting drug which acts as an inhibitor or inducer of CYP enzymes. The 2006 FDA draft guidance classified the inhibitors of CYP enzymes based on their *in vivo* fold-change in the plasma AUC of the substrate. A new study drug is a strong inhibitor of CYP enzymes if, given at the highest dose and shortest dosage interval, it can increase the plasma AUC of the sensitive CYP substrates by more than 5-fold or higher or more than 80% decrease in clearance of CYP substrates. A moderate inhibitor is the one for which the increase of the plasma AUC of the CYP substrate is at least 2-fold but no more than 5-fold. Furthermore, a weak inhibitor increases the plasma AUC of the CYP substrate by at least 1.25-fold but no more than 2-fold. An inducer is the one that decreases plasma AUC values of substrates for that CYP enzyme by 30% or higher. On the other hand, a new study drug could also be a substrate of CYP enzymes which can be inhibited or induced by other medications. In addition, a new study drug can also act as an inhibitor, inducer, or a substrate of P-gp transporter or other transporters.

As suggested by the 2006 FDA draft guidance, clinical drug-to-drug interaction studies are generally conducted in healthy volunteers or volunteers drawn from the general population based on the assumption that the results from this population can be extrapolated to the patient population for which the new study drug is intended. However, sometimes, the use of patients may offer advantages for studying the safety and pharmacodynamic (PD) endpoints. However, the extent of drug interactions may be different due to subjects' genotype for the specific enzymes being evaluated. In addition, it is well known that CYP2D6, CYP2C19, and CYP2C9 are the known valid biomarkers. It is, therefore, very important to have diagnostic devices with good performance of phenotype or genotype determinations to identify the study subjects with genetically determined metabolic polymorphisms.

With respect to the 2006 FDA draft guidance recommends that the following measures of parameters of substrate PK be obtained in every *in vivo* drug interaction studies:

1. Exposure measures such as AUC, $C_{\max}$, $T_{\max}$, and others as appropriate; and
2. PK parameters such as clearance, volumes of distribution, and half-lives.

18.2.3 Designs of *In Vivo* Drug Interaction Studies

Table 18.2.1 presents the design for *in vivo* drug-to-drug interaction studies recommended by the 2006 FDA draft guidance. The dose regimen combinations of a substrate and interacting drug suggested by the 2006 FDA draft guidance is given in Table 18.2.2. In both Tables 18.2.1 and 18.2.2, the new study drug can be the substrate or interacting drug and the other medication can also serve as a substrate or an interacting drug. The first design at the one-sequence crossover design in which the substrate is always administered in the first period and both of the substrate and interacting drug are co-administered in the second period. Strictly speaking, one-sequence crossover design is not a good design for the unbiased statistical inference about the fold-change with respect to the plasma AUC as compared to the two-sequence and two-period crossover design. The 2006 FDA draft guidance provides an example for both the substrate and interacting drug given chronically over an extended period of time. In the first period, the substrate is administrated to the steady state with collection of blood samples over one or more dosing intervals. During the second period, both the substrate and interacting drug are co-administered in a multiple-dose manner with collection of blood samples for measurements of both the substrate and interacting drug. This is not only an example of one-sequence crossover design but also an illustration of dosing regimen of multiple doses for both the substrate and interacting drug. From the above description, there is no washout period between the two treatment periods in the one-sequence crossover design. The objectives of the first period are to let the substrate to reach its steady state and to collect the blood samples at the steady state. Once the substrate reaches the steady state, the multiple doses of the interaction drug are immediately co-administered with collecting blood samples of the substrate and interacting drug. Therefore, for one-sequence crossover design, attainment of steady state is very important. On the other hand, when either the substrate or interacting drug and their metabolites have long half-lives, then the two-group parallel design may be a better choice than the traditional two-sequence and two-period crossover design.

If both the substrate and interacting drug do not have long half-lives and are given in a single-dose fashion, then the traditional two-sequence, two-period crossover design with a washout period with sufficient length is an appropriate design to investigate the impact of the interacting drug on the fold-change in the plasma

TABLE 18.2.1: Designs for *in vivo* drug interaction studies.

Design C1: One-Sequence Crossover Design

	Period	
Sequence	**I**	**II**
1	S	S + I

Design C2: Two-Group Parallel Design

Group	**Treatment**
1	S
2	S + I

Design C3: Two-Sequence and Two-Period Crossover Design

	Period	
Sequence	**I**	**II**
1	S	S + I
2	S + I	S

Design C4: Williams Design

		Period	
Sequence	**I**	**II**	**III**
1	I	S	I + S
2	I + S	I	S
3	S	I + S	I
4	I + S	S	I
5	S	I	I + S
6	I	I + S	S

Note: S = Substrate; I = Interacting drug.

AUC of the substrate because it can not only provide an unbiased statistical inference but also can reduce the variability of the estimated fold-change. If the objective of the study is to investigate the impact of the new study drug on the other approved drug, then the new study drug is the interacting drug and the other approved drug is the substrate. On the other hand, if the objective of the study is to assess the influence of

TABLE 18.2.2: Dosing regimen combinations.

Substrate	**Interacting Drug**
Single dose	Single dose
Single does	Multiple dose
Multiple doses	Single doses
Multiple doses	Multiple doses

an approved drug on the new study drug, then the approved drug is the interacting drug and the new study drug is the substrate.

However, Designs C1, C2, and C3 can only be employed to investigate the effect of the interacting drug on the fold-change of the plasma AUC of the substrate. Therefore, the primary endpoints for these three designs are the exposure measures and PK parameters associated with the substrate. If the drug interaction effects are to be assessed for both the substrate and interacting drug and PK characteristics of both agents make it feasible, then dual assessment can be done in a single study. One of possible designs for the dual assessment is the Williams design given in Table 18.2.1. Under Design C4, basically, there are three treatments to be compared; namely, I (interacting drug), S (substrate), and I + S (co-administration of I and S). The comparisons of primary interest are I versus I + S (the effect of S on I) and S versus I + S (the effect of I on S). In addition, it can be seen that the assessment of the effect of S on I is based on the data from periods where I and I + S are administered. Similarly, the assessment of the effect of I on S is based on the data from periods where S and I + S are administered.

18.2.4 Evaluation of Drug Interaction

As mentioned above, the primary objective of a drug-to-drug interaction study is to investigate whether co-administration of the substrate and an interacting drug can change the magnitude of exposure measures such as the AUC and $C_{\max}$ or other PK parameters of the substrate when it is administered alone. Furthermore, when the interacting drug inhibits or induces the activities of CYP enzymes, and depends upon the magnitude of the fold-change, the 2006 FDA draft guidance classified the interacting drug as strong, moderate, weak inhibitor, no interaction, or inducer. Then the corresponding statistical hypotheses can be formulated with specific limits. Let $\mu_S = \mu + F_S$ and $\mu_{IS} = \mu + F_{IS}$ are the population treatment means for the log-transformed exposure measure of S and I + S, respectively. The parameter of interest on the log-scale is $\theta_S = \mu_{IS} - \mu_S = F_{IS} - F_S$. Therefore, on the original scale, the parameter of interest is

$$\delta_S = \exp(\mu_{IS} - \mu_S) = \frac{\widetilde{\mu}_{IS}}{\widetilde{\mu}_S}.$$

It follows that the hypotheses for the interacting drug being a strong inhibitor is given as below:

$$\begin{aligned} &\mathrm{H_{U50}}\colon\ \delta_S \le 5 \\ \text{versus}\quad &\mathrm{H_{U5a}}\colon\ \delta_S > 5, \end{aligned}$$

or equivalently on the log-scale

$$\begin{aligned} &\mathrm{H_{U50}}\colon\ \theta_S \le 1.6094 \\ \text{versus}\quad &\mathrm{H_{U5a}}\colon\ \theta_S > 1.6094. \end{aligned} \tag{18.2.1}$$

On the other hand, the hypotheses for the interacting drug being an inducer can be formulated as

$$\begin{aligned} &H_{U10}\colon\ \delta_S \geq 0.70 \\ \text{versus}\quad &H_{U1a}\colon\ \delta_S < 0.7, \end{aligned}$$

or equivalently on the log-scale

$$\begin{aligned} &H_{U10}\colon\ \theta_S \leq -0.3567 \\ \text{versus}\quad &H_{U1a}\colon\ \theta_S > -0.3567. \end{aligned} \tag{18.2.2}$$

For the other types of inhibitor, the hypotheses can be formulated as the two-sided equivalence hypotheses as follows:

$$\begin{aligned} &H_{i0}\colon\ \delta_S \leq \delta_{iL} \text{ or } \delta_S \geq \delta_{iU} \\ \text{versus}\quad &H_{ia}\colon\ \delta_{iL} < \delta_S < \delta_{iU}, \end{aligned} \tag{18.2.3}$$

where $i = 2, 3, 4$ correspond to no interaction, weak, and moderate inhibitor, respectively.

Table 18.2.3 provides the lower and upper limits for each of the above hypotheses of inducer, no interaction, weak, moderate, and strong inhibitor. The equivalence limits of 0.8 and 1.25 are referred to as the default no effect boundaries when the no effect boundaries can be defined from population average dose or concentration–dose relationship or pharmacokinetic/pharmacodynamic (PK/PD) models.

Let $\widehat{\theta}_S$ be the best linear unbiased estimator of θ_S obtained under a particular design in Table 18.2.1 and S_{θ_F} be its corresponding standard error with ν degrees of freedom. Then, a $100(1-2\alpha)\%$ confidence interval for θ is given by

$$(L, U) = \widehat{\theta}_S \pm S_{\theta_F}\, t(\alpha, \nu) \tag{18.2.4}$$

where $t(\alpha, \nu)$ is the α upper quantile of a central t distribution with ν degrees of freedom.

Co-administration of the substrate and the interacting drug can be concluded to have no drug interaction at the α significance level if the corresponding $100\,(1-2\alpha)\%$ confidence interval for θ_S is completely contained within the no

TABLE 18.2.3: Equivalence limits for drug interaction studies.

	Equivalence Limits			
	Lower		**Upper**	
Interaction	**Original**	**Logarithmic**	**Original**	**Logarithmic**
Inducer	—	—	0.7	−0.3567
No interaction	0.80	−0.2231	1.25	0.2231
Weak	1.25	0.2231	2	0.6931
Moderate	2	0.6931	5	1.6094
Strong	5	1.6094	—	—

effect boundaries or (−0.2231, 0.2231). On the other hand, an interacting drug is concluded as an inducer for the substrate drug at the α significance level if the upper limit of the $(1-2\alpha)\times 100\%$ confidence interval for θ_S is less than −0.3567. In addition, one can claim an interacting drug is a strong inhibitor for the substrate drug if the lower limit of the $(1-2\alpha)\times 100\%$ confidence interval for θ_S is greater than 1.6094. For other types of inhibitors, the traditional confidence interval approach for equivalence is adopted here too. In other words, an interacting drug is concluded either a moderate (or weak) inhibitor at the α significance level if the corresponding $(1-2\alpha)\times 100\%$ confidence interval for θ_S is completely contained within the equivalence limits for the moderate (or weak) inhibitor.

In some cases, the information on the PK properties of the study drug may be available when it is administered alone. However, its characteristics in presence of other drugs may not be known. Therefore, in drug interaction studies, it is important not only that a sufficient length of washout must be given, but also that the presence of the carryover effect be examined. Although, in practice, the standard two-sequence, two-period crossover design is commonly used in a drug interaction study because of its simplicity, it is recommended that an optimal crossover design for comparing two treatments as discussed in Chapters 2 and 9 are used because it provides the best linear unbiased estimates for both treatment and carryover effects.

In addition to evaluation of the existence of change or difference in PK responses between substrate S and co-administration of I + S, it is also important to examine the change in intra-subject variability of the substrate S in the presence of the interacting drug I. This can be examined by testing the following hypotheses:

$$\begin{aligned} &\text{H}_0\colon\ \sigma_S^2 = \sigma_{IS}^2 \\ \text{versus}\quad &\text{H}_a\colon\ \sigma_S^2 \neq \sigma_{IS}^2. \end{aligned} \tag{18.2.5}$$

For a standard two-sequence, two-period crossover design, Pitman–Morgan's test for equality of intra-subject variability, given in Equation 7.4.9 or 7.4.11, can be used. For an optimal design comparing two treatments, since the design provides independent, unbiased estimates of $\widehat{\sigma}_S^2$ and $\widehat{\sigma}_{IS}^2$, the test statistic given in Equation 9.3.26 can be directly applied by simply replacing $\widehat{\sigma}_1^2$ and $\widehat{\sigma}_2^2$ with

$$\begin{aligned} \widehat{\sigma}_1^2 &= \max\left(\widehat{\sigma}_S^2, \widehat{\sigma}_{IS}^2\right), \\ \widehat{\sigma}_2^2 &= \min\left(\widehat{\sigma}_S^2, \widehat{\sigma}_{IS}^2\right), \end{aligned}$$

and the corresponding degrees of freedom with ν_1 and ν_2, respectively.

18.2.5 Joint Assessment of Interaction

As indicated in the 2006 FDA draft guidance, if the drug interactions are to be evaluated for both substrate and interacting drug in a combination regimen, the evaluation can be performed in two separate trials. However, if the PK characteristics of the agents make it feasible, the dual assessment can be done in a single study. In this case, basically, there are three treatments to be compared: namely, I (interacting drug), S (substrate), and I + S (co-administration of I and S). The comparisons

TABLE 18.2.4: Expected values of sequence-by-period means for comparing I and I + S.

	Period		
Sequence	I	II	III
1	$\mu+G_1+P_1+F_I$	—	$\mu+G_1+P_3+F_{IS}$
2	$\mu+G_2+P_1+F_{IS}$	$\mu+G_2+P_2+F_I+C_{IS}$	—
3	—	$\mu+G_3+P_2+F_{IS}$	$\mu+G_3+P_3+F_I+C_{IS}$
4	$\mu+G_4+P_1+F_{IS}$	—	$\mu+G_4+P_3+F_I$
5	—	$\mu+G_5+P_2+F_I$	$\mu+G_5+P_3+F_{IS}+C_I$
6	$\mu+G_6+P_1+F_I$	$\mu+G_6+P_2+F_{IS}+C_I$	—

of primary interest are S versus I + S (the effect of I on S) and I versus I + S (the effect of S on I). In this section, we discuss statistical methods for assessment of the effect of I on S and that of S on I using the Williams design for comparing three treatments. Design C4 in Table 18.2.1 is the Williams design for drug interaction study. It can be seen that the assessment of the effect of S on I is based on the data from periods where I and I + S are administered. Similarly, the assessment of the effect of I on S is based on the data from periods where S and I + S are administered.

Table 18.2.4 provides the expected values of sequence by period means. The analysis of variance table in terms of degrees of freedom is given in Table 18.2.5. The expected values of period differences are given in Table 18.2.6. Let θ_I be the treatment effect between I + S and I (or the effect of S on I). Then,

$$\theta_I = F_{IS} - F_I \qquad (18.2.6)$$

An unbiased estimate of θ_I can also be expressed as a linear contrast of sequence-by-period means; for example,

$$\widehat{\theta}_I = \tfrac{1}{2}[(\overline{Y}_{\cdot 31} - \overline{Y}_{\cdot 11}) + (\overline{Y}_{\cdot 14} - \overline{Y}_{\cdot 34})],$$

TABLE 18.2.5: Analysis of variance table for the Williams design for drug interaction study.

Source of Variation	Degrees of Freedom
Inter-subject	$N^a - 1$
Sequence	5
Residual	$N-6$
Intra-subject	N
Period	2
Formulation	1
Carryover	1
Residual	$N-4$
Total	$2N-1$

[a] $N=\Sigma_k n_k$.

TABLE 18.2.6: Expected values of period differences for comparison between I and I + S.

Sequence	Period Differences	Expected Value	$\Sigma_k C_{jk}^2$
1	$\frac{1}{2}(\overline{Y}_{\cdot 31} - \overline{Y}_{\cdot 11})$	$\frac{1}{2}[(F_{IS} - F_I) + (P_3 - P_1)]$	$\frac{1}{2}$
2	$\frac{1}{2}(\overline{Y}_{\cdot 12} - \overline{Y}_{\cdot 22})$	$\frac{1}{2}[(F_{IS} - F_I) + (P_1 - P_2) - C_{IS}]$	$\frac{1}{2}$
3	$\frac{1}{2}(\overline{Y}_{\cdot 33} - \overline{Y}_{\cdot 23})$	$\frac{1}{2}[(F_I - F_{IS}) + (P_3 - P_2) + C_{IS}]$	$\frac{1}{2}$
4	$\frac{1}{2}(\overline{Y}_{\cdot 14} - \overline{Y}_{\cdot 34})$	$\frac{1}{2}[(F_{IS} - F_I) + (P_1 - P_3)]$	$\frac{1}{2}$
5	$\frac{1}{2}(\overline{Y}_{\cdot 25} - \overline{Y}_{\cdot 35})$	$\frac{1}{2}[(F_I - F_{IS}) + (P_2 - P_3) - C_I]$	$\frac{1}{2}$
6	$\frac{1}{2}(\overline{Y}_{\cdot 26} - \overline{Y}_{\cdot 16})$	$\frac{1}{2}[(F_{IS} - F_I) + (P_2 - P_1) + C_I]$	$\frac{1}{2}$

which is the sum of period differences from sequences 1 and 4. The variance of $\widehat{\theta}_I$ is given by

$$\text{Var}(\widehat{\theta}_I) = \frac{1}{n}\sigma_e^2, \tag{18.2.7}$$

where σ_e^2 can be estimated unbiasedly by the intra-subject mean-squared error from the analysis of variance table with $N-4$ degrees of freedom. Therefore, the treatment effect θ_I can be assessed using either the confidence interval Equation 18.2.4 or hypothesis testing procedures described above for θ_S.

For the comparison of S and S + I, Tables 18.2.7 and 18.2.8 summarize the excepted values of sequence-by-period means and the expected values of period differences for each sequence. In a similar manner, a statistical test for the effect of I on S, denoted by θ_S, can also be obtained.

Note that the design and analysis for drug interaction studies discussed in this section can also be directly applied to bioavailability/bioequivalence (BA/BE) studies for a fixed-dose combination drug (Yeh and Chiang, 1991) because I and S represent two drugs and I + S is their combination.

TABLE 18.2.7: Expected values of sequence-by-period means for comparing S and I + S.

	Period		
Sequence	I	II	III
1	—	$\mu + G_1 + P_2 + F_S$	$\mu + G_1 + P_3 + F_{IS} + C_S$
2	$\mu + G_2 + P_1 + F_{IS}$	—	$\mu + G_2 + P_3 + F_S$
3	$\mu + G_3 + P_1 + F_S$	$\mu + G_3 + P_2 + F_{IS} + C_S$	—
4	$\mu + G_4 + P_1 + F_{IS}$	$\mu + G_4 + P_2 + F_S + C_{IS}$	—
5	$\mu + G_5 + P_1 + F_S$	—	$\mu + G_5 + P_3 + F_{IS}$
6	—	$\mu + G_6 + P_2 + F_{IS}$	$\mu + G_6 + P_3 + F_S + C_{IS}$

TABLE 18.2.8: Expected values of period differences for comparison between S and I + S.

Sequence	Period Differences	Expected Value	$\Sigma_k C_{jk}^2$
1	$\frac{1}{2}(\bar{Y}_{\cdot 31} - \bar{Y}_{\cdot 21})$	$\frac{1}{2}[(F_{IS} - F_S) + (P_3 - P_2) + C_S]$	$\frac{1}{2}$
2	$\frac{1}{2}(\bar{Y}_{\cdot 12} - \bar{Y}_{\cdot 32})$	$\frac{1}{2}[(F_{IS} - F_S) + (P_1 - P_3)]$	$\frac{1}{2}$
3	$\frac{1}{2}(\bar{Y}_{\cdot 13} - \bar{Y}_{\cdot 23})$	$\frac{1}{2}[(F_S - F_{IS}) + (P_1 - P_2) - C_S]$	$\frac{1}{2}$
4	$\frac{1}{2}(\bar{Y}_{\cdot 24} - \bar{Y}_{\cdot 14})$	$\frac{1}{2}[(F_S - F_{IS}) + (P_2 - P_1) + C_{IS}]$	$\frac{1}{2}$
5	$\frac{1}{2}(\bar{Y}_{\cdot 35} - \bar{Y}_{\cdot 15})$	$\frac{1}{2}[(F_{IS} - F_S) + (P_3 - P_1)]$	$\frac{1}{2}$
6	$\frac{1}{2}(\bar{Y}_{\cdot 26} - \bar{Y}_{\cdot 36})$	$\frac{1}{2}[(F_{IS} - F_S) + (P_2 - P_3) - C_{IS}]$	$\frac{1}{2}$

18.3 Dose Proportionality Study

How to characterize the PK profile of an active (or potentially active) compound is always of interest to researcher. The dose relation of a therapeutic compound is important in studying the PK effect of dose range within a given dose range. For this purpose, a crossover experiment at several predetermined dose levels is usually conducted with some healthy human subjects. Each dosing period is preceded by a fasting period and followed by a washout period. Blood samples are collected before dosing and at various time points after dosing. On the basis of these collected blood samples, the relation between the PK parameters, such as AUC or $C_{\max}$, and the dose levels is then evaluated within the dose range tested.

Frequently, it is of particular interest to determine whether the relation between the PK parameters and dose levels is linear (or log linear). If the relation is linear, the rate of change in PK effect over a given dose range is a constant. Here, the PK effect of a dose change can be easily predicted, and the dose can be adjusted accordingly to achieve the desired magnitude of effect. In the following, we will characterize the dose proportionality and introduce the classic methods, the confidence interval criteria for assessment of dose linearity.

18.3.1 Dose Linearity Model

Let Y be AUC or $C_{\max}$ and X be the dose level. Because, often, the standard deviation of Y increases as the dose increases, the primary assumption of dose proportionality is that the standard deviation of Y is proportional to X; that is,

$$\text{Var}(Y) = X^2\sigma^2,$$

where σ^2 usually consists of inter- and intra-subject variability. Under this assumption, the following models are usually considered to evaluate the relation between the response Y and the dose X.

$$\text{Model 1: } E(Y) = \beta X.$$

$$\text{Model 2: } E(Y) = \alpha + \beta X \quad \text{where } \alpha \neq 0.$$

$$\text{Model 3: } E(Y) = \alpha \cdot X^{\beta} \quad \text{where } \alpha > 0 \text{ and } \beta \neq 0.$$

$$\text{Model 4: } E(Y) = \alpha + \lambda X^{\beta} \quad \text{where } \alpha \neq 0 \text{ and/or } \beta \neq 1.$$

Model 1 indicates that the relation between AUC and the dose is linear. The dose–response curve is a straight line, which goes through the origin. This indicates that a double dose will result in a double AUC. Model 1 is usually referred to as dose proportionality. It can be seen that model 1 can be used to evaluate dose proportionality by testing the following hypotheses:

$$\begin{aligned} &\text{H}_{01}\colon\ \beta = 0 \\ \text{versus}\quad &\text{H}_{a1}\colon\ \beta \neq 0. \end{aligned}$$

This can be done using a weighted linear regression with weights equal to X^{-1} based on the original data (X, Y). It also can be tested examining the 95% confidence interval for the slope β. Note that failure to reject H_{01} may indicate that the AUC is independent of the dose level.

Model 2 indicates that the relation between AUC and the dose is a straight line with nonzero intercept, α. Again, it can be tested using a weighted linear regression with weights equal to X^{-1} and with the original data (X, Y). The hypotheses of primary interest are given as

$$\begin{aligned} &\text{H}_{02}\colon\ \alpha = 0 \\ \text{versus}\quad &\text{H}_{a2}\colon\ \alpha \neq 0. \end{aligned}$$

Similarly, model 2 can also be evaluated by examining the 95% confidence interval for the intercept α.

Model 3 can be equivalently expressed in terms of the following logarithmic form:

$$\text{Log}(E(Y)) = \log(\alpha) + \beta \log X.$$

Therefore, similar to model 2, model 3 can be tested using a weighted linear regression with log-transformed data ($\log X$, $\log Y$). The hypotheses of primary interest are

$$\begin{aligned} &\mathrm{H}_{03}\colon\ \beta = 0 \\ \text{versus}\quad &\mathrm{H}_{a3}\colon\ \beta \neq 0. \end{aligned}$$

Again, it can be tested indirectly by examining the 95% confidence interval for the exponent β.

Model 4 is, in fact, the combination of models 2 and 3 and requires nonlinear-weighted regression techniques to evaluate. This can be done using PROC GLM of SAS.

Let $X_1 < X_2 < \cdots < X_k$ be the k dose levels and Y_i, $i = 1, \ldots, k$, be the corresponding responses. Under the assumption of $\mathrm{Var}(Y) = X^2\sigma^2$, the ratio Y_i/X_i is approximately equal to the slope β for all doses. Usually the ratio Y_i/X_i is commonly used as normalized responses. Draper and Smith (1981), however, indicated that the average of these ratios

$$\widehat{R} = \frac{1}{k}\sum_{i=1}^{k}\frac{Y_i}{X_i} \tag{18.3.1}$$

is the best-weighted linear estimate of β. Therefore, the ratio $Y_i/\widehat{R}$ is sometimes considered as the normalized responses of Y_i. Note that, under models 1 and 2 (linear), the normalized response should be approximately equal to the dose X_i. Moreover, the linear regression of the normalized response versus X_i should result approximately in a straight line through the origin with slope equal to 1. This, however, is not true for models 3 and 4 (nonlinear). Linear regression of the normalized responses X_i will result in a straight line with slope not necessarily equal to 1. It is then of interest to measure the departure from dose linearity under models 3 and 4 when the model is incorrectly assumed to be linear (i.e., models 1 or 2).

18.3.2 Departure from Dose Linearity

In this section, we compare the relation between model 2 (linear) and model 3 (nonlinear) and the effects of curvature and normalization. Suppose model 3 is the true model for the data. Then there is a relation between estimates obtained assuming model 3 and estimates obtained assuming (incorrectly) model 2. This relation can be examined in terms of the difference between $Y = \alpha X^\beta$ and a least squares linear approximation (Smith, 1986), which is given by

$$Y_l \approx \alpha_l + \beta_l X,$$

where

$$\alpha_l = \frac{2(1-\beta)}{(\beta+1)(\beta+2)}\alpha \quad \text{and} \quad \beta_l = \frac{6\beta}{(\beta+1)(\beta+2)}\alpha. \tag{18.3.2}$$

From Equation 18.3.2, we note that $\alpha_l < 0$ if, and only if, $\beta > 1$. If model 2 is assumed to be the true model and a weighted linear regression is fitted to the data, what results is the following estimated regression equation:

$$Y = a + bX,$$

then we have

$$E(a) \gg \alpha_l \quad \text{and} \quad E(b) = \beta_l.$$

This indicates that the estimated regression equation is an estimator of the linearized form of true response. We would expect a negative (positive) intercept if the data is convex (concave). To measure the degree of curvature, we first normalize the domain of X so that $X = 1$ corresponds to the highest dose under study. Therefore, the ratio of Y and Y_l at $X = 1$ compares the true response to its linearized response, which is given as

$$\kappa = Y/Y_l = \frac{(\beta + 1)(\beta + 2)}{4\beta + 2}. \tag{18.3.3}$$

From Equation 18.3.3, it can be seen that κ ranges from 0.98 to 1.05 for $\beta \in (0.75, 1.25)$. Therefore, the true response is within 5% of the linearized response at the highest dose. This indicates that a lack of dose linearity with β within (0.75, 1.25) has little practical significance.

For the normalized response, under model 3, if we assumed that $X = 1$ corresponds to the highest dose, then $\widehat{R}$ in Equation 18.3.1 is an estimator of the following parameter:

$$\sum_{i=1}^{k} \frac{1}{k} \frac{Y_i}{X_i} = \sum_{i=1}^{k} \frac{1}{k} \frac{\alpha \cdot X_i^{\beta}}{X_i} = \int_0^1 \alpha \cdot x^{\beta - 1}\, \mathrm{d}x = \frac{\alpha}{\beta}$$

Therefore, the normalized dose response is

$$Y_n = \frac{Y}{(\alpha/\beta)} = \beta \cdot X^{\beta}$$

Hence, the normalized linearized response is given by

$$Y_{\text{nl}} = \frac{Y_l}{(\alpha/\beta)} = \frac{2\beta(1-\beta)}{(\beta + 1)(\beta + 2)} + \frac{6\beta^2}{(\beta + 1)(\beta + 2)} X.$$

Thus, the normalized response Y_{nl} can also given some indication of departures from dose linearity because

$$\frac{Y_{\text{n}}}{Y_{\text{nl}}} = \frac{(\beta + 1)(\beta + 2)}{4\beta + 2} = \kappa.$$

From these results, Smith (1986) proposed some decision criteria using the 95% confidence interval of the slope to determine the departure from dose linearity. If the confidence interval (L, U) satisfies

$$0.75 < L < 1 < U < 1.25,$$

then we conclude that there is no departure from dose linearity. If the confidence interval satisfy

1. $1 < L < U < 1.25$, and
2. $0.75 < L < U < 1.0$.

then we conclude that there is a slight departure but no practical significance from dose linearity. Finally, if $L > 1.25$ or $U < 0.75$, then reject the hypothesis of dose linearity.

Note that the departure from dose linearity can also be examined by a lack of fit test through stepwise polynomial regression (Draper and Smith, 1981), which will not be further discussed here. However, it is recommended that the mean response versus dose level be plotted before an appropriate model is chosen for analysis.

18.3.3 Traditional Evaluation of Dose Proportionality

In the interest of balance for carryover effects, a dose proportionality study is usually conducted with a Latin squares or a balanced incomplete block design. Let Y_{ijk} be the responses for the ith subject at the jth dose from a $K \times K$ Latin squares with n_k subjects in each sequence. Then, under the assumption that the standard deviation of the response is proportional to the dose, dose proportionality can be assessed using the following statistical models based on the normalized responses:

$$\text{Model 1: } \frac{Y_{ijk}}{X_j} = G_k S_{ik} X_j^{\beta_j} C_{(j-1,k)} P_{(j,k)} e_{ijk};$$

$$\text{Model 2: } \frac{Y_{ijk}}{X_j} = G_k + S_{ik} + \beta_j X_j + C_{(j-1,k)} + P_{(j,k)} + e_{ijk},$$

where

G_k is the fixed effect of the kth sequences
S_{ik}, $C_{(j-1,k)}$, $P_{(j,k)}$, and e_{ijk} are as defined in Equation 4.2
$i = 1, 2, \ldots, n_k$
$j = 1, 2, \ldots, K$
$k = 1, 2, \ldots, K$

It is assumed that $\{S_{ik}\}$ are i.i.d. with mean 0 and variance σ_S^2 and $\{e_{ij}\}$ are independently identically distributed with mean 0 and variance σ_e^2. $\{S_{ik}\}$ and $\{e_{ijk}\}$ are mutually independent. The analysis of variance table in terms of degrees of freedom for a Latin squares is given in Table 18.3.1.

TABLE 18.3.1: Analysis of variance table for the $K \times K$ Latin squares.

Source of Variation	Degrees of Freedom
Inter-subject	$N-1$
Sequence	$K-1$
Residual	$N-K$
Intra-subject	$(K-1)N$
Period	$K-1$
Carryover	$K-1$
Dose	$K-1$
Linear	1
Quadratic	1
Cubic	1
⋮	⋮
Residual	$(K-1)(N-3)$
Total	$KN-1$

Note that a long-transformation on model 1 (multiplicative) leads to model 2 (additive). For model 2, the variance of Y_{ijk} is given by

$$\mathrm{Var}(Y_{ijk}) = X_j^2\left(\sigma_S^2 + \sigma_e^2\right).$$

Therefore, the assumption that the standard deviation of Y_{ijk} is proportional to X_j is met.

Under either model 1 or model 2, we first test whether the model is adequate before the assessment of dose proportionality. This can be done by testing the following hypotheses:

$$\begin{aligned} &\mathrm{H_0}\colon\ \beta_j = \beta \quad \text{for all } j \\ \text{versus}\quad &\mathrm{H_a}\colon\ \beta_j \neq \beta \quad \text{for at least one } j. \end{aligned} \tag{18.3.4}$$

We then conclude that the model is adequate if we fail to reject the null hypothesis. Here, dose proportionality can be assessed by testing the following hypotheses:

$$\begin{aligned} &\mathrm{H_0}\colon\ \beta = 0 \\ \text{versus}\quad &\mathrm{H_a}\colon\ \beta \neq 0. \end{aligned} \tag{18.3.5}$$

A dose proportionality relation between Y and X is concluded if we fail to reject the null hypothesis.

For assessment of dose linearity, the following models based on the original data may be useful:

$$\text{Model 3: } Y_{ijk} = G_k S_{ik} X_j^{\beta j} C_{(j-1,k)} P_{(j,k)} e_{ijk};$$

$$\text{Model 4: } Y_{ijk} = G_k + S_{ik} + \beta_j X_j + C_{(j-1,k)} + P_{(j,k)} + e_{ijk}.$$

In a similar manner, we first test whether the model is adequate. If the model is adequate, then test hypothesis 18.3.5 for dose linearity.

Note that tests for hypotheses 18.3.4 and 18.3.5 under each of models 1 through 4 can be easily performed using PROC GLM of SAS.

18.3.4 Confidence Interval Approach to Assessment of Dose Proportionality

The dose proportionality is proved by the traditional evaluation when we fail to reject both null hypotheses in Equations 18.3.4 and 18.3.5 as described in Section 18.3.3. However, from a statistical viewpoint, the null hypothesis can never be proven (Colton, 1974). Hence, the objective of the hypotheses in Equations 18.3.4 and 18.3.5 is to prove that the PK profile of the active ingredient for a drug product does not exhibit dose proportionality. Therefore, based on the concept of average BE, Smith et al. (2000) proposed to use the confidence interval approach to evaluation of dose proportionality. They considered the simple regression model, the power model (regression of log-transformation data), and the saturated elimination model (quadratic regression model with no intercept). For simplicity, the power model is elected to illustrate the concept and the method.

The power model considered in Smith et al. (2000) is in fact model 3 introduced in Section 18.3.1. One of the key assumptions of the power model is that the logarithm of the average exposure measure is linearly related to the logarithm of dose. In other words

$$\mu_j = \log(\alpha) + \beta \log(X_j), \quad j = 1, \ldots, K, \tag{18.3.6}$$

where μ_j is the average exposure measure on log-scale.

Let r be the ratio of the highest dose to the lowest dose in the study. Under model 18.3.6, the predicted average exposure measures at the highest dose and lowest dose are $e^{\alpha}X_K^{\beta}$ and $e^{\alpha}X_1^{\beta}$, respectively. Therefore the dose proportionality implies that

$$\begin{aligned} \frac{e^{\alpha}X_K^{\beta}}{e^{\alpha}X_1^{\beta}} &= \frac{X_K}{X_1} = r, \quad \text{and} \\ \left(\frac{X_K}{X_1}\right)^{\beta-1} &= r^{\beta-1} = 1. \end{aligned} \tag{18.3.7}$$

It follows that the parameter of interest is $r^{\beta-1}$ which is referred to as the ratio of dose-normalized geometric means, R_{dnm}, by Smith et al. (2000). The dose proportionality is defined if $r^{\beta-1}$ is within some predefined acceptable limits (θ_L, θ_U). Since

R_{dnm} is a function of the slope, therefore, evaluation of dose proportionality can then be performed through β with the following upper and lower equivalence limits:

$$\theta'_{\text{L}} = 1 + \frac{\log(\theta_{\text{L}})}{\log(r)}, \quad \text{and} \qquad \theta'_{\text{U}} = 1 + \frac{\log(\theta_{\text{U}})}{\log(r)}. \tag{18.3.8}$$

Consequently, the dose proportionality of a certain exposure measure of the active ingredient for a given drug product can be concluded at the α significance level if the $100(1-2\alpha)\%$ confidence interval for β is completely contained within $(\theta'_{\text{L}}, \theta'_{\text{U}})$. One of the advantages offered by the confidence interval approach is that only the ratio of the highest dose to the lowest dose, not the actual doses, is required for determination of the equivalence limits. For example, if $\theta_{\text{U}} = 1/\theta_{\text{L}} = 1.25$ and $r = 10$, then the acceptable interval for β is (0.9031, 1.0969). Therefore, under these conditions, the dose proportionality is proved at the α significance level if the $100(1-2\alpha)\%$ confidence interval for β is completely contained within (0.9031, 1.0969).

18.3.5 Adjacent Slope Approach to Assessment of Dose Proportionality

If the dose proportionality is true, then the relationship between the average exposure measures and dose levels can be adequately described by a simple linear regression, either on the original scale or log-scale. Therefore, the slopes between adjacent doses should be equal or similar. On the basis of this concept, Cheng et al. (2006) proposed a procedure for assessment of dose proportionality based on the two slope approach. For the purpose of illustration, the method for the simple linear regression model on the original scale (model 2) in Section 18.3.1 is presented here. However, as mentioned early in Section 18.3.1, the standard deviation of exposure measure is proportional to the dose level.

Let μ_j denote the average exposure measure at dose level X_j, $j = 1, \ldots, K$. The adjacent slopes is defined as

$$\beta_j = \frac{\mu_j - \mu_{j-1}}{X_j - X_{j-1}}, \quad j = 2, \ldots, K. \tag{18.3.9}$$

Let $\boldsymbol{\mu} = (\mu_1, \ldots, \mu_K)'$, $\boldsymbol{\beta} = (\beta_2, \ldots, \beta_K)'$, and

$$\mathbf{B} = \begin{pmatrix} -\frac{1}{X_2 - X_1} & \frac{1}{X_2 - X_1} & 0 & \cdots & 0 \\ 0 & -\frac{1}{X_3 - X_2} & \frac{1}{X_3 - X_2} & \cdots & 0 \\ \cdot & \cdot & \cdot & \cdots & \cdot \\ \cdot & \cdot & \cdot & \cdots & \cdot \\ 0 & 0 & \cdot & -\frac{1}{X_K - X_{K-1}} & \frac{1}{X_K - X_{K-1}} \end{pmatrix}.$$

Then it is easy to verify that $\boldsymbol{\beta} = \mathbf{B}\boldsymbol{\mu}$. Cheng et al. (2006) suggested the following hypothesis for assessment of dose proportionality:

$$\begin{aligned} & \mathrm{H_0}\colon \ \beta_2 = \cdots = \beta_K \\ \text{versus} \quad & \mathrm{H_a}\colon \ \beta_j \neq \beta_{j'}, \quad 2 \leq j \neq j' \leq K. \end{aligned} \tag{18.3.10}$$

Denote $\mathbf{A}$ as a $(k-2)\times(K-1)$ matrix such that $\mathbf{A1}_{k-1} = 0$, where $\mathbf{1}_{k-1}$ is the $k-1\times 1$ vector of ones. Cheng et al. (2006) show that hypothesis 18.3.10 can also be expressed as

$$\begin{aligned} & \mathrm{H_0}\colon \ \mathbf{A}\boldsymbol{\beta} = 0 \\ \text{versus} \quad & \mathrm{H_a}\colon \ \mathbf{A}\boldsymbol{\beta} \neq 0 \end{aligned}$$

Let $\overline{Y}_j$ and s_j^2 be the observed mean and within-sample variance at dose level X_j, respectively. Then μ_j and σ^2 can be estimated unbiasedly by $\overline{Y}_j$ and

$$\widehat{\sigma}^2 = \frac{1}{K}\sum_{j=j}^{K} \frac{s_j^2}{X_j^2}. \tag{18.3.11}$$

The null hypothesis in Equation 18.3.10 is rejected at the α significance level if

$$F = \frac{n\widehat{\boldsymbol{\mu}}\mathbf{B}'\mathbf{A}(\mathbf{ABDD}'\mathbf{B}'\mathbf{A}')^{-1}\mathbf{A}'\mathbf{B}\widehat{\boldsymbol{\mu}}/(K-2)}{\widehat{\sigma}^2} > F(\alpha, K-2, K(n-1)), \tag{18.3.12}$$

where

n is the number of subjects received dose X_j

$\mathbf{D}$ is a $K \times K$ diagonal matrix with X_j on the diagonal

$F(\alpha,\ K-2,\ K(n-1))$ is the α upper quantile of a central F distribution with degrees of freedom $K-2$ and $K(n-1)$.

Although the F test given in Equation 18.3.12 is uniformly most powerful invariant test to reject the null hypothesis of dose proportionality, it is not the test to prove the dose proportionality. On the other hand, one of choices for $\mathbf{A}\boldsymbol{\beta}$ can be written as $\mathbf{A}\boldsymbol{\beta} = \mathbf{AB}\boldsymbol{\mu} = (\beta_3 - \beta_2, \ldots, \beta_K - \beta_{K-1})'$. If dose proportionality holds, then the magnitudes of the $K-1$ adjacent slopes should be similar and differences between two adjacent slopes are within some acceptable range, say $(-\delta_\mathrm{L}, \delta_\mathrm{U})$, which has no significant impact of applications of dose proportionality to clinical practice. One method for determination of the acceptable range is to modify the method described in Section 18.3.4. Because the ideal slope for the dose proportionality under Equation 18.3.6 is 1, it follows from Equation 18.3.8 that

$$\begin{aligned} \delta_\mathrm{L} &= \frac{\log(\theta_\mathrm{L})}{\log(r)}, \quad \text{and} \\ \delta_\mathrm{U} &= \frac{\log(\theta_\mathrm{U})}{\log(r)}. \end{aligned} \tag{18.3.13}$$

If $\theta_U = 1/\theta_L$, then $\delta_U = -\delta_L = \delta$ and the acceptable range is symmetric about 0. Consequently, a hypothesis for verification of dose proportionality can be written as

$$\begin{aligned} &\text{H}_0\text{: } \boldsymbol{\beta}'\mathbf{A}'\mathbf{A}\boldsymbol{\beta} \geq (k-2)\delta^2 \\ \text{versus } &\text{H}_0\text{: } \boldsymbol{\beta}'\mathbf{A}'\mathbf{A}\boldsymbol{\beta} < (k-2)\delta^2. \end{aligned} \tag{18.3.14}$$

We can reject the null hypothesis in Equation 18.3.14 at the α significance level if

$$F < F(1-\alpha, K-2, K(n-1), \text{NC}), \tag{18.3.15}$$

where NC is the noncentrality parameter given as

$$F = \frac{2n\delta^2\mathbf{1}'(\mathbf{ABDD}'\mathbf{B}'\mathbf{A}')^{-1}1/(K-2)}{\sigma^2}.$$

Although the test given in Equation 18.3.15 is the correct test to prove the dose proportionality, the noncentrality parameters involve an unknown parameter σ^2 which require estimation and introduce additional variability. One way to resolve this issue is to specify the maximum variability for the observed exposure measures allowed in the dose proportionality study, say, σ_M^2. Then in this case, the noncentrality parameter becomes

$$F = \frac{2n\delta^2\mathbf{1}'(\mathbf{ABDD}'\mathbf{B}'\mathbf{A}')^{-1}1/(K-2)}{\sigma_M^2}.$$

However, the area for development of statistical methodology in proving the dose proportionality requires further research.

18.3.6 Discussion

As indicated earlier, a weighted linear regression is often used to evaluate dose linearity. The coefficient of correlation obtained from the model is always misused as an indicator of linearity. It should be noted that if the relation between Y and X is linear, the coefficient of correlation is close to 1. However, a high coefficient of correlation does not necessarily imply a linear relation between Y and X.

In model 1, under the assumption of $\text{Var}(Y) = X^2\sigma^2$, we have $\text{Var}(\log(Y)) \approx E(Y)^{-2}\text{Var}(Y) = \sigma^2/\beta^2$, which is the square of the coefficient of variation of Y. This indicates that log-transformation is a variance stabilizing transformation for Y if the standard deviation of Y is proportional to X.

In many applications, each subject may be bled serially. The AUC and C_{max} are obtained for each subject at each dose. In this case, weighted linear regression techniques can be applied either to the individual data $\{(X_j, Y_{ij}), j = 1, 2, \ldots, k; i = 1, \ldots, n_i\}$ or to the mean data $\{(X_j, \overline{Y}_j), j = 1, 2, \ldots, k\}$. Smith (1986) developed a computer program for assessing dose linearity in animal experiments with serial and nonserial collection of blood samples. However, narrower confidence intervals are often obtained with the individual data than with the mean data because the individual data provides more degrees of freedom for error.

The evaluation of model 4 requires a nonlinear weighted regression statistical package such as PROC NLIN of SAS. This procedure sometimes is very sensitive to the selected initial values. To characterize a nonlinear dose–response curve, a nonparametric test procedure by comparing the mean rate of change (slope) in response among adjacent dose intervals may be used. Although this method does not provide an exact test for the dose–response curve, it is more sensible and easier to implement in practice.

Frequently, a dose–response curve is assumed to be linear with zero intercept (dose proportionality, i.e., $E(Y|X)=\alpha+\beta X$ with $\alpha=0$). However, there are situations when the dose–response curve is nonlinear at the first pass. In practice, it is generally very difficult to verify that $\alpha=0$ if the lowest dose included in the study is not small enough, even though the response is zero at zero dose. A reasonable approach is to assume that there is a simple linear relation between Y an X over the range (X_1, X_k), with an arbitrary intercept at dose zero, and test its significance against the hypothesis of a nonlinear dose–response curve.

18.4 Steady-State Analysis

For a multiple-dose regimen, the amount of drug in the body is said to have reached a steady-state level if the amount or average concentration of the drug in the body remains stable. To determine whether the steady state has been reached, the PK parameter AUC from zero to infinity is usually considered because it measures the extent of absorption. AUC from zero to infinity is probably the most reliable PK response for determination of steady state. However, it requires many blood samples from each subject over a period that investigators feel that steady state might be reached. Therefore, in practice, the use of AUC from zero to infinity for determination of a steady state of a drug may not be totally feasible.

As an alternative, if the preliminary information of the PK profile of the active ingredient is available, then the trough and peak values of plasma concentrations are usually used to determine whether the steady state has been reached. In a multiple dose regimen, the trough values are defined as the plasma concentrations at the lowest dose level, which is usually measured at the time immediately prior to dosing. Peak plasma concentration, which is measured at the estimated T_{max} obtained from previous studies, provides information for determination of whether the plasma concentration exceeds the toxicity level. On the other hand, trough value is an indication of whether the plasma concentration is above the efficacious therapeutic level. The peak to trough ratio is usually used as an indicator of fluctuation of drug efficacy and safety. For example, a large peak to trough value may indicate that either the drug is not effective (trough concentration is too low), or the drug has harmful adverse effects (peak concentration is too high), or both. Therefore, an effective and safe drug should have a relatively small peak to trough ratio.

18.4.1 Univariate Analysis

Let Y_{ij} be the trough value of the ith subject at the jth dose. Then, the following model can be used to evaluate changes in trough values:

$$\begin{aligned} Y_{ij} &= \mu + S_i + F_j + e_{ij} \\ &= \alpha_j + S_i + e_{ij}, \end{aligned} \tag{18.4.1}$$

where
μ is the overall mean
S_i is the random effect of subject i, $i = 1, 2, \ldots, N$
F_j is the fixed effect of the jth dose, $j = 1, 2, \ldots, d$
e_{ij} is the random error

Under assumptions of normality and compound symmetry of S_i and e_{ij}, the maximum likelihood estimators of α_j, σ_e^2, and σ_S^2 are given by

$$\begin{aligned} \widehat{\alpha}_j &= \overline{Y}_{\cdot j}, \\ \widehat{\sigma}_e^2 &= \text{MSE}, \\ \widehat{\sigma}_S^2 &= \frac{(\text{MSB} - \text{MSE})}{d}, \end{aligned}$$

where $\overline{Y}_{\cdot j}$, MSB, and MSE are as defined in Section 8.5.

For a total of d doses, the Helmert transformation (Searle, 1971) consists of the following $d - 1$ row vectors:

$$\begin{aligned} \mathbf{C}_1' &= \left(-1, \frac{1}{d-1}, \ldots, \frac{1}{d-1}\right), \\ \mathbf{C}_2' &= \left(0, -1, \frac{1}{d-2}, \ldots, \frac{1}{d-2}\right), \\ \mathbf{C}_{d-1}' &= (0, 0, \ldots, -1, 1). \end{aligned} \tag{18.4.2}$$

Note that $\mathbf{C}'_j \mathbf{C}_{j'} = 0$. Let

$$\begin{aligned} \widehat{\alpha} &= (\widehat{\alpha}_1, \widehat{\alpha}_2, \ldots, \widehat{\alpha}_d) \\ &= (\overline{Y}_{\cdot 1}, \overline{Y}_{\cdot 2}, \ldots, \overline{Y}_{\cdot d})', \end{aligned}$$

and

$$t_j = \frac{\mathbf{C}_j'\widehat{\alpha}}{[\text{MSE } \mathbf{C}_j'\mathbf{C}_j]^{1/2}}. \tag{18.4.3}$$

Then, we conclude that the steady state is reached at the jth dose if

$$|t_j| \leq t[\alpha/2, (N-1)(d-1)] \tag{18.4.4}$$

provided that $|t_1|, \ldots, |t_{j-1}|$ are greater than $t[\alpha/2, (N-1)(d-1)]$.

18.4.2 Multivariate Analysis

If the assumption of compound symmetry is not satisfied, one can either apply a log-transformation of the trough plasma concentrations, or use a multivariate analysis based on the one-sample Hotelling T^2 statistic to determine whether the steady state is reached.

Let $\mathbf{Y}_i = (Y_{i1}, \ldots, Y_{id})'$ be $d \times 1$ vector of the trough plasma concentrations at d different dosing times observed on subject i. Also, let $\mathbf{S}$ be the sample covariance matrix computed from $\mathbf{Y}_i$; that is

$$\mathbf{S} = \frac{1}{N-1} \sum_{i=1}^{N} [\mathbf{Y}_i - \hat{\boldsymbol{\alpha}}]\,[\mathbf{Y}_i - \hat{\boldsymbol{\alpha}}]'. \tag{18.4.5}$$

Then, the steady state is considered to be reached at the jth dose if

$$T_j^2 \leq T^2(1-\alpha, d-1, N-d+1) \tag{18.4.6}$$

provided that $T_1{}^2, \ldots, T_{j-1}^2 > T^2(\alpha, d-1, N-d+1)$, where

$$T_j^2 = \frac{N(\mathbf{C}_j'\hat{\boldsymbol{\alpha}})^2}{\mathbf{C}_j'\mathbf{S}\mathbf{C}_j}, \tag{18.4.7}$$

and

$$T^2(\alpha, d-1, N-d+1) = \left[\frac{(N-1)(d-1)}{N-d+1}\right] F(\alpha, d-1, N-d+1). \tag{18.4.8}$$

18.4.3 Discussion

The procedure for determination of the steady state, either univariate or multivariate, is to search the first dose (time) where $T_j(t_j)$ is not rejected at the α significance level. However, although $T_j(t_j)$ is not rejected, $T_j'(t_j')$ might be rejected for $j' > j$. This indicates that the trough plasma concentrations still fluctuate after the jth dose. Although $T_j(t_j)$ and $T_j'(t_j')$ are independent of each other ($j' \neq j$), to have an overall α-type I error rate, an adjustment for the test significance level is necessary.

As indicated earlier, peak to trough ratios can also be used to determine whether the steady state is reached. A relatively small peak to trough ratio indicates that the study drug is relatively effective and safe. Analysis of peak to trough values is very important for assessing efficacy and safety of the drug in antihypertensive, antiangina, and antiarrhythmia therapies. However, the procedure discussed in the above cannot be applied directly because the peak to trough ratios may not satisfy normality assumptions. In fact, even when the peak values and the trough values follow normal distributions, the peak/trough ratios,

$$R_i = \frac{Y_{pi}}{Y_{ti}}, \quad i = 1, 2, \ldots, N.$$

R_i may follow a Cauchy distribution, which does not have first and any higher moments (e.g., mean and variance) where Y_{pi} and Y_{ti} are the peak and trough values for subject i. As an alternative, one may consider analyzing the peak to trough ratios using nonparametric summary statistics, such as median and interquantile range, or apply Fieller's theorem discussed in Chapter 4 to construct a confidence interval for the true population peak to trough ratio.

18.5 Evaluation of Food Effects

For orally administrated drugs, one of the important dosing issues is whether the drugs can be taken together with food. In other words, does there exist food–drug interaction? There two types of food–drug interaction studies. The first type of the food–drug interaction studies is to investigate the effect of food on the change in magnitudes of exposure measures or other PK parameters. This type of the food–drug interaction studies is referred to as the food-effect BA study. Second type of food–drug interaction studies is to evaluate whether the food can have an impact on the BE between the generic test formulation and innovative reference formulation. This type of the food–drug interaction studies is called the fed BE study. As a result, the U.S. FDA in December, 2002 issued guidance on *Food-Effect bioavailability and Fed Bioequivalence Studies* which provides recommendations to sponsors planning to conduct food-effect BA and BE studies for orally administrated drug products for investigational new drug applications (INDs), NDAs, and ANDAs.

As pointed out, the 2002 FDA guidance, there are many ways that food can alter the BA of a drug product, including

1. Delay gastric emptying
2. Stimulate bile flow
3. Change gastrointestinal (GI) flow
4. Increase splanchnic blood flow
5. Change luminal metabolism of a drug product
6. Physically or chemically interact with a dosage form or a drug substance.

As a result, for both orally administered immediate-release and modified-release drug products, the 2002 FDA draft guidance recommends that a food-effect BA study be conducted during the IND period. On the other hand, for ANDA, in addition to a BE study conducted under fasting conditions, additional BE study under fed conditions also should be conducted for all orally administered immediate-release and modified-release drug products.

18.5.1 General Considerations

Both food-effect BA and fed BE studies should be conducted in health volunteers drawn from the general population. The 2002 FDA guidance recommends that a minimum of 12 subjects or a sufficient number of subjects should complete the food-effect BA and fed BE studies to provide adequate power for the assessment of food effects on BA or claim BE in a fed BE study. On the other hand, the highest strength of a drug product should be investigated in food-effect BA and fed BE studies. In addition, if the highest strength is employed in a fed BE study, then *in vivo* BE evaluation for one or more lower doses can be waived based on *in vitro* dissolution profile comparisons.

The 2002 FDA guidance recommends that meal conductions expected to provide the greatest effect on GI physiology with maximal effect of systemic drug availability be employed for both food-effect BA and fed BE studies. A high-fat and high-calorie meal is recommended. A high-fat meal is defined as a meal that fat provides approximately 50% of total calorie content of the meal. A high-calorie meal is the meal with approximately 800–1000 calories. In addition, the test meal should derive approximately 150, 250, and 500–600 calories from protein, carbohydrate, and fat, respectively. The fasted treatments recommended by the 2002 FDA include the following:

1. Overnight fast of at least 10 hours
2. Subjects should be administrated the drug product with 8 fluid ounces of water
3. No food is allowed for at least 4 hours postdose
4. Water is not allowed within 1 hour before and after the dose
5. Standard meals should be scheduled at the same time in each period of the study

The fed treatments include the following:

1. Overnight fast of at least 10 hours
2. Meal should be served 30 minutes prior to administration of the drug product
3. Subject should complete the meal within 30 minutes
4. Subjects should be administrated the drug product with 8 fluid ounces of water
5. No food is allowed for at least 4 hour postdose

6. Water is not allowed within 1 hour before and after the dose
7. Standard meals should be scheduled at the same time in each period of the study

18.5.2 Evaluation Procedures

For food-effect BA studies, the 2002 FDA guidance recommends the use of a randomized, balanced, single-dose, two-treatment, two-sequence, and two-period crossover design as described in Design C3 of Section 18.2.3. In Design C3, S is the reference fasting conditions, I is the food, and I + S denotes the test fed conditions. For fed BE studies, again, the same standard two-treatment, two-sequence and two-period crossover design is employed for which both generic test and innovative reference formulations are administrated under fed conditions. The 2002 FDA guidance suggests the following exposure measures and PK parameters be obtained from the concentration–time curves for both food-effect BA and fed BE conditions:

1. Total exposure: AUC(0–∞) and AUC(0–t)
2. Peak exposure (C_{max})
3. Time to peak exposure (T_{max})
4. Lag-time (t_{lag}) for modified-release products, if present
5. Terminal elimination half-life
6. Other relevant PK parameters

For food-effect BA studies, let $\mu_{fast} = \mu + F_{fast}$ and $\mu_{fed} = \mu + F_{fed}$ be the population treatment means for the log-transformed exposure measure under fasting and fed conditions, respectively. The parameter of interest on the log-scale is $\theta_F = \mu_{fed} - \mu_{fast} = F_{fed} - F_{fast}$. The 2002 FDA guidance recommends the use of an equivalence approach for sponsors to make a claim of no food effect which is based on the following hypothesis:

$$\begin{aligned} & \text{H}_0\text{: } \theta_F \leq -0.2231 \quad \text{or} \quad \theta_F \geq 0.2231 \\ \text{versus} \quad & \text{H}_a\text{: } -0.2231 < \theta_F < 0.2231. \end{aligned}$$

It follows that the confidence interval approach described in Section 4.2 can be used to verify no food effect. The exposure measures for evaluation of an absence of food effect include AUC(0−∞), AUC(0−t), and peak exposure (C_{max}). No food effect can be concluded at the 5% significance level if the 90% confidence interval for the difference in population means on the log-scale between fed and fasted treatments is totally contained within (−0.2231, 0.2231). In this case, For an NDA, a sponsor can make a specific claim in the clinical pharmacology or dosage and administration section of the label that no food effect on BA is expected (FDA, 2002). On the other hand, an absence of food effect cannot be concluded at the 5% significance level if the 90% confidence interval for the difference in population means on the log-scale between fed and fasted treatments is not totally contained within $(-0.2231, 0.2231)$. Under this situation, the sponsor should provide specific recommendations on the clinical significance of the food effect. The 2002 FDA guidance indicates that the results of the food-effect BA study be reported factually in the clinical pharmacology section of the label and should address whether the drug product should be taken only on an empty stomach in the dosage and administration section of the label.

The traditional Schuirmann's two one-sided tests procedure in the form of confidence approach is recommended by the 2002 FDA guidance for evaluation of BE between the generic test formulation and the innovative reference formulation under fed conditions. In other words, for an ANDA, BE between the generic test formulation and the innovative reference formulation under fed conditions is concluded at the 5% significance level if the 90% confidence interval for the difference in population means on the log-scale between is totally contained within $(-0.2231, 0.2231)$. Consequently, the language in the package insert of the generic test formulation with regard to food can be the same as the innovative reference formulation.

18.6 Discussion

For development of a new study drug, it is very important to understand whether it can affect other approved drug products or can be affected by approved drugs by in terms of the clinically relevant changes in exposure measures or other PK parameters. In addition, it is of equal importance to determine whether the exposure measures is linearly related to the dose levels so that the change in exposure measures due to a change in dose can be reliably predicted and dose can be adjusted if necessarily. Another simple but important question is whether the new study drug should or should not be taken with food. To address the above questions, drug interaction studies, dose proportionality studies, and food-effect BA studies are conducted to obtain the specific information. These studies are usually conducted in the early stage of the drug development so that the cumulative information from these studies can be used for administration of the new study drug and selection and adjustment of doses in the later phase II and III studies. Although these studies are conducted in the early stage of drug development, randomized crossover designs described in Chapter 3 are mostly commonly employed and the equivalence approach using the confidence interval reviewed in Chapter 4 is used to evaluate the absence of drug-to-drug interactions and food effects, and dose proportionality. As mentioned above, the information, knowledge, and results from these studies also should be provided in the drug interactions, warnings and precautions, clinical pharmacology, and dosage and administration sections of the drug label.

Recently, for easy administration of the drug products, there is an increasing trend to develop fixed-dose combination drugs where both components were approved by the regulatory agencies. Section 300.50 in Part 21 of CFR states that "Two or more drugs may be combined in a single dosage form when each component makes a contribution to the claimed effects." Therefore, according to the U.S. FDA, a fixed-dose combination drugs belong to a class of drug products in which different drugs are formulated into one dosage form. During the development of fixed-dose combination drugs, if BE of each component in the fixed-dose combination drug to each component at the same dose, administrated as co-administration of the free combination, can be established, then phase III confirmatory clinical studies with the fixed-dose combination may be waived by regulatory authorities if the efficacy and safety of the co-administration of the free combination have been established and approved by the regulatory authorities. Therefore, BE studies comparing the fixed-dose combination product and the co-administration of the free combination can be served as bridging studies if the co-administration of the free combination is approved.

Because the co-administration of the free combination has been approved, component-to-component interactions in the free combination have been evaluated in drug interaction studies, therefore, the objective of the BE studies of the fixed-dose and free combinations is to assess BE with respect to each individual component. In this case, the fixed-dose combination drug is the test formulation and free combination is the reference formulation. In general, a randomized, balanced, single-dose, two-treatment, two-sequence, and two-period crossover design is often employed too. Let θ_i be the difference in population average exposure measures between the fixed-dose combination and free-dose combination on the log-scale with respect to component i, $i = 1, \ldots, H$. Then the hypotheses for evaluation of BE between the fixed-dose combination and free combination are given as

$$\begin{aligned} &\mathrm{H}_{0i}\colon\ \theta_i \le -0.2231 \quad \text{or} \quad \theta_i \ge 0.2231 \\ \text{versus}\quad &\mathrm{H}_{ai}\colon\ -0.2231 < \theta_i < 0.2231, \quad i = 1, \ldots, H. \end{aligned}$$

As a result, the BE between the fixed-dose and free combinations is concluded at the 5% significance level if 90% confidence intervals for θ_i for all components are totally contained within (−0.2231, 0.2231) for AUC(0−∞), AUC(0−t), and $C_{\max}$. This approach is conservative because it requires all exposure measures for all components meet the equivalence requirements at the same 5% level.

If the free combination has not been approved by the regulatory agencies, then the fixed-dose combination is considered as a new drug product and the interaction studies employed Design C4 of Section 18.2.3 should be conducted to assess jointly the interaction effects of the fixed-dose combination using the methods described in Section 18.2.5. However, for this case, phase III confirmatory trials should be conducted to provide necessary efficacy and safety information to meet the regulatory requirements. For more details about the clinical evaluation of fixed-dose combination, see Chow and Liu (2004).

Chapter 19

Review of Regulatory Guidances on Bioequivalence

19.1 Introduction

When an innovator (brand-name) drug product is going off patent, the innovator drug company may develop a new dosage form (formulation) of the innovator drug product with the same active ingredient to extend its market exclusivity of this product. At the same time, generic drug companies may file an abbreviated new drug application (ANDA) to obtain generic approval of the innovator drug product. For approval of a new dosage form or a generic copy of an innovator drug product, most regulatory agencies including the U.S. Food and Drug Administration (FDA) require only that evidence of equivalence in average bioavailabilities be provided through a bioequivalence trial. As a result, the design, conduct, analysis, report, and presentation of bioequivalence trials are extremely important to ensure the validity of bioequivalence between a test drug product (e.g., a new dosage form or a generic copy) and the reference drug product (e.g., the innovator drug product) under the current regulations of bioequivalence. For this purpose, most regulatory agencies have developed several guidelines or guidances, including both general guidances and drug-specific guidances to assist the sponsors in conducting a valid bioequivalence trial for good pharmaceutical practice.

In this chapter, we provide a comprehensive review of important guidances or draft guidances issued by the U.S. FDA, EMEA, and WHO (World Health Organization). These guidances can generally be classified into three classes. The first class is the recommendations of the statistical methods on the design and analysis for evaluation of bioequivalence between the test and reference formulations. Almost all of these guidances were issued by the U.S. FDA over the past 25 years. These include *Guidance on Statistical Procedures for Bioequivalence Studies Using a Standard Two-Treatment Crossover Design* (July, 1992), *Draft Guidance on In Vivo Bioequivalence Studies Based on Population and Individual Bioequivalence Approaches* (October, 1997), and *Statistical Approaches to Establishing Bioequivalence* (January, 2001). The second group of the guidances is on the general considerations for bioavailability and bioequivalence studies. These include the EMEA *Guidance on the Investigation of Bioavailability and Bioequivalence* (July, 2001), the U.S. FDA *Guidance on Bioavailability and Bioequivalence Studies for Orally Administrated Drug Products—General Considerations* (March, 2003), and the WHO draft *Guidance on Multisource (Generic) Pharmaceutical Products: Guidelines on Registration Requirements to Establish Interchangeability* (October, 2005a). The last category of the guidances includes guidelines, notes, or concept paper on assessment of bioequivalence for special drug products. These include the U.S. FDA guidances on slow-release potassium chloride and clozapine tablets, and EMEA notes on modified release oral and transdermal dosage forms. In addition, on May 1, 2007, the U.S. FDA issued a document on critical path opportunities for generic drugs which outlines the challenges and opportunities for the generic drug development process. Evolution and development of the guidances on statistical procedures for evaluation of bioequivalence is reviewed in Section 19.2. Review of the guidances on bioequivalence for orally administrated drug products by the U.S. FDA, EMEA, and WHO are provided in Section 19.3. Section 19.4 presents the review of guidances on assessment of bioequivalence of specific drug products. The U.S. FDA critical path opportunities for generic drugs are examined in Section 19.5. Final remarks and discussion are provided in Section 19.6.

19.2 Guidances on Statistical Procedures

As more generic drug products become available in the marketplace, the quality, efficacy, and safety of generic drug products have become a public concern. As a result, a public hearing was conducted by the FDA in 1986. At the public hearing, several scientific issues were raised. A bioequivalence task force was then formed to investigate these issues. On the basis of the report released by the bioequivalence task force in 1989, the Division of Bioequivalence, Office of Generic Drugs of the FDA issued the guidance on *Statistical Procedure for Bioequivalence Studies Using a Standard Two-Treatment Crossover Design*, in July 1992.

In the medical community, as more generic drug products become available in the marketplace, it is of great concern whether various generic drug products of the same brand-name drug can be used safely and interchangeably. As indicated in Chapter 11, drug interchangeability can be classified as drug prescribability or drug switchability. The underlying assumption of drug prescribability is that the brand-name drug product and its generic copies can be used interchangeably in terms of the efficacy and safety of the drug product. Drug switchability is considered more critical than drug prescribability in the study of drug interchangeability for patients who have been taking a medication for some time. The concept of IBE has attracted FDA's attention since introduced by Anderson and Hauck (1990), which has led to a significant change in regulatory requirement for assessment of bioequivalence. In October 1997, a draft guidance, *In Vivo Bioequivalence Studies Based on Population and Individual Bioequivalence Approaches* was distributed by the FDA for public comments (FDA, 1997). As a result, a special issue of *Statistics in Medicine* devoted to individual bioequivalence was published on October 30, 2000. This issue, edited by Chow and Liu, consists of 13 papers contributed by the authors from academia, industry, and regulatory agencies, including the U.S. FDA. In consolidation of the comments and viewpoints by different concerning parties, guidance on *Statistical Approaches to Establishing Bioequivalence* was published by the U.S. FDA in January 2001. For evaluation of average bioequivalence (ABE), we review the issues of the logarithmic transformation of pharmacokinetic (PK) responses, sequence effect, and the detection and treatment of outlying data. With respect to assessment of PBE and IBE, we focus on the issues of criteria for PBE and IBE, masking effect, power and sample size determination, statistical procedures, and study design.

19.2.1 Logarithmic Transformation

Both the 1992 and 2001 FDA guidances provide the PK rationale as the clinical rationale for use of logarithmic transformation of exposure measures. In addition, the 2001 FDA guidance also states that the limited sample size in a typical BE study precludes a reliable determination of the distribution of the data. In addition, it also does not encourage the sponsors to test for normality of error distribution after log-transformation, nor to use normality of error distribution as a reason for carrying out the statistical analysis on the original scale.

With respect to the PK rationale, deterministic multiplicative PK models are used to justify the routine use of logarithmic transformation for AUC(0–∞) and C_{max}. However, the deterministic PK models are theoretical derivations of AUC(0–∞) and C_{max} for a single object. The guidances suggest that AUC(0–∞) be calculated from the observed plasma–blood concentration–time curve using the trapezoidal rule, and that C_{max} be obtained directly from the curve, without interpolation. It is not known whether the observed AUC(0–∞) and C_{max} can provide good approximations to those under the theoretical models if the models are correct.

On the other hand, assessment of bioequivalence requires statistical models that take into consideration the design features and the random components caused by inter- and intra-subject variations. The validity of the statistical inferences, such as confidence intervals and hypotheses testing, relies on the normality assumption of the random components in the statistical models. Consequently, determination of a scale of the exposure responses for assessment of bioequivalence also should be based solely on whether the random components in the statistical models satisfy the normality assumption.

The AUC(0–∞) and C_{max} are calculated from the observed plasma–blood concentrations. Therefore, the distributions of the observed AUC(0–∞) and C_{max} depend on the distributions of plasma–blood concentrations. Liu and Weng (1994) showed that the log-transformed AUC(0–∞) and C_{max} do not generally follow a normal distribution, even when either the plasma concentrations or log-plasma concentrations are normally distributed. This argues against the routine use of the logarithmic transformation in assessment of bioequivalence. Moreover, Patel (1994) also pointed out that performing a routine log-transformation of data and then applying normal, theory-based methods is not a scientific approach. In addition, the sample size of a typical BE study is generally too small to allow an adequate large-sample normal approximation.

Because current statistical methods for evaluation of bioequivalence are based on the normality assumption on the inter- and intra-subject variabilities, the examination of the normal probability plots for the studentized inter- and intra-subject residuals should always be carried out for the scale intended to be used in the analysis. In addition, formal statistical tests for normality of the inter- and intra-subject variabilities can also be carried out through Shapiro–Wilk's method. Contrary to the misconception of many people, Shapiro–Wilk's method is an exact method for small samples, such as bioequivalence studies. It is then scientifically imperative that tests for normality be routinely performed for the sale used in analysis, such as log-scale, suggested in the guidances. If normality cannot be satisfied by both original scale and log-scale, nonparametric methods should be employed.

Other issues concerning the routine use of the logarithmic transformation of exposure responses are the equivalence limits and presentation of the results on the original scale. The guidances recommend that the bioequivalence limits of (80%, 125%) on the original scale for assessment of ABE be used. On the log-scale, they are $[\log(0.8), \log(1.25)] = (-0.2331, 0.2331)$, where log denotes the natural logarithm. This set of limits is symmetrical about zero on the log-scale but it is not symmetrical about on the original scale. It should be noted that the rejection region of Schuirmann's two one-sided tests procedure associated with the new limits of (80%, 125%) is larger than that with the limits of (80%, 120%). As a result, a 90% confidence interval of (82%, 122%), for the ratio of averages of AUC(0–∞) between the test and reference formulations, will pass the bioequivalence test by the new limits, but not by the old limits. The new bioequivalence limits are 12.5% wider and 25% more liberal in the upper limit than the old limits. A new, wider upper bioequivalence limit may have an influence on the safety of the test formulation, which should be carefully examined if the new bioequivalence limits are adopted.

The FDA guidance requires that the results of analyses be presented on the log-scale as well as on the original scale, which can be obtained by taking the inverse transformation. Because the logarithmic transformation is not linear, the inverse transformation of the results to the original scale is not straightforward (Liu and Weng, 1992). For example, the point estimator of the ratio of averages on the original scale obtained from the antilog of the estimator of difference in averages on the log-scale is biased and is always overestimated. Furthermore, the antilog of the standard deviation of the difference in averages on the log-scale is not the standard deviation for the point estimator of the ratio of the averages on the original scale. Further research is needed for the presentation of the results on the original scale, especially the estimation of variability after the analyses are performed on the log-scale.

19.2.2 Sequence Effect

For a standard two-sequence, two-period crossover design, the sequence effect is confounded with the carryover effect and the formulation-by-period interaction.

Therefore, a statistically significant sequence effect could indicate that there is (1) a true sequence effect, (2) a true carryover effect, (3) there is a true formulation-by-period interaction, or (4) a failure of randomization. Therefore, assessment of bioequivalence based on averages might be contaminated with the unknown confounded effects. For example, if the true cause of a statistically significant sequence effect is due to the persistent effect of the formulation administered in the previous period, then the estimated ratio of averages and its associated 90% confidence interval are biased and are contaminated with the carryover effect. On the other hand, if a statistically significant sequence effect is caused, for some reasons, by a true difference between the two sequence groups, then the estimated ratio of averages and its associated 90% confidence interval are unbiased. The 2001 FDA guidance lists those conditions for which the possibility of unequal carryover effects is unlikely and claim of bioequivalence may be acceptable in the presence of a statistically significant sequence effect. These conditions are those from which the possibility of a true carryover effect or a formulation-by-period interaction can be eliminated. It is suggested that a diagnostic plot be added to the list of conditions, that is, the plot of sequence-by-period means. The parallelism might indicate that a statistically significant sequence effect is a true sequence effect (Jones and Kenward, 1989).

In general, a test for the sequence effect is performed at a 10% nominal level of significance. The reason for the test of the sequence effect being carried out at the 10% level is that the test is based on the sum of the inter- and intra-subject variabilities. Hence, this test is not as powerful as the test for the formulation effect. The use of a 10% nominal level of significance for the sequence effect, however, may not be justifiable because it can only create confusion between the true or false sequence and carryover effects. On the other hand, it is extremely difficult to distinguish a true carryover effect from a true sequence effect. As an alternative, a higher-order crossover design for comparing two formulations is recommended.

As indicated in Chapter 9, one of the advantages of a higher-order crossover design over the standard two-sequence, two-period crossover design is that the formulation, carryover and sequence effects are not confounded with one another. Therefore, bioequivalence on average bioavailability can be assessed based on the intra-subject variability in the presence of both the sequence and carryover effects. Moreover, the statistical inference of the carryover effect is also based on the intra-subject variability. In addition, some subjects in a higher-order crossover design may receive the same formulation more than once. As a result, independent estimates and statistical inference of intra-subject variabilities for each formulation can also be obtained. Because a higher-order crossover design has either more sequences or more periods than the standard two-sequence, two-period crossover design, complications in randomization and the conduct of the study are expected. Moreover, it requires a much longer time to complete the study. Subjects are likely to drop out from a higher-order crossover design than from the standard two-sequence, two-period design. Therefore, in spite of the relative merits, a higher-order crossover design for comparing two formulations might not be cost effective.

19.2.3 Outlying Data

The 1992 FDA guidance provides a PK definition of subject outliers and provides possible causes for their occurrence. The 1992 FDA guidance suggests that Lund's method (Lund, 1975) be used for outlier detection. Although Lund's method is useful in a linear regression setting that requires statistical independence of all PK responses, this method may not be appropriate for a crossover design in which the PK responses from the same subject are correlated. Although Lund's method may be applied to the difference of the PK responses between the test and the reference formulations from the same subject in a standard two-sequence, two-period crossover design, it does not take into account the feature of the study design. Moreover, it does not eliminate other nuisance effects; hence, it cannot be applied to other crossover designs.

As an alternative, Chow and Tse (1990a) first proposed two formal statistical test procedures for detection of a subject outlier in any crossover designs for assessment of bioequivalence. Their methods are the extension of Cook's likelihood distance (Cook and Weisberg, 1982). Their methods are valid for large samples. For small samples, Liu and Weng (1991) proposed the use of Hotelling T^2 for detection of multiple subject outliers. Wang and Chow (2003) proposed a procedure for detection of outliers under a mean-shift model. Although Liu and Weng's method is an exact method for small samples, it requires some special tables for critical values. Frequently, a subject may be considered an outlier based on the difference between the test and reference formulations. This subject, however, may not be considered an outlier based on the ratio. The reason for this conflict is that the design structure, statistical model, and scale for analysis are not taken into account for outlier detection. As a result, it is recommended that the detection of subject outliers should be carried out with a scale (original scale or the log-scale) intended from analysis under an appropriate statistical model for the design employed. In summary, Lund's method cannot take all of these factors into account for detecting subject outliers. Chow and Tse's method, Liu and Weng's procedures, and Wang and Chow test can accommodate the design, scale, and statistical models for detection of subject outliers. Ramsay and Elkum (2005) conducted a simulation study to compare the above four methods.

The 2001 FDA guidance suggests that product failure and subject-by-formulation interaction are the two causes of outliers in a BE study. In addition, it discourages any deletion of outliers. Although statistical procedures for detection of outliers are available, these methods are derived from the model for assessment of ABE. Consequently, they are inadequate for identification of outliers in assessment of either PBE or ABE. More research on this topic is urgently needed.

19.2.4 Criteria for PBE and IBE

To address drug prescribability, the 2001 FDA guidance proposed the following aggregated, scaled moment-based one-sided criterion:

$$\frac{(\mu_T - \mu_R)^2 + \left(\sigma_{TT}^2 - \sigma_{TR}^2\right)}{\max\left(\sigma_{TR}^2, \sigma_{T0}^2\right)} \leq \theta_P,$$

where

μ_T and μ_R are the mean of the test drug product and the reference drug product
σ_{TT}^2 and σ_{TR}^2 are total variance of the test drug product and the reference drug product, respectively
σ_{T0}^2 is a constant that can be adjusted to control the probability of passing PBE
θ_P is the bioequivalence limit

The numerator on the left-hand side of the criterion is the sum of the squared difference of the traditional population averages and the difference between total variance between the test and reference drug products that measures the similarity for the marginal population distribution between the test and reference drug products. The denominator on the left-hand side of the criterion is a scaled factor depending on the variability of the drug class of the reference drug product. The guidance suggests that θ_P be chosen as

$$\theta_P = \frac{(\log 1.25)^2 + \varepsilon_P}{\sigma_{T0}^2},$$

where ε_P is guided by the consideration of the variability term $\sigma_{TT}^2 - \sigma_{TR}^2$ added to the ABE criterion. However, the 2001 FDA guidance asks the sponsor to check with the FDA for further information on θ_P and ε_P if applicants wish to use PBE. For the determination of σ_{T0}^2, the guidance recommends the use of population difference ratio (PDR), which is defined as

$$\begin{aligned}
\text{PDR} &= \left[\frac{E(T-R)^2}{E(R-R')^2}\right]^{1/2} \\
&= \left[\frac{(\mu_T - \mu_R)^2 + \sigma_{TT}^2 + \sigma_{TR}^2}{2\sigma_{TR}^2}\right]^{1/2} \\
&= \left[\frac{\text{PBC}}{2} + 1\right]^{1/2}.
\end{aligned}$$

Therefore, assuming that the maximum allowable PDR is 1.25, substitution of $(\log 1.25)^2/\sigma_{T0}^2$ for PBC without adjustment of the variance term yields approximately $\sigma_{T0} = 0.2$. Again the 2001 FDA guidance recommends consulting with the agency for further information about σ_{T0}.

To address drug switchability, the 2001 FDA proposed the following aggregated, scaled moment-based one-sided criterion:

$$\frac{(\mu_T - \mu_R)^2 + \sigma_D^2 + \left(\sigma_{WT}^2 - \sigma_{WR}^2\right)}{\max\left(\sigma_{WR}^2, \sigma_{W0}^2\right)} \leq \theta_I,$$

where

σ_{WT}^2 and σ_{WR}^2 are the within-subject variance for the test drug product and the reference drug product, respectively

σ_D^2 is the variance of the subject-by-formulation interaction

σ_{W0}^2 is a constant that can be adjusted to control the probability of passing IBE

θ_I is the bioequivalence limit

The guidance suggests that θ_I be chosen as follows:

$$\theta_I = \frac{(\log 1.25)^2 + \varepsilon_I}{\sigma_{W0}^2},$$

where ε_I is set as 0.05 by the guidance. For the determination of σ_{W0}^2, the guidance recommends the use of individual difference ratio (IDR) which is defined as

$$\begin{aligned}
\text{IDR} &= \left[\frac{E(T-R)^2}{E(R-R')^2}\right]^{1/2} \\
&= \left[\frac{(\mu_T-\mu_R)^2 + \sigma_D^2 + \left(\sigma_{WT}^2 + \sigma_{WR}^2\right)}{2\sigma_{WR}^2}\right]^{1/2} \\
&= \left[\frac{\text{IBC}}{2} + 1\right]^{1/2}.
\end{aligned}$$

Therefore, assuming that the maximum allowable IDR is 1.25, substitution of $(\log 1.25)^2/\sigma_{W0}^2$ for IBC without adjustment of the variance term approximately yields $\sigma_{W0} = 0.2$. Furthermore, the 2001 FDA guidance recommends a value of 0.3 for σ_D^2 and a value for allowance in difference between σ_{WT}^2 and σ_{WR}^2 However, the selection of σ_{W0}^2, σ_D^2, and difference between σ_{WT}^2 and σ_{WR}^2 do not have any clinical and PK justification and interpretation and lack of statistical reasoning too.

19.2.5 Aggregate versus Disaggregate

The 2001 FDA guidance recommends aggregate criteria, as described earlier, for assessment of both PBE and IBE. The PBE criterion accounts for average of bioavailability and variability of bioavailability, whereas, in addition, the IBE criterion takes into account the variability caused by subject-by-formulation interaction. Under the proposed aggregate criteria, however, it is unclear whether the IBE criterion is superior to those of the ABE or PBE for assessment of drug interchangeability. In other words, it is unclear whether or not IBE implies PBE and PBE implies ABE under aggregate criteria. Hence, the question of particular interest to pharmaceutical scientists is, "Does the proposed aggregate PBE or IBE criterion really address drug interchangeability (i.e., prescribability and switchability)?"

Liu and Chow (1997a) suggested disaggregate criteria be implemented for assessment of drug interchangeability. The concept of disaggregate criteria for assessment of PBE and IBE are described in the following. In addition to ABE, we may consider the following hypotheses testing for assessment of bioequivalence in variability of bioavailabilities:

$$\begin{aligned} &\mathrm{H_0}: \sigma^2_{\mathrm{WT}}/\sigma^2_{\mathrm{WR}} \geq \lambda_{30} \\ \text{versus} \quad &\mathrm{H_a}: \sigma^2_{\mathrm{WT}}/\sigma^2_{\mathrm{WR}} < \lambda_{30}, \end{aligned}$$

where λ_{30} is bioequivalence limit for the ratio of intra-subject variabilities. We conclude PBE if $100(1-\alpha)\%$ upper confidence limit $\sigma^2_{\mathrm{WT}}/\sigma^2_{\mathrm{WR}}$ is less than λ_{30}. For assessment of IBE, we further consider the following hypotheses:

$$\begin{aligned} &\mathrm{H_0}: \sigma^2_{\mathrm{D}} \geq \lambda'_{20} \\ \text{versus} \quad &\mathrm{H_a}: \sigma^2_{\mathrm{D}} < \lambda'_{20}, \end{aligned}$$

where λ'_{20} is an acceptable limit for variability owing to subject-by-formulation interaction. We conclude IBE if both $100(1-\alpha)\%$ upper confidence limit for $\sigma^2_{\mathrm{WT}}/\sigma^2_{\mathrm{WR}}$ is less than λ_{30} and $100(1-\alpha)\%$ upper confidence limit for σ^2_{D} is less than λ'_{20}. Under the above disaggregate criteria, it is clear that IBE implies PBE, and PBE implies ABE.

In practice, it is then of interest to examine the relative merits and disadvantages between the FDA proposed aggregate criteria and the disaggregate criteria described in the above for assessment of drug interchangeability. In addition, it is also of interest to compare the aggregate and disaggregate criteria of PBE and IBE with the current ABE criterion in terms of the consistencies and inconsistencies in concluding bioequivalence for regulatory approval.

19.2.6 Interpretation of the Criteria

The 2001 FDA guidance suggests that a logarithmic transformation be performed for PK metrics except for $T_{\max}$ and the degree of fluctuation. For ABE, the interpretation on both original and log-scale is straightforward and easily understood because the difference in arithmetic means on the log-scale is the ratio of geometric means on the original scale. For log transformation, two drug products are concluded ABE if the ratio of the average bioavailabilities on the original scale is between 80% and 125%. This statement is the same as that the two drug products are concluded ABE if the difference between the arithmetic means on the log-scale is between −0.2231 [=log 0.8] and 0.2231 [=log 1.25]. However, the interpretation of the aggregate criteria for both PBE and IBE is not straightforward and clear on the original scale. For example, the exponential of subject-by-formulation interaction and intra-subject variability on the log-scale are not the corresponding subject-by-formulation and intra-subject variability on the original scale. In addition, the guidance needs to provide an explanation of the criteria on the original scale for PBE and IBE and their corresponding bioequivalence limits θ_{P} and θ_{I}.

19.2.7 Masking Effect

The goal for evaluation of bioequivalence is to assess the similarity of the distributions of the PK metrics obtained either from the population or from individuals in the population. However, under aggregate criteria, different combinations of values for the components of the aggregate criterion can yield the same value. In other words, bioequivalence can be reached by two totally different distributions of PK metrics. This is another artifact of the aggregate criteria. At the 1996 Advisory Committee meeting, it was reported that the data sets from the FDA's files showed that a 14% increase in the average (ABEs only allow 80%–125%) is offset by a 48% in the variability and the test passes IBE but fails ABE. As a result, the 2001 FDA guidance recommends that the point estimate of the ratio of geometric means on the original scale fall within 80%–125% if PBE or IBE approach is employed to assess bioequivalence. However, a point estimate of the ratio of geometric means being within 0.8 and 1.25 on the original scale does not imply the corresponding 90% confidence interval is also within 0.8 and 1.25. It follows that the masking effect remains and two different distributions of exposure measures can be concluded PBE or IBE.

19.2.8 Power and Sample Size Determination

For the proposed aggregated criterion, it is desirable to have sufficient statistical power to declare IBE (or PBE) if the value of the aggregated criterion is small. On the other hand, we would not want to declare IBE or PBE if the value is large. In other words, a desirable property for assessment of bioequivalence is that the power function of the statistical procedure is a monotonic decreasing function of individual bioequivalence criterion (IBC). However, because different combinations of values of the components in the aggregated criteria may reach the same value, the power function for any statistical procedure, based on the proposed aggregated criteria, is not a monotonic decreasing function of IBC. The experience for implementing the aggregate criteria in regulatory approval of generic drugs is still lacking.

Another major concern is how the proposed criteria for PBE and IBE will affect the sample size determination based on powder analysis. Although the 2001 FDA guidance did not provide a close-form formula for sample size determination and recommends that the sample size be determined based only on the method of bootstrap through a Monte Carlo simulation study. However, as mentioned in Chapter 12, Chow et al. (2003a,b) proposed a method for the sample size determination based on the modified large-simple (MLS) method. Because the formula for sample size was based on the aggregate criteria, the drawbacks described above still remain.

19.2.9 Normality Assumptions

The criteria for both PBE and IBE are functions of second-moments of the distribution. For ABE, the criterion is based on average, which is the first moment.

As a result, statistical inference for ABE is quite robust against normality. On the contrary, the statistical inference for IBE or PBE aggregate second-moment criteria may be very sensitive to any mild violation of normality. In addition, the MLS upper confidence limit for evaluation of PBE and IBE proposed by Hyslop et al. (2000), and adopted in the 2001 FDA guidance are derived from the normality assumption. Furthermore, it is not known the impact of departure from the normality on conclusion of PBE or IBE when the aggregate criteria are employed. Therefore, theoretical and empirical research are urgently needed.

19.2.10 Two-Stage Test Procedure

To apply the proposed criteria for assessment of PBE or IBE, the 2001 FDA guidance suggests that a constant scale be used if the observed estimator of σ_{TR} or σ_{WR} is smaller than σ_{T0} or σ_{W0}. However, statistically, the observed estimator of σ_{TR} or σ_{WR} being smaller than σ_{T0} or σ_{W0} does not mean that σ_{TR} or σ_{WR} is smaller than σ_{T0} or σ_{W0}. A test on the null hypothesis that σ_{TR} or σ_{WR} is smaller than σ_{T0} or σ_{W0} is necessarily performed. As a result, the proposed statistical procedure for assessment of PBE or IBE becomes a two-stage test procedure. It is then recommended that the overall type I error rate and the calculation of power be adjusted accordingly.

19.2.11 Study Design

The 2001 FDA guidance recommends that two replicated designs—(TRTR, RTRT) and (TRT, RTR)—be used for assessment of individual bioequivalence. Although some justifications were provided in the guidance, it is unclear whether the two replicated crossover designs are the optimal design in terms of power in 2×4 and 2×3 replicated crossover designs relative to the aggregate criterion. In addition, the 2001 FDA guidance indicates that the 2×4 design is recommended, whereas the 2×3 design is preferred as an alternative. Several questions are raised. First, it is unclear what the relative efficiency of the two designs is if the total number of observations is to be fixed. Second, it is unclear how these two designs compare with other 2×4 and 2×3 replicated designs, such as (TRRT, RTTR) and (TTRR, RRTT) designs, and (TRR, RTT) and (TTR, RRT) designs. Finally, it may be of interest to study the relative merits and disadvantages of these two designs as compared with other designs, such as Latin square designs and four-sequence and four-period designs.

Other issues on the proposed replicated designs include (1) it will take a longer time to complete, (2) subject's compliance may be a concern, (3) it is likely to have a higher dropout rate and missing values especially in 2×4 designs, and (4) there is little literature on statistical methods dealing with dropouts and missing values in a replicated crossover design setting, especially in the context of evaluation of PBE and IBE.

19.3 Guidances on General Considerations for Bioequivalence

As shown in Chapters 11 and 12, the research on population bioequivalence and individual bioequivalence was quite active in 1990s. However, despite of all the research, regulatory implementation of IBE and PBE has been hindered by the masking effect, inability for PK and clinical interpretation, additional cost and feasibility of conducting replicated crossover designs as described in Section 19.2. As a result, at the beginning of the twenty-first century, the *Note for Guidance on the Investigation of Bioequivalence and Bioequivalence* issued by the Committee for Proprietary Medicinal Products (CPMP) of EMEA in January 2002 still recommends the ABE for approval of generic drug products citing the reason of limited experience with IBE and PBE. Then again in March 2003, the U.S. FDA *Guidance on Bioavailability and Bioequivalence Studies for Orally Administered Drug Products—General Considerations* also suggests the use of ABE for approval of generic drugs under ANDA. In addition, inexpensive and affordable generic drugs are vital to the welfare and public health of the people for the developing third world countries. To ensure the safety, efficacy, quality, and exchangeability of the generic drugs, the WHO also issues a draft guideline *Multi-source (Generic) Pharmaceutical Products: Guidelines on Registrations to Establish Interchangeability* in July 2005. The WHO draft guideline also proposes to employ the ABE as the criterion of approving generic drug products. In what follows, we review these three regulatory requirements and provide some comments on the relevant statistical issues.

19.3.1 Design

The 2003 FDA guidance recommends the use of nonreplicate crossover designs for bioequivalence studies of immediate-release and modified-release dosage forms. On the other hand, both 2002 EMEA guidance and the 2005 WHO draft guideline suggest the two-sequence and two-period crossover design is the design of choice for comparison of a test formulation and a reference formulation. Because of a greater sensitivity in assessing release of drug substance from the drug product into the systemic circulation, all three regulatory agencies suggest a single-dose PK bioequivalence studies for both immediate-release and modified-release drug products. On the other hand, for the long half-life drugs, all three regulatory agencies recommend that a parallel-group design can be considered.

In addition, the 2003 FDA guidance requires a washout period of at least 5 half-lives of the moieties to separate two adjacent treatment periods. However, the 2005 WHO draft guideline requests that the duration of the washout be at least 7 days. However, to avoid any ambiguity and misinterpretation, it is very important to clearly specify the beginning and end of a washout period for any bioequivalence study using a crossover design in the regulatory guidelines. We would like to suggest the beginning of a washout period to be the day after the last sampling time point of the previous treatment period. In addition, the end of a washout period is the day before the day of the first sampling time point of the current treatment period.

The 2005 WHO draft guideline also suggests that if the predose concentration of the current treatment period is less than 5% of C_{max}, then the washout period is considered adequate. On the other hand, the 2003 FDA guidance recommends that the PK responses of a subject be deleted from all bioequivalence evaluations if the predose concentration is greater than 5% of C_{max}. In addition, the PK data of subject (s) should be deleted if this subject vomited at or before two times median C_{max}.

19.3.2 Study Population

All three guidelines generally recommend that the PK bioequivalence studies be conducted in healthy normal volunteers to minimize variability and allow detection of differences between the test and reference formulations. In addition, the 2003 FDA guidance requires that the subjects recruited in a BE study represent the general population, taking into consideration age, gender, and race. In addition, the FDA sets the minimum age for enrolment into a BE study is 18 years of age. However, both the EMEA and WHO guidelines set the range of age from 18 to 55 years old for a BE study. Although the sample size for any BE study should provide sufficient power, all three regulatory agencies suggest that the minimum number of subjects for a BE study be 12. In both the EMEA and WHO guidelines, the subjects should preferably be nonsmokers without a history of alcohol or drug abuse and of weight within the normal range.

The 2003 FDA guidance recommends that in general blood, instead of urine or tissue be used for description of the absorption, distribution, and elimination of the drug. To obtain reliable estimates of exposure measures, the 2003 FDA recommends 12–18 samples, including a predose. In addition, the sampling times should continue for at least three or more terminal half-lives of the drug. In order to avoid the situation of first point C_{max}, the FDA suggests that the sampling time points include an early time point between 5 and 15 minutes and additional 2–5 time points in the first hour for evaluation of early peak concentration. However, on the other hand, the 2005 WHO draft guideline recommends a predose time point, at least 1–2 time points around C_{max}, and 3–4 time points during the elimination phase. Therefore, there are a total of at least 7 time points for estimation of the PK parameters which are 5 fewer than what the U.S. FDA requires. In addition, the 2005 WHO draft guideline also suggests that sampling time period should be sufficiently long to ensure than 80% of AUC(0–∞) can be accrued. To protect the safety of the subjects and to avoid excessive sampling, all three regulatory agencies are against sampling beyond 72 hours. The information about the sampling time points is not provided in the 2002 EMEA guidance.

19.3.3 Pharmacokinetic Measures

All three regulatory guidelines suggest the following PK parameters for assessment of ABE in a single dose study between the test and reference formulations: AUC(0–t_k), AUC(0–∞), C_{max}, T_{max}, and half-life. However, the 2003 FDA guidance also requires the elimination rate constant to be included in the report for ANDA submission. For steady-state studies, all three guidelines require the following PK responses:

AUC(0–τ): the area under the concentration–time curve from time 0 to τ over a dosing time interval at steady state

C_{min}: the concentration at the end of a dosing interval

C_{av}: average concentration during a dosing interval

$(C_{max}-C_{min})/C_{av}$: degree of fluctuation

$(C_{max}-C_{min})/C_{min}$: swing

Although the same PK parameters like AUC and C_{max} are employed to evaluate the ABE between the test and reference formulations, the 2003 FDA guidance provides a change in focus from these direct or indirect measures of absorption rate to measures of systematic exposure. Therefore, AUC and C_{max} are used for BE evaluation in terms of their capacity to assess exposure rather than their capacity to reflect the rate and extent of absorption. Furthermore, the 2003 FDA guidance classifies the exposure measures into early, peak and total portions of the concentration–time curve. C_{max}, AUC(0–t_k), and AUC(0–∞) are the measures for the peak and total exposures, respectively. To avoid an excessive hypotensive active of an antihypertensive, one needs to understand the early exposure of the drug for a better control of drug absorption into systemic circulation. In this situation, an early exposure measure may provide useful information than the peak and total exposures. The 2003 FDA guidance recommends the use of the partial AUC for the measure of early exposure. In addition, it also suggest that the partial AUC be truncated at the population mean T_{max} values for the reference formulations and at least two quantifiable samples be collected before the expected C_{max} for an adequate estimation of the partial AUC.

19.3.4 Statistical Analysis

Because in 2001 the U.S. FDA issued guidance on *Statistical Approaches to Establishing Bioequivalence*, the 2003 FDA guidance on general considerations did not emphasize specific statistical methods for evaluation of bioequivalence. However, it mentions that an equivalence approach be recommended and it includes (1) a criterion for comparison, (2) a confidence interval for the criterion, and (3) a bioequivalence limit. As indicated above, the average bioequivalence is the BE criterion adapted by the U.S. FDA, EMEA, and WHO. In addition, all three guidelines recommend that the 90% confidence interval for the ratio of the population averages (Test/Reference) be employed to test the two one-sided tests procedure at the 5% significance level. To establish the ABE, the 90% confidence interval should be within the prespecified limits for ABE. In addition, the 2005 WHO draft guideline also indicates that the statistical procedures leading to a decision scheme be symmetrical with respect to the two formulations under investigation. Furthermore, logarithmic transformation of AUC(0–t_k), AUC(0–∞), and C_{max} is recommended by all three guidelines.

The 2002 EMEA guidance indicates that the log-transformed PK measures should be analyzed by the ANOVA method taking into consideration appropriate sources of variation. The 2005 WHO draft guideline is clearer than the 2002 EMEA guidance and 2003 FDA guidance in that the ANOVA model under the standard 2×2 crossover design should include the formulation, period, sequence (carryover), and subject effects. As indicated in Section 19.2.1, the U.S. FDA does not encourage the sponsors to test for normality of error distribution after log-transformation, nor to use normality of error distribution as a reason for carrying out the statistical analysis on the original scale. Therefore, in general, the analysis for evaluation of ABE is based on parametric methods using normal theory. On the other hand, both the 2002 EMEA guidance and 2005 WHO draft guideline allow alternative approach such nonparametric procedures if the logarithmic transformation of the PK measures is not normally distributed. However, special care should be exercised if the nonparametric methods are used to assess ABE on the original scale. First, the nonparametric approach should take the design feature into account. Second, if the bioequivalence limit is expressed in terms of the ratio of the population means between the test and reference formulations, then the equivalence limit on the original scale is expressed as a percentage of the population reference average which has to be estimated from the data. Therefore, the variability of the estimated reference average is not considered in the equivalence limit, Liu and Weng (1995) show that under the standard two-sequence and two-period crossover design, the size for the two one-sided tests procedure can be inflated to 50%. As a result, Liu and Weng (1995) proposed a modified two one-sided tests procedure on the original scale which can be easily extended to a nonparametric method for evaluation of ABE on the original scale if the normality assumption is violated. Simulation results showed that the nonparametric modified two one-sided tests procedure can adequately control the size at the nominal level (Liu and Weng, 1995).

Due to a longer duration of the crossover design, sometimes, dropouts are inevitable for bioequivalence studies. All three guidances generally discourage replacement of dropouts because of complication of the statistical models and analysis. In addition, all guidelines require that the reasons for early withdrawals and the available data from the dropouts should be fully documented in the report. However, the 2001 FDA guidance on statistical approaches recommends modification of the statistical analysis if the dropout rate is high and sponsors want to add more subjects. If a sponsor wishes to use an add-on design for the bioequivalence study, this should be preplanned in the protocol. The 2005 WHO draft guideline suggests the following considerations for an add-on subject study:

1. Add-on study can be performed using not fewer than half the number of subjects in the initial study.

2. Combining the data from the initial study and add-on study is allowed only if the same protocol is used and the test and reference formulations are from the same batches.

3. It must be carried out strictly according to the study protocol and standard operating procedures.

However, as mentioned in both the 2001 FDA guidance and the 2005 WHO draft guideline, an add-on study is conducted after the initial study was carried out according to the sample size of the protocol and it failed to demonstrate the ABE due to a larger than expected variability or difference. In other words, the add-on study is conducted after the results of the initial study are unblinded. Therefore, bias may be introduced in the add-on study and the type I error rate of falsely declaring ABE will be inflated even though the add-on study is preplanned in the protocol. We would suggest that a group-sequential method for the add-on study be employed. First, the analysis of the initial study is considered as an interim analysis, if the results of the interim analysis meet the requirements of equivalence limits. The study is terminated and the test formulation is concluded to be average bioequivalent to the reference formulation. However, if the results of the interim analysis based on the data from the initial study fail to establish ABE, then sample size should be re-estimated according to the method specified in the protocol and the add-on study is carried out with the additional number of subjects from the sample size re-estimation. However, the interim results should not be disseminated to any personnel involved with the study and sample size estimation should be conducted in a blinded fashion. After the add-on study is completed, the ABE can be assessed with the data from both the initial and add-on studies. However, most importantly, the significance levels for the interim and final analyses should be properly adjusted to control the overall type I error rate at the nominal level. For application of the group sequential method to bioequivalence evaluation, see Gould (1995).

19.3.5 Equivalence Limits

The 2003 FDA guidance requires that the evaluation of ABE should be based on the exposure measures AUC(0–t_k), AUC(0–∞), and $C_{\max}$. Therefore, for these three measures of systemic exposure, geometric average, arithmetic averages, ratio of the averages, and 90% confidence interval should be provided. In addition, ABE between the test and reference formulations is concluded at the 0.05 significance level if the 90% confidence intervals for the ratios of the population averages for the three measures of systemic exposure are completely within 80% and 125%. In addition, the traditional limits of 80% and 125% for the non-narrow therapeutic range drugs remained unchanged for the three exposure measures of narrow therapeutic range drugs. Furthermore, the 2003 FDA guidance does not allow the rounding off of the lower and upper limits of the 90% confidence intervals. In other words, to conclude ABE at the 5% significance level, the lower limit should be at least 80% and the upper limit should be no more than 125%.

Both the 2002 EMEA guidance and the 2005 WHO draft guideline employed the same equivalence limits of 80% and 125% for AUC(0–t_k) and AUC(0–∞). However, for $C_{\max}$, lenient equivalence limits of 75% and 133% can be employed if it is prospectively specified in the protocol and justifications should be given based on efficacy and safety considerations. Both the 2002 EMEA guidance and the 2005 WHO draft guideline recommend the use of nonparametric method to construct the confidence interval for the difference in $T_{\max}$ if there is clinically relevant

TABLE 19.3.1: Comparisons of the U.S. FDA, EMEA, and WHO bioequivalence guidances.

Features	FDA	EMEA	WHO
Date published	March 2003	January 2002	July 2005
Design	Nonreplicate	2×2	2×2
Dose	Single	Single	Single
Duration of washout period	≥ 5 half-lives	—	≥ 7 days
Age	≥ 18	18–55	18–55
Sample size	≥ 12	≥ 12	≥ 12
BE limit			
AUC(0–t_k) and AUC(0–∞)	0.8–1.25	0.8–1.25	0.8–1.25
$C_{\max}$	0.8–1.25	0.75–1.33	0.75–1.33
Analysis for AUC and C_{max}			
CI approach	Yes	Yes	Yes
Log-transformation	Required	Required	Required
Original scale	Not allowed	Allowed	Allowed

claim for rapid onset of action or concerns of adverse reactions. However, no specific bioequivalence limits were provided in the guidance other than the confidence interval should lie within a clinical relevant range. The 2002 EMEA guidance suggests use of tighter equivalence limits for narrow therapeutic range drugs. Table 19.3.1 provides a comparison of the U.S. FDA, EMEA, and WHO bioequivalence guidances.

A highly variable drug is defined as the drug product with the within-subject variability obtained from the within-subject residual mean-squared error of the ANOVA table and expressed in terms of CV is greater than 30%. The 2005 WHO draft guideline does not recommend any suggestions but mentioned the following three approaches used by different drug regulatory jurisdictions:

1. Relax the equivalence limits from 80%–125% to 75%–133%,
2. Use of scaling to relax the equivalence limit. The scale can be the within-subject residual mean-squared error for the standard 2×2 crossover design or the estimated within-subject variability of the reference formulation for the replicated design, and
3. 90% confidence interval fails to lie within 80% and 125% and the ABE can be claimed if the following three conditions are satisfied:
   (i) Total sample size of the initial bioequivalence study is greater than 20 or the total sample size of the initial study and the add-on study is at least 30,
   (ii) Point estimate of the ratio of the geometric averages is within 90% and 111%, and
   (iii) Dissolution profiles of the test and reference formulations are evaluated to be similar using the method described in Chapter 15.

The first approach may be acceptable as long as it is prespecified in the protocol and clinically relevant reasons in terms of efficacy and safety should be provided. The second approach tries to scale the equivalence limit by the estimated within-subject variability. This approach is currently stated in a concept paper on highly variable drug products by the EMEA (2006). The parameter of interest in this approach is

$$(\mu_T - \mu_R)/\sigma, \tag{19.3.1}$$

where

- μ_T and μ_R are the population average of the test and reference formulations on the log-scale
- σ is either the square root of the within-subject residual mean-squared error obtained from the ANOVA table for a nonreplicate design or the with-subject variability of the reference formulation σ_{WR}

Therefore, the criterion for evaluation of ABE is not on the difference in the population averages but on the coefficient of variation. Similar to individual and population bioequivalence, its PK and clinical interpretation on the original scale will be an issue. Furthermore, Tothfalushi and Endrenyi (2003) suggested the methods for the scaled and mixed-scaled ABE and proposed an exact procedure using noncentral *t* distribution. However, their paper used the estimated standard deviation to estimate the unknown noncentrality parameter of the noncentral *t* distribution. On the other hand, Karallis et al. (2004) proposed another type of the scaled ABE based on geometric mean ratio and variability considerations. However, the equivalence limits for the scaled ABE involve the unknown intra-subject variability. As a result, the equivalence limits become random variables and are not fixed constants and the variability introduced by scaling will have an impact on the type I error rate. Therefore, the attempt to use the scaled ABE for resolution of high variable drug products will face the similar issues and challenges that the individual and population bioequivalence encountered in the 1990s as described in Section 19.2. These issues must be satisfactorily addressed before the scaled ABE can be implemented into regulatory framework.

The third approach was suggested by the 1997 Japanese guideline for bioequivalence studies of generic products. It relies on the correlation between the *in vitro* dissolution similarity and *in vivo* bioequivalence. However, this assumption is very difficult to verify. In addition, no theoretical and empirical evidence on the type I error rate of this approach were provided. Further research on the third approach is urgently required.

19.4 Guidances on Bioequivalence for Special Drug Products

In this section, guidances on bioequivalence studies for some special drug products are reviewed. The first is the clozapine tablets for indication of the management of patients with severe schizophrenia who fail to respond adequately to the standard antipsychotic drug treatment. Because clozapine can cause serious adverse events such as hypotension, bradycardia, syncope, and asystole, the U.S. FDA recommends that bioequivalence be conducted in patients but not in health volunteers. On the other hand, the 1994 FDA guideline suggests that the measures of the systemic exposure for evaluation of ABE for slow-release potassium chloride tablets should be those derived from urine in a three-sequence and three-period crossover design. Finally, the 2000 EMEA guidance addressed some special issues on evaluation of ABE for modified-release oral and transdermal dosage forms. In the following sections, these three guidances are reviewed and comments regarding statistical issues are provided.

19.4.1 Clozapine Tablets

The original 1996 FDA guidance on bioequivalence studies for clozapine tablets recommended a single-dose study using 12.5 mg dose in healthy volunteers. However, due to the serious adverse events described above, in January 2005, the U.S. FDA issued a new guidance in which a single-dose study using 12.5 mg dose in healthy volunteers is no longer recommended. Instead, the 2005 FDA guidance suggests multiple-dose steady studies for evaluation of clozapine drug products at the highest dosage strength of 100 mg tablets in patients who are already receiving an established maintenance dose of an approved clozapine drug and have failed to respond adequately to the standard antipsychotic drug treatment.

As for any research, one has to clearly understand the PK characteristics of the drug to design an adequate bioequivalence studies. Table 19.4.1 provides some PK properties of clozapine. From these PK characteristics of clozapine and patient's

TABLE 19.4.1: Pharmacokinetic characteristics of clozapine.

Parameter	Characteristic
C_{max} at steady-state for 100 mg	
Average	2.5 hours
Range	1–6 hours
Elimination half-life for 75 mg	
Average	8 hours
Range	4–12 hours
Steady-state half-life for 100 mg	
Average	12 hours
Range	4–66 hours
Food effect	No
Dose proportionality	Yes

need, the 2005 FDA recommends the design for evaluation of bioequivalence for clozapine is the standard two-sequence and two-period crossover design. However, in order to reach steady state, the duration of each treatment period is 10 days without a washout period between the two treatment periods. Because severe schizophrenia is a very serious illness, patients should not be off the appropriate therapy. Therefore, one important inclusion criterion of the patients is that patients should be appropriate candidates for clozapine therapy and have been taking a stable dose of clozapine for at least 3 months. In addition, patients are eligible for the study of 100 mg by continuing their established maintenance dose if they are receiving multiples of 100 mg every 12 hours. As a result, half of the patients will be randomized to each of the two sequences of the standard 2×2 crossover design. Either the test or reference formulation will be administrated at 100 mg every 12 hours for 10 days. After the study is completed, the patients should be continued on their current dose using an approved clozapine drug product as prescribed by their physicians.

Patients should be hospitalized for at least two days to collect PK samples. To confirm steady-state blood plasma/serum levels, the predose blood samples at three successive trough levels should be collected on days 7, 8, and 9. After fasting for at least 8 hours prior to and 4 hours after the administration of morning dose on day 10 of each period, venous blood samples should be collected at 0.25, 0.5, 1.0, 2.0, 2.5, 3.0, 3.5, 4.0, 5.0, 6.0, 8.0, 10.0, and 12.0 hours. The PK measures for the steady-state studies described in Section 19.3.3 should be provided. However, evaluation of ABE is based on AUC(0–τ) and $C_{\max}$ on the log-scale with the same equivalence limits of 80% and 125%.

From the above depiction, the bioequivalence studies for clozapine are of high degree of difficulty. First, the duration of the study is very long and the patients have to be hospitalized for at least two days. Consequently, it is anticipated that dropout rates will be higher than the traditional single-dose bioequivalence studies. Second, to be eligible for the study, patients must have been taking a stable dose of clozapine and after the completion of the study patients will continue their current dose using an approved clozapine. What will happen if the current maintenance dose is from an approved clozapine drug product which is different from the reference formulation used in the bioequivalence study? Of course, switch between two approved drugs of clozapine is clinically feasible and allowable. However, in an experiment setting for evaluation of bioequivalence, this switch in conjunction with no washout period between two treatment periods will certainly have an impact on the conclusion of bioequivalence. The 2005 FDA guidance on clozapine requires that the trough concentration data be statistically analyzed to verify that steady state is reached before PK sampling. However, the duration of each treatment period is based on the average PK characteristics of clozapine. In addition, from Table 19.4.1, the ranges in the PK measures such as $C_{\max}$ at steady state for 100 mg or steady-state half-life for 100 mg are quite wide. Therefore, it is quite possible that the steady state is not reached for some patients in either or both treatment periods. How to handle the data for the patients who fail to reach steady state is another statistical issue. See Section 18.4 for the statistical methods of verifying the steady state.

19.4.2 Slow-Release Potassium Chloride Tablets

Potassium chloride (KCL) tablet is indicated for K^+ depletion or hypokalemia which can occur during prolonged diuretic therapy, hyperaldosteronism, diabetic ketoacidosis, or gastrointestinal loss through vomiting or diarrhea. The guidance on bioequivalence studies for slow-release (SR) potassium chloride tablets was initially issued in May 1987. The original 1987 FDA guidance suggests a single-dose, three-sequence and three-period crossover design, including an approved KCL liquid product served as the immediate-release reference, for evaluation of bioequivalence of SR potassium chloride tablets. However, in June 1994, in answering the questions about the design and analysis of bioequivalence studies for ER KCL tablets by a sponsor, the U.S. FDA responded that a single-dose, fasting study using the standard two-treatment, two-sequence and two-period crossover design without an approved KCL liquid product should be employed for evaluation of ER KCL tablets. The special characteristic of the bioequivalence studies for evaluation of ER KCL tablets is that the measures of systemic exposure are not derived from the plasma, serum, or blood concentration–time profile but from urine for amounts of excretion of K^+. Because evaluation of bioequivalence of ER KCL tablets is based on excretion of K^+ and people normally also excrete K^+ through urine and sweat, special considerations in design must be taken to control this known but different variation.

The 1994 FDA guidance recommend that the bioequivalence study be conducted with at least 24 healthy normal male subjects with age between 20 and 40 years, within $\pm 10\%$ of ideal body weight, and without serious renal, gastrointestinal, cardiovascular, hepatic, or adrenal–pituitary disorders. The experimental condition should be a climate-controlled environment such that the subjects do not lose potassium through sweat. The other special considerations in design of bioequivalence studies for ER KCL are that the subjects should receive definite amount of potassium, sodium, water, and calories in daily diet throughout the study; and they have to be adequately hydrated at regular time intervals throughout the study so that sufficient amount of urine can be obtained. Therefore, Table 19.4.2 provides some information about the amount of daily intakes for potassium, sodium, calories, and fluid as suggested in the 1994 FDA guidance. Subjects are strongly advised to ingest the required amounts and only those amounts in Table 19.4.2 and to avoid unnecessary physical activities. In addition subjects are required to report any prolong episodes of diarrhea or excessive sweating. The 1994 FDA guidance also suggest that the dose of ER KCL in the bioequivalence study be 80 mEq.

TABLE 19.4.2: Amount of daily intakes of potassium, sodium, calories, and fluids.

Item	Amount
Potassium	50–60 mEg/day
Sodium	160–180 mEg/day
Calorie	2500–3000 calories/day
Fluids	3000–5000 mL/day

Each treatment period is further divided into three cycles: diet equilibration days, baseline days, and drug dosing days. Diet equilibration days are from day 1 to day 4 in which standard amount of sodium, potassium, calories and fluids are administrated according to the intake amounts given in Table 19.4.2. 500 mL of the fluids should be given at 7 AM and then 200 mL every hour for 12 hours. No urine will be collected during the diet equilibration days. Baseline days are from day 5 to day 6. During the baseline day, sodium, potassium, calories, and fluids are administrated as the diet equilibration days. In addition, the urine is collected each day according to the following schedules:

Day 5: 7 AM, 0–1, 1–2, 2–4, 4–6, 6–8, 8–12, 12–16, and 16–24 hours after 7 AM
Day 6: same as day 5 except voiding 7 AM sample

The objective of collecting the urine samples during the baseline days is to establish each subject's baseline level of potassium excretion.

The drug dosing days are from day 7 to day 8. The subjects are administrated 80 mEq dose of ER KCL at 7 AM on day 7. Sodium, potassium, calories, fluids, and diets are administrated as the diet equilibration days. However, subjects should remain upright for 3 hours following dosing. Urine samples are collected at 0–1, 1–2, 2–4, 4–6, 6–8, 8–12, 12–16, and 16–24 hours on day 7 and day 8. There is no actual washout period between two treatment periods. Day 1 to day 4 of the second treatment period (day 9 to day 12) serves as the diet equilibration days of period II as well as the washout period.

The measures of interest for evaluation of bioequivalence for ER KCL are cumulative urinary excretion of K^+ from 0 to 24 hours, maximal rate of excretion (R_{max}), the time of maximal urinary excretion (T_{max}) and a rate profile (rates at 0–1, 1–2, 2–4, 4–6, 6–8, 8–12, 12–16, and 16–24 hours). The urinary measures at each time interval of the dosing days should be subtracted by the corresponding average baseline excretion of K^+. In addition, the baseline amount of excretion of K^+ should be subject-specific and period-specific. In other words, the urinary measures of each period for each subject should be subtracted by the subject's baseline amount of the same period. The 1994 FDA guidance also requests the following statistical quantities for cumulative urinary excretion from 0 to 24 hours, R_{max}, and T_{max}:

1. Power of the study to detect difference of 20% of the reference means
2. 90% confidence interval using the two one-sided t test
3. Westlake's 95% symmetrical confidence intervals

Since the original guidance was issued in 1987, it did not incorporate the latest development of statistical methodology for evaluation of ABE. In addition, there is some inconsistency between the 1987 original guidance and the 1994 comments. For example, the 1987 original guidance require urine collection only for one day after dosing on day 6. However, the 1994 comments suggest a two-day urine collection (day 7 and day 8) after dosing on day 7. It is not clear that how the urine excretion on day 7 and day 8 are adjusted by the baseline data on day 5 and day 6. In addition, the urinary measures for evaluation of bioequivalence for ER KCL tablets are based on an interval from 0 to 24 hours. Therefore, it needs to clarify how the cumulative urinary excretion from 0 to 24 hours, R_{max}, and T_{max} are computed.

Unlike the 2003 FDA guidance on general considerations for bioequivalence studies, the 1994 FDA guidance for evaluation of bioequivalence for ER KCL tablets does not specify whether the analyses should be performed on the original or log-scale. In addition, the power to detect difference of 20% of the reference means is only applicable only when the power approach described in Section 5.3.4 is employed. However, from Section 5.3.4, the power approach has lots of drawbacks and currently is no longer used to evaluation of ABE. Both 90% classical confidence interval and Westlake's 95% symmetrical confidence interval are required by the 1994 FDA guidance. However, Section 4.2.2 points out that Westlake's 95% symmetrical confidence interval is not symmetrical about the observed average difference and shifts from a two-sided to a one-sided approach. As a result, as in line with the current state of art, we suggest the use of the classic confidence interval for evaluation of bioequivalence for ER KCL tablets. In addition, if the analysis is performed on the original scale, then the modified two one-sided tests procedure (Liu and Weng, 1995) should be used to avoid excessive type I error rate.

19.4.3 Modified Release Oral and Transdermal Dosage Form

The EMEA issued a note on guidance on modified release oral and transdermal dosage forms in 1999. It classifies modified release oral dosage forms into two classes. The first class is the prolonged release formulation and the second class is the delayed release formulation. The advantages of a prolonged release formulation, as pointed in the EMEA 1999 guidance include (1) unnecessary repetitions of high concentrations to produce and maintain full efficacy and (2) a desirable clinical effect at a lower dose without a high level of adverse events. On the other hand, the objectives of a delayed release formulation consists of (1) protection of the active ingredients from the acid environment of the stomach and vice versa and (2) releasing the active ingredient in a defined segment of the intestine to decrease drug absorption and to yield local action.

The 1999 EMEA guidance recommends that bioavailability and bioequivalence should provide the following information of characterization of modified release dosage forms:

1. Rate and extent of absorption.
2. Fluctuations in drug concentrations.
3. Variability in PKs arising from the drug formulation.
4. Dose proportionality.
5. Factors impacting the performance of the modified drug formulation.
6. Risk of unexpected release characteristics (e.g., dose dumping).

In addition the factors considered for influencing the performance of the modified drug formulation include food, gastrointestinal function, diurnal rhythms, and site of application. If a test modified release formulation is different from the reference formulation in release controlling excipients or mechanism but has the similar *in vitro* dissolution profile, then only the PK bioequivalence studies are required for approval. However, if the *in vitro* dissolution profiles are also different from the reference formulation, then clinical trials should be considered for bioequivalence. Therefore, for a prolonged release formulation, at least one fasting bioequivalence study and one fed bioequivalence study are required. The standard two-treatment, two-sequence, and two-period crossover design should be employed in both studies. The results of both studies should demonstrate that the test formulation exhibits the similar prolonged release characteristics as the reference formulation. In addition, ABE must be demonstrated after single dose and at the steady state. However, as requested in the 1999 EMEA guidance, if the prolonged release dosage forms are in the single-unit formulation with multiple strengths, then a single-dose fasting bioequivalence study is required for each strength. The steady-state studies may be conducted at the highest strength.

Similar to the prolonged release formulations, ABE of the test transdermal formulation must be shown after single dose and after multiple dose administration. In addition, the site of application for the bioequivalence study should be in the same body area for both the test and reference formulation. Unlike the prolonged release formulations, the bioequivalence study may be required only at the highest strength if there are multiple strengths for approval. In addition to the traditional measures of systemic exposures, for transdermal dosage form, the test formulation should demonstrate similar or less degree of local irritation, adhesiveness to the skin, phototoxicity, sensitization, and systemic adverse events. Because most of transdermal patches are highly variable rug products due to their route of absorption, the 1999 EMEA guidance recommend the use of replicate design to estimate the intra-subject variability. On the other hand, if the test formulation has a different release mechanism, for example, matrix versus reservoir, then a replicate design can be used to detect the existence of subject-by-formulation interaction.

The traditional measures of systemic exposure for the single dose and steady state described in the Section 19.3.3 are recommended by the EMEA for evaluation of ABE of modified release and transdermal dosage forms.

The guidelines provided in the 1999 EMEA guidance are quite general and flexible for evaluation of ABE of modified release and transdermal dosage forms. However, it can be more specific on design for transdermal dosage form because the patch is applied on the individual. In addition, the guidance for the duration of the washout period of the prolonged release formulation and transdermal formulation should be provided. Replicate designs may provide important information about the intra-subject variability or subject-by-formulation interactions. However, the durations of replicate designs will be much longer especially for the prolonged release formulations and transdermal dosage form with the requirement of ABE at the steady state after multiple dosing. Since the 1999 EMEA guidance requires that local reactions and systemic adverse event profiles be compared between the test and reference formulations, they are in general correlated categorical data under crossover designs. As a result, appropriate statistical methods for correlated categorical data should be applied (Agresti, 2002).

19.5 Critical Path Opportunities for Generic Drugs

In 2004, the U.S. FDA announced the critical path initiatives (2004, 2006a, 2006b) which basically focused on the challenges involved in the research and development of novel and cutting-edge innovative drugs, biologics, and devices. As indicated in Chapter 1, to obtain approval, generic drug products must be pharmaceutical equivalent of the same active ingredients in the same strength in the same dosage form and must also demonstrate average bioequivalent to the reference list drug. For most of drug products, ABE can be demonstrated using the measures of systemic exposure derived from the plasma drug concentrations in health normal volunteers. However, as shown in the previous sections of this chapter, examples of ER KCL, clozapine, and transdermal patches, alternative methodology is applied although the concept and principles of ABE remain the same. Another is example is *in vivo* bioequivalence studies for topical dermatologic corticosteroids. The 1995 FDA guidance suggests the use of the area under effect curve derived from pharmacodynamic measurements of the skin blanching response with a chromameter (FDA, 1995). Application of the 1995 FDA guidance to the Japanese population received mixed results. (Keida et al., 2006) Therefore, in May 2007 the U.S. FDA issued a document on the critical path opportunities for generic drugs that provides the opportunities as well as challenges to the attention of interested parties for facilitating generic drug product development.

Table 19.5.1 presents the critical path opportunity areas for generic drug products identified by the U.S. FDA. From Table 19.5.1, The U.S. FDA classifies the critical path opportunities for generic drug into four areas: quality by design, systemically acting drugs, locally acting and target delivery drugs, and complex drug substances and products. Within each area, there are several topics for different opportunities. The first area is quality by design. As pointed out by the U.S. FDA critical path opportunities for generic drugs, quality is built into the final product by understanding controlling formulation and manufacturing variables and testing is used to verify the quality of the final product. This concept of formulation and manufacturing process control is not new but exists in many years. Chow and Liu (1995b) provide some fundamental statistical understanding and methods for controlling the variables in formulation and manufacturing process so that there is a high probability that the final product will meet the required quality for the drug product.

Another opportunity for quality by design is to develop some methods for *in vitro vivo* correlation (IVIVC). Because large amounts of results of dissolution tests and ABE studies based on PK measures of generic products have accumulated over years. One way to develop such correlation is to use the results of f_2 and 90% confidence intervals for the ratio of geometric averages based on AUC and $C_{\max}$. For each product, the value of f_2 can be further classified as smaller than 50 or greater than or equal to 50 and the results of bioequivalence studies can be groups whether they meet the criterion of (80%, 125%) as shown in Table 19.5.2. If there is a good IVIVC, a and d should be large and b and c should be

TABLE 19.5.1: Critical path opportunity areas for generic drug products.

Area	Topic	Opportunity
Quality by design	Model development and *in vitro*/*in vivo* correlations	Better absorption models Development of *in vitro vivo* correlations
	Formulation and manufacture of generic drugs	Formulation expert systems *In vitro* tests to test formulation Development of process simulation tools
Systemic acting drugs	Expanding BCS biowaivers	Biowaivers for BCS class II drugs Biowaivers for BCS class III drugs Development of biorelevant dissolution
	Fed bioequivalence studies Novel delivery technologies Highly variables drugs Inhalation products	Food and drug interactions PK profiles with multiple peaks Transdermal products Molecular level imaging Novel pharmacodynamic study designs Study design for combination products

		Study designs for COPD
		Evaluation of difference in formulation composition
		Modeling and simulation of dry powder inhaler performance and drug delivery
Locally acting and targeted delivery drugs	Nasal sprays	Computation modeling of drug delivery
		Direct measure of particle size equivalence
	Topical dermatological products	Design bioequivalence trials with clinical endpoints
		In vitro characterization of topical dermatological products
		Local delivery of topical dermatological products
	Gastrointestinal acting products	Biowaivers for low solubility drugs
		In vivo drug release for GI acting products
		Establishment of biomarkers for local delivery to GI tract
Complex drug substance and products	Liposome formulations	Methods for liposome-based formulations
	Natural source drugs	Improve analytical methods for identity
		Statistical methods for profile comparisons

Source: Adapted from the U.S. Food and Drug Administration Critical Path Opportunities for Generic Drugs, 2007.

TABLE 19.5.2: *In vitro/in vivo* correlation.

Results of *In Vitro* Dissolution Test of f_2	Results of Bioequivalence Studies		
	BE	NBE	Total
≥ 50	a	b	$a+b$
≤ 50	c	d	$c \pm d$
Total	$a+c$	$b+d$	$a+b+c+d$

smaller. In Table 19.5.2, b represents the number of false positive in which the generic drug product passes the *in vitro* dissolution f_2 test but fails to meet the *in vivo* ABE. On the other hand, c is the amount of generic products that fails to show similarity in dissolution profiles but meets the ABE. We anticipate c should be small. To have a better understanding of the relationship between f_2 and success rate of ABE, the receiver's operating characteristic (ROC) curve can be constructed with different value of f_2 for the cutoff points and the area under the ROC curve can be used to evaluate the predicting probability of f_2 (Feinstein, 2002).

The 2007 FDA critical path opportunities for generic drugs also identify novel modified release formulation with multiple peaks, transdermal products and highly variable drugs as additional opportunities. However, these issues are not really new as we just reviewed in Section 19.4. Apparently, no satisfactorily regulatory solution is currently available and the U.S. FDA puts these issues as the challenges for the generic drug development. However, before the possible solutions are proposed, one has to really understand the functions and characteristics of the novel formulation. For example, what are the functions of multiple peaks for modified release formulations? If it is required to show bioequivalence for each peak, then multivariate approaches or some adjustment of multiple comparisons may be applied. In addition, as mentioned in Section 19.4.3, clinical outcomes such as skin irritation, sensitization potential, and adhesive performance currently are recorded in either binary data or ordered categorical data. Therefore, a large number of subjects are required to compare the test transdermal formulation to the reference formulation. For the design efficiency, new measures with much improved sensitivity and less variability must be developed for skin irritation, sensitization potential, or adhesive performance.

For inhalation drug products, three different types of bioequivalence studies are required to obtain approval of generic copies. The first type is the *in vitro* test for device performance. The second type is the pharmacodynamic bioequivalence study based on the performance of lung function for local delivery and the last type is the traditional PK bioequivalence study for systemic exposure. In Chapter 14, some statistical methods for *in vitro* bioequivalence tests were presented for nasal sprays. On the other hand, statistical designs and methods for the pharmacodynamic bioequivalence study based on FEV1 are provided in Chapter 13. As indicated in the 2007 FDA critical path opportunities for generic drugs, despite the facts that statistical methods are available and many of the older MDI products currently on the market do not have protection of patents, few applications were filed because the difficulty of demonstration of bioequivalence in three types of studies. These three types of bioequivalence studies can be thought as another translation research: translation from equivalence in product performance to equivalence in PK measures and then to equivalence in pharmacodynamic parameters. As any type of the translation research, the variability increases as it moves from *in vitro* testing in device to *in vivo* testing in human. To have a high probability of success in translation, it is very important to keep the variability under control or develop new assays or outcome measures with high sensitivity and low variability.

For MDI products, there are in fact a total of two stages of translations: one from *in vitro* device performance to PK bioequivalence and another from PK bioequivalence to pharmacodynamic bioequivalence. In each stage, one can build a translation calibration curve to find the correlation in two states of the translation and compute the probability of success of translation from one state to another state. The IVIVC mentioned above is another type of translation. If for a certain product, the probability of a success from a previous state to a subsequent state is very high, then from a regulatory point of view, the testing at the subsequent state may be waived. This is extremely important for development of generic drug products if costly and time consuming *in vivo* PK, pharmacodynamic, or clinical bioequivalence trials can be waived due to high correlations between each pair of adjacent states. However, statistical strategies and methodology for assessment of correlations between translation states are urgently required.

19.6 Discussion

Back to 1997, the U.S. FDA issued the draft guidance on *in vivo* bioequivalence studies based on population and individual bioequivalence approaches with the attempt to replace the ABE with individual bioequivalence or population bioequivalence as the criteria for regulatory approval of generic drug products. (FDA, 1997c). However, the draft guidance on population and individual bioequivalence, the rationale for switching from ABE to PBE or IBE lacks (1) convincing clinical evidence of the limitations of ABE for addressing drug interchangeability and (2) a valid scientific/statistical justification of PBE and IBE. It is, then, recommended that clinical evidence for the limitations of ABE and scientific/statistical justification of PBE or IBE be carefully evaluated before the proposed PBE and IBE criteria and the corresponding approaches are implemented as standard requirement for assessment of bioequivalence. To provide convincing clinical evidence of the limitations of ABE for addressing drug interchangeability, it would be helpful to study the incidence rates of the failure or critical safety issue of approved generic drug products in the past decade. A high incidence rate may indicate that there is a deficiency in the current regulation of ABE. If the incidence rate is relatively low and considered clinically acceptable, then there is no need to switch from ABE to

PBE or IBE, especially because their clinical performance is unknown. On the other hand, to provide scientific/statistical justification for the use of PBE or IBE, it is suggested that the probabilities of consistencies and inconsistencies for bioequivalence assessment based on ABE, PBE, and IBE be evaluated (Liu and Chow, 1997a). If the probability of consistency between ABE and PBE or IBE is high, and the probability of inconsistency is small, then there is no need to switch from ABE to PBE or IBE because ABE, PBE, and IBE will basically reach the same conclusion for bioequivalence. If there is a relatively high probability of inconsistency between ABE and PBE or IBE, with a relatively low probability of consistency between ABE and PBE or IBE, then the influence on clinical performance for the switch from ABE to PBE or IBE is necessarily provided. In this case, instead of switching from ABE to PBE or IBE, we might tighten the bioequivalence limits for ABE to achieve the same result for IBE. Due to issues described above and difficulties of regulatory implementation of IBE or PBE mentioned in Section 19.2, the 2003 FDA guidance on the general considerations for bioequivalence studies still recommends the ABE as the criterion for regulatory requirement although IBE or PBE remain as the optional criteria in the 2001 FDA guidance on statistical approaches to establishing bioequivalence.

In addition to the efficacy and safety, the identity, strength, quality, purity, and stability of approved generic drug products are also important drug characteristics that have an effect on average bioavailability, variability of bioavailability, and variability due to subject-by-formulation interaction and, consequently, drug interchangeability. As a result, it is suggested that regulatory requirements for post-approval equivalence in laboratory development and the manufacturing process be established, regardless of the switch from ABE to PBE or IBE.

In this chapter, we have reviewed the currently available guidances for evaluation of bioequivalence issued by regulatory agencies such as the U.S. FDA, EMEA, and WHO. These guidelines include general considerations for orally administrated dosage forms, statistical methods for evaluation of bioequivalence, and special guidelines for some particular drug products for which the methods for evaluation of bioequivalence are not covered by the guidance on general considerations. Only the U.S. FDA issued guidance on statistical approaches and most of guidelines for special drug products. In addition, in May 2007 the U.S. FDA also issued the critical path opportunities for generic drugs although some of the challenges issued in the critical path opportunities are not new. However, some areas with emerging importance are not addressed in the critical path opportunities for generic drugs. These new areas include the use of genomic data to facilitating evaluation of bioequivalence, methodological issues in evaluation of bioequivalence of biologic products, concept and evaluation of substantial equivalence for medical devices, and bridging bioequivalence studies for developing countries. These issues are some future challenges that will be covered in Chapter 20.

Chapter 20

Frequently Asked Questions and Future Challenges

20.1 Introduction

According to Saul (2007), the United States spends about 275 billion dollars annually on prescription drug products. In addition, she also pointed out that in the next 5 years, a series of innovative drug products with a total combined sale of 60 billion dollars per year are going off patents. This opens a door of tidal wave of generic drug products that are 30%–80% cheaper. In addition, despite that the number of prescriptions is increasing due to an aging population in the United States, the spending is even slower than before. This has led to the passage of the Drug Price Competition and Patent Term Restoration Act in 1984, which allows a regulatory framework for low-cost pathway for generic drug products to enter the market (Frank, 2007). However, as pointed out by Saul (2007), a survey conducted in 2002 by the Association of American Retire People (AARP) indicated that 22% of the responders considered that generic drug products are less effective or of poor quality than the innovator drug products. This shows that a sizable portion of the public in the United States still lacks confidence in generic drug products even they are approved by the regulatory authorities based on the criterion of average bioequivalence. Therefore, in May 2007, the U.S. FDA added generic drugs in the critical path opportunities to use latest breakthroughs in technique to assure that the efficacy and safety of the generic drug products are same as those of the innovator drug products.

However, the U.S. FDA critical path opportunities for generic drugs do not cover all important emerging challenges for generic drugs. The first one is how to use the currently genomic information into assessment of bioequivalence of generic products. In Section 20.2, we review a method proposed by Chow et al. (2004) to incorporate the genomic data into assessment of average, population, and individual bioequivalence (IBE). The second challenge occurs in most of the developing countries in which almost all available drugs are generic drug products because of high costs of the innovator drug products. Therefore, if a local generic sponsor is to develop a generic product, selection of the comparator then becomes an issue for approval. This is because the innovator drug product on the WHO list (2005b) is not approved in the developing countries and hence, it cannot be used as a comparator in the bioequivalence study for evaluation of the generic copy of the local sponsor. We refer this challenge as bridging bioequivalence problem which is discussed in Section 20.3. Another important but yet still unresolved issue is evaluation of bioequivalence for biosimilar or follow-on biological drug products. Because most of the biological products are complicated large molecules, the question lies on whether one can actually manufacture a biosimilar drug product that is truly, biologically and functionally equivalent to the innovator biological product. In addition, the patents of most of the first generation of biological products approved in 1980s will expire in the next 5 years. Therefore, there is an urgent need to address this critical issue of evaluation of bioequivalence of follow-on biological drug products which is discussed in Section 20.4. In Section 20.5, a list of frequently asked questions (FAQ) in assessment of bioequivalence is provided. We address some of these issues and make some suggestions whether more research is required or some of current regulation can be modified. Discussion and final remarks are provided in Section 20.6.

20.2 Assessment of Bioequivalence Using Genomic Information

As discussed in Chapter 15, for some drug products, the FDA indicates that an *in vitro* dissolution testing may serve as a surrogate for an *in vivo* bioequivalence testing by comparing the dissolution profiles between drug products. Two drug products are considered to have a similar drug absorption profile if their dissolution profiles are similar. These drug products include (1) pre-1962 classified "AA" drug products, (2) lower strength products, (3) scale-up and postapproval change, and (4) products demonstrating *in vitro* and *in vivo* correlation (Chow and Shao, 2002). Along this line, Chow et al. (2004) proposed assessing bioequivalence using genomic data. In other words, under the assumption that two drug products will have a similar drug absorption profile if their genomic profiles are similar provided that there is a well-established relationship between the pharmacokinetic (PK) parameters and the genomic data. This concept is useful in establishing bioequivalence especially between a new (or modified) formulation and a reference formulation of an innovative drug product going off patent protection if it is accepted by the regulatory agencies.

Let x be a genomic prediction of a PK response under consideration. Typically, x is a function of genomic data such as genetic markers, DNA sequence, mRNA transcription profiling, linkage and physical maps, gene location, and quantitative trait loci (QTL) mapping. Chow et al. (2004) attempted to use the genomic prediction x as a surrogate for the PK response in assessing bioequivalence. More specifically, if we can claim bioequivalence between two drug products using x in place of the PK response but the same statistical test designed for PK data, can we claim bioequivalence between the two drug products without a bioavailability/bioequivalence study?

The answer is affirmative if x is a perfect prediction of the PK response. In practice, however, genomic prediction is usually not perfect, because of the existence of variability, model misspecification, and missing important genomic variables. The idea of Chow et al. (2004) is to evaluate the impact of the differences between the distribution of the genomic prediction and PK response on the assessment of bioequivalence. For ABE, a tolerance limit for this difference is derived so that if the difference is within the tolerance limit, then ABE can be assessed by using the genomic prediction. For PBE and IBE, Chow et al. (2004) consider a sensitivity analysis of prediction bias and variation difference within some predetermined limits.

20.2.1 Bioequivalence Criteria, Design, and Model

Bioequivalence is usually assessed through a statistical test for the following hypotheses:

$$\begin{aligned} &\mathrm{H_0}:\ \theta \geq \eta \\ \text{versus}\quad &\mathrm{H_1}:\ \theta < \eta, \end{aligned} \tag{20.2.1}$$

where
θ is a parameter measuring the bioequivalence between two drug products
η is a given equivalence limit set by regulatory agencies

If $\mathrm{H_0}$ is rejected at the 5% level, then the two drug products under consideration are bioequivalent. Let y_T and y_R be log-transformed PK responses under drug treatment T (test formulation) and R (reference formulation), respectively. If

$$\theta = |E(y_\mathrm{T} - y_\mathrm{R})|,$$

then testing hypotheses 20.2.1 is referred to as assessing average bioequivalence (ABE). If

$$\theta = \frac{E(y_\mathrm{T} - y_\mathrm{R})^2 - E(y_\mathrm{R} - y'_\mathrm{R})^2}{E(y_\mathrm{R} - y'_\mathrm{R})^2/2}, \tag{20.2.2}$$

where y'_R is an independent replicate of y_R (from a different patient), then testing hypotheses 20.2.1 is referred to as assessing population bioequivalence (PBE). If θ is given by Equation 20.2.2 but y_R and y'_R are repeated measurements from the same patient, then testing hypotheses 20.2.1 is referred to as assessing IBE. For different types of bioequivalence, the limit η takes different values.

In a bioequivalence study, pharmacokinetic (PK) data are usually obtained from a standard 2×2 or a 2×4 replicated crossover design. Let y_{ijkl} be the log-transformed PK response from the kth subject ($k = 1, \ldots, n_j$) in the jth sequence ($j = 1, 2$) under the lth replicate ($l=1$, 2) of treatment i ($i=$T, R). As indicated earlier, the usual model under this replicated design is the one given by Chinchilli and Esinhart (1996):

$$y_{ijkl} = \mu_i + \gamma_{ijl} + S_{ijk} + e_{ijkl}, \tag{20.2.3}$$

where

μ_i is the treatment effect

γ_{ijl} is the fixed effect of the lth replicate on treatment i in sequence j with the constraint $\sum_j \sum_l \gamma_{ijl} = 0$ for each i

(S_{Tjk}; S_{Rjk}) values are the random effect of the kth subject in the jth sequence that are i.i.d. bivariate normal random vectors (with mean 0, $\text{Var}(S_{ijk})=\sigma_{Bi}^2$, $i=$T, R), and $\text{Cov}(S_{Tjk}, S_{Rjk})=\rho\,\sigma_{BT}\sigma_{BR}$, e_{ijkl} values are independent normal random errors (with mean 0 and $\text{Var}(e_{ijkl})=\sigma_{Wi}^2$, $i=$T, R), and (S_{Tjk}; S_{Rjk}) and e_{ijkl} values are independent. Under model 20.2.3, $\theta=|\delta|$ for ABE, where $\delta=\mu_T-\mu_R$, $\theta=(\delta^2+\sigma_T^2-\sigma_R^2)/\sigma_R^2$ for PBE, where $\sigma_i^2=\sigma_{Bi}^2+\sigma_{Wi}^2$, $i=$T, R, and $\theta=(\delta^2+\sigma_D^2+\sigma_{WT}^2-\sigma_{WR}^2)/\sigma_{WR}^2$ for IBE, where $\sigma_D^2=\sigma_{BT}^2+\sigma_{BR}^2-2\rho\sigma_{BT}\sigma_{BR}$.

Our concern is to test hypotheses 20.2.1 by using x_{ijkl}, the genomic prediction of y_{ijkl}. We assume that x_{ijkl} values follow the model in Equation 20.2.3 but with all parameters changed. In particular, treatment effects, μ values are changed to ν values and variance components σ^2's are changed to τ^2 values. Define

$$\varepsilon = (\mu_T - \mu_R) - (\nu_T - \nu_R). \tag{20.2.4}$$

Note that $\varepsilon=0$ if the genomic predictions are unbiased. Because of possible model misspecification and missing important genomic variables, however, ε may not be 0.

20.2.2 Assessment of ABE

ABE can be assessed under the standard 2×2 crossover design. Thus, the subscript l in y_{ijkl} can be dropped (i.e., $y_{ijkl}=y_{ijk}$). Let $\bar{y}$ or $\bar{x}$ be the average of y-values or x-values with a dot in the subscript indicating which index is averaging over:

$$\widehat{\delta}_y = \bar{y}_{T\cdot\cdot} - \bar{y}_{R\cdot\cdot},$$

and

$$s_y^2 = \frac{1}{n_1+n_2-2}\sum_{j,k}(y_{Tjk} - y_{Rjk} - \bar{y}_{Tj\cdot} + \bar{y}_{Rj\cdot})^2.$$

Then, $\widehat{\delta}_y$ is normally distributed with mean $\delta=\mu_T-\mu_R$, $(n_1+n_2-2)s_y^2/\sigma^2$ is chi-square distributed with degrees (n_1+n_2-2) of freedom, where

$$\sigma^2 = \sigma_{BT}^2 + \sigma_{BR}^2 - 2\rho\sigma_{BT}\sigma_{BR} + \sigma_{WT}^2 + \sigma_{WR}^2, \tag{20.2.5}$$

and $\widehat{\delta}_y$ and s_y^2 are independent. According to FDA (2003b), ABE is claimed (i.e., the null hypothesis H_0 in hypotheses 20.2.1 with $\theta = |\delta|$ is rejected at the 5% level of significance) if the 90% confidence interval for δ, $(\widehat{\delta}_{y-}, \widehat{\delta}_{y+})$ falls within $(-\eta, \eta)$, where

$$\widehat{\delta}_{y\pm} = \widehat{\delta}_y \pm t_{0.95,\, n_1+n_2-2} \frac{s_y}{2} \sqrt{\frac{1}{n_1} + \frac{1}{n_2}},$$

and $t_{a,m}$ denotes the ath quantile of the central t distribution with m degrees of freedom.

Let $\widehat{\delta}_{x\pm}$ be the same as $\widehat{\delta}_{y\pm}$ but calculated with y-data replaced by x-values. If $(\widehat{\delta}_{x-}, \widehat{\delta}_{x+})$ is within $(-\eta, \eta)$, can we claim ABE? If the genomic prediction x is a perfect prediction of y, then the answer is affirmative. However, there is a difference between the distributions of y and x. Let ε be defined in Equation 20.2.4. If ε is known, then a 90% confidence interval for $\delta = \mu_T - \mu_R$ is $(\widehat{\delta}_{x-} + \varepsilon, \widehat{\delta}_{x+} + \varepsilon)$. Consequently, ABE can be claimed if

$$-\eta < \widehat{\delta}_{x-} + \varepsilon \quad \text{and} \quad \widehat{\delta}_{x+} + \varepsilon < \eta.$$

The parameter ε is typically unknown. If $\varepsilon_- \leq \varepsilon \leq \varepsilon_+$ and the bounds $\varepsilon_\pm$ are known, then ABE can be claimed if

$$-\eta < \widehat{\delta}_{x-} + \varepsilon_- \quad \text{and} \quad \widehat{\delta}_{x+} + \varepsilon_+ < \eta. \tag{20.2.6}$$

The tolerance limits for ε to claim ABE are then

$$\widehat{\varepsilon}_- = -\eta - \widehat{\delta}_{x-} \quad \text{and} \quad \widehat{\varepsilon}_+ = \eta - \widehat{\delta}_{x+}.$$

The difference in variability of y and x, together with ε, plays an important role in the power of claiming ABE. Let $\mathfrak{I}_m(\cdot|\vartheta)$ be the distribution function of the noncentral t distribution with degrees of freedom m and the noncentrality parameter ϑ. Then the power of claiming ABE (when $|\delta| < \eta$ holds) using PK data is given by

$$1 - \mathfrak{I}_{n_1+n_2-2}\left(t_{0.95,\, n_1+n_2-2} \left| \frac{\eta - \delta}{\sigma\sqrt{n_1^{-1} + n_2^{-1}}}\right.\right) - \mathfrak{I}_{n_1+n_2-2}\left(t_{0.95,\, n_1+n_2-2} \left| \frac{\eta + \delta}{\sigma\sqrt{n_1^{-1} + n_2^{-1}}}\right.\right).$$

Let

$$C = \sigma/\tau,$$

where τ^2 is the same as σ^2 defined in Equation 20.2.5 but with y replaced by x. If we adopt the rule in Equation 20.2.6 to test ABE using genomic data, then the power of claiming ABE is

$$1 - \Im_{n_1+n_2-2}\left(t_{0.95,\,n_1+n_2-2}\middle|\frac{C[\eta - (\varepsilon_+ - \varepsilon) - \delta]}{\sigma\sqrt{n_1^{-1} + n_2^{-1}}}\right)$$
$$- \Im_{n_1+n_2-2}\left(t_{0.95,\,n_1+n_2-2}\middle|\frac{C[\eta - (\varepsilon - \varepsilon_-) + \delta]}{\sigma\sqrt{n_1^{-1} + n_2^{-1}}}\right). \qquad (20.2.7)$$

This power is strictly increasing in C, because $\Im_{n_1+n_2-2}(t|\vartheta)$ is strictly decreasing in ϑ. This finding indicates that if x is more variable than y, then the power based on genomic data is smaller. The power based on genomic data is also decreasing in $\varepsilon_+ - \varepsilon < 0$ and $\varepsilon - \varepsilon_- > 0$, which means that the loser the bounds for ε, the less power we can have by using genomic data.

The derived power function provides a way of determining the required sample size for genomic data to achieve certain power in claiming ABE. Assume that $\varepsilon_- = -\varepsilon_+$ and $\varepsilon_+ < \eta$. When $n = n_1 = n_2$ is large, the power function in Equation 20.2.7 is approximately

$$2\Phi\left(\frac{C(\eta - \varepsilon_+ - |\delta - \varepsilon|)\sqrt{n}}{\sigma\sqrt{2}} z_{0.95}\right) - 1,$$

where

Φ is the standard normal distribution function

$z_a = \Phi^{-1}(a)$

Then, to achieve approximately $1 - \beta$ power, n should be at least

$$n_* = \frac{2C^2\sigma^2\left(z_{0.95} + z_{1-\beta/2}\right)^2}{(\eta - \varepsilon_+ - |\delta - \varepsilon|)^2} = \frac{2\tau^2\left(z_{0.95} + z_{1-\beta/2}\right)^2}{(\eta - \varepsilon_+ - |\nu_T - \nu_R|)^2}$$

if initial values of $|\nu_T - \nu_R|$ and τ are provided.

20.2.3 Assessment of PBE

For PBE, we consider the standard 2×2 crossover design. Other designs can be similarly treated. We use the same notations as those in Equation 20.2.2. From the result in Lee et al. (2004), a 95% upper confidence bound for $(\nu_T - \nu_R)^2 + \tau_T^2 - (1 + \eta)\tau_R^2$ is

$$\hat{\gamma} = \hat{\delta}_x^2 + \hat{\tau}_T^2 - (1 + \eta)\hat{\tau}_R^2 + \sqrt{\bar{\nu}},$$

where

$$\hat{\tau}_i^2 = \frac{1}{n_1 + n_2 - 2}\sum_{j,k}(x_{ijk} - \bar{x}_{ij\cdot})^2,$$

$$\nu = \left(u^2 - \widehat{\delta}_x^2\right)^2 + \widehat{\lambda}_+^2\left(\frac{n_1 + n_2 - 2}{x^2_{0.05,\, n_1+n_2-2}} - 1\right)^2 + \widehat{\lambda}_-^2\left(\frac{n_1 + n_2 - 2}{x^2_{0.05,\, n_1+n_2-2}} - 1\right)^2,$$

$x^2_{a,m}$ is the ath quantile of the chi-square distribution with m degrees of freedom,

$$u = |\widehat{\delta}_x| + t_{0.95,\, n_1+n_2-2}\frac{s_x}{2}\sqrt{\frac{1}{n_1} + \frac{1}{n_2}}$$

with

$$s_x^2 = \frac{1}{n_1 + n_2 - 2}\sum_{j,k}(x_{\mathrm{T}jk} - x_{\mathrm{R}jk} - \bar{x}_{\mathrm{T}j\cdot} + \bar{x}_{\mathrm{R}j\cdot})^2,$$

and

$$\widehat{\lambda}_\pm = \frac{\widehat{\tau}_\mathrm{T}^2 - (1+\eta)\widehat{\tau}_\mathrm{R}^2 \pm \sqrt{\left[\widehat{\tau}_\mathrm{T}^2 + (1+\eta)\widehat{\tau}_\mathrm{R}^2\right]^2 - 4(1+\eta)\widehat{\tau}_c^2}}{2}$$

with

$$\widehat{\tau}_c = \frac{1}{n_1 + n_2 - 2}\sum_{j,k}(x_{\mathrm{T}jk} - \bar{x}_{\mathrm{T}j\cdot})(x_{\mathrm{R}jk} - \bar{x}_{\mathrm{R}j\cdot}).$$

If the distribution of the PK data are the same as its genomic prediction, then H_0 in hypotheses 20.2.1 is rejected (i.e., PBE can be claimed) with 95% statistical assurance if $\widehat{\gamma} < 0$ (FDA, 2001; Lee et al., 2004).

For PBE, the difference between the distributions of y and x can be characterized by the parameter ε defined in Equation 20.2.4 and

$$C_i = \sigma_i/\tau_i, \quad i = \mathrm{T}, \mathrm{R},$$

where C_T and C_R may be different. Let

$$\Delta = \frac{1 + \varepsilon/(\nu_\mathrm{T} - \nu_\mathrm{R})}{C_\mathrm{T}} = \frac{\mu_\mathrm{T} - \mu_\mathrm{R}}{C_\mathrm{T}(\nu_\mathrm{T} - \nu_\mathrm{R})}, \tag{20.2.8}$$

and

$$\rho = C_\mathrm{R}^2/C_\mathrm{T}^2.$$

Suppose first that Δ and ρ are known. Then, PBE can be claimed at 95% assurance if

$$\widehat{\gamma}(\Delta, \rho) < 0,$$

where

$$\widehat{\gamma}(\Delta, \rho) = \Delta^2\widehat{\delta}_x^2 + \widehat{\tau}_T^2 - (1+\eta)\rho\widehat{\tau}_R^2 + \sqrt{\nu(\Delta, \rho)},$$

$$\nu(\Delta, \rho) = \Delta^2\left(u^2 - \widehat{\delta}_x^2\right)^2 + \widehat{\lambda}_+^2(\rho)\left(\frac{n_1+n_2-2}{\chi^2_{0.05,\, n_1+n_2-2}} - 1\right)^2 + \widehat{\lambda}_-^2(\rho)\left(\frac{n_1+n_2-2}{\chi^2_{0.05,\, n_1+n_2-2}} - 1\right)^2,$$

and

$$\widehat{\lambda}_\pm(\rho) = \frac{\widehat{\tau}_T^2 - (1+\eta)\rho\widehat{\tau}_R^2 \pm \sqrt{[\widehat{\tau}_T^2 + (1+\eta)\rho\widehat{\tau}_R^2]^2 - 4(1+\eta)\rho\widehat{\tau}_c^2}}{2}.$$

When Δ and ρ are unknown, we may consider a sensitivity analysis by finding the ranges of Δ and ρ for which PBE will be preserved, (i.e., the region $\{(\Delta^2, \rho)\colon \widehat{\gamma}(\Delta,\rho) < 0\}$). This region can be explicitly obtained as follows. Let $a = \widehat{\delta}_x^2$, $b(\rho) = \widehat{\tau}_T^2 - (1+\eta)\rho\widehat{\tau}_R^2$, $c = (u^2 - \widehat{\delta}_x^2)^2$, and $d(\rho) = \widehat{\lambda}_+^2(\rho)\left(\frac{n_1+n_2-2}{\chi^2_{0.05,n_1+n_2-2}} - 1\right)^2 + \widehat{\lambda}_-^2(\rho)\left(\frac{n_1+n_2-2}{\chi^2_{0.05,n_1+n_2-2}} - 1\right)^2$. Then,

$$\widehat{\gamma}(\Delta, \rho) = a\Delta^2 + b(\rho) + \sqrt{c\Delta^2 + d(\rho)}.$$

For every fixed $\rho > 0$, $\widehat{\gamma}(\Delta, \rho)$ is a strictly increasing function of Δ^2 so that for any fixed ρ, the equation

$$az + b(\rho) + \sqrt{cz + d(\rho)} = 0$$

has at most one solution

$$z(\rho) = \frac{c - 2ab(\rho) - \sqrt{c^2 - 2acb(\rho) + 4a^2d(\rho)}}{2a^2}. \tag{20.2.9}$$

Thus,

$$\{(\Delta^2, \rho)\colon\ \widehat{\gamma}(\Delta, \rho) < 0\} = \left\{(\Delta^2, \rho)\colon\ -\sqrt{z(\rho)} < \Delta < \sqrt{z(\rho)}\right\}.$$

Note that if for a fixed $\rho > 0$, $z(\rho) < 0$ or $z(\rho)$ is not real, then PBE cannot be claimed for any Δ.

20.2.4 Assessment of IBE

Unlike the assessment of ABE or PBE, the assessment of IBE requires a crossover design with order higher than 2×2. We focus on the standard 2×4 crossover design recommended by FDA (2001). From the result in Hyslop et al. (2000), a 95% upper confidence bound for the parameter $(\nu_T - \nu_R)^2 + \tau_D^2 + \tau_{WT}^2 - (1+\eta)\tau_{WR}^2$ is

$$\widehat{\gamma} = \widehat{\delta}_x^2 + s_x^2 + 0.5\widehat{\tau}_{WT}^2 - (1.5+\eta)\widehat{\tau}_{WR}^2 + \sqrt{\nu},$$

where $\widehat{\delta}^2$ and s_x^2 are the same as those in Section 20.2.3 but calculated with x_{ijkl} replaced by x_{ijkl},

$$\widehat{\tau}_{Wi}^2 = \frac{1}{2(n_1+n_2-2)} \sum_{j,k} (x_{ijk1} - x_{ijk2} - \bar{x}_{ij\cdot 1} + \bar{x}_{ij\cdot 2})^2,$$

$$\nu = (u^2 - \widehat{\delta}_x^2)^2 + s_x^4\left(\frac{n_1+n_2-2}{\chi^2_{0.05,\,n_1+n_2-2}} - 1\right)^2 + \frac{\widehat{\tau}_{WT}^4}{4}\left(\frac{n_1+n_2-2}{\chi^2_{0.05,\,n_1+n_2-2}} - 1\right)^2 + \frac{\widehat{\tau}_{WR}^4}{(1.5+\eta)^2}\left(\frac{n_1+n_2-2}{\chi^2_{0.05,\,n_1+n_2-2}} - 1\right)^2,$$

and u is the same as that in Section 20.2.3.

For IBE, the difference between the distributions of y and x can be characterized by the parameter ε defined in Equation 20.2.4 and

$$C_i = \sigma_{Wi}/\tau_{Wi}, \quad i = \mathrm{T}, \mathrm{R},$$

and

$$D = \sigma_D^2/(\tau_D^2 C_T^2).$$

Let Δ be as defined in Equation 20.2.8 and $\rho = C_R^2/C_T^2$. If Δ, ρ, and D are known, then IBE can be claimed at 95% assurance if $\widehat{\gamma}(\Delta, \rho, D) < 0$, where

$$\widehat{\gamma}(\Delta, \rho, D) = \Delta^2\widehat{\delta}_x^2 + Ds_x^2 + 0.5\widehat{\tau}_{WT}^2 - (1.5+\eta)^2\rho\widehat{\tau}_{WR}^2 + \sqrt{\nu(\Delta, \rho, D)},$$

and

$$\nu(\Delta, \rho, D) = \Delta^2\left(u^2 - \widehat{\delta}_{x^2}\right)^2 + Ds_x^4\left(\frac{n_1+n_2-2}{\chi^2_{0.05,\,n_1+n_2-2}} - 1\right)^2 + \frac{\widehat{\tau}_{WT}^4}{4}\left(\frac{n_1+n_2-2}{\chi^2_{0.05,\,n_1+n_2-2}} - 1\right)^2 + \frac{\rho\widehat{\tau}_{WR}^4}{(1.5+\eta)^2}\left(\frac{n_1+n_2-2}{\chi^2_{0.05,\,n_1+n_2-2}} - 1\right)^2.$$

When Δ, ρ, and D are unknown, we may consider a sensitivity analysis by finding the ranges of these parameters for which $\widehat{\gamma}(\Delta, \rho, D) < 0$. Let $a = \widehat{\delta}_x^2$,

$$b(\rho, D) = Ds_x^2 + 0.5\hat{\tau}_{\mathrm{WT}}^2 - (1.5+\eta)^2\rho\hat{\tau}_{\mathrm{WR}}^2, \quad c = \left(u^2 - \hat{\delta}_x^2\right)^2,$$

$$d(\rho, D) = Ds_x^4\left(\frac{n_1+n_2-2}{x_{0.05,n_1+n_2-2}^2} - 1\right)^2 + \frac{\hat{\tau}_{\mathrm{WT}}^4}{4}\left(\frac{n_1+n_2-2}{x_{0.05,n_1+n_2-2}^2} - 1\right)^2$$
$$+ \frac{\rho\hat{\tau}_{\mathrm{WR}}^4}{(1.5+\eta)^2}\left(\frac{n_1+n_2-2}{x_{0.05,n_1+n_2-2}^2} - 1\right)^2,$$

and

$$z(\rho, D) = \frac{c - 2ab(\rho, D) - \sqrt{c^2 - 2acb(\rho, D) + 4a^2 d(\rho, D)}}{2a^2}. \quad (20.2.10)$$

Then

$$\left\{(\Delta^2, \rho, D)\colon\ \hat{\gamma}(\Delta, \rho, D) < 0\right\} = \left\{(\Delta^2, \rho, D)\colon\ -\sqrt{z(\rho, D)} < \Delta < \sqrt{z(\rho, D)}\right\}.$$

20.2.5 Example

Landowski et al. (2003) evaluated the correlations of PK parameters following oral valacyclovir or acyclovir administration with expression levels of intestinal genes in humans by employing microarray techniques. Positively significant correlations between the AUC (area under the curve from 0 to the last concentration) and the expression intensities of HPT1 peptide transporters were observed (correlation coefficient 0.794, p-value = 0.011). Let y be the AUC and z be the expression intensities of HPT1. The linear regression fitting between y and z is $y = 0.0005z - 0.4578$. Therefore, we can assess bioequivalence by using HPT1 expression intensities data $x = 0.0005z - 0.4578$ instead of PK data y.

For illustration, a data set was generated based on Landowski et al. (2003). Subjects were randomly assigned to receive either the sequence of *TR* or *RT* in a 2×2 crossover design, where T is 500 mg oral valacyclovir and R is 400 mg oral acyclovir. For example, those subjects who were assigned to the sequence of *TR* receive 500 mg oral valacyclovir (regimen T) at the first dosing period. After a sufficient length of washout, these subjects were crossed over to receive 400 mg oral acyclovir (regimen R). The data are listed in columns 3, 4, 7, and 8 of Table 20.2.1.

If we use the log-transformed AUC for the ABE test, the following 90% confidence interval for d is obtained: (−0.040, 0.026). Because this interval is within the interval (−0.2231; 0.2231), according to FDA (2003b), ABE is claimed between T and R. Using the genomic prediction x to replace y, we obtain the following 90% confidence interval: (−0.039; 0.025), which is within (−0.2231; 0.2231). Hence, the approach of using genomic data for assessing ABE is consistent with the approach of using the AUC data. According to the discussion in Section 20.2.2, the tolerance limits for the ε in Equation 20.2.4 to claim ABE are

TABLE 20.2.1: AUC (ng·h/mL) and expression intensities of HPT1 of acyclovir (2 × 4 crossover design).

Subject	Sequence	AUC				HPT1			
1	TRTR	20.29	20.70	17.29	17.99	41490	42310	35491	36902
2	RTRT	23.34	25.28	16.78	28.22	47588	51475	34469	57354
3	TRTR	21.12	19.89	26.05	34.81	43146	40687	53015	70542
4	RTRT	26.58	26.84	20.49	27.39	54067	54601	41898	55686
5	TRTR	23.57	25.03	16.12	22.2	48057	50972	33154	45312
6	RTRT	28.22	28.79	23.34	20.29	57354	58493	47588	41490
7	RTRT	29.37	31.19	19.11	24.05	59657	63290	39128	49009
8	TRTR	19.11	21.12	22.42	28.5	39128	43146	45758	57921
9	RTRT	25.28	24.29	30.27	20.9	51475	49492	61446	42726
10	TRTR	19.89	21.54	17.81	16.28	40687	43999	36544	33478

$$\hat{\varepsilon}_{-} = -0.184 \quad \text{and} \quad \hat{\varepsilon}_{+} = 0.198$$

For the PBE, according to the formula in Section 20.2.3, $\hat{\gamma} = -0.0026$ based on the log-transformed AUC. Hence, PBE can be claimed based on AUC data. Using the genomic prediction x to replace y, we obtain that $\hat{\gamma}(\Delta, \rho) = -0.0025$ with $\Delta = 1$ and $\rho = 1$. For the sensitivity analysis suggested in Section 20.2.3, values of $\sqrt{z(\rho)}$ with $z(\rho)$ defined by Equation 20.2.9 are 8.40, 9.72, 10.87, 11.91, and 12.85, for $\rho = 0.8$, 0.9, 1.0, 1.1, and 1.2, respectively.

For illustration, a data set was generated from a 2 × 4 crossover design with sequences TRTR and RTRT. The data are listed in Table 20.2.1. According to the formula in assessment of IBE, $\hat{\gamma} = -0.089$, based on the log-transformed AUC. Hence, IBE can be claimed based on AUC data. Using the genomic prediction x to replace y, we obtain that $\hat{\gamma}\ (\Delta, \rho, D) = -0.086$ with $\Delta = 1$, $\rho = 1$, and $D = 1$. For the sensitivity analysis suggested in assessment of IBE, values of $\sqrt{z(\rho, D)}$ with $z(\rho, D)$ defined in Equation 20.2.10 are listed in Table 20.2.2.

20.3 Bridging Bioequivalence Studies

Generic drugs are very crucial for the health and welfare of the people of developing countries. For example, in some countries, generic drugs in fact account for more than 70% of total prescriptions. To ensure efficacy, safety, and quality of the generic drugs, approval of generic drugs is a very important task for the regulatory authorities in developing countries. However, the generic drugs in these countries are either from foreign countries or from local generic sponsors of their own countries. As a result, approval of generic copies is a very complicated and challenging issue that the regulatory authorities of the developing countries have to face.

TABLE 20.2.2: Values of $\sqrt{z(\rho, D)}$ based on data in Table 20.1.

ρ	D	$\sqrt{z(\rho, D)}$
0.8	0.8	18.26
	0.9	18.20
	1.0	18.15
	1.1	18.09
	1.2	18.04
0.9	0.8	19.59
	0.9	19.53
	1.0	19.48
	1.1	19.43
	1.2	19.38
1.0	0.8	20.84
	0.9	20.79
	1.0	20.75
	1.1	20.70
	1.2	20.65
1.1	0.8	22.04
	0.9	21.99
	1.0	21.95
	1.1	21.90
	1.2	21.85
1.2	0.8	23.18
	0.9	23.14
	1.0	23.09
	1.1	23.05
	1.2	23.00

In this section we describe one of the situations often encountered for approval of generic drugs in developing countries. In what follows, we use new region as a generic name for the developing countries. Suppose that for some reasons such as the price of the innovative drug or the market size of the new region, the innovative drug product of the original region was not marketed in the new region. After the patent of the innovative drug product was expired in the original region, a generic copy manufactured in the original region was approved by the regulatory authority of the original region. However, because of its affordability this generic copy of the original region was introduced and approved by the regulatory authority for marketing in the new region. Another generic copy of the innovative drug manufactured by the local sponsor is seeking for marketing approval in the new region. However, equivalence between two generic copies does not imply bioequivalence between the local generic copy by and the innovative drug (Chow and Liu, 1997; Fleming, 2000). To ensure the equivalent efficacy and safety of the local generic copy, therefore, the regulatory authority in the new region may still require the evidence of average bioequivalence between the local generic copy and the innovative drug despite the fact that it is not available in the new region.

Because the generic copy from the original region has been approved by both the original and new regions, following the bridging concept suggested in the ICH E5 guideline on *Ethnic Factors in the Acceptability of Foreign Clinical Data* (ICH, 1998), one could utilize the data provided by the bioequivalence study conducted in the original region to evaluate average bioequivalence between the local generic copy of the new region and the innovative drug of the original region. This problem is referred to as bridging bioequivalence problem as illustrated in Figure 20.3.1 and the innovative drug of the original region is called the original reference formulation. Suppose that a local bioequivalence study is conducted to compare the local generic copy to the generic copy of the original region. In this local bioequivalence study, the generic copy of the original region is served as the reference formulation. On the other hand, the generic copy of the original region is the test formulation in the bioequivalence study conducted in the original region. As a result, average bioequivalence of the generic copy manufactured by the local sponsor in the new region to the original reference formulation in the original region can be evaluated through the generic copy of the original region. Therefore, the local bioequivalence study in the new region is referred to as the bridging bioequivalence study (BBES). The generic copy made by the local sponsor in the new region is designated as the test formulation, and the generic copy of the original region is referred to as the bridging reference formulation. We also called the bioequivalence study conducted in the original region for comparing the bridging reference formulation with the original reference formulations as the original bioequivalence study (OBES). However, to avoid bias, it is very crucial that both bioequivalence studies have the same inclusion/exclusion criteria, the same design, the same sampling time point, the same amount of blood drawn at each time point, and

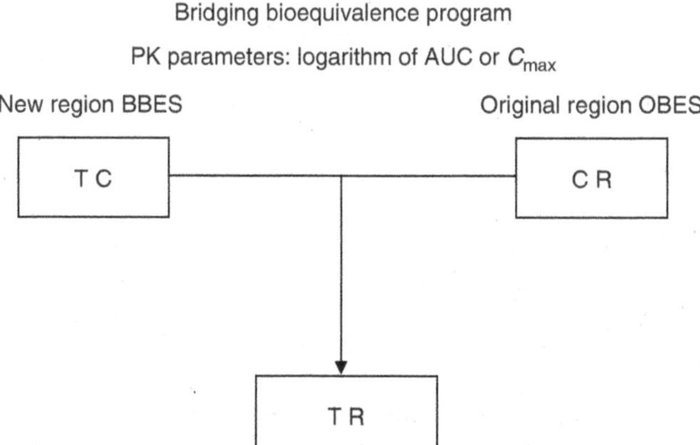

FIGURE 20.3.1: Bridging bioequivalence problem. (From Liu, J.P., *J. Biopharm. Stat.*, 14, 857, 2004.)

most important of all, the same analytical procedures for determination of the plasma concentration of active ingredients (Wang et al., 2002).

20.3.1 Hypothesis

Under the assumption that the standard two-sequence, two-period (2×2) crossover design for the BBES and OBES, let μ_T, μ_C, and μ_R be the population average of some PK response such as area under plasma concentration–time curve (AUC) or peak response (C_{max}) on the log-scale for test (T), bridging reference (*C*), and original reference formulations (R), respectively. Denote $\theta = \mu_T - \mu_R$. Then the interval hypothesis for average bioequivalence between the test formulation and the original reference formulation is given as

$$\begin{aligned} &\mathrm{H_0}: \mu_T - \mu_R \geq -\delta \quad \text{or} \quad \mu_T - \mu_R \leq \delta \\ \text{versus} \quad &\mathrm{H_A}: -\delta < \mu_T - \mu_R < \delta, \end{aligned} \tag{20.3.1}$$

where δ is the bioequivalence limit which is usually set as $\ln(1.25) = 0.2231$ by the regulatory authorities (FDA, 2003b). However, the difference in average between the test and original reference formulations can be reformulated as the sum of the difference in average between test and bridging reference formulations and that between the bridging reference and original reference formulations, i.e., $\mu_T - \mu_R = (\mu_T - \mu_C) + (\mu_C - \mu_R)$. If follows that the interval hypothesis in (20.3.1) can be expressed as

$$\begin{aligned} &\mathrm{H_0}: (\mu_T - \mu_C) + (\mu_C - \mu_R) \geq -\delta \quad \text{or} \quad (\mu_T - \mu_C) + (\mu_C - \mu_R) \leq \delta \\ \text{versus} \quad &\mathrm{H_A}: -\delta < (\mu_T - \mu_C) + (\mu_C - \mu_R) < \delta. \end{aligned} \tag{20.3.2}$$

The estimate of $(\mu_C - \mu_R)$ cannot be obtained from BBES in the new region because it does not include the original reference formulation but must be extrapolated from OBES in the original region. However, this extrapolation from the original reference formulation is based on a very strong constancy assumption that the effect of the bridging reference formulation is the same for both BBES in the new region and OBES in the original region. However, in practice, the constancy assumption not only may not be true but also is not testable (Wang et al., 2002). As a result, adjustment for the effect of the bridging reference formulation in the BBES may be required.

Let μ_{C2} and μ_{R2} be the population averages of the PK responses (AUC or C_{max}) on the log-scale of the bridging reference formulation (C_2) and the original reference formulation (R_2) which are included in BBES conducted in the new region. In addition, let μ_{C1} and μ_R be the population average of the PK (AUC or C_{max}) responses of the bridging reference formulation (C_1) and the original reference formulation (R) for OBES in the original region. A possible adjustment is that the assumed effect of the bridging reference formulation for the local BBES maintains at least a certain fraction of its effect from OBES in the original study (Rothman et al., 2003). In other words,

$$(\mu_{C2} - \mu_{R2}) = \lambda(\mu_{C1} - \mu_R) \quad \text{for some fixed } \lambda > 0. \tag{20.3.3}$$

Therefore, the interval hypothesis for comparing the test formulation to the putative original reference formulation is given as

$$\begin{aligned} &H_0: (\mu_T - \mu_{C2}) + (\mu_{C2} - \mu_{R2}) \geq -\delta \quad \text{or} \quad (\mu_T - \mu_{C2}) + (\mu_{C2} - \mu_{R2}) \leq \delta \\ \text{versus} \quad &H_A: -\delta < (\mu_T - \mu_{C2}) + (\mu_{C2} - \mu_{R2}) < \delta. \end{aligned} \tag{20.3.4}$$

When it is reasonable to assume that $(\mu_{C2} - \mu_{R2}) = \lambda(\mu_{C1} - \mu_R)$, then the interval hypothesis can be re-expressed as

$$\begin{aligned} &H_0: (\mu_T - \mu_{C2}) + \lambda(\mu_{C1} - \mu_R) \geq -\delta \quad \text{or} \quad (\mu_T - \mu_{C2}) + \lambda(\mu_{C1} - \mu_R) \leq \delta \\ \text{versus} \quad &H_a: -\delta < (\mu_T - \mu_{C2}) + \lambda(\mu_{C1} - \mu_R) < \delta. \end{aligned} \tag{20.3.5}$$

However, the effect of ethnic factors in the new region on the PK responses for the bridging reference formulation should be the same for the original reference formulation. In other words, although the magnitudes of μ_{C2} and μ_{R2} are different from those of μ_{C1} and μ_R, $\mu_{C2} - \mu_{R2}$ should be approximately equal to $\mu_{C1} - \mu_R$. Otherwise, a possible region-by-formulation interaction exists and the test formulation is not average bioequivalent to the original reference formulation. This is what the regulatory agency in the new region is interested in. Therefore, setting $\lambda = 1$ is reasonable from a regulatory viewpoint in the new region and the interval hypothesis in Equation 20.3.5 then reduces to

$$\begin{aligned} &H_0: (\mu_T - \mu_{C_2}) + (\mu_{C_1} - \mu_R) \geq -\delta \quad \text{or} \quad (\mu_T - \mu_{C_2}) + (\mu_{C_1} - \mu_R) \leq \delta \\ \text{versus} \quad &H_a: -\delta < (\mu_T - \mu_{C_2}) + (\mu_{C_1} - \mu_R) < \delta. \end{aligned} \tag{20.3.6}$$

Because the original reference formulation is not included in the local bioequivalence bridging study, the estimate of $(\mu_{C_2} - \mu_{R_2})$ cannot be obtained. However, the estimate of $(\mu_{C_1} - \mu_R)$ is available from the bioequivalence study in the original region. Average bioequivalence between the test formulation and the original reference formulation can be evaluated by hypotheses 20.3.6 and the results can then be extrapolated to hypothesis 20.3.4. For this reason, interval hypothesis 20.3.6 is referred to as a surrogate hypothesis (Rothman et al., 2003).

20.3.2 Methods

Let Y_{ijk} denote the log PK responses of subject k receiving formulation i in sequence j from BBES employing the standard 2×2 crossover design comparing the test formulation with the bridging reference drug conducted in the new region, $k = 1, \ldots, n_{Nj}$, $j = 1, 2$, $i = \text{T}, \text{C}_2$. Also let $\theta_N = \mu_T - \mu_{C_2}$ and $\theta_O = \mu_{C_1} - \mu_R$. The parameter of interest for hypothesis 20.3.6 in evaluation of average bioequivalence is $\theta = \theta_N + \theta_O$. It is assumed that the log PK responses are normally distributed and their covariance under the standard 2×2 crossover design has a compound symmetry structure. Under the assumption of no unequal carryover effects, the least square estimates (LSE) for θ_N is $\overline{Y}_T - \overline{Y}_{C_2}$, where $\overline{Y}_i = (\overline{Y}_{i1} + \overline{Y}_{i2})/2$ and $\overline{Y}_{ij}$ is the sample mean of log PK responses of formulation i in sequence j; $j = 1, 2$ and $i = \mathrm{T}, \mathrm{C}_2$. An unbiased estimator for the variance of $\overline{Y}_T - \overline{Y}_{C_2}$ is given as $s_N^2 = s_{Nd}^2[(1/n_{N1}) + (1/n_{N2})]$, where s_{Nd}^2 is the pooled sample variance of period differences from both sequences and is an unbiased estimator for the intra-subject variability of BBES in the new region, σ_{Nd}^2. Similarly, $\overline{Y}_{C1} - \overline{Y}_R$ and s_O^2 denote the LSE for θ_O and its estimated variance for OBES in the original region comparing the bridging reference formulation with the original reference formulation under the standard 2×2 crossover design, where $\overline{Y}_i = (\overline{Y}_{i1} + \overline{Y}_{i2})/2$, $i = \mathrm{C}_1, \mathrm{R}$; $s_O^2 = s_{Od}^2[(1/n_{O1}) + (1/n_{O2})]$; and s_{Od}^2 is an unbiased estimator for the intra-subject variability σ_{Od}^2.

It follows that an unbiased estimator for θ is $\overline{Y} = [(\overline{Y}_T - \overline{Y}_{C_2}) + (\overline{Y}_{C_1} - \overline{Y}_R)]/2$. If $\sigma_{Od}^2 = \sigma_{Nd}^2$, then an unbiased estimator for the variance of $\overline{Y}$ is given as

$$s^2 = s_P^2\{[(1/n_{N1}) + (1/n_{N2})] + [(1/n_{O1}) + (1/n_{O2})]\},$$

where s_P^2 is the pooled sample variance computed from period differences of both sequences from both bioequivalence studies.

The lower and upper limits of a $(1 - 2\alpha)100\%$ confidence interval for θ is given as

$$U(L) = \overline{Y} \pm t(\alpha, \mathrm{df}P)s, \tag{20.3.7}$$

where

$t(\alpha, \mathrm{df}P)$ is the αth upper percentile of a central distribution with degrees of freedom $\mathrm{df}P$

$\mathrm{df}P = n_{N1} + n_{N2} + n_{O1} + n_{O2} - 4$

If (L, U) is completely contained within $(-\delta, \delta)$, then average bioequivalence between the test formulation and the original formulation is concluded at the α significance level. If $\sigma_{Od}^2 \neq \sigma_{Nd}^2$, a weighted t statistic can be used to construct an approximate $(1 - 2\alpha)$ 100% confidence interval for θ (Cochran and Cox, 1957) which is given as

$$U(L) = \overline{Y} \pm t'\sqrt{s_{Nd}^2 + s_{Od}^2}, \tag{20.3.8}$$

where

$$t' = \frac{t(\alpha, \mathrm{df_O})s_{Od}^2(n_{O1} + n_{O2}) + t(\alpha, \mathrm{df})s_{Nd}^2(n_{N1} + n_{N2})}{s_{Od}^2(n_{O1} + n_{O2}) + s_{Nd}^2(n_{N1} + n_{N2})},$$

$$\mathrm{df_N} = n_{N1} + n_{N2} - 2, \text{ and } \mathrm{df_O} = n_{O1} + n_{O2} - 2.$$

Under the assumption that $\sigma_{Od}^2 = \sigma_{Nd}^2 = \sigma_d^2$, the minimum sample size per sequence for BBES to provide $(1 - \beta)$ power at the α significance level when $\mu_T - \mu_{R2} = 0$ is given as

$$n = 1/\{[\Delta^2/2\sigma_d^2]/[t(\alpha, 2n_O + 2n - 4) + t(\beta/2, 2n_O + 2n - 4)]^2 - (1/n_O)\}, \tag{20.3.9}$$

where

$\Delta = \log 1.25 = 0.2231$, the average bioequivalence limit on the log-scale
$n_O = n_{O1} = n_{O2}$ is the number of subjects per sequence for OBES in the original study

Since average bioequivalence limit Δ is set at 0.2231 for AUC and C_{max} by most of regulatory agencies, the sample size for BBES in the new region is an increasing function of σ_d^2 and a decreasing function of n_O. In addition, from Equation 20.3.9, the required sample size per sequence for the BBES in the new region n is positive only if

$$\left[\Delta^2/2\sigma_d^2\right]/[t(\alpha, 2n_O + 2n - 4) + t(\beta/2, 2n_O + 2n - 4)]^2 \geq 1/n_O. \qquad (20.3.10)$$

However, the requirement in Equation 20.3.10 is not unreasonable because BBES is conducted only when the bridging reference formulation was proven to be average bioequivalent to the original reference formulation in OBES in the original region. It follows that the sample size of the bioequivalence study in the original region is large enough to provide at least $(1 - \beta)$ power at the α significance level. In other words,

$$\begin{aligned} n_O &\geq 2\left[\sigma_d^2/\Delta^2\right][t(\alpha, 2n_O - 2) + t(\beta/2, 2n_O - 2)]^2 \\ &\geq 2\left[\sigma_d^2/\Delta^2\right][t(\alpha, 2n_O + 2n - 4) + t(\beta/2, 2n_O + 2n - 4)]^2. \end{aligned}$$

Therefore condition in Equation 20.3.10 is satisfied. Table 20.3.1 presents the required sample sizes per sequence (n_O) of OBES for various values of σ_d^2 to achieve

TABLE 20.3.1: Sample size per sequence for the bioequivalence bridging study for $\Delta = 0.2231$, $\alpha = 0.05$.

β	σ_d	n_O	n
0.2	0.10	5	14
	0.15	9	61
	0.20	15	177
	0.25	23	344
0.1	0.10	6	19
	0.15	11	97
	0.20	19	216
	0.25	29	447

n_O is the sample size required for OBES to achieve $1 - \beta$ at the 5% significance level and n is the sample size required for BBES to achieve $1 - \beta$ at the 5% significance level.

80% or 90% power at the 5% significance level. In addition, the required sample sizes per sequence (n) of BBES are also given next to n_O. For example, when $\sigma_d = 0.15$, the sample size per sequence required is 9 to achieve 80% power at the 5% significance level for OBES in the original region comparing the bridging reference formulation with the original reference formulation. However the required sample size for the BBES is 61 per sequence to achieve 80% power at the 5% significance level to compare the test formulation with the original reference formulation. This sample size for BBES is almost seven times as large as that required for OBES. However, if the sample size for OBES is fewer than 9, no sample size for the BBES in the new region can achieve 80% power for testing hypothesis 20.3.6 at the 5% significance level. From Table 20.3.1, the sample size requirement for BBES seems formidable. However, on the other hand, when $\sigma_d = 0.15$ if the sample size for OBES increases to 12 per sequence, then the sample size for BBES decreases to 24. Therefore, for this particular situation, if the sample size of OBES increases only 6 subjects (about one-third), the sample size for BBES decreases by more than 37 subjects (about 61% reduction). Although a sample size of 24 subjects per sequence for BBES is considered large, it is feasible and manageable. On the other hand, when the actual sample size for OBES is far more than the minimal required sample size to provide $(1 - \beta)$ power, then the sample size for BBES can dramatically be reduced and could be fewer than that for OBES. However, to assure the sample design features between OBES and BBES, we recommend that the minimal required sample size for BBES be at least as many as that for OBES.

20.3.3 Example

Suppose that a bioequivalence study using the standard 2×2 crossover design was conducted in the original region to compare the bridging reference formulation with the original reference formulation. The sample size for this OBES is 12 subjects per sequence. Summary statistics for the log AUC(0$-\infty$) for this OBES are given in Part A of Table 20.3.2. On the log-scale, the mean difference between the two formulations is -0.02838 with an estimated intra-subject variability s_{Od} of 0.15. It follows that a 90% confidence interval for $\mu_{C1} - \mu_R$ is $(-0.1335, 0.07676)$. Because the point estimate for the ratio of the mean of the bridging reference formulation to that of the original reference formulation on the original scale is 102.88% with a 90% confidence interval on the original scale is (87.50%, 107.98%), therefore, based on AUC(0$-\infty$) the bridging reference formulation is claimed to be average bioequivalent to the original reference formulation at the 5% significance level. With the evidence of average bioequivalence from other PK responses, the bridging reference formulation was approved in the original region.

Suppose that the original reference formulation was not marketed in the new region but the bridging reference formulation was approved in the new region after it obtained the approval from the original region. Now a BBES was conducted in the new region to compare the test formulation of the local sponsor with the bridging reference formulation. To avoid bias, the BBES in the new region also employed the same 2×2 crossover design with the same number of subjects (12) per sequence, the

TABLE 20.3.2: Summary of results of the logarithmic AUC($0-\infty$) for the OBES and BBES.

Part A: Original Bioequivalence Study	
Bridging reference mean	4.66836
Original reference mean	4.69674
Estimated intra-subject variability s_{Od}	0.15
Difference in means	−0.02838
Lower 90% CI limit	−0.1335
Upper 90% CI limit	0.07676
CI in original scale	(87.50%, 107.98%)
Part B: Bridging Bioequivalence Study	
Test mean	4.49479
Bridging reference mean	4.56637
Estimated intra-subject variability s_{Nd}	0.18371
Difference in means	−0.07158
Lower 90% CI limit	−0.20035
Upper 90% CI limit	0.05719
CI in original scale	(81.84%, 105.89%)

same inclusion/exclusion criteria, and the same validated analytical procedure to assay the plasma concentration of active ingredients. Summary statistics for the logarithmic AUC($0-\infty$) for this BBES are given in Part B of Table 20.3.2. From Table 20.3.2, the mean difference between the test formulation and bridging reference formulation is −0.07158 with an estimated intra-subject variability s_{Nd} of 0.18371. Hence a 90% confidence interval for $\mu_{\mathrm{T}} - \mu_{\mathrm{C2}}$ is (−0.20035, 0.05719). Therefore, the test formulation is average bioequivalent to the bridging reference formulation since the 90% confidence interval for the ratio of the mean of the test formulation to that of the bridging reference formulation is (81.84%, 105.89%). However, this result does not provide the evidence of average bioequivalence between the test formulation and the original reference formulation.

Because $s_{\mathrm{Nd}}^2/s_{\mathrm{Od}}^2 = 1.5 < F(0.05, 22, 22) = 2.06$, no evidence shows that the intra-subject variability of the BBES is different from that of the OBES. It follows that the pooled sample variance s_{P}^2 is 0.028125. On the log-scale, an unbiased estimate for $(\mu_{\mathrm{T}} - \mu_{\mathrm{C}_2}) + (\mu_{\mathrm{C}_1} - \mu_{\mathrm{R}})$ is given as $-0.07158 - 0.02238 = -0.09996$. From Equation 20.3.7 a 90% confidence interval is found to be (−0.26291, 1.06502). Since the 90% confidence interval on the original scale is (76.88%, 106.50%), then the test formulation is not average bioequivalent to the original reference formulation at the 5% significance level. On the basis of the pooled sample variance s_{P}^2 for σ_{P}^2 and Equation 20.3.10, the required sample for BBES in the new region to provide 80% power at the 5% significance level is 52 per sequence. This example illustrates that bioequivalence between the local generic and bridging reference formulations does not provide the evidence that the local generic formulation is bioequivalent to the innovative drug product of the original region.

20.4 Bioequivalence for Biological Products

20.4.1 Importance of Biological Products

Biological products, as defined by Public Health Service (PHS) Act, is a virus, therapeutic serum, toxin, antitoxin, vaccine, blood, blood components, or derivative, allergenic product, or analogous product, or arsphenamine or derivative of arsphenamine (or any other trivalent organic arsenic compound), applicable to the prevention, treatment, or cure of a disease or condition of human beings (section 3519 (i), PHSA, 42, U.S.C. & 262(i)). However, many biological products are also drugs which are broadly defined in the Food, Drug, and Cosmetic (FD&C) Act. On the other hand, the EMEA defines a biological product as the drug product containing a biological substance which has the following two important characteristics: (1) it is produced by or extracted from a biological resource and (2) a combination of physico–chemical–biological testing, together with process control, is required to define its quality and characteristics. As a result, the definition by the EMEA makes a clear distinction between a biological product and a chemically synthesized drug product.

Most of biological drug products are proteins developed by the following biotechnological processes: (1) recombinant DNA technology, (2) controlled expression of genes coding for biological active proteins in prokaryotes and eukaryotes, and (3) hybridoma and monoclonal antibody methods. Antibodies, vaccines, cytokines, interleukins, hormones, and *in vivo* diagnostic allergenic products represent the largest proteins derived from the above mentioned biotechnology. These therapeutic proteins include recombinant human (rh) insulin for the treatment of diabetes, human growth hormone for the treatment of hypopituitary dwarfism, interferon for cancer therapy, colony stimulating factors (CSF) for treatment of neutropenia caused by the chemotherapy for cancer patients and hepatitis, erythroproietin (EPO) for the treatment of anemia in cases of chronic renal failure, various blotting factors and many other conditions. In 2003, there were over 100 approved biological products in the United States with a total of revenues about 40 billions U.S. dollars. These biological products provide efficacious and safe treatment of some of the important and devastating diseases. In addition, the biological products are crucial in the treatment of rare illnesses. It is estimated that 50% of all biological products in the U.S. market are intended for use in orphan diseases affecting fewer than 200,000 people. Furthermore, 20% of all marketed orphan drug products are biological products.

On the other hand, most of orphan biological products are also biological products that are manufactured by only one biopharmaceutical or biotechnology company. As a result, critical shortage of several lifesaving biological products has been experienced because the sole manufacturer cannot make enough products or has had problems with production. For example, in the United States, there have been repeated occurrences of shortages of recombinant factor III for hemophilia, trigging rationing of the treatment. This phenomenon seems unacceptable because the biotechnology industry appears to be so vulnerable to manufacturing limitation. As a result, access to the needed biological products is severely hampered by the monopoly of the manufacturer for the biological products. On the other hand, affordability is also another crucial issue of biological products. Costs of biological products to consumers and their insurers, on average, tend to be significantly higher than those of conventional drug products. For example, the cost of conventional drug products to a major health management organization has nearly doubled during a period of 5 years, while the cost of biological products has tripled and is expected to double again in the next two years. Inability to access to lifesaving biological products is primarily due to high cost of biological products. However, a biological product that is not affordable is neither safe nor efficacious.

In the next few years, the patents of the early biological products which reached the market in the United States and Europe will be soon expired. This represents a total of 10 billion dollars worth of biological products, including rh insulin, rh growth hormone, interferon, and EPO. It provides the opportunity for generic version of biologic products to reach the regulated market in the North America and Europe as early as 2007. Introduction of generic copies of biologic products to the market will not only provide affordability and accessibility to the patients but also nurture a healthy environment for competition and innovation to the biopharmaceutical industry. For the conventional drug products, since the enactment of the Hatch-Waxman Amendments in 1984, over 10,000 generic drugs have entered the U.S. market and generic drugs now account for close to 50% of prescriptions filled in the United States. Generic drugs typically cost 50% to 70% less than their innovator counterparts and can save consumers an estimated 8–10 billion dollars a year at retailed pharmacies. Currently, the U.S. FDA approves generic drugs at an average rate of one per day. The improvement of access to generic drugs and lowering prescription drug costs will save American over 35 billion dollars in drug costs for the next 10 years and will also provide billions in savings for the Medicare and Medicaid programs. If the generic copies of the biological products with equivalent safety and efficacy can entered the U.S. market, affordability, accessibility, and savings of the similar magnitude with conventional drug products can also be achieved.

20.4.2 Differences between Biological and Conventional Products

Biological products are very different from conventional chemical drug products in many ways. First, the molecules of biological products are much large. For example, aspirin has a molecular weight of 180.2 Dalton while Epogen has a molecular weight of 30,400 Dalton Second, biological products have much more complex spatial structure and are more diverse and heterogeneous. Typically, a biological product is a protein made of chain of several hundred amino acids which has primary, secondary, tertiary, and quaternary structures. For example, erythropoietin is a glycoprotein of medium size. It is glycosylated, having four glycol chains and sialic acid at the end of these chains, making it a complex molecule. In fact, it is a family of molecules in one product, consisting of isoforms. Due to the size and complexity of structure, the manufacture of a biological product is a highly complicated process which usually consists of more than 250 critical tests in contrast to fewer than 50 tests for conventional chemical drug products.

In addition, a small change to the manufacturing process or formulation of a biological product may have detrimental effects. For example, it has been reported that more patients receiving one version of erythropoietin developed pure red cell aplasia and required blood transfusion. This may be due to the differential immune response (immunogenicity) to different versions of erythropoietin that may results in changes in protein structure, glycosylation, contaminants, formulations, and degradation products. In addition, current analytical technology and tools available are not sufficient to fully characterize the attributes of a biological product. As a result, the traditional approach to testing the finished product in terms of pharmaceutical equivalent and bioequivalence based on PK characteristics may not be sufficient to ensure the equivalent safety and efficacy of the follow-on biological products.

As indicated in Chapter 1, for conventional chemical drug products, in the United States, the abbreviated new drug application (ANDA) was established through the 1984 Hatch-Waxman Amendments for approval of generic drugs. A generic drug must contain the same active ingredient and must have the same dosage form, strength, route of administration, labeling, and condition of use as an innovator product. In addition, it must demonstrate its bioequivalence to the innovator product. However, the ANDA process does not require the generic sponsor to repeat costly and time-consuming animal and clinical research on ingredients or dosage forms already for safety and efficacy by the U.S. FDA. Because no requirement for submission of substantial evidence on efficacy and safety from clinical trials and animal studies, generic drugs are sold at substantial discounts from the price of the innovator drugs.

Just like conventional chemical drug products, follow-on biological products will have to demonstrate profiles of identity, purity, potency, quality, safety, and efficacy that are equivalent to innovative biological products and hence that can be used interchangeably for the innovator biological products. However, due to complicated structure and heterogeneity, a full characterization of biological products for active ingredients, dose, purity, stability and immunogenicity may turn out to be very difficult using the current state-of-the-art technology, In addition, equivalence in structure of active ingredients and biological activity, and bioequivalence based on PK profiles may not be extrapolated to equivalence in efficacy and safety. Recognizing this fundamental difference and difficulty of biological products, a series of guidelines, draft guidelines and concept papers were issued by the U.S. FDA, EMEA (EMEA, 2003a,b, 2005a–g), and International Conference on Harmonization (ICH, 1996, 1999, 2005) for comparability of biological products subject to changes in manufacturing process and for similar biological medicinal products. However, because of complexity of the large molecules for the biological product, the Drug Price Competition and Patent Term Restoration Act passed by the U.S. Congress in 1984 is not sufficient and a new regulatory structure for approval of biosimilar or follow-on biological drug products is required. (Frank, 2007.)

As stated before, traditional approach to bioequivalence based on PK responses such as the area under the plasma–concentration curve (AUC) and peak concentration level ($C_{\max}$) may not be sufficient for therapeutic equivalence and interchangeability of the follow-on biological products with the innovator product. On the other hand, if a full clinical development with conventional phase I, II, and III trials is required to demonstrate the efficacy and safety of the follow-on biological products, then equal financial resources and time as that of the innovator product will be invested and they are not follow-on biological products anymore. Consequently, accessibility and affordability of biological products is severely hampered even after the patents of many innovator biological products expired.

20.4.3 Possible Approaches

Because of this dilemma, although a series of guidelines or draft guidelines were published by the regulatory agencies, no statistical methodology was proposed or specified for clinical evaluation of equivalence between follow-on biological products and innovator biological products. Therefore, this section will state the challenges of establishing equivalence of generic biological products. Hopefully, it may address and resolve this quandary on clinical studies for assessment of equivalence. Due to the complexity, heterogeneity, and complication mechanisms of biological drug products, difference in variability between follow-on and innovator biological products in PK, PD, and clinical responses will be much larger than the difference observed between the conventional generic and innovator chemical drug product. Therefore, average bioequivalence alone is not sufficient to establish equivalence between the follow-on and innovator biological products. On the other hand, because of masking effect, the aggregate metrics for PBE and IBE may fail to address the closeness of the distributions of the responses between the follow-on and innovator biological products. Disaggregate metrics can address the masking effect suffered by the aggregate metrics and find the sources of inequivalence. However, determination of individual equivalence margins with different interpretations is not an easy task. In addition, because of multiparameters, any procedures based on disaggregate metric for evaluation of equivalence between follow-on and innovator biological products will tend to be conservative, especially in the small samples. To resolve this dilemma between the aggregate and disaggregate metrics for evaluation of equivalence, we consider the concept of stochastic equivalence or stochastic noninferiority in our proposal.

Let $F(x)$ and $G(y)$ be the cumulative distribution functions of the responses for follow-on and innovator biological products, respectively. Assuming that a large response value indicates a better efficacy, the follow-on and innovator biological products are said to be stochastically equivalent (two-sided) if the absolute difference between $F(x)$ and $G(x)$ is within some prespecific margins for all x. In other words, metric $\theta = \sup|F(x) - G(x)|$ and hypothesis for equivalence becomes to

$$\begin{aligned} &\mathrm{H_0}:\ \sup|F(x) - G(x)| \geq \eta, \quad \text{for some } x \\ \text{versus}\ &\mathrm{H_1}:\ \sup|F(x) - G(x)| < \eta, \quad \text{for all } x. \end{aligned} \tag{20.4.1}$$

Similarly, the follow-on biological product is said to be stochastically noninferior to the innovator counterpart if the difference between $F(x)$ and $G(x)$ is greater than $-\eta$. The corresponding hypotheses are given follows

$$\begin{aligned} &\mathrm{H}_0: \sup[F(x) - G(x)] \leq -\eta, \quad \text{for some } x \\ \text{versus} \quad &\mathrm{H}_1: \sup[F(x) - G(x)] > -\eta, \quad \text{for all } x. \end{aligned} \tag{20.4.2}$$

Since some of the biological products such as therapeutic antibody or pegylated proteins have a long half-life and equivalence in terms of absorption/bioavailability may not be sufficient, demonstration of equivalence on clearance and half-life may be required to assess the risk of difference in elimination rate. As a result, the traditional crossover designs may not be optimal for evaluation of equivalence between follow-on and innovator biological products. On the other hand, it is very important to investigate the extrapolation ability of equivalence in PK responses to equivalence in PD, and efficacy responses. In order to ensure the internal validity of treatment comparisons, PK, PD, and efficacy response should be evaluated simultaneously in the same trials. We will consider the following design proposed in Figure 20.4.1.

The design in Figure 20.4.1 is a two group parallel design in patients for the comparability bridging study with the disease for which the innovator biological product indicates. After meeting the inclusion and exclusion criteria, patients are randomly divided into two groups. PD/efficacy/safety will be evaluated for the first group of the patients (validation set). Additional PK responses will be assessed for the second group of the patients (training set). A randomization in a 1:1 ratio will be performed separately for each group. The sample size of the second group will be large enough to provide sufficient power for evaluation of bioequivalence based on PK responses. Calibration models will be built based on the PK/PD/efficacy response obtained from the patients in the training set. The PD/efficacy data from the validation set will be used to provide independent assessment of extrapolation ability of equivalence in PK responses to equivalence in PD/efficacy responses.

Although the methods based on Kolmogorov–Simirnov type of statistics have extensively investigated (Serfling, 1980), relatively few literature exists on the statistical tests for stochastic equivalence or noninferiority. First, we suggest using the naïve asymptotic confidence band for $\theta = \sup|F(x) - G(x)|$ or $\theta = \sup[F(x) - G(x)]$ as the test statistics for hypotheses in Equations 20.4.1 and 20.4.2. The test statistics for the parameters in hypotheses in Equations 20.4.1 and 20.4.2 at the boundary

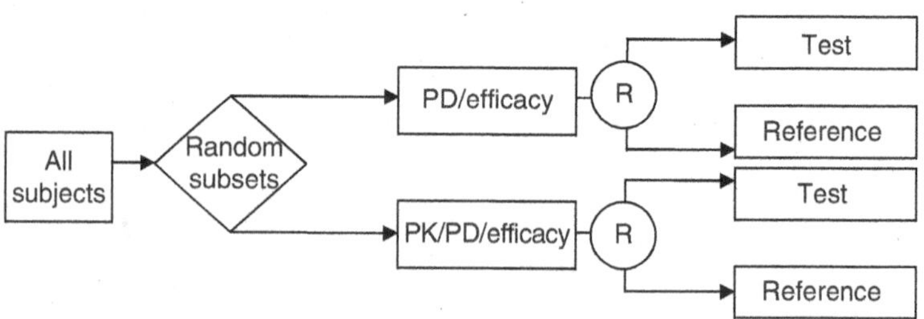

FIGURE 20.4.1: A design for evaluation of equivalence for generic biological products.

margins of the null hypothesis and the corresponding confidence interval may be obtained. If the distribution of the test statistics at the equivalence limits cannot be derived theoretically, permutation and bootstrap techniques can be used to find the distribution of the test statistics and the corresponding confidence intervals.

Because of the nature of the design proposed in Figure 20.4.1, it is in fact an active control trial without a placebo control arm where the follow-on biological product is the test treatment and its innovator counterpart is the active control treatment. Assuming that the innovator biological product was approved due to its superior efficacy over placebo, the equivalence in PD/efficacy is in fact the equivalence in relative efficacy as compared to the (putative) placebo of the follow-on biological product with the innovator counterpart. On the other hand, the prior information of the comparison of the innovator biological product to the placebo can be incorporated into the determination of equivalence margins and the evaluation of equivalence between the follow-on and innovator biological products. The Bayesian design proposed by Simon (1999) will be considered to derive the procedures for assessment of equivalence based on PD/efficacy endpoints.

Calibration models have been used to correlate the surrogate responses with the definitive endpoints (Sargent et al., 2005). Because PK, PD, and efficacy responses are random variables, mixed models were suggested to assessing surrogates as trial endpoints (Korn et al., 2005). We can use the measurement error models to establish calibration models (Cheng and Van Ness, 1999). With the established calibration model obtained from the data of the training set from the design in Figure 20.4.1,

$$P_{\text{efpk}} = \text{Pr(equivalence in efficacy responses} \mid \text{equivalence in PK responses)},$$

and

$$P_{\text{pdpk}} = \text{Pr(equivalence in PD responses} \mid \text{equivalence in PK responses)} \tag{20.4.3}$$

may be estimated for evaluation extrapolation ability of the PK responses using the data from the validation set provided by design in Figure 20.4.1. If P_{efpk} is sufficiently high, then the equivalence in PK responses can be extrapolated to the equivalence in efficacy, then no further phase III clinical evaluation of the follow-on biological product based on efficacy responses may not be required. On the other hand, if P_{efpk} is low, then equivalence in PK responses cannot predict the equivalence in efficacy responses and phase III clinical trials for evaluation of follow-on biological product is required.

If a validated biochip diagnostic device is available for detection of clinically relevant antibody, then each patient in the study under the design described in Figure 20.4.1 should be given two diagnostic tests, one before the randomization and another at the end of the study, to characterize the within-subject change in immune responses. Statistical methods can then be derived for estimation of the within-subject immune changes as well as the procedures for assessment of equivalence in within-subject immune changes between the follow-on and innovator biological products. This allows the short-term evaluation of immunogenicity and its relationship with PK/PD/efficacy responses. However, it should be noted that postmarketing monitoring of antibodies be required for definitive evaluation of clinical significance of the immune responses of follow-on biological products.

20.5 Frequently Asked Questions in Bioequivalence

As noted before, current FDA's position regarding the assessment of bioequivalence is that average bioequivalence is required and IBE/PBE may be considered. However, the FDA encourages that medical/statistical reviewers be consulted if IBE/PBE is to be used. For assessment of bioequivalence, some questions are frequently asked during the regulatory submission and review. In what follows, frequently asked questions in bioequivalence assessment are briefly described below.

20.5.1 What if We Pass Raw Data Model but Fail Log-Transformed Data Model?

As indicated in the FDA guidance, the EMEA, and WHO guideline, all these guidelines recommend that a log-transformation of AUC($0-t_k$), AUC($0-\infty$), and $C_{\max}$ be performed before analysis. No assumption checking or verification of the log-transformed data is encouraged. However, the sponsors often conduct analysis based on both raw data and log-transformed data and submit the one passes bioequivalence testing. If the sponsor passes BE testing under the log-transformed data model, then there is no problem because it meets regulatory requirement. In practice, however, the sponsor may fail BE testing under the log-transformed data model but pass under the raw data model. In this case, the sponsor often provides scientific/statistical justification for the use of raw data model. One of the most commonly seen scientific/statistical justifications is that the raw data model is a more appropriate statistical model than that of the log-transformed data model because all of the assumptions for the raw data model are met. In addition, as pointed out in Section 19.3.3 for the raw data, the bioequivalence limit is expressed in terms of the ratio of the population means between the test and reference formulations, then the equivalence limit is expressed as a percentage of the population reference average which has to be estimated from the data. Therefore, the variability of the estimated reference average is not considered in the equivalence limit. Hence, the false positive rate for claiming average bioequivalence for the two one-sided tests procedure can be inflated to 50%. As a result, one should apply the modified two one-sided tests procedure using the raw data proposed by Liu and Weng (1995) to control the size at the nominal level.

Many researchers have criticized that the use of log-transformed data are not scientifically/statistically justifiable. Liu and Weng (1992) studied the distribution of log-transformed PK data assuming that the hourly concentrations are normally distributed. The results indicated that the log-transformed data are not normally distributed.

Their findings argue against the use of log-transformed data since the primary normality assumption is not met and consequently the assurance of the obtained statistical inference is questionable. In this case, it is suggested that either other transformation such as Box–Cox transformation or a nonparametric method be considered. However, the interpretation of such a transformation is challenging to both pharmacokinetist and biostatisticians.

20.5.2 What If We Pass AUC but Fail C_{max}?

On the basis of log-transformed data, the U.S. FDA requires that both AUC and C_{max} meet the (80%, 125%) bioequivalence criterion for establishment of average bioequivalence. In practice, however, it is not uncommon to pass AUC (the extent of absorption) but fail C_{max} (the rate of absorption). In this case, average bioequivalence cannot be claimed according to the FDA guidance on bioequivalence. However, for C_{max}, the EMEA and WHO guideline use a more relaxed equivalence margin of (70%, 133%).

As indicated by Endrenyi et al. (1991), C_{max}/AUC could be used as an alternative bioequivalence measure for the rate of absorption. Thus, it is suggested that we may look at C_{max}/AUC as an alternative measure of bioequivalence if we fail to pass BE testing based on C_{max}. On the other hand, it is very likely that we may pass C_{max} but fail AUC. In this case, it is suggested that we may look at partial AUC as an alternative measure of bioequivalence (Chen et al., 2001) if we fail to pass BE testing based on AUC from 0 to the last time point or AUC from zero to infinity. However, C_{max}/AUC is not currently selected as the required PK responses for approval of generic drug products by any of the regulatory authorities in the world including the U.S. FDA, EMEA, and WHO. It should be noted that no alpha adjustment for multiple comparisons is required by the regulatory agencies such as the U.S. FDA.

20.5.3 What if We Fail by a Relatively Small Margin?

In practice, it is very possible that we fail BE testing for either AUC or C_{max} by a relatively small margin. For example, the 90% confidence interval for AUC, say (79.5%, 120%) is slightly outside the lower limit of (80%, 125%). In this case, the FDA's position is very clear that "rule is rule and you fail." As a matter of fact, the U.S. FDA is very strict about this rule, the equivalence margin is (80%, 125%) in the 2003 FDA guidance. However, the sponsor usually performs either an outlier detection analysis or a sensitivity analysis to resolve the issue. In other words, if a subject is found to be an outlier statistically, it may be excluded from the analysis with appropriate clinical justification. Once the identified outlier is excluded from the analysis, a 90% confidence interval is recalculated. If the 90% confidence interval after excluding the identified outlier is totally within the bioequivalence limit of (80%, 125%), the sponsor then argues to claim bioequivalence.

It should be noted that the FDA uses one-fits-all criterion, that is, (80%, 125%) for all PK parameters. But some other countries allow flexible bioequivalence limits for some PK parameters such as for C_{max}. For example, as mentioned in Sections 19.3.3 and 20.5.3, for C_{max}, the 2002 EMEA guidance and the 2005 WHO draft guideline employ lenient equivalence limits of 75% and 133% if it is prospectively specified in the protocol and justifications should be given based on efficacy and safety considerations.

20.5.4 Can We Still Assess Bioequivalence if There Is a Significant Sequence Effect?

As indicated in Section 19.2.2, a significant sequence effect is an indication of possible (1) failure of randomization, (2) true sequence effect, (3) true carry-over effect, and (4) true formulation-by-period effect. Under the standard two-sequence and two-period crossover design, the sequence effect is confounded with the carry-over effect. Therefore, if a significant sequence effect is found, the treatment effect and its corresponding 90% confidence interval cannot be estimated unbiasedly due to possible unequal carryover effects. However, in the 2001 U.S. FDA guidance on *Statistical Approaches to Establishing Bioequivalence*, a list of conditions is provided to rule out the possibility of unequal carryover effects:

1. It is a single-dose study.
2. Drug is not an endogenous entity.
3. More than an adequate washout period has been allowed between periods of the study and in the subsequent periods the predose biological matrix samples do not exhibit a detectable drug level in any of the subjects.
4. Study meets all scientific criteria (e.g., it is based on an acceptable study protocol and it contains a validated assay methodology).

The 2001 FDA guidance also recommends that sponsors conduct a bioequivalence study with parallel designs if unequal carryover effects become an issue.

20.5.5 What Should We Do When We Have Almost Identical Means but Still Fail to Meet the Bioequivalence Criterion?

It is not uncommon to run into the situation that we have almost identical means but still fail to meet bioequivalence criterion. This indicates that (1) the variation of the reference product is too large to establish bioequivalence between the test product and the reference product, (2) the bioequivalence study was poorly conducted, and (3) analytical assay methodology is inadequate and not fully validated. The concept of IBE and PBE is an attempt to overcome this problem. As a result, it is suggested that either PBE or IBE be considered to establish bioequivalence.

However, in our experience, unless the variability of the test formulation is much smaller than that of the reference formulation, it is still unlikely to pass either PBE or IBE. In addition to avoid masking effect of PBE or IBE, the 2001 FDA guidance requires that the geometric test/reference averages be within (80%, 125%) as well.

20.5.6 Bioequivalence Does Not Necessarily Imply Therapeutic Equivalence

To protect the exclusivity of a brand-name drug product, the sponsor of innovator drug products will usually make every attempt to prevent generic drug products from being approved by the regulatory agencies such as the U.S. FDA. One of the strategies is to convince regulatory agency that the generic copy of the brand name drug will not achieve therapeutic equivalence as compared to the brand-name drug even it has been shown to be bioequivalent to the brand-name drug. For this purpose, the sponsor may file a *Citizen Petition* with scientific/clinical justification. The FDA has legal obligation to respond within 180 days after the receipt of the petition.

It should be noted that bioequivalence assessment is performed under the *Fundamental Bioequivalence Assumption,* which constitutes legal basis for regulatory approval. As a result, the FDA will not suspend the review/approval process of generic submission of a given brand-name drug even a citizen petition is under review within the FDA. In addition, as mentioned in Section 20.1, tremendous saving and reduction of costs for prescription drugs are achieved because of availability of generic drug products. Therefore, the Drug Price Competition and Patent Term Restoration Act is widely considered as a success (Frank, 2007). On the other hand, a therapeutic equivalence may not imply bioequivalence either.

20.5.7 Inconsistency between Test Statistics under a 2×2 Crossover Design and a $2 \times 2m$ Replicated Crossover Design

A commonly asked question in the assessment of average bioequivalence is that there is an inconsistency between test statistics given in this book (second edition) and the one as described in the FDA draft guidance. It should be noted that test statistic for assessment of ABE given in this book was derived under a 2×2 crossover design and the test statistic as described in the FDA guidance was derived under a replicated $2 \times 2m$ crossover design. However, the test statistics derived under a replicated 2×2 crossover design is reduced to the test statistics derived under a 2×2 crossover design given in our book if $m = 1$. In addition, the current regulatory requirement for approval of generic drug is still average bioequivalence. As a result, the 2003 FDA guidance for general considerations recommends nonreplicate 2×2 crossover design for bioequivalence studies of immediate-release and modified-release dosage forms (p. 7 of the guidance). It follows that the test statistics given in Chapter 4 should be used for evaluation of average bioequivalence under the standard 2×2 crossover design.

To address the inconsistency, first we would like to point out that the assessment of ABE is usually done under a 2×2 crossover design under certain assumptions (e.g.,

$\sigma_{BT} = \sigma_{BR} = \sigma_S$, where σ_{BT} and σ_{BR} are between subject variability for the test product and the reference product, respectively, and $\sigma_{WT} = \sigma_{WR} = \sigma$, where σ_{WT} and σ_{WR} are within subject variability for the test product and the reference product, respectively. For convenience's sake, we will refer to the statistical model under the 2×2 crossover design with these assumptions as the classical model (Chow and Liu, 2000). However, in practice, these assumptions may not hold. If there are replicates, we will be able to provide independent estimates for σ_{BT}, σ_{BR}, σ_{WT}, and σ_{WR}. In this case, the FDA suggests a mixed effects model be used. We will refer to the statistical model with the assumption that (1) σ_{BT} and σ_{BR} are not necessarily the same and (2) σ_{WT} and σ_{WR} are not necessarily the same as the FDA's model. The difference between the classical model and the FDA's model is summarized below.

20.5.7.1 FDA's Model

As an example, consider a 2×6 crossover design, i.e., (ABABAB, BABABA), the following mixed effect model is considered:

$$y_{ijkl} = \mu_k + \gamma_{ik} + s_{ik} + e_{ijkl},$$

where

y_{ijkl} is the PK response from the jth ($j = 1, \ldots, n$) subject in the ith ($i = 1, 2$) sequence under the lth ($l = 1, 2, 3$) replicate of treatment k ($k = 1$: test; 2: reference)
μ_k is the kth formulation effect such that $\mu_1 - \mu_2 = \delta$
γ_{ik} is the fixed effect of the ith sequence under treatment k
s_{ik} is the random effect of the ith subject under treatment
k, (s_{i1}, s_{i2}), $i = 1, \ldots, n$ are assumed to be i.i.d. as bivariate normal random variable with mean 0 and covariance matrix

$$\begin{pmatrix} \sigma_{BT}^2 & \rho\sigma_{BT}\sigma_{BR} \\ \rho\sigma_{BT}\sigma_{BR} & \sigma_{BR}^2 \end{pmatrix};$$

e_{ij1l}'s are assumed to be i.i.d normal random variables with mean 0 and variance σ_{WT}^2, and e_{ij2l}'s are assumed to be i.i.d normal random variables with mean 0 and variance σ_{WR}^2.

20.5.7.2 Classical Model Under a 2 × 2 Crossover Design

The classical model in Chapter 4 is essentially the same as FDA's model under the assumption that $s_{i1} = s_{i2}$, $i = 1, \ldots, n$, which implies that $\sigma_{BT} = \sigma_{BR}$ and $\rho = 1$. Consequently, the variability due to formulation-by-subject interaction

$$\sigma_D^2 = \sigma_{BT}^2 + \sigma_{BR}^2 - 2\rho\sigma_{BT}\sigma_{BR} = 0.$$

This may not be true under the FDA's model. As a result, under different models with different assumptions, test statistics for assessment of ABE could be different.

For example, under the 2×2 design, the unbiased estimates for δ and σ^2_{WT}, σ^2_{WR} are given by $\widehat{\delta} = \frac{1}{2n}\sum_{i=1}^{2}\sum_{j=1}^{n}(y_{ij11} - y_{ij21})$, which follows a normal distribution

$$\widehat{\delta} \sim N\left(\delta, \frac{\sigma^2_{\text{WT}} + \sigma^2_{\text{WR}}}{2n}\right).$$

On the other hand, under the FDA's model, we have

$$\widehat{\delta} \sim N\left(\delta, \frac{\sigma^2_{\text{D}} + \sigma^2_{\text{WT}} + \sigma^2_{\text{WR}}}{2n}\right).$$

Now, under a $2 \times m$ design (e.g., $m = 4, 6$), let

$$\bar{y}_{ijk\cdot} = \frac{1}{m}(y_{ijk1} + \cdots + y_{ijkm}).$$

Then the unbiased estimates for δ is given by

$$\widehat{\delta} = \frac{1}{2n}\sum_{i=1}^{2}\sum_{j=1}^{n}(\bar{y}_{ij1\cdot} - \bar{y}_{ij2\cdot})$$

Under the classical model, we have

$$\widehat{\delta} \sim N\left(\delta, \frac{(\sigma^2_{\text{WT}} + \sigma^2_{\text{WR}})/m}{2n}\right).$$

On the other hand, under the FDA's model,

$$\widehat{\delta} \sim N\left(\delta, \frac{\sigma^2_{\text{D}} + (\sigma^2_{\text{WT}} + \sigma^2_{\text{WR}})/m}{2n}\right).$$

As discussed above, we have the following observations. First, the ABE is established based on $\widehat{\delta}$. According to the above discussion, it is clear that based on the FDA's model, increasing the number of replicates does not decrease the variability due to the subject-by-formulation interaction. Especially in our simulation study, we choose $\rho = 0.75$ and σ^2_{BT} and σ^2_{BR} are not necessarily equal to each other. Therefore, $\sigma^2_{\text{D}} \neq 0$, which prevent the further improvement of ABE. Second, for assessment of ABE under a 2×2 crossover design, the methods described in Chapter 4, which assumes $\sigma^2_{\text{D}} = 0$, has been widely used and accepted in practice. The reason is multi-fold. First, under the 2×2 crossover design, ρ, σ^2_{BT}, and σ^2_{BR} are confounded with σ^2_{WR} and σ^2_{WR} and thus cannot be separated. As a result, the assumption that $\sigma_D^2 = 0$ is necessarily made for a valid statistical assessment of ABE. In addition, the 2×2 crossover design considered in Chapter 4 is the non-replicate design recommended by the 2003 FDA guidance on general considerations for bioequivalence studies. However, as indicated in the 2001 FDA guidance, the assumption of $\sigma_D^2 = 0$ may not hold. In addition, replicated crossover designs provide independent estimates of ρ and all variance components.

20.5.8 Power and Sample Size Calculation Based on Raw Data Model and Log-Transformed Model Are Different

Power analysis and sample size calculation based on the raw data model are different from those under the log-transformed model due to the fact that they are different models. Under different models, means, standard deviations, and coefficients of variation are different. As mentioned before, for assessment of bioequivalence, all regulatory authorities including the U.S. FDA, EMEA, WHO, and Japan require log-transformation of AUC($0-t_k$), AUC($0-\infty$), and C_{max} be done before analysis and evaluation of bioequivalence. As a result, one should use differences in mean and standard deviation or coefficient of variation for power analysis and sample size calculation based on the method for the log-transformed model as given in Chapter 5.

Note that sponsors should make decision as to which model (the raw data model or the log-transformed data model) will be used for bioequivalence assessment. Once the model is chosen, appropriate formulas can be used to determine the sample size. Fishing around for obtaining the smallest sample size is not a good clinical practice.

20.5.9 Adjustment for Multiplicity

The 2003 FDA guidance for general considerations requires that for AUC($0-t_k$), AUC($0-\infty$) and C_{max}, the following information be provided

1. Geometric means
2. Arithmetic means
3. Ratio of means
4. 90% Confidence interval

In addition, the 2003 FDA guidance recommends that logarithmic transformation be provided for measures for bioequivalence demonstration using a bioequivalence limit of 80.00% to 125.00%. Therefore, to pass the average bioequivalence, each 90% confidence interval of AUC($0-t_k$), AUC($0-\infty$), and C_{max} must fall within 80.00% and 125.00%. It follows that according to the intersection-union principle (Berger, 1982), the type I error rate of average bioequivalence is still controlled under the nominal level of 5%. Therefore, there is no need for adjustment due to multiple PK measures.

20.5.10 Why Log-Transformation? Why Nonparametric Method Is Not Encouraged? Any Scientific Justification?

As mentioned in Section 19.2.1, the 2001 FDA guidance uses the deterministic multiplicative PK models as the PK rationale for the logarithmic transformation of exposure measures such as AUC$(0 - t_k)$, AUC$(0 - \infty)$, and C_{max}. The EMEA and WHO guidelines also have the similar requirement for log-transformation of AUC $(0 - t_k)$, AUC$(0 - \infty)$, and C_{max}. However, the EMEA and WHO guidelines suggest that the analysis of T_{max} should be nonparametric and be applied to the untransformed data. Therefore, the nonparametric confidence interval for difference in averages should be constructed for T_{max} (WHO, 2005a). However, as indicated in Section 19.3.4, for the untransformed data, the equivalence limit is a function of the unknown reference population average and has to be estimated from the data. If the variability of the estimated equivalence limit is not considered, Liu and Weng (1995) showed that the type I error rate can be inflated as high as 50% if the correlation of the observed T_{max} from the same subject approaches to 1. It is suggested that the modified two-sided tests procedure proposed by Liu and Weng (1995) be used for evaluation of average bioequivalence based on T_{max}. It should be noted that unlike AUC$(0 - t_k)$, AUC $(0 - \infty)$ and C_{max}, neither the EMEA guidance nor the WHO draft guidance recommend bioequivalence limits for T_{max}.

20.5.11 Challenges in Population PK Modeling

In the past decade, several challenges in population PK have been discussed in the literature. These challenges include (1) appropriate fitting methods, (2) accuracy of approximations and asymptotics, (3) the need for stable and well-documented software, (4) the need for development of diagnostic tools such as outlier and influence analysis, robust and resistant fitting methods, and (5) incorporation of time-dependent covariates.

Note that Edler (1998) provided a list of PK–PD software packages currently available in the marketplace. The list includes 72 software packages. Most of these software packages were developed based on maximum likelihood approach. These software packages include, but are not limited to, NONMEM (Sheiner and Beal, 1980, 1981, 1983), SAS macros NLINMIX and NLMEN, PROC NLMIXED of SAS, NLME of S-Plus, WnNonlin or WinNonlinMix of Pharsight. Software packages based on nonparametric maximum likelihood approach are also available. For example, NPLM (Mallet, 1986), and SAS macros for Bayesian EM Algorithm (Racine-Poon and Smith, 1990).

20.6 Discussion

From Chapters 1 through 12, the concept and statistical methodology of ABE, PBE, and IBE were introduced by using the oral formulations, for example, tablets or capsules, of the traditional chemical drug products with a low molecular weight for which the concentrations of the active ingredients can be quantified from blood samples. In other chapters, statistical methodology were either extended or modified to evaluation of the drug products other than the oral formulations with special characteristics or under special conditions, or drug products with alternative administrating routes. In addition, we also demonstrated the procedures for assessment of equivalence based on dissolution profiles between two formulations. In Chapter 19, we have reviewed almost all important guidance or guidelines on bioequivalence issued by regulatory authorities in the world. However, extension or modification of current methodology to evaluation of bioequivalence to other drug products may not be so straightforward and requires more innovations on technology. This is one of the reasons why in May 2007, the U.S. FDA issued the critical path opportunities for generic drugs which lay out the opportunities as well as the challenges that are unique to the generic drug products. However, the critical path opportunities for generic drugs were issued by the Office of Generic Drugs, Center for Drug Evaluation and Research. Consequently, the critical path opportunities for generic drugs are only confined to the traditional chemical drug products. Therefore, in this chapter, we introduce the issues and challenges of bioequivalence in other areas of emerging importance. These include using genomic data to facilitate evaluation of bioequivalence, bridging bioequivalence studies in developing countries, assessment of bioequivalence for biological products. In addition, we provide a list of most frequently asked questions in bioequivalence.

However, the concept of equivalence is not limited only to bioequivalence for approval of generic drug products. On the basis of the risk of medical devices posed to the patient and user, the U.S. FDA categorized medical devices into three classes, Regulations for Class I devices require the general controls while the Class II devices require both general controls and special controls. On the other hand, because of higher risks, in addition to the general controls and special controls, the U.S. FDA requests that Class III devices require a premarket approval (PMA) to obtain marketing clearance (FDA, 2006c). However, for Class I and II devices, the sponsor can make a premarket notification through a 510 (k) submission to the U.S. FDA (FDA, 2006d). Under 510 (k), the new device must demonstrate that it is at least safe and effective as a legally U.S. market device or a predicate device. This concept of equivalence for approval of medical devices under 510 (k) is referred to *substantial equivalence*. According to the U.S. FDA, a device is substantially equivalent if, in comparison to a predicate it

- Has the same intended use as the predicate,
- Has the same technological characteristics as the predicate

or

- Has the same intended use as the predicate,
- Has different technological characteristics and the information submitted to FDA.

Does not raise new questions of safety and effectiveness, and
Demonstrates that the device is at least as safe and effective as the legally market device.

Therefore, the under 510 (k) submission, as compared to the predicate, a device must demonstrate or a two-sided equivalence in technological characteristics or a one-sided equivalence or non-inferiority in safety and effectiveness. However, very scarce literature on statistical methods of substantial equivalence for approval of medical devices can be found. In addition, even the selection of equivalence limits for evaluation of substantial equivalence has not been fully investigated or mentioned in the regulatory guidelines. Therefore more research on these two areas is urgently required.

Recently, the concept of substantial equivalence has been extended to evaluation and approval of genetic modified crops or food (GMO) (Hothorn and Oberdoerfer, 2006), According to Organization for Economic Cooperation and Development (OECD) the concept of substantial equivalence relies upon that the characteristics of the existing food/feed source can serve as the references for the comparison in assessment of the safety of human and animal consumption of a food or feed that is genetically modified. For example, OECD Consensus Documents provided a set of key nutrients and toxicants in low erucic acid rapeseed (canola) for evaluation of substantial equivalence. However, application of either substantial equivalence for medical devices or bioequivalence for generic drug products to GMOs may require some modification. For example, it is impossible to insert a washout period without food for the feed experiments using the standard 2×2 crossover design where the test formulation is the GM feed and reference is the conventional feed. As a result, carryover effects can not be avoided under the standard 2×2 crossover design. Therefore, for feed experiments must employ higher-order crossover designs reviewed in Chapter 9. (Tempelman, 2004). On the other hand, the impact of the GM crops or food is at least two-fold. First, they may be the food products from which human directly consume, for example, the GM papaya, GM meat or milk. Secondly, they may be the products derived from the GM organisms, e.g., cooking oil or soybean milk from soybean or flour made from GM wheat. Another example is the beef from the genetically unmodified cattle which were fed with the GM feeds. In addition, the objective of substantial equivalence in the context of GM food/feed is to demonstrate that the GM food/feed is as safe as its conventional counterpart. These differences from the generic drugs must be taken into consideration in designing the experiment for evaluation of substantial equivalence of GM food.

As indicated by Hothorn and Oberdoerfer, 2006, the parameters used for assessment of substantial equivalence between the GM food/feed and its conventional counterpart consist of measurements of agronomic and phenotypic characteristics, compositional analyses and animal feeding tests. It follows that the number of parameters for establishment of substantial equivalence are usually in hundreds. These characteristics can be classified into at least two groups. The first group represents the traits introduced through genetically alteration of the traditional crops or organisms. The second class is those characteristics which should not be affected by genetically alteration. For the first class of the measurements, one must show that the differences between the GM food/feed and their conventional counterpart must exceed some threshold to be declared as genetic modification. Let μ_{Ti} and μ_{Ci} be the population averages of trait i for the GM food/feed and their conventional counterpart, respectively, $i = 1, \ldots, a$. Then the hypothesis for testing whether the trait i is truly introduced to the GM food can be formulated into the following hypothesis:

$$\begin{aligned} &\mathrm{H_0}: -C_i' \leq \mu_{\mathrm{T}_i} - \mu_{\mathrm{C}_i} \leq C_i \\ \text{versus} \quad &\mathrm{H_1}: \mu_{\mathrm{T}_i} - \mu_{\mathrm{C}_i} < -C_i' \quad \text{or} \quad \mu_{\mathrm{T}_i} - \mu_{\mathrm{C}_i} > C_i \\ &i = 1, \ldots, a \end{aligned} \tag{20.6.1}$$

where

C_i is the minimal biologically meaningful upper threshold
$-C_i'$ is the maximal biological meaningful lower threshold
C_i and $-C_i'$ are positive

For other class of characteristics, the GM food/feed must demonstrate equivalence to its conventional counterpart. Therefore the traditional two one-sided hypotheses can be employed:

$$\begin{aligned} &\mathrm{H_{0U}}: \mu_{\mathrm{T}_i} - \mu_{\mathrm{C}_i} > C_i \\ \text{versus} \quad &\mathrm{H_{aU}}: \mu_{\mathrm{T}_i} - \mu_{\mathrm{C}_i} < C_i \\ \text{and} \quad & \\ &\mathrm{H_{0L}}: \mu_{\mathrm{T}_i} - \mu_{\mathrm{C}_i} < -C_i' \\ \text{versus} \quad &\mathrm{H_{1L}}: \mu_{\mathrm{T}_i} - \mu_{\mathrm{C}_i} > -C_i', \quad i = a + 1, \ldots, b \end{aligned} \tag{20.6.2}$$

If the objective is to prove that the GM food/feed is at least as safe as the conventional counterpart, then the noninferiority hypothesis of the two one-sided hypotheses in Equation 20.6.2 can be used. However, main issues of evaluation of substantial equivalence for GM food/feed lie upon the adequate control or type I error rate induced by multiplicity due to hundreds of characteristics and the determination of thresholds for each characteristic either for differentiation of inserted genetic traits or for equivalence in other unaltered characteristics. Of course, based on the intersection–union principle, an overall type I error rate will be less than the α significance level if each of b hypotheses in Equations 20.6.1 and 20.6.2 is tested at the α level. However, this approach is extremely conservative and may not be practically feasible. On the other hand, the normal ranges of agronomic and phenotypic characteristics, compositional analyses and animal feeding tests for the conventional crop/food/feed must first be established to determine the thresholds in hypotheses 20.6.1 and 20.6.2. Currently, few consensuses about the normal ranges of characteristics even for the conventional crops or food have been reached. Therefore, the issues on the multiplicity and determination of threshold for assessment of substantial equivalence require further research.

References

Aarons, L. 1991. Population pharmacokinetics: theory and practice. *Br. J. Clin. Pharmacol.*, 32, 669–670.

Agresti, A. 1990. *Categorical Data Analysis*. 1st ed., John Wiley & Sons, New York.

Agresti, A. 2002. *Categorical Data Analysis*. 2nd ed., John Wiley & Sons, New York.

Al-Banna, M.K., Kelman, A.W., and Whiting, B. 1990. Experimental design and efficient parameter estimation in population pharmacokinetics. *Journal of Pharmacokinetics and Biopharmaceutics*, 18, 347–360.

Albert, K.S. and Smith, R.B. 1980. Bioavailability assessment as influenced by variations in drug absorption. In: *Drug Absorption and Disposition: Statistical Considerations*, Albert, K.S. (Ed.), American Pharmaceutical Association, Washington, DC, pp. 87–113.

Altham, P.M.E. 1971. The analysis of matched proportions. *Biometrika*, 58, 561–576.

Amidon, G.L., Lennernas, H., Shah, V.P., and Crison, J.R. 1995. A theoretical basis for a biopharmaceutic drug classification: The correlation of in vitro drug product dissolution and in vivo bioavailability. *Pharmaceutical Research*, 12, 413–420.

Anderson, R.L. 1982. *Analysis of Variance Components, Unpublished Lecture Notes*. University of Kentucky, Lexington, KY.

Anderson, S. 1993. Individual bioequivalence: A problem of switchability [with discussion]. *Biopharmaceutical Report*, 2, 1–11.

Anderson, S. and Hauck, W.W. 1983. A new procedure for testing equivalence in comparative bioavailability and other clinical trials. *Communications in Statistics—Theory and Methods*, 12, 2663–2692.

Anderson, S. and Hauck, W.W. 1990. Consideration of individual bioequivalence. *Journal of Pharmacokinetics and Biopharmaceutics*, 18, 259–273.

Armitage, P. and Berry, G. 1987. *Statistical Methods in Medical Research*. 2nd ed., Blackwell Scientific, Oxford, UK.

Balaam, L.N. 1968. A two-period design with t^2 experimental units. *Biometrics*, 24, 61–73.

Balant, L.P. 1991. Is there a need for more precise definitions of bioavailability? *European Journal of Clinical Pharmacology*, 40, 123–126.

Beal, S.L. and Sheiner, L.B. 1980. The NONMEM system. *American Statistician*, 34, 118–119.

Beal, S.L. and Sheiner, L.B. 1982. Estimating population pharmacokinetics. *Critical Reviews in Biomedical Engineering*, 8, 195–222.

Beal, S.L. and Sheiner, L.B. 1989. *NONMEM, User's Guide*. NONMEM Project Group, University of California, San Francisco, CA.

Beckhofer, R.E., Dunnett, C.W., and Sobel, M. 1954. A two sample multiple decision procedure for linking means of normal populations with a common unknown variance. *Biometrika*, 41, 170–176.

Bellavance, F. and Tardif, S. 1995. A nonparametric approach to the analysis of three-treatment three-period crossover design. *Biometrika*, 82, 865–875.

Benet, L.Z. and Goyan, J.E. 1995. Bioequivalence and narrow therapeutic index drugs. *Pharmacotherapy*, 15, 433–440.

Berger, R.L. 1982. Multiparametric hypothesis testing and acceptance sampling. *Technometrics*, 24, 295–300.

Bickel, P.J. and Doksum, A.D. 1977. *Mathematical Statistics*. Holden-Day, San Francisco, CA.

Blackwelder, W.C. 1982. Proving the null hypothesis in clinical trials. *Controlled Clinical Trials*, 3, 345–353.

Blume, H.H. and Midha, K.K. 1993a. Conference Report. In: *Bio-International: Bioavailability, Bioequivalence and Pharmacokinetics*, Blume, H.H. and Midha, K.K. (Eds.), Medpharm, Stuttgart, Germany, pp. 13–23.

Blume, H.H. and Midha, K.K. 1993b. Bio-international 92, conference on bioavailability, bioequivalence and pharmacokinetic studies. *Pharmaceutical Research*, 10, 1806–1811.

Boardman, T.J. 1974. Confidence intervals for variance components—a comparative Monte Carlo study. *Biometrics*, 30, 251–262.

Bose, R.C., Clatworthy, W.H., and Shrinkhande, S. 1954. Tables of partially balanced incomplete block design with two associate classes. *Journal of the American Statistical Association*, 47, 151–184.

Box, G.E.P. and Tiao, G.C. 1973. *Bayesian Inference in Statistical Analysis*. Addison-Wesley, Reading, MA.

Bradu, D. and Mundlak, Y. 1970. Estimation in lognormal linear model. *Journal of the American Statistical Association*, 65, 198–211.

Brown, B.W. 1980. The crossover experiment for clinical trials. *Biometrics*, 36, 69–79.

Brown, L.D., Hwang, J.T.G., and Munk, A. 1998. An unbiased test for the bioequivalence problem. *Annals of Statistics*, 25, 2345–2367.

Buonaccorsi, J.P. and Gatsonis, C.A. 1988. Bayesian inference for ratios of coefficients in a linear model. *Biometrics*, 44, 87–101.

Carrasco, J.L. and Jover, L. 2002. Assessing individual bioequivalence using the structural equation model. *Statistics in Medicine*, 22, 901–912.

Chen, K.W., Li, G., Sun, Y., and Chow, S.C. 1996. A confidence region approach for assessing equivalence in variability of bioavailability. *Biometrical Journal*, 38, 475–487.

Chen, K.W., Li, G., Sun, Y., and Chow, S.C. 1997a. Internal estimation for ratios in bioequivalence trials. *Biometrical Journal*, 39, 989–1002.

Chen, K.W., Li, G., and Chow, S.C. 1997b. A note on sample size determination for bioequivalence studies with higher-order crossover designs. *Journal of Pharmacokinetics and Pharmacodynamics*, 25, 753–765.

Chen, M.L. 1995. Individual bioequivalence. Invited presentation at International Workshop: Statistical and Regulatory Issues on the Assessment of Bioequivalence. Dusseldorf, Germany, October 19–20.

Chen, M.L. 1996. Individual bioequivalence criterion. Presented at the meeting of the Advisory Committee for Pharmaceutical Sciences. Gaitherburg, Maryland, August 15–16.

Chen, M.L. 1997. Individual bioequivalence—a regulatory update. *Journal of Biopharmaceutical Statistics*, 7, 5–11.

Chen, M.L. and Pelsor, F.R. 1991. Half-life revisited: Implication in clinical trials and bioavailability/bioequivalence evaluation. *Journal of the American Pharmacists Association*, 80, 406–408.

Chen, M.L., Patnaik, R., Hauck, W.W., Schuirmann, D.F., Hyslop, T., and Williams, R. 2000. An individual bioequivalence criterion—regulatory considerations. *Statistics in Medicine*, 19, 2821–2842.

Chen, M.L., Patnaik, R., Hauck, W.W., Schuirmann, D.J., Hyslop, T., and Williams, R. 2000. An individual bioequivalence criterion: Regulatory considerations. *Statistics in Medicine*, 19, 2821–2842.

Chen, M.L., Shah, V., Patnaik, R., Adams, W., Hussain, A., Conner, D., Mehta, M., Malinowski, H., Lazor, J., Huang, S.M., Hare, D., Lesko, L., Sporn, D., and Williams, R. 2001a. Bioavailability and bioequivalence: An FDA regulatory overview. *Pharmaceutical Research*, 18, 1645–1650.

Chen, M.L., Lesko, L., and Williams, R.L. 2001b. Measures of exposure versus measures of rate and extent of absorption. *Clinical Pharmacokinetics*, 40, 565–572.

Cheng, C.L. and Van Ness, J.W. 1999. *Statistical Regression with Measurement Error*. Arnold, London.

Cheng, C.S. and Wu, C.F. 1980. Balanced repeated measurements designs. *Annals of Statistics*, 8, 1272–1283 (Corrigendum, 11, p. 349 [1983]).

Chinchilli, V.M. 1996. The assessment of individual and population bioequivalence. *Journal of Biopharmaceutical Statistics*, 6, 6–14.

Chinchilli, V.M. and Durham, B.S. 1989. Testing for bioequivalence via R-estimation. Presented at the 45th Conference on Applied Statistics, Atlantic City, NJ.

Chinchilli, V.M. and Esinhart, J.D. 1994. Extension to the use of tolerance interval for the assessment of individual bioequivalence. *Journal of Biopharmaceutical Statistics*, 4, 39–52.

Chinchilli, V.M. and Esinhart, J.D. 1996. Design and analysis of intra-subject variability in cross-over experiments. *Statistics in Medicine*, 15, 1619–1634.

Chow, S.C. 1985. Resampling procedures for the estimation of non-linear functions of parameters. Ph.D. Thesis. University of Wisconsin, Madison, WI.

Chow, S.C. 1989. Some results on bioavailability/bioequivalence studies. Proceedings of the Biopharmaceutical section of the American Statistical Association, Washington, D.C., pp. 260–268.

Chow, S.C. 1990. Alternative approaches for assessing bioequivalence regarding normality assumptions. *Drug Information Journal*, 24, 753–762 (Corrigendum, 25, p. 161 [1991]).

Chow, S.C. 1995. Ed. Bioavailability and bioequivalence. *Drug Information Journal*, 29 (3; special issue), 793–1068.

Chow, S.C. 1996a. Issues in bioequivalence. *Biopharmaceutical Report*, 4, 1–12.

Chow, S.C. 1996b. Statistical considerations for replicated design. In: *Bioavailability, Bioequivalence and Pharmacokinetic Studies*. Proceedings of FIP Bio-International'96. Midha, K.K. and Nagai, T. (Eds.), Business Center for Academic Societies, Tokyo, Japan, pp. 107–112.

Chow, S.C. 1997a. Ed. Recent issues in bioequivalence trials. *Journal of Biopharmaceutical Statistics*, 7 (1; special issue), 1–204.

Chow, S.C. 1999. Individual bioequivalence—a review of the FDA draft guidance. *Drug Informational Journal*, 33, 435–444.

Chow, S.C. and Ju, H.L. 1994. Bioequivalence: A review and prospects for the future. *Journal of Chinese Statistical Association*, 32, 179–196.

Chow, S.C. and Ki, F. 1997. Statistical comparison between dissolution profiles of drug products. *Journal of Biopharmaceutical Statistics*, 7, 241–258.

Chow, S.C. and Liu, J.P. 1992. On assessment of bioequivalence under a higher-order crossover design. *Journal of Biopharmaceutical Statistics*, 2, 239–256.

Chow, S.C. and Liu, J.P. 1994a. Statistical considerations in bioequivalence trials. *Communications in Statistics—Theory and Methods*, 23, 289–304.

Chow, S.C. and Liu, J.P. 1994b. Recent statistical development in bioequivalence trials—a review of FDA guidance. *Drug Information Journal*, 28, 851–864.

Chow, S.C. and Liu, J.P. 1995a. Current issues in bioequivalence trials. *Drug Information Journal*, 29, 795–804.

Chow, S.C. and Liu, J.P. 1995b. *Statistical Design and Analysis in Pharmaceutical Science*. Marcel Dekker, New York.

Chow, S.C. and Liu, J.P. 1997. Meta-analysis for bioequivalence review. *Journal of Biopharmaceutical Statistics*, 7, 97–111.

Chow, S.C. and Liu, J.P 2000. *Design and Analysis of Bioavailability and Bioequivalence Studies*, 2nd Ed., Marcel Dekker, New York.

Chow, S.C. and Liu, J.P. 2004. *Design and Analysis of Clinical Trials*. 2nd edn. John Wiley & Sons, New York.

Chow, S.C. and Shao, J. 1988. A new procedure for the estimation of variance components. *Statistics and Probability Letters*, 6, 349–355.

Chow, S.C. and Shao, J. 1989. Tests for batch-to-batch variation in stability analysis. *Statistics in Medicine*, 8, 883–890.

Chow, S.C. and Shao, J. 1990. An alternative approach for the assessment of bioequivalence between two formulation of a drug. *Biometrical Journal*, 32, 969–976.

Chow, S.C. and Shao, J. 1991. A note on decision rules in bioequivalence studies. Unpublished manuscript.

Chow, S.C. and Shao, J. 1997. Statistical methods for two-sequence three-period cross-over designs with incomplete data. *Statistics in Medicine*, 16, 1031–1039.

Chow, S.C. and Shao, J. 1999. Bioequivalence review for drug interchangeability. *Journal of Biopharmaceutical Statistics*, 9, 485–497.

Chow, S.C. and Shao, J. 2002. *Statistics in Drug Research–Methodologies and Recent Developments*. Marcel Dekker, New York.

Chow, S.C., Cheng, J., and Shao, J. 1990. A nonparametric bootstrap approach for assessing bioequivalence. Unpublished manuscript.

Chow, S.C., Peace, K., and Shao, J. 1991. Assessment of bioequivalence using multiplicative model. *Journal of Biopharmaceutical Statistics*, 1, 193–203.

Chow, S.C., Shao, J., and Wang, H. 2002a. Individual bioequivalence testing under 2×3 designs. *Statistics in Medicine*, 21, 629–648.

Chow, S.C., Shao, J., and Wang, H. 2002b. Statistical tests for population bioequivalence. *Statistica Sinica*, 13, 539–554.

Chow, S.C., Shao, J., and Wang, H. 2003a. In vitro bioequivalence testing. *Statistics in Medicine*, 22, 55–68.

Chow, S.C., Shao, J., and Wang, H. 2003b. *Sample Size Calculation in Clinical Research*. Marcel Dekker, New York.

Chow, S.C., Shao, J., and Li, L. 2004. Assessing bioequivalence using genomic data. *Journal of Biopharmaceutical Statistics*, 14, 869–880.

Chow, S.C. and Tse, S.K. 1988. Intrasubject variability estimation in bioavailability/bioequivalence studies. Proceedings of the Biopharmaceutical Section of the American Statistical Association, pp. 142–147, Chicago, Illinois.

Chow, S.C. and Tse, S.K. 1990a. Outlier detection in bioavailability/bioequivalence studies. *Statistics in Medicine*, 9, 549–558.

Chow, S.C. and Tse, S.K. 1990b. A related problem in bioavailability/bioequivalence studies—estimation of intrasubject variability with a common CV. *Biometrical Journal*, 32, 597–607.

Clayton, D. and Leslie, A. 1981. The bioavailability of erythromycin stearate versus enteric-coated erythromycin based when taken immediately before and after food. *Journal of International Medical Research*, 9, 470–477.

Cochran, W.G. and Cox, G.M. 1957. *Experimental Designs*. 2nd ed., John Wiley & Sons, New York.

Colton, T. 1974. *Statistics in Medicine*. Little, Brown, and Company, Boston, MA.

Cook, R.D. and Weisberg, S. 1982. *Residuals and Influence in Regression*. Chapman & Hall, New York and London.

Cornell, R.G. 1980. Evaluation of bioavailability data using nonparametric statistics. In: *Drug Absorption and Disposition: Statistical Considerations*, Albert, K.S. (Ed.), American Pharmaceutical Association, Academy of Pharmaceutical Sciences, Washington DC, pp. 51–57.

Cornell, R.G. 1990. The evaluation of bioequivalence using nonparametric procedures. *Communications in Statistics—Theory and Methods*, 19, 4153–4165.

Cox, D.R. and Reid, N. 2000. *The Theory of the Design of Experiments*. Chapman & Hall/CRC, New York.

Crow, E.L. and Shimizu, K. 1988. *Lognormal Distribution*. Marcel Dekker, New York.

Dare, J.G. 1964. Particle size in relation to formulation. *Australian Journal of Pharmacology*, 45, S58.

Davidian, M. 2003. What's in between dose and response? Lecture notes. Myrto Lefkopoulou Lecture.

Davidian, M. and Gallant, A.R. 1993. The nonlinear mixed effects model with a smooth random effects density. *Biometrika*, 80, 475–488.

Davidian, M. and Giltinan, D.M. 1995. *Nonlinear Models for Repeated Measurement Data*. Chapman & Hall, London, UK.

Dempster, A.P., Laird, N.M., and Rubin, D.B. 1977. Maximum likelihood from incomplete data via EM algorithm. *Journal of the Royal Statistical Society Series B*, 39, 1–38.

DerSimonian, R. and Laird, N. 1986. Meta-analysis in clinical trials. *Controlled Clinical Trials*, 7, 177–188.

Diggle, P.J., Liang, K.Y. and Zeger, S.L. 1994. *Analysis of Longitudinal Data*. Oxford Science, Oxford, UK.

Diletti, E., Hauschke, D., and Steinijans, V.W. 1991. Sample size determination for bioequivalence assessment by means of confidence interval. *International Journal of Clinical Pharmacology, Therapy and Toxicology*, 29, 1–8.

Draglin, V., Fedorov., V., Patterson, S., and Jones, B. 2003. Kullback–Leibler divergence for evaluation bioequivalence. *Statistics in Medicine*, 22, 913–930.

Draper, N.R. and Smith, H. 1981. *Applied Regression Analysis*. 2nd ed., John Wiley & Sons, New York.

Drug Bioequivalence Study Panel 1974. Drug Bioequivalence. A report from the Drug Bioequivalence Study Panel to the Office of Technology Assessment, Congress of the United States, prepared by Family Health Care, Inc., Washington, DC under contract OTAC-1 with the Office of Technology Assessment, Congress of the United States.

Dubey, S. 1988. Regulatory considerations on meta-analysis, dentifrice studies and multicenter trials. Proceedings of the Biopharmaceutical Section of the American Statistical Association, pp. 18–27 Chicago, Illinois.

Dunnett, C.W. and Gent, M. 1977. Significance testing to establish equivalence between treatments, with special reference to data in the form of 2×2 tables. *Biometrics*, 33, 593–602.

Eaton, M.L., Muirhead, R.J., and Steeno, G.S. 2003. Aspects of the dissolution profile testing problem. *Biopharmaceutical Report*, 11, 2–7.

Edler, L. 1998. List of PK–PD software packages. http://www.dkfz-heidelberg.de/biostatistics/pkpd/pkcomp1/html, Heidelberg, Germany.

Edwards, W., Lindman, H., and Savage, L.J. 1963. Bayesian statistical inference for psychological research. *Psychological Review*, 70, 193.

Efron, B. 1982. *The Jackknife, Bootstrap and Other Resampling Plans*. SIAM, Philadelphia, PA.

Efron, B. and Tibshirani, R.J. 1993. *An Introduction to the Bootstrap*. Chapman & Hall, New York.

Ekbohm, G. and Melander, H. 1989. The subject-by-formulation interaction as a criterion of interchangeability of drugs. *Biometrics*, 45, 1249–1254.

Endrenyi, L. 1981. Design of experiments for estimating enzyme and pharmacokinetic experiments. In: *Kinetic Data Analysis of Enzyme and Pharmacokinetic Experiments*, Endrenyi, L. (Ed.), Plenum Press, New York.

Endrenyi, L. 1994. A method for the evaluation of individual bioequivalence. *International Journal of Clinical Pharmacology and Therapeutics*, 32, 497–508.

Endrenyi, L. and Hao, Y. 1998. Asymmetry of the mean-variability tradeoff raises question about the model in investigations of individual bioequivalence. *International Journal of Clinical Pharmacology, Therapy and Toxicology*, 36, 1–8.

Endrenyi, L. and Midha, K.K. 1998. Individual bioequivalence—has its time come? *European Journal of Pharmaceutical Sciences*, 6, 271–277.

Endrenyi, L. and Tothfalusi, L. 1999. Subject-by-formulation interaction in determination of individual bioequivalence: Bias and prevalence. *Pharmaceutical Research*, 16, 186–190.

Endrenyi, L., Fritsch, S., and Yan, W. 1991. (C_{max})/AUC is a clearer measure than (C_{max}) for absorption rates in investigations of bioequivalence. *International Journal of Clinical Pharmcology, Therapy and Toxicology*, 29, 394–399.

Endrenyi, L., Amidon, G.L., Midha, K.K., and Skelly, J.P. 1998. Individual bioequivalence: Attractive in principle, difficulty in practice. *Pharmaceutical Research*, 15, 1321–1325.

Endrenyi, L., Taback, N., and Tothfalusi, L. 2000. Properties of the estimated variance component for subject-by-formulation interaction in studies of individual bioequivalence. *Statistics in Medicine*, 19, 2867–2878.

Esinhart, J.D. and Chinchilli, V.M. 1990. Statistical inference on intra-subject variability in bioequivalence studies. Proceedings of the Biopharmaceutical Section of the American Statistical Association, pp. 37–42, Anaheim, California.

Esinhart, J.D. and Chinchilli, V.M. 1991. The analysis of bioequivalence studies using generalized estimating equations. Presented at the 1991 ENAR Meeting of the Biometric Society, Houston, TX.

Esinhart, J.D. and Chinchilli, V.M. 1994a. Extension to the use of the tolerance intervals for the assessment of individual bioequivalence. *Journal of Biopharmaceutical Statistics*, 4, 39–52.

Esinhart, J.D. and Chinchilli, V.M. 1994b. Sample size considerations for assessing of individual bioequivalence on the method of tolerance intervals. *International Journal of Clinical Pharmacology and Therapeutics*, 32, 26–32.

Ette, E.L., Sun, H., and Ludden, T.M. 1994. Design of population pharmacokinetic studies. Proceedings of the Biopharmaceutical Section of the American Statistical Association, Alexandria, VA, pp. 487–492.

The European Agency for the Evaluation of Medicinal Products (EMEA) 2001. Note for Guidance on the Investigation of Bioavailability and Bioequivalence, London, UK.

EMEA 2003a. Note for Guidance on Comparability of Medicinal Products Containing Biotechnology-Derived Proteins as Drug Substance—Non Clinical and Clinical Issues. The European Medicines Agency Evaluation of Medicines for Human Use. EMEA/CHMP/3097/02, London, UK.

EMEA 2003b. Revision 1 Guideline on Comparability of Medicinal Products Containing Biotechnology-Derived Proteins as Drug Substance—Quality Issues. The European Medicines Agency Evaluation of Medicines for Human Use. EMEA/CHMP/BWP/3207/00/Rev 1, London, UK.

EMEA 2005a. Guideline on Similar Biological Medicinal Products. The European Medicines Agency Evaluation of Medicines for Human Use. EMEA/CHMP/437/04, London, UK.

EMEA 2005b. Draft Guideline on Similar Biological Medicinal Products Containing Biotechnology-Derived Proteins as Drug Substance: Quality Issues. The European Medicines Agency Evaluation of Medicines for Human Use. EMEA/CHMP/49348/05, London, UK.

EMEA 2005c. Draft Annex Guideline on Similar Biological Medicinal Products Containing Biotechnology-Derived Proteins as Drug Substance—Non Clinical and Clinical Issues—Guidance on Biosimilar Medicinal Products Containing Recombinant Erythropoietins. The European Medicines Agency Evaluation of Medicines for Human Use. EMEA/CHMP/94526/05, London, UK.

EMEA 2005d. Draft Annex Guideline on Similar Biological Medicinal Products Containing Biotechnology-Derived Proteins as Drug Substance—Non Clinical and Clinical Issues—Guidance on Biosimilar Medicinal Products Containing Recombinant Granulocyte-Colony Stimulating Factor. The European Medicines Agency Evaluation of Medicines for Human Use. EMEA/CHMP/31329/05, London, UK.

EMEA 2005e. Draft Annex Guideline on Similar Biological Medicinal Products Containing Biotechnology-Derived Proteins as Drug Substance—Non Clinical and Clinical Issues—Guidance on Biosimilar Medicinal Products Containing Somatropin. The European Medicines Agency Evaluation of Medicines for Human Use. EMEA/CHMP/94528/05, London, UK.

EMEA 2005f. Draft Annex Guideline on Similar Biological Medicinal Products Containing Biotechnology-Derived Proteins as Drug Substance—Non Clinical and Clinical Issues—Guidance on Biosimilar Medicinal Products Containing Recombinant Human Insulin. The European Medicines Agency Evaluation of Medicines for Human Use. EMEA/CHMP/32775/05, London, UK.

EMEA 2005g. Guideline on the Clinical Investigating of the Pharmacokinetics of Therapeutic proteins. The European Medicines Agency Evaluation of Medicines for Human Use. EMEA/CHMP/89249/04, London, UK.

EMEA 2006. Concept Paper for an Addendum to the Note for Guidance on the Investigation of Bioavailability and Bioequivalence: Evaluation of Bioequivalence of Highly Variable Drugs and Drug Products, London, UK.

FDA 1992. Guidance on Statistical Procedures for Bioequivalence Using a Standard Two-treatment Crossover Design, Division of Bioequivalence, Office of Generic Drugs, Center for Drug Evaluation and Research, U.S. Food and Drug Administration, Rockville, MD.

FDA 1995a. SUPAC-IR: Guidance on Immediate Release Solid Dosage Forms, Scale-up and Post-Approval Changes: Chemistry, Manufacturing and Controls, In Vitro Dissolution Testing, and In Vivo Bioequivalence Documentation, Center for Drug Evaluation and Research, U.S. Food and Drug Administration, Rockville, MD.

FDA 1995b. Guidance on Topical Dermatologic Corticosteriods: In Vivo Bioequivalence, Center for Drug Evaluation and Research, U.S. Food and Drug Administration, Rockville, MD.

FDA 1997a. SUPAC-MR: Guidance on Modified Release Solid Dosage Forms, Scale-up and Post-Approval Changes: Chemistry, Manufacturing and Controls, In Vitro Dissolution Testing, and In Vivo Bioequivalence Documentation, Center for Drug Evaluation and Research, U.S. Food and Drug Administration, Rockville, MD.

FDA 1997b. Dissolution Testing of Immediate Release Solid Oral Dosage Forms, Center for Drug Evaluation and Research, U.S. Food and Drug Administration, Rockville, MD.

FDA 1997c. Draft Guidance on In Vivo Bioequivalence Studies Based on Population and Individual Bioequivalence Approaches, Center for Drug Evaluation and Research, U.S. Food and Drug Administration, Rockville, MD.

FDA 1998. Data Sets of Bioequivalence for Individual and Population Bioequivalence. Published on Internet: www.fda.gov/cder/bioeuivdata/ index.htm.

FDA 1999a, Guidance for Industry on *Average Population and Individual Approaches to Establishing Bioequivalence*. Center for Drug Evaluation and Research, U.S. Food and Drug Administration, Rockville, Maryland.

FDA 1999b. Guidance for Industry—Population Pharmacokinetics. Center for Drug Research and Evaluation, the United States Food and Drug Administration, Rockville, Maryland.

FDA 1999c, Guidance for Industry on *Bioavailability and Bioequivalence Studies for Nasal Aerosols and Nasal Sprays for Local Action*. Center for Drug Evaluation and Research, U.S. Food and Drug Administration, Rockville, Maryland.

FDA 1999d, Guidance for Industry on *Nasal Spray and Inhalation Solution, Suspension and Spray Drug Products*. Center for Drug Evaluation and Research, U.S. Food and Drug Administration, Rockville, Maryland.

FDA 2000. Guidance on Waiver of In Vivo Bioavailability and Bioequivalence Studies for Immediate-Release Solid Oral Dosage Forms Based on a Biopharmaceutics Classification System, Center for Drug Evaluation and Research, U.S. Food and Drug Administration, Rockville, MD.

FDA 2001. Guidance on Statistical Approaches to Establishing Bioequivalence, Center for Drug Evaluation and Research, U.S. Food and Drug Administration, Rockville, MD.

FDA 2003a. Guidance on Food-Effect Bioavailability and Fed Bioequivalence Studies, Center for Drug Evaluation and Research, U.S. Food and Drug Administration, Rockville, MD.

FDA 2003b. Guidance on Bioavailability and Bioequivalence Studies for Orally Administrated Drug Products—General Considerations, Center for Drug Evaluation and Research, U.S. Food and Drug Administration, Rockville, MD.

FDA 2003c. Second Draft Guidance on Bioavailability and Bioequivalence Studies for Nasal Aerosols and Nasal Sprays for Local Action, Center for Drug Evaluation and Research, U.S. Food and Drug Administration, Rockville, MD.

FDA 2003d. Statistical Information from the June 1999 Draft Guidance and Statistical Information for In Vitro Bioequivalence Data Posted on August 18, 1999, Center for Drug Evaluation and Research, U.S. Food and Drug Administration, Rockville, MD.

FDA 2003e. Guidance on Clozapine Tablets: In Vivo Bioequivalence and In Vitro Dissolution Testing, Center for Drug Evaluation and Research, U.S. Food and Drug Administration, Rockville, MD.

FDA 2004. Challenge and Opportunity on the Critical Path to New Medicinal Products. http://www.fda.gov/oc/initiatives/criticalpath/whitepaper.pdf.

FDA 2006a. Challenge and Opportunity on the Critical Path to New Medicinal Products. http://www.fda.gov/oc/initiatives/criticalpath/whitepaper.pdf.

FDA 2006b. Critical Path Opportunities List. http://www.fda.gov/oc/initiatives/criticalpath/reports/opp_list.pdf.

FDA 2006c. Premarket Approval. http://www.fda.gov/cdrh/devadvice/pma.

FDA 2006d. Premarket Notification 510 (k). http://www.fda.gov/CDRH/DEVADVICE/314.html.

FDA 2007. Critical Path Opportunities for Generic Drugs. http://www.fda.gov/oc/initiatives/criticalpath/reports/generic/html.

Feingold, M. and Gillespie, B.W. 1996. Cross-over trials with censored data. *Statistics in Medicine*, 15, 953–967.

Feinstein, A.R. 2002. *Principles of Medical Statistics*. Chapman & Hall/CRC, New York.

Ferguson, T.S. 1967. On the rejection of outliers. Proceedings of the Fourth Berkeley Symposium on Mathematical Statistics and Probability, Vol. 1, 253–287, Berkeley and Los Angeles: University of California Press, Berkeley, California.

Fieller, E. 1954. Some problems in interval estimation. *Journal of Royal Statistical Society Series B*, 16, 175–185.

Fisher, R.A. and Yates, F. 1953. *Statistical Tables for Biological, Agricultural, and Medical Research*. 4th ed., Oliver and Boyd, Edinburgh, UK.

Fleming, T.R. 2000. Design and interpretation of equivalence trials. *American Heart Journal*, 139, S172–S176.

Fluehler, H., Grieve, A.P., Mandallaz, D., Mau, J., and Moser, H.A. 1983. Bayesian approach to bioequivalent assessment: An example. *Journal of Pharmaceutical Science*, 72, 1178–1181.

Fluehler, H., Hirtz, J., and Moser, H.A. 1981. An aid to decision-making in bioequivalence assessment. *Journal of Pharmacokinetics and Pharmacodynamics*, 9, 235–243.

France, L.A., Lewis, J.A., and Kay, R. 1991. The analysis of failure time data in crossover studies. *Statistics in Medicine*, 10, 1099–1113.

Frank, R.G. 2007. Regulation of follow-on biologics. *New England Journal of Medicine*, 357, 841–843.

Frick, H. 1987. On level and power of Anderson and Hauck's procedure for testing equivalence in comparative bioavailability. *Communications in Statistics—Theory and Methods*, 16, 2771–2778.

Gibaldi, M. and Perrier, D. 1982. *Pharmacokinetics*. Marcel Dekker, New York.

Ghosh, P. and Khattree, R. 2003. Bayesian approach to average bioequivalence using Bayes' factor. *Journal of Biopharmaceutical Statistics*, 13, 719–734.

Gill, J.L. 1998. Repeated measurement: Split-plot trend analysis versus analysis of first differences. *Biometrics*, 44, 289–297.

Gould, A.L. 1995. Group sequential extensions of standard bioequivalence testing procedure. *Journal of Pharmacokinetics and Biopharmaceutics*, 23, 57–85.

Grahnen, A., Hammerlund, M., and Lundquist, T. 1980. Implication of intrasubject variability in bioavailability studies of furosemide. *European Journal of Clinical Pharmacology*, 27, 595–602.

Graybill, F.A. 1961. *An Introduction to Linear Statistical Models*. McGraw-Hill, New York.

Graybill, F.A. 1976. *Theory and Application of the Linear Model*. Duxbury, Boston.

Graybill, F.A. and Wang, C.M. 1980. Confidence intervals on nonnegative linear combinations of variances. *Journal of the American Statistical Association*, 75, 869–873.

Grieve, A.P. 1985. A Bayesian analysis of the two-period crossover design for clinical trials. *Biometrics*, 21, 467–480.

Grizzle, J.E. 1965. The two-period changeover design and its use in clinical trials. *Biometrics*, 21, 467–480.

Grizzle, J.E. and Allen, D.M. 1969. Analysis of growth and dose response curves. *Biometrics*, 25, 357–480.

Guidelines for Biopharmaceutical Studies in Man, American Pharmaceutical Association, Academy of Pharmaceutical Sciences, Washington, DC, 1972, Appendix I, p. 17.

Guilbaud, O. 1993. Exact inference about the within-subject variability in 2×2 crossover study. *Journal of the American Statistical Association*, 88, 939–946.

Halperin, M. 1961. Almost linearly-optimum combination of unbiased estimates. *Journal of the American Statistical Association*, 56, 36–43.

Hashimoto, Y. and Sheiner, L.B. 1991. Designs for population pharmacodynamics: Value of pharmacokinetic data and population analysis. *Journal of Pharmacokinetics and Biopharmaceutics*, 19, 333–353.

Hauck, W.W. 1996a. Mean difference vs. variability reduction: Tradeoffs in aggregate measures for individual bioequivalence. *International Journal of Clinical Pharmacology, Therapy and Toxicology*, 34, 535–541.

Hauck, W.W. 1996b. Individual bioequivalence: Concepts. Presented at the Meeting of the Advisory Meeting for Pharmaceutical Science, Holiday Inn, Gaithersburg, Maryland, August 15.

Hauck, W.W. and Anderson, S. 1984. A new statistical procedure for testing equivalence in two-group comparative bioavailability trials. *Journal of Pharmacokinetics and Biopharmaceutics*, 12, 83–91.

Hauck, W.W. and Anderson, S. 1992. Types of bioequivalence and related statistical considerations. *International Journal of Clinical Pharmacology, Therapy and Toxicology*, 30, 181–187.

Hauck, W.W. and Anderson, S. 1994. Measuring switchability and prescriptability: When is average bioequivalence sufficient? *Journal of Pharmacokinetics and Biopharmaceutics*, 22, 551–564.

Hauck, W.W., Bois, F.Y., Hyslop, T., Gee, L., and Anderson, S. 1997. A parametric approach to population bioequivalence. *Statistics in Medicine*, 16, 441–454.

Hauck, W.W., Chen, M.L., Tyslop, T., Patnaik, R., Schuirmann, D., and Williams, R. 1996. Mean difference vs. variability reduction: Tradeoff in aggregate measures for individual bioequivalence? *International Journal of Clinical Pharmacology, Therapy and Toxicology*, 30, 181–187.

Hauck, W.W., Tyslop, T., Chen, M.L., Patnaik, R., Williams, R., and the FDA Population/Individual Bioequivalence Working Group. 2000. Subject-by-formulation interaction in bioequivalence: Concept and statistical issues, *Pharmaceutical Research*, 375–380.

Hauschke, D., Steinijans, V.W., and Diletti, E. 1990. A distribution-free procedure for the statistical analyses of bioequivalence studies. *International Journal of Clinical Pharmacology, Therapy and Toxicology*, 28, 72–78.

Hawkins, P.M. 1980. *Identification of Outliers*. Chapman & Hall, New York.

Haynes, J.D. 1981. Statistical simulation study of new proposed uniformity requirements for bioequivalency studies. *Journal of Pharmaceutical Sciences*, 70, 673–675.

Herson, J. 1991. Statistical controversies in design and analysis of bioequivalence trials for pharmaceuticals with negligible blood levels: The metered dose inhaler trial. Presented at the 14th Midwest Biopharmaceutical Statistics Workshop, Muncie, IN.

Hills, M. and Armitage, P. 1979. The two-period cross-over clinical trial. *British Journal of Clinical Pharmacology*, 8, 7–20.

Hinkley, D.V. 1969. On the ratio of two correlated normal variables. *Biometrika*, 56, 635–639.

Ho, I. and Patel, H.I. 1988. Comparison of variances in a bioequivalence study. Presented at the American College of Clinical Pharmacology. 17th Annual Meeting Orlando, FL.

Hochberg, Y. and Tamhane, A.C. 1987. *Multiple Comparison Procedures*. John Wiley & Sons, New York.

Hocking, R.P. 1985. *The Analysis of Linear Models*. Brooks/Cole, Monterey, CA.

Hodges, J.L. and Lehmann, E.L. 1963. Estimates of location based on rank tests. *The Annals of Mathematical Statistics*, 34, 598–611.

Holder, D.J. and Hsuan, F. 1993. Moment-based criteria for determining bioequivalence. *Biometrika*, 80, 835–846.

Hollander, M. and Wolfe, D.A. 1973. *Nonparametrics Statistical Methods*. John Wiley & Sons, New York.

Holt, J.D. and Prentice, R.L. 1974. Survival analysis in twin studies and matched-pair experiments. *Biometrika*, 61, 17–30.

Hothorn, L. and Oberdoerfer, R. 2006. Statistical analysis used in the nutritional assessment of novel food using the proof of safety. *Regulatory Toxicology and Pharmacology*, 44, 125–135.

Howe, W.G. 1974. Approximate confidence limit on mean of X + Y where X and Y are two tabled independent random variables. *Journal of the American Statistical Association*, 69, 789–794.

Hoyle, M.H. 1968. The estimation of variances after using a Gaussinating transformation. *The Annals of Mathematical Statistics*, 39, 1125–1143.

Hsu, H.C. and Lu, H.L. 1997. On confidence limits associated with Chow and Shao's joint confidence region approach for assessment of bioequivalence. *Journal of Biopharmaceutical Statistics*, 7, 125–134.

Hsuan, F.C. and Reeve, R. 2003. Assessing individual bioequivalence with higher-order cross-over designs: A unified procedure. *Statistics in Medicine*, 22, 2847–2860.

Hsu, J.C., Hwang, J.T.G., Liu, H.K., and Ruberg, S.J. 1994. Confidence intervals associated with tests for bioequivalence. *Biometrika*, 81, 103–114.

Huitson, A., Poloniecki, J., Hews, R., and Barker, N. 1982. A review of cross-over trials. *Statistician*, 31, 71–80.

Huque, M. and Dubey, S.D. 1990. A three arm design and analysis for clinical trials in establishing therapeutic equivalence with clinical endpoints. Proceedings of the Biopharmaceutical Section of the American Statistical Association, Anaheim, California, pp. 91–98.

Huster, W.J., Brookmeyer, R., and Self, S.G. 1989. Model paired survival data with covariates. *Biometrics*, 45, 145–156.

Hwang, J.T.G. and Wang, W. 1997. The validity of the test of individual bioequivalence ratios. *Biometrika*, 84, 893–900.

Hyslop, T., Hsuan, F., and Holder, D.J. 2000. A small sample confidence interval approach to assess individual bioequivalence. *Statistics in Medicine*, 19, 2885–2897.

ICH 1996. Q5C Guideline on Quality of Biotechnological Products: Stability Testing of Biotechnological/Biological Products. Center for Drug Evaluation and Research, Center for Biologics Evaluation and Research, the US Food and Drug Administration, Rockville, MD.

ICH E5 1998. International Conference on Harmonization Tripartite Guidance E5, *Ethnic Factors in the Acceptability of Foreign Data*; the U.S. Federal Register, 83, 31790–31796.

ICH 1999. Q6B Guideline on Test Procedures and Acceptance Criteria for aBiotechnological/Biological Products. Center for Drug Evaluation and Research, Center for Biologics Evaluation and Research, the U.S. Food and Drug Administration, Rockville, MD.

ICH 2005. Q5E Guideline on Comparability of Biotechnological/Biological Products Subject to Changes in Their Manufacturing Process. Center for Drug Evaluation and Research, Center for Biologics Evaluation and Research, the U.S. Food and Drug Administration, Rockville, MD.

Jacques, J.A. 1972. *Compartmental Analysis in Biology and Medicine*. Elsevier, New York.

The Japanese National Institute of Health Sciences 1997. Guideline for Bioequivalence Studies of Generic Drugs.

Jelliffe, R.W., Gomis, P., and Schumitzky, A. 1990. A population model of gentamicin made with a new nonparametric EM algorithm. Technical Report 90-4, USC.

Jennrich, R.I. and Schluchter, M.D. 1986. Unbalanced repeated measures models with structural covariance matrices. *Biometrics*, 42, 805–820.

John, P.W.M. 1971. *Statistical Design and Analysis of Experiments*. Macmillan, New York.

Johnson, R.A. and Wichern, D.W. 1982. *Applied Multivariate Statistical Analysis*. Prentice Hall, Englewood Cliffs, NJ.

Johnson, N.E., Wade, J.R., and Karlson, M.O. 1996. Comparison of some practical sampling strategies for population pharmacokinetic studies. *J. Pharmacokinet. Biopharm.*, 24, 245–272.

Jones, B. and Kenward, M.G. 1989. *Design and Analysis of Crossover Trials*. 1st edn., Chapman & Hall, London, UK.

Jones, B. and Kenward, M.G. 2003. *Design and Analysis of Crossover Trials*. 2nd ed., Chapman & Hall, London, UK.

Jung, S.H. and Su, J.Q. 1995. Non-parametric estimation for the difference or ratio of median failure times for period observations. *Statistics in Medicine*, 14, 275–281.

Kalbfleisch, J.P. and Prentice, R.L. 1980. *The Statistical Analysis of Failure Time Data*. John Wiley & Sons, New York.

Karalis, V., Symillides, M., and Macheras, P. 2004. Novel scaled average bioequivalence limits based on GMR and variability considerations. *Pharmaceutical Research*, 21, 1933–1942.

Karlson, M.O. and Sheiner, L.B. 1993. The importance of modeling interoccasion variability in population pharmacokinetic analyses. *J. Pharmacokinet. Biopharm.*, 21, 735–750.

Keida, T., Hayashi, N., and Kawashima, M. 2006. Application of the food and drug administration (FDA) bioequivalent guidance of topical dermatologic corticosteroids in yell-skinned Japanese population: Validation study using a chromameter. *Journal of Dermatology*, 33, 684–691.

Kendall, M.G. and Stuart, A. 1979. *The Advance Theory of Statistics*. Vol. II, Griffen, London, UK.

Kershner, R.P. and Federer, W.T. 1981. Two-treatment crossover design for estimating a variety of effects. *Journal of the American Statistical Association*, 76, 612–618.

Ki, F.Y., Liu, J.P., Wang, W., and Chow, S.C. 1995. The impact of outlying subjects on decision of bioequivalence. *Journal of Biopharmaceutical Statistics*, 5, 71–94.

Kimanani, E.K. and Potvin, D. 1997. A parametric confidence interval for a moment-based scaled criterion for individual bioequivalence. *Journal of Pharmacokinetics and Biopharmaceutics*, 25, 595–614.

Kirkwood, T.B.L. 1981. Bioequivalence testing—a need to rethink. *Biometrics*, 37, 589–591.

Koch, G.G. 1972. The use of nonparametric methods in the statistical analysis of the two-period change-over design. *Biometrics*, 28, 577–584.

Koch, G.G. and Edwards, S. 1988. Clinical efficacy trials with categorical data. In: *Biopharmaceutical Statistical for Drug Development*, Peace, K. (Ed.), Marcel Dekker, New York, pp. 403–457.

Korn, E.L., Alber, P.S., and McShane, L.M. 2005. Assessing surrogated as trial endpoints using mixed models. *Statistics in Medicine*, 24, 163–182.

Kunin, C.M. 1966. Absorption, distribution, excretion and fate of kanamycin. *Annals of the New York Academy of Sciences*, 132, 811.

Laird, N.M. and Ware, J.H. 1982. Random effects models for longitudinal data. *Biometrics*, 38, 963–974.

Land, C.E. 1988. Hypothesis tests for interval estimates. In: *Lognormal Distribution*, Crow, E.L. and Shimizu, K. (Eds.), Marcel Dekker, New York, pp. 87–112.

Landowski, C.P., Sun, D., Foster, D.R., Menon, S.S., Barnett, J.L., Welage, L.S., Ramachandran, C., and Amidon, G.L. 2003. Gene expression in the human intestine and correlation with oral valacyclovir pharmacokinetic parameters. *Journal of Pharmacology and Experimental Therapeutics*, 306, 778–786.

Laska, E.M. and Meisner, M. 1985. A variational approach to optimal two-treatment crossover designs: Applications to carryover effect methods. *Journal of the American Statistical Association*, 80, 704–710.

Laska, E.M., Meisner, M., and Kushner, H.B. 1983. Optimal crossover designs in the presence of carryover effects. *Biometrics*, 39, 1089–1091.

Lasserre, V. 1991. Determination of optimal designs using linear models in crossover trials. *Statistics in Medicine*, 10, 909–924.

Lee, A.F.S. and Fineberg, N.S. 1991. A fitted test for the Behrens–Fisher problem. *Communications in Statistics—Theory and Methods*, 20, 653–666.

Lee, Y., Shao, J., Chow, S.C., and Wang, H. 2002. Tests for inter-subject and total variabilities under crossover designs. *Journal of Biopharmaceutical Statistics*, 12, 503–534.

Lee, Y., Shao, J., and Chow, S.C. 2004. Modified large-sample confidence intervals for linear combinations of variance components: Extension, theory and application. *Journal of the American Statistical Association*, 99, 467–478.

Leeson, L.J. 1995. In vitro/vivo correlation. *Drug Information Journal*, 29, 903–915.

Lehmann, E.L. 1975. *Nonparametrics: Statistical Methods Based on Ranks*. Holden-Day, San Francisco, CA.

Lehmann, E.L. and Romano, J.P. 2005. *Testing Statistical Hypotheses*. Springer, New York.

Levy, N.W. 1986. Bioequivalence of solid oral dosage forms. A presentation to the U.S. Food and Drug Administration Hearing on Bioequivalence of Solid Oral Dosage Forms, September 29–October 1, Pharmaceutical Manufacturer Association, Section II, 9–11.

Liang, K.Y. and Zeger, S.L. 1986. Longitudinal data analysis using generalized linear models. *Biometrika*, 73, 13–22.

Lin, J.S., Chow, S.C., and Tse, S.K. 1991. A SAS procedure for outlier detection in bioavailability/bioequivalence studies. Proceedings of the 16th SAS Users Group International Conference, New Orleans, Louisiana, pp. 1433–1437.

Lin, T.L. and Tsong, Y. 1990. Removal of a statistical outlier—impact on the subsequent statistical test. Presented at Joint Statistical Meetings, Anaheim, CA.

Lindley, D.V. 1965. *Introduction to Probability and Statistics for a Bayesian Viewpoint, Part II Inference*. Cambridge University Press, Cambridge, UK.

Lindsey, J.K. 1993. *Models of Repeated Measurements*. Oxford University Press, Oxford, UK.

Lindstrom, M.J. and Bates, D.M. 1990. Nonlinear mixed effects models for repeated measures data. *Biometrics*, 46, 673–687.

Liu, J.P. 1991. Bioequivalence and intrasubject variability. *Journal of Biopharmaceutical Statistics*, 1, 205–219.

Liu, J.P. 1995. Use of the repeated cross-over designs in assessing bioequivalence. *Statistics in Medicine*, 14, 1067–1078.

Liu, J.P. 1998. Statistical evaluation of individual bioequivalence. *Communications in Statistics—Theory and Methods*, 27, 1433–1451.

Liu, J.P. 2004. Bridging bioequivalence studies. *Journal of Biopharmaceutical Statistics*, 14, 857–867.

Liu, J.P. and Chow, S.C. 1992a. On power calculation of Schuirmann's two one-sided tests procedure in bioequivalence. *Journal of Pharmacokinetics and Biopharmaceutics*, 20, 101–104.

Liu, J.P. and Chow, S.C. 1992b. On assessment of bioequivalence in variability of bioavailability. *Communications in Statistics—Theory and Methods*, 21, 2591–2608.

Liu, J.P. and Chow, S.C. 1993. On assessment of bioequivalence for drugs with negligible plasma levels. *Biometrical Journal*, 35, 109–123.

Liu, J.P. and Chow, S.C. 1995. Replicated cross-over designs in bioavailability and bioequivalence trials. *Drug Information Journal*, 29, 871–884.

Liu, J.P. and Chow, S.C. 1996. Discussion of bioequivalence trials, intersection—union tests, and equivalence confidence sets, by Berger and Hsu. *Statistical Science*, 11, 306–312.

Liu, J.P. and Chow, S.C. 1997a. Some thoughts on individual bioequivalence. *Journal of Biopharmaceutical Statistics*, 7, 41–48.

Liu, J.P. and Chow, S.C. 1997b. A two one-sided tests procedure for assessing individual bioequivalence. *Journal of Biopharmaceutical Statistics*, 7, 49–61.

Liu, J.P. and Chow, S.C. 2005a. Minimum therapeutically effective dose. In: *Encyclopedia of Biostatistics*, Armitage, P. and Colton, T. (Eds.), 2nd ed., Vol. 5. John Wiley & Sons, New York, pp. 3249–3251.

Liu, J.P. and Chow, S.C. 2005b. Median effective dose. In: *Encyclopedia of Biostatistics*, Armitage, P. and Colton, T. (Eds.), 2nd ed., Vol. 5. John Wiley & Sons, New York, pp. 3104–3117.

Liu, J.P. and Weng, C.S. 1991. Detection of outlying data in bioavailability/bioequivalence studies. *Statistics in Medicine*, 10, 1375–1389.

Liu, J.P. and Weng, C.S. 1992. Estimation of direct formulation effect under log-normal distribution in bioavailability/bioequivalence studies. *Statistics in Medicine*, 11, 881–896.

Liu, J.P. and Weng, C.S. 1993. Evaluation of parametric and nonparametric two one-sided tests procedures for assessing bioequivalence of average bioavailability, *Journal of Biopharmaceutical Statistics*, 3, 85–102.

Liu, J.P. and Weng, C.S. 1994. Estimation of log-transformation in assessing bioequivalence. *Communications in Statistics—Theory and Methods*, 23, 421–434.

Liu, J.P. and Weng, C.S. 1995. Bias of two one-sided tests procedures in assessment of bioequivalence. *Statistics in Medicine*, 14, 853–861.

Liu, J.P., Ma, M.C., and Chow, S.C. 1997. Statistical evaluation of similarity factor f_2 as a criterion for assessment of similarity between dissolution profiles. *Drug Information Journal*, 31, 1255–1271.

Locke, C.S. 1984. An exact confidence interval for untransformed data for the ratio of two formulation means. *Journal of Pharmacokinetics and Biopharmaceutics*, 12, 649–655.

Lund, R.E. 1975. Tables for an approximate test for outliers in linear models. *Technometrics*, 17, 473–476.

Ma, M.C., Lin, R.P., and Liu, J.P. 1999. Statistical evaluation of dissolution similarity. *Statistica Sinica*, 9, 1011–1027.

Ma, M.C., Wang, B.B.C, Liu, J.P., and Tsong, Y. 2000. On assessment of similarity between dissolution profiles. *Journal of Biopharmaceutical Statistics*, 10, 229–249.

Mallet, A. 1986. A maximum likelihood estimation method for random coefficient regression models. *Biometrika*, 73, 645–656.

Mandallaz, D. and Mau, J. 1981. Comparison of different methods for decision-making in bioequivalence assessment. *Biometrics*, 37, 213–222.

Mann, H.B. and Whitney, D.R. 1947. On a test of whether one or two random variables is stochastically larger than the other. *The Annals of Mathematical Statistics*, 18, 50–60.

Mantel, N. 1977. Do we want confidence interval symmetric about the null value? *Biometrics*, 33, 759–760.

Martinez, M.N. and Jackson, A.J. 1991. Suitability of various noninfinity area under the plasma concentration–time curve (AUC) estimates for use in bioequivalence determination: Relationship to AUC from zero to time infinity (AUC0-inf). *Pharmaceutical Research*, 18, 512–517.

McCulloch, C.E. 1987. Tests for equality of variances with paired data. *Communications in Statistics—Theory and Methods*, 16, 1377–1391.

McNally, R.J., Iyer, H., and Mathew, T. 2003. Tests for individual and population bioequivalence based on generalized *p*-values. *Statistics in Medicine*, 22, 31–53.

McQuarrie, D.A. 1967. Stochastic approach to chemical kinetics. *Journal of Applied Probability*, 4, 413–478.

Meeting transcript of the U.S. FDA Advisory Committee for Pharmaceutical Science, August 15–16, 1996, Gaithersburg, MD.

Mehran, F. 1973. Variance of the MVUE for the lognormal mean. *Journal of the American Statistical Association*, 67, 726–727.

Mentre, F., Mallet, A., and Baccar, D. 1997. Optimal design in random-effects regression models. *Biometrika*, 84, 429–442.

Metzler, C.M. 1974. Bioavailability: A problem in equivalence. *Biometrics*, 30, 309–317.

Metzler, C.M. 1988. Statistical methods for deciding bioequivalence of formulations. In: *Oral Substained Released Formulations: Design and Evaluation*, Yacobi, A. and Halperin-Walega, E. (Eds.), Pergamon Press, New York, pp. 217–238.

Metzler, C.M. and Huang, D.C. 1983. Statistical methods for bioavailability and bioequivalence. *Clinical Research Practices and Drug Regulatory Affairs*, 1, 109–132.

Midha, K.K., Rawson, M.I., and Hubbard, J.W. 1997. Individual and average bioequivalence of high variability drugs and drug products. *Journal of Pharmaceutical Sciences*, 86, 1193–1197.

Mohandoss, E. and Chow, S.C. 1995. A SAS macro for assessment of variability in bioequivalence trials. Proceedings of the 20th SAS User Group International Conference, pp. 1263–1267, Orlando, Florida.

Mohandoss, E., Chow, S.C., and Ki, F.Y.C. 1995. Application of Williams' design for bioequivalence trials. *Drug Information Journal*, 29, 1029–1038.

Moore, J.W. and Flanner, H.H. 1996. Mathematical comparison of curves with an emphasis on dissolution profiles. *Pharmaceutical Technology*, 20, 64–74.

Morgan, W.A. 1939. A test for the significance of the difference between the two variances in a sample from a normal bivariate population. *Biometrika*, 31, 13–19.

Müller, P. and Rosner, G.L. 1997. A Bayesian population model with hierarchical mixture priors applied to blood count data. *Journal of American Statistical Association*, 92, 1279–1292.

Müller-Cohrs, J. 1990. The power of the Anderson–Hauck test and the double t-test. *Biometrical Journal*, 32, 259–266.

Munk, A., Hwang, J.T.G., and Brown, L.D. 2000. Testing average equivalence—finding a compromise between theory and practice. *Biometrical Journal*, 42, 531–552.

Nedelman, J.R. 2005. On some disadvantages of the population approach. *The AAPS Journal*, 7, E374–E382.

Neyman, J. and Scott, E.L. 1960. Correction for bias introduced by a transformation of variables. *The Annals of Mathematical Statistics*, 31, 643–655.

O'Brien, P.C. and Fleming, T.R. 1987. A paired Prentice–Wilcoxon test for censored paired data. *Biometrics*, 43, 169–180.

Organization for Economic Cooperation and Development (OECD) 2001. Consensus Document on Key Nutrients and Key Toxicants in Low Erucic Acid Rapeseed (Canola), Series of the Safety of Novel Foods and Feeds No. 1, ENV/JM/MONO(2001)13.

Oser, B.L., Melnick, D., and Hochberg, M. 1945. Physiological availability of the vitamins—study of methods for determining availability in pharmaceutical products. *Industrial and Engineering Chemistry, Analytical Edition*, 17, 401–411.

OTA 1974. *Drug Bioequivalence*. A report of the Office of Technology Assessment Drug Bioequivalence Study Panel. United States Congress. Washington, D.C.

Ott, L. 1984. *An Introduction to Statistical Method and Data Analysis*. 2nd ed., Duxbury Press, Boston.

Owen, D.B. 1965. A special case of a noncentral *t* distribution. *Biometrika*, 52, 437–446.

Patel, H.I. 1994. Dose–response in pharmacokinetics. *Communications in Statistics—Theory and Methods*, 23, 451–465.

Patil, V.H. 1965. Approximation to the Behrens–Fisher distributions. *Biometrika*, 52, 267–271.

Patnaik, R.N. 1996. Individual bioequivalence: Pharmacokinetic data—replicated designs. Presented at the Meeting of the Advisory Meeting for Pharmaceutical Science, Holiday Inn, Gaithersburg, MD, August 15, 1996.

Patnaik, R.N., Lesko, L.J., Chen, M.L., Williams, R.L., and the FDA Individual Bioequivalence Working Group. 1997. Individual bioequivalence—new concepts in the statistical assessment of bioequivalence metrics. *Clinical Pharmacokinetics*, 33, 1–6.

Peace, K.E. 1986. Estimating the degree of equivalence and non-equivalence: An alternative to bioequivalence testing. Proceedings of the Biopharmaceutical section of the American Statistical Association, St. Louis, Missouri, pp. 63–69.

Peace, K.E. 1990. *Statistical Issues in Drug Research and Development*. Marcel Dekker, New York.

Phillips, K.F. 1990. Power of the two one-sided tests procedure in bioequivalence. *Journal of Pharmacokinetics and Biopharmaceutics*, 18, 137–144.

Phillips, K.F. 1993. A log-normal model for individual bioequivalence. *Journal of Biopharmaceutical Statistics*, 3, 185–201.

Pinheiro, J.C. and Bates, D.M. 1995. Approximations to the log-likelihood function in the nonlinear mixed effects model. *Journal of Computational and Graphical Statistics*, 4, 12–35.

Pinheiro, J.C. and Bates, D.M. 2000. *Mixed Effects Models in S and S-Plus*. Springer, New York.

Pitman, E.J.G. 1939. A note on normal correlation. *Biometrika*, 31, 9–12.

Pocock, S.J. 1983. *Clinical Trials—A Practical Approach*. John Wiley & Sons, New York.

Poli, J.E. and McLean, A.M. 2001. Novel direct curve comparison metrics for bioequivalence. *Pharmaceutical Research*, 18, 734–741.

Pong, A.P. and Chow, S.C. 1996. A SAS program for the assessment of unbalanced data in two-sequence, three-period crossover trials. Proceedings of the 21st SAS User Group International Conference, Chicago, Illinois, pp. 1420–1425.

Purich, E. 1980. Bioavailability/bioequivalence regulations: An FDA perspective. In: *Drug Absorption and Disposition: Statistical Considerations*, Albert, K.S. (Ed.), American Pharmaceutical Association, Academy of Pharmaceutical Sciences, Washington, DC, pp. 115–137.

Quiroz, J., Ting, N., Wei, G.C., and Burdick, R.K. 2002. Alternative confidence intervals for the assessment of bioequivalence in four-period cross-over designs. *Statistics in Medicine*, 21, 1825–1847.

Racine-Poon, A. 1985. A Bayesian approach to nonlinear random effects models. *Biometrics*, 41, 1015–1023.

Racine-Poon, A. and Smith, A.M.F. 1990. Population models. In: *Statistical Methodology in Pharmaceutical Sciences*, Berry, D.A. (Ed.), Dekker, New York, pp. 139–162.

Racine-Poon, A., Grieve, A.P., Fluehler, H., and Smith, A.F. 1986. Bayesian methods in practice experiences in the pharmaceutical industry (with discussion). *Applied Statistics*, 35, 93–150.

Racine-Poon, A., Grieve, A.P., Fluehler, H., and Smith, A.F. 1987. A two-stage procedure for bioequivalence studies. *Biometrics*, 43, 847–856.

Ramsay, T. and Elkum, N. 2005. A comparison of four different methods for outlier detection in bioequivalence studies. *Journal of Biopharmaceutical Statistics*, 15, 43–52.

Randles, R.H. and Wolfe, D.A. 1979. *Introduction to the Theory of Nonparametric Statistics*. John Wiley & Sons, New York.

Ratkowsky, D.A., Evans, M.A., and Alldredge, I.R. 1993. *Cross-Over Experiments*. Marcel Dekker, New York.

Retout, S. and Mentre, F. 2003. Further development of the Fisher information matrix in nonlinear mixed effects models with evaluation in population pharmacokinetics. *Journal of Biopharmaceutical Statistics*, 13, 209–227.

Richardson, B.A. and Flack, V.F. 1996. The analysis of incomplete data in the three-period two-treatment cross-over design for clinical trials. *Statistics in Medicine*, 15, 127–143.

Rocke, D.M. 1984. On testing for bioequivalence. *Biometrics*, 40, 225–230.

Rodda, B.E. 1986. Bioequivalence of solid oral dosage forms. A presentation to the U.S. Food and Drug Administration Hearing on Bioequivalence of Solid Oral Dosage Forms, September 29–October 1, Pharmaceutical Manufacturers Association, Section III, pp. 12–15.

Rodda, B.E. and Davis, R.L. 1980. Determining the probability of an important difference in bioavailability. *Clinical Pharmacology and Therapeutics*, 28, 247–252.

Rothmann, M., Li, N., Chen, G., Chi, G.Y.H., Temple, R., and Tsou, H.H. 2003. Design and analysis of non-inferiority mortality trials in oncology. *Statistics in Medicine*, 22, 239–264.

Rowland, M. and Tozer, T.N. 1980. *Clinical Pharmacokinetics Concepts and Applications*. Lea & Febiger, Philadelphia, PA.

Roy, A. and Ette, E.I. 2005. A pragmatic approach to the design of population pharmacokinetic studies. *The AAPS Journal*, 7, E408–E419.

Ryde, M., Huitfeldt, B., and Pettersson, R. 1991. Relative bioavailability of Olsalazine from tables and capsules: A drug targeted for local effect in the colon. *Biopharmaceutics and Drug Disposition*, 12, 233–246.

Saranadasa, H. and Krishnamoorthy, K. 2005. A multivariate test for similarity of two dissolution profile. *Journal of Biopharmaceutical Statistics*, 15, 265–278.

Sargent, D.J., Weiand, H.S., Haller, D.G., Gray, R., Beneditti, J.K., Buyre, M., Labianca, Roberto, Seitz, J.F., O'Callaghan, C.J., Francini, G., Grothey, A., O'Connel, M., Catalano, P.J., Blaube, C.D., Kerr, D., Green, E., Wolmark, N., Andre, T., Goldberg, R.M., and Gramont, A.De. 2005. Disease-free survival versus overall survival as a primary end point for adjuvant colon cancer studies. *Journal of Clinical Oncology*, 23, 8864–8870.

SAS 2005. Statistical Analysis System. *SAS User's Guide: Statistics*, Version 9. SAS Institute, Cary, NC.

Saul, S. 2007. More generics slow rias in drug prices, August 8, 2007, The New York Times.

Schall, R. 1995. Assessment of individual and population bioequivalence using the probability that bioavailabilities are similar. *Biometrics*, 51, 615–626.

Schall, R. and Luus, H.G. 1993. On population and individual bioequivalence. *Statistics in Medicine*, 12, 1109–1124.

Schuirmann, D.J. 1981. On hypothesis testing to determine if the mean of a normal distribution is continued in a known interval. *Biometrics*, 37, 617 [abstract].

Schuirmann, D.J. 1987. A comparison of the two one-sided tests procedure and the power approach for assessing the equivalence of average bioavailability. *Journal of Pharmacokinetics and Biopharmaceutics*, 15, 657–680.

Schuirmann, D.J. 1989. Confidence intervals for the ratio of two means from a cross-over study. Proceedings of the Biopharmaceutical Section of the American Statistical Association, Washington, DC, pp. 121–126.

Schumitzky, A. 1990. Nonparametric EM algorithms for estimating prior distributions. Technical Reports, 90-2, USC.

Searle, S.R. 1971. *Linear Models*. John Wiley & Sons, New York.

Searle, S.R., Casella, G., and McCulloch, C.E. 1992, *Variance Components*. John Wiley & Sons, New York.

Selwyn, M.R. and Hall, N.R. 1984. On Bayesian methods for bioequivalence. *Biometrics*, 40, 1103–1108.

Selwyn, M.R., Dempster, A.P., and Hall, N.R. 1981. A Bayesian approach to bioequivalence for the 2×2 changeover design. *Biometrics*, 37, 11–21.

Senn, S. 1993. *Cross-over Trials in Clinical Research*. John Wiley & Sons, New York.

Serfling, R.J. 1980. *Approximation Theorems of Mathematical Statistics*, Wiley, New York.

Shah, V.P., Tsong, Y., Sathe, P., and Liu, J.P. 1998. In vitro dissolution profile comparison-statistics and analysis of the similarity factor, f_2. *Pharmaceutical Research*, 15, 889–896.

Shao, J., Chow, S.C., and Ju, H.L. 1995. Analysis of missing data for replicated crossover design. *Journal of China Statistical Association*, 33, 215–233.

Shao, J., Chow, S.C., and Wang, B. 2000. Bootstrap methods for individual bioequivalence. *Statistics in Medicine*, 19, 2741–2754.

Shapiro, S.S. and Wilk, M.B. 1965. An analysis of variance test for normality (complete samples). *Biometrika*, 52, 591–611.

Sheiner, L.B. 1992. Bioequivalence revisited. *Statistics in Medicine*, 11, 1777–1788.

Sheiner, L.B. 1997. Learning vs confirming in clinical drug development. *Clin. Pharmacol. Ther.*, 61, 275–291.

Sheiner, L.B. and Beal, S.L. 1980. Evaluation of methods for estimating population pharmacokinetic parameters, I. Michaelis–Menten model: Routine clinical data. *Journal of Pharmacokinetics and Biopharmaceutics*, 8, 553–571.

Sheiner, L.B. and Beal, S.L. 1981. Evaluation of methods for estimating population pharmacokinetic parameters, II. Biexponential model and experimental pharmacokinetic data. *Journal of Pharmacokinetics and Biopharmaceutics*, 9, 635–651.

Sheiner, L.B. and Beal, S.L. 1983. Evaluation of methods for estimating population pharmacokinetic parameters, III. Monoexponential model and routine clinical data. *Journal of Pharmacokinetics and Biopharmaceutics*, 11, 303–319.

Sheiner, L.B., Beal, S.L. and Dunne, A. 1997. Analysis of nonrandomly censored ordered categorical longitudinal data from analgesic trials. *Journal of American Statistical Association*, 92, 1235–1244.

Sheiner, L.B., Rosenberg, B., and Melmon, K.L. 1972. Modelling of individual pharmacokinetics for computer-aided drug dosage. *Computer and Biomedical Research*, 5, 441–459.

Sheiner, L.B., Rosenberg, B., and Marathe, V.V. 1977. Estimation of population characteristics of pharmacokinetic parameters from routine clinical data. *Journal of Pharmacokinetics and Biopharmaceutics*, 5, 445–479.

Shimizu, K. 1988. Point estimation. In: *Lognormal Distribution*, Crow, E.L. and Shimizu, K. (Eds.), Marcel Dekker, New York, pp. 27–86.

Shirley, E. 1976. The use of confidence intervals in biopharmaceutics. *Journal of Pharmacy and Pharmacology*, 28, 312–313.

Simon, R. 1999. Bayesian design and analysis of active control clinical trials. *Biometrics*, 55, 484–487.

Smith, S.J. 1988. Evaluating the efficiency of the Δ distribution mean estimator. *Biometics*, 44, 485–493.

Smith, T. 1986. Statistical methods—dose proportionality. Technical Report, Ayerst Laboratories, New York.

Smith, B.P., Vandenhende, F.R., deSante, K.A., Welch, P.A., Callaghan, J.T., and Forgne, S.T. 2000. Confidence interval criteria for assessment of dose proportionality. *Pharmaceutical Research*, 17, 1278–1283.

Snedecor, G.W. and Cochran, W.G. 1980. *Statistical Methods*. 7th ed., Iowa State University Press, Ames, IA.

Snee, R.D. 1972. On the analysis of response curve data. *Technometrics*, 14, 47–62.

Srikantan, K.S. 1961. Testing a single outlier in a regression model. *Sankhyá*, A, 23, 251–260.

Srinivasan, R. and Langenberg, P. 1986. A two-stage procedure with controlled error probabilities for testing bioequivalence. *Biometrical Journal*, 28, 825–833.

Steimer, J.L., Mallet, A., Golmard, J.F., and Boisvieux, J.F. 1984. Alternative approaches to estimation of population pharmacokinetic parameters; comparison with the nonlinear mixed effect model. *Drug Metabolism Reviews*, 15, 265–292.

Steinijans, V.W. and Diletti, E. 1983. Statistical analysis of bioavailability studies: Parametric and nonparametric confidence intervals. *European Journal of Clinical Pharmacology*, 24, 127–136.

Steinijans, V.W. and Diletti, E. 1985. Generalization of distribution-free confidence intervals for bioavailability ratios. *European Journal of Clinical Pharmacology*, 28, 85–88.

Steinijans, V.W. and Shulz, H.U. 1992. Bioequivalence Assessment: Methods and Applications of the International Journal of Clinical Pharmacology Therapy and Toxicology, 30, Suppl. 1, S1-6.

Sun, H., Ette, E.L., and Ludden, T.M. 1996. On the recording of sampling times and parameter estimation from repeated measures of pharmacokinetic data. *Journal of Pharmacokinetics and Biopharmaceutics*, 24, 637–650.

Tempelman, R.J. 2004. Experimental design and statistical model for classical and bioequivalence hypothesis testing with an application to dairy nutrition studies, *Journal of Animal Science*, 82(E. Suppl.), E162–E172.

The Numerical Algorithm Group. 2008. Oxford, U.K. website: www.nag.co.uk.

Thiyagarajan, B. and Dobbins, T.W. 1987. An assessment of the 75/75 rule in bioequivalence. Proceedings of the Biopharmaceutical section of the American Statistical Association, San Francisco, California. pp. 143–148.

Thompson, C.M. 1941. Tables of percent points of the χ^2-distribution, *Biometrica*, 32, 188–189.

Ting, N., Burdick, R.K., Graybill, F.A., Jeyaratnam, S., and Lu, T.-F.C. 1990. Confidence intervals on linear combinations of variance components that are unrestricted in sign. *Journal of Statistical Computation and Simulation*, 35, 135–143.

Tothfalusi, L. and Endrenyi, L. 2003. Limits for the scaled average bioequivalence of highly variable drugs and drug products. *Pharmaceutical Research*, 20, 382–389.

Tse, S.K. 1990. A comparison of interval estimation procedures in bioavailability/ bioequivalence. Proceedings of the Biopharmaceutical section of the American Statistical Association, Anaheim, California, pp. 43–46.

Tsong, Y. 1995. Statistical assessment of mean differences between two dissolution data sets. Presented at the 1995 Drug Information Association Dissolution Workshop, Rockville, MD.

Tsong, Y., Hammerstorm, T., Sathe, P., and Shah, V.P. 1996. Statistical assessment of mean differences between two dissolution data sets. *Drug Information Journal*, 30, 1105–1112.

Tsui, K.W. and Weeranhandi, S. 1989. Generalized p-values in significance testing of hypotheses in the presence of nuisance parameters. *Journal of American Statistical Association*, 84, 602–607.

Turkey, J.W. 1951. Components in regression. *Biometrics*, 7, 33–69.

Vonesh, E.F. 1996. A note on the use of Laplace's approximation for nonlinear mixed-effects models. *Biometrika*, 83, 447–452.

Vonesh, E.F. and Chinchilli, V.M. 1997. *Linear and Nonlinear Models for the Analysis of Repeated Measurements*. Marcel Dekker, New York.

Vuorinen, J. 1997. A practical approach for the assessment of bioequivalence under selected higher-order cross-over designs. *Statistics in Medicine*, 16, 2229–2243.

Vuorinen, J. and Turunen, J. 1996. A three-step procedure for assessing bioequivalence in the general mixed linear framework. *Statistics in Medicine*, 15, 2635–2655.

Wagner, J.G. 1971. *Biopharmaceutics and Relevant Pharmacokinetics*. Drug Intelligence Publications, Hamilton, IL.

Wagner, J.G. 1975. *Fundamentals of Clinical Pharmacokinetics*. Drug Intelligence Publications, Hamilton, IL.

Wakefield, J. 1996. The Bayesian analysis of population pharmacokinetic models. *Journal of American Statistical Association*, 91, 62–75.

Walsh, J.E. 1949. Some significance tests for the median which are valid under very general conditions. *The Annals of Mathematical Statistics*, 20, 64–81.

Wang, C.M. 1990. On the lower bound of confidence coefficients for a confidence interval on variance components. *Biometrics*, 46, 187–192.

Wang, H., Zhang, Y., Shao, J., and Chow, S.C. 2000. In vitro bioequivalence testing. In: *Encyclopedia of Biopharmaceutical Statistics*, Chow, S.C. (Ed.), 2nd ed., Marcel Dekker, New York.

Wang, J. and Endrenyi, L. 1992. A computationally efficient approach for the design of population pharmacokinetic studies. *Journal of Pharmacokinetics and Biopharmaceutics*, 20, 279–294.

Wang, S.J., Hung, J.H.M., and Tsong, Y. 2002. Utility and pitfalls of some statistical methods in active control trials. *Controlled Clinical Trials*, 23, 15–28.

Wang, S.J. and Hung, J.H.M. 2003. TACT method for noninferiority testing in active controlled trials. *Statistics in Medicine*, 22, 227–238.

Wang, W. 1997. Optimal unbiased tests for equivalence in intrasubject variability. *Journal of the American Statistical Association*, 88, 939–946.

Wang, W. and Chow, S.C. 2003. Examining outlying subjects and outlying records in bioequivalence trials. *Journal of Biopharmaceutical Statistics*, 13, 43–56.

Wang, W., Hwang, J.T., and DasGupta, A. 1999. Statistical tests for multivariate bioequivalence. *Biometrika*, 86, 395–402.

Wang, W.P., Chow, S.C., and Wei, W. 1995. On likelihood distance for outliers detection. *Journal of Biopharmaceutical Statistics*, 5, 307–322.

Wang, W.P., Hsuan, F., and Chow, S.C. 1996. Patient compliance and fluctuation of the serum drug concentration. *Statistics in Medicine*, 15, 659–669.

Wang, W.P., Hsuan, F., and Chow, S.C. 1997. An adjusted two one-sided *t*-test for bioequivalence trials with multiple doses. *Journal of Biopharmaceutical Statistics*, 7, 157–170.

Ware, J.H. 1985. Linear models for the analysis of longitudinal studies. *American Statistical Association*, 39, 95–101.

Ware, J.H., Mosteller, F., and Ingelfinger, J.A. 1986. *p*-Values. In: *Medical Use of Statistics*, Bailar, J.C. and Mosteller, F. (Eds.), NEJM Books, Waltham, MA.

Wearahandi, S. 1995. *Exact Statistical Method for Data Analysis*. Springer, New York.

Weiner, D. 1989. Bioavailability. Notes on the training course for new clinical statisticians sponsored by the Biostatistics Subsections of Pharmaceutical Manufacture Association, March, 1989, Washington, DC.

Wellek, S. 1993. Basing the analysis of comparative bioavailability trials on an individualized statistical definition of equivalence. *Biometrical Journal*, 35, 47–55.

Westlake, W.J. 1972. Use of confidence intervals in analysis of comparative bioavailability trials. *Journal of Pharmaceutical Science*, 61, 1340–1341.

Westlake, W.J. 1973. The design and analysis of comparative blood-level trials. In: *Current Concepts in the Pharmaceutical Sciences*, Swarbrick, J. (Ed.), Lea & Febiger, Philadelphia.

Westlake, W.J. 1974. The use of balanced incomplete block designs in comparative bioavailability trials. *Biometrics*, 30, 319–327.

Westlake, W.J. 1976. Symmetrical confidence intervals for bioequivalence trials. *Biometrics*, 32, 741–744.

Westlake, W.J. 1979. Statistical aspects of comparative bioavailability trials. *Biometrics*, 35, 273–280.

Westlake, W.J. 1981. Bioequivalence testing—a need to rethink [reader reaction response]. *Biometrics*, 37, 591–593.

Westlake, W.J. 1986. Bioavailability and bioequivalence of pharmaceutical formulations. In: *Biopharmaceutical Statistics for Drug Development*, Peace, K. (Ed.), Marcel Dekker, New York, pp. 329–352.

Wijnard, H.P. and Timmer, C.J. 1983. Mini-computer programs for bioequivalence testing for pharmaceutical drug formulations in two-way crossover studies. *Computer Programs in Biomedicine*, 17, 73–88.

Wilcoxon, F. 1945. Individual comparisons by ranking methods. *Biometrics*, 1, 80–83.

Williams, E.J. 1949. Experimental designs balanced for the residual effects of treatment. *Australian Journal of Science and Research*, 2, 149–168.

Williams, J.S. 1962. A confidence interval for variance components. *Biometrika*, 49, 278–281.

Wolfinger, R. 1993. Covariance structure selection in general mixed models. *Communication in Statistics*, B, 22, 1079–2006.

WHO 2005a. World Health Organization Draft Revision on Multisource (Generic) Pharmaceutical Products: Guidelines on Registration Requirements to Establish Interchangeability, Geneva, Switzerland.

WHO 2005b. World Health Organization Revision/Update of the Guidance on the Selection of Comparator Pharmaceutical Products for Equivalence Assessment of Interchangeable Multisource (Generic) Products, Geneva, Switzerland.

Yee, K.F. 1986. The calculation of probabilities in rejecting bioequivalence. *Biometrics*, 42, 961–965.

Yeh, C.M. and Chiang, T. 1991. Bioavailability in a 3 × 3 crossover study of a combination drug. Presented at 1991 Drug Information Association Statistics Workship. Hilton Head, SC.

Yeh, K.C. and Kwan, K.C. 1978. A comparison of numerical integrating algorithms by trapezoidal, Lagrange, and spline approximations. *Journal of Pharmacokinetics and Biopharmaceutics*, 6, 79–81.

Zeger, S. and Liang, K.Y. 1986. Longitudinal data analysis for discrete and continuous outcomes. *Biometrics*, 42, 121–130.

Appendix A

Statistical Tables

TABLE A.1: Areas of upper tail of the standard normal distribution.

z	**0.00**	**0.01**	**0.02**	**0.03**	**0.04**	**0.05**	**0.06**	**0.07**	**0.08**	**0.09**
0.0	0.5000	0.4960	0.4920	0.4880	0.4840	0.4801	0.4761	0.4721	0.4681	0.4641
0.1	0.4602	0.4562	0.4522	0.4483	0.4443	0.4404	0.4364	0.4325	0.4286	0.4247
0.2	0.4207	0.4168	0.4129	0.4090	0.4052	0.403	0.3974	0.3936	0.3897	0.3859
0.3	0.3821	0.3783	0.3745	0.3707	0.3669	0.3632	0.3594	0.3557	0.3520	0.3483
0.4	0.3446	0.3409	0.3372	0.3336	0.3300	0.3264	0.3228	0.3192	0.3156	0.3121
0.5	0.3085	0.3050	0.3015	0.2981	0.2946	0.2912	0.2877	0.2843	0.2810	0.2776
0.6	0.2743	0.2709	0.2676	0.2643	0.2611	0.2578	0.2546	0.2514	0.2483	0.2451
0.7	0.2420	0.2389	0.2358	0.2327	0.2296	0.2266	0.2236	0.2206	0.2177	0.2148
0.8	0.2119	0.2090	0.2061	0.2033	0.2005	0.1977	0.1949	0.1922	0.1894	0.1867
0.9	0.1841	0.1814	0.1788	0.1762	0.1736	0.1711	0.1685	0.1660	0.1635	0.1611
1.0	0.1587	0.1562	0.1539	0.1515	0.1492	0.1469	0.1446	0.1423	0.1401	0.1379
1.1	0.1357	0.1335	0.1314	0.1292	0.1271	0.1251	0.1230	0.1210	0.1190	0.1170
1.2	0.1151	0.1131	0.1112	0.1093	0.1075	0.1056	0.1038	0.1020	0.1003	0.0985
1.3	0.0968	0.0951	0.0934	0.0918	0.0901	0.0885	0.0869	0.0853	0.0838	0.0823
1.4	0.0808	0.0793	0.0778	0.0764	0.0749	0.0735	0.0721	0.0708	0.0694	0.0681

1.5	0.0668	0.0655	0.0643	0.0630	0.0618	0.0606	0.0594	0.0582	0.0571	0.0559
1.6	0.0548	0.0537	0.0526	0.0516	0.0505	0.0495	0.0485	0.0475	0.0465	0.0455
1.7	0.0446	0.0436	0.0427	0.0418	0.0409	0.0401	0.0392	0.0384	0.0375	0.0367
1.8	0.0359	0.0351	0.0344	0.0336	0.0329	0.0322	0.0314	0.0307	0.0301	0.0294
1.9	0.0287	0.0281	0.0274	0.0268	0.0262	0.0256	0.0250	0.0244	0.0239	0.0233
2.0	0.02275	0.02222	0.02169	0.02118	0.02068	0.02018	0.01970	0.01923	0.01876	0.01831
2.1	0.01786	0.01743	0.01700	0.01659	0.01618	0.01578	0.01539	0.01500	0.01463	0.01426
2.2	0.01390	0.01355	0.01321	0.01287	0.01255	0.01222	0.01191	0.01160	0.01130	0.01101
2.3	0.01072	0.01044	0.01017	0.00990	0.00964	0.00939	0.00914	0.00889	0.00866	0.00842
2.4	0.00820	0.00798	0.00776	0.00755	0.00734	0.00714	0.00695	0.00676	0.00657	0.00639
2.5	0.00621	0.00604	0.00587	0.00570	0.00554	0.00539	0.00523	0.00508	0.00494	0.00480
2.6	0.00466	0.00453	0.00440	0.00427	0.00415	0.00402	0.00391	0.00379	0.00368	0.00357
2.7	0.00347	0.00336	0.00326	0.00317	0.00307	0.00298	0.00289	0.00280	0.00272	0.00264
2.8	0.00256	0.00248	0.00240	0.00233	0.00226	0.00219	0.00212	0.00205	0.00199	0.00193
2.9	0.00187	0.00181	0.00175	0.00169	0.00164	0.00159	0.00154	0.00149	0.00144	0.00139

Source: From Murdock, J. and Barnes, J.A., *Statistical Tables for Science, Engineering and Management* (Table 3), Macmillian, London, 1968.

TABLE A.2: Upper quantiles of a χ^2 distribution.

ν/α	0.995	0.990	0.975	0.950	0.900	0.100	0.050	0.025	0.010	0.005
1	392704.10^{-10}	157088.10^{-9}	982069.10^{-9}	393214.10^{-8}	0.0157908	2.70554	3.84146	5.02389	6.63490	7.87944
2	0.0100251	0.0201007	0.0506356	0.102587	0.210720	4.60517	5.99147	7.37776	9.21034	10.5966
3	0.0717212	0.114832	0.215795	0.351846	0.584375	6.25139	7.81473	9.34840	11.3449	12.8381
4	0.206990	0.297110	0.484419	0.710721	1.063623	7.77944	9.48773	11.1433	13.2767	14.8602
5	0.411740	0.54300	0.831211	1.145476	1.61031	9.23635	11.0705	12.8325	15.063	16.7496
6	0.675727	0.872085	1.237347	1.63539	2.20413	10.6446	12.5916	14.4494	16.8119	18.5476
7	0.989265	1.239043	1.68987	2.16735	2.83311	12.0170	14.0671	16.0128	18.4753	20.2777
8	1.344419	1.646482	2.17973	2.73264	3.48954	13.3616	15.5073	17.5346	20.0902	21.9550
9	1.734926	2.087912	2.70039	3.32511	4.16816	14.6837	16.9190	19.0228	21.6660	23.5893
10	2.15585	2.55821	3.24697	3.94030	4.86518	15.9871	18.3070	20.4831	23.2093	25.1882
11	2.60321	3.05347	3.81575	4.57481	5.57779	17.2750	19.6751	21.9200	24.7250	26.7569
12	3.07382	3.57056	4.40379	5.22603	6.30380	18.5494	21.0261	23.3367	26.2170	28.2995
13	3.56503	4.10691	5.00874	5.89186	7.04150	19.8119	22.3621	24.7356	27.6883	29.8194
14	4.07468	4.66043	5.62872	6.57063	7.78953	21.0642	23.6848	26.1190	29.1413	31.3193
15	4.60094	5.22935	6.26214	7.26094	8.54675	22.3072	24.9958	27.4884	30.5779	32.8013
16	5.14224	5.812321	6.90766	7.96164	9.31223	23.5418	26.2962	28.8454	31.9999	34.2672
17	5.69724	6.40776	7.56418	8.67176	10.0852	24.7690	27.5871	30.1910	33.4087	35.7185
18	6.26481	7.01491	8.23075	9.39046	10.8649	25.9894	28.8693	31.5264	34.8053	37.1564

19	6.84398	7.63273	8.90655	10.1170	11.6509	27.2036	30.1435	32.8523	36.1908	38.5822
20	7.43386	8.26040	9.59083	10.8508	12.4426	28.4120	31.4104	34.1696	37.5662	39.9968
21	8.03366	8.89720	10.28293	11.5913	13.2396	29.6151	32.6705	35.4789	38.9321	41.4010
22	8.64272	9.54249	10.9823	12.3380	14.0415	30.8133	33.9244	36.7807	40.2894	42.7956
23	9.26042	10.19567	11.6885	13.0905	14.8479	32.0069	35.1725	38.0757	41.6384	44.1813
24	9.88623	10.8564	12.4011	13.8484	15.6587	33.1963	36.4151	39.3641	42.9798	45.5585
25	10.5197	11.5240	13.1197	14.6114	16.4734	34.3816	37.6525	40.6465	44.3141	46.9278
26	11.1603	12.1981	13.8439	15.3791	17.2919	35.5631	38.8852	41.9232	45.6417	48.2899
27	14.8076	12.8786	14.5733	16.1513	18.1138	36.7412	40.1133	43.1944	46.9630	49.6449
28	12.4613	13.5648	15.3079	16.9279	18.9392	37.9159	41.3372	44.4607	48.2782	50.9933
29	13.1211	14.2565	16.0471	17.7083	19.7677	39.0875	42.5569	45.7222	49.5879	52.3356
30	13.7867	14.9535	16.7908	18.4926	20.5992	40.2560	43.7729	46.9792	50.8922	53.6720
40	20.7065	22.1643	24.4331	26.5093	29.0505	51.8050	55.7585	59.3417	63.6907	66.7659
50	27.9907	29.7067	32.3574	34.7642	37.6886	63.1671	67.5048	71.4202	76.1539	79.4900
60	35.5346	37.4848	40.4817	43.1879	46.4589	74.3970	79.0819	83.2976	88.3794	91.9517
70	43.2752	45.4418	48.7576	51.7393	55.3290	85.5271	90.5321	95.0231	100.425	104.215
80	51.1720	53.5400	57.1532	60.3915	64.2778	96.5782	101.879	106.629	112.329	116.321
90	59.1963	61.7541	65.6466	69.1260	73.2912	107.565	113.145	118.136	124.116	128.299
100	67.3276	70.0648	74.2219	77.9295	82.3581	118.498	224.342	129.561	135.807	140.169

Source: From Thompson, C.M., *Biometrika* (Tables of Percentage Points of the χ^2-Distribution), 32, 188, 1941.

TABLE A.3: Upper quantiles of a central t distribution.

ν/α	0.050	0.025	0.010	0.005
1	6.3138	12.706	25.452	63.657
2	2.9200	4.3027	6.2053	9.9248
3	2.3534	3.1825	4.1765	5.8409
4	2.1318	2.7764	3.4954	4.6041
5	2.0150	2.5706	3.1634	4.0321
6	1.9432	2.4469	2.9687	3.7074
7	1.8946	2.3646	2.8412	3.4995
8	1.8595	2.3060	2.7515	3.3554
9	1.8331	2.2622	2.6850	3.2498
10	1.8125	2.2281	2.6338	3.1693
11	1.7959	2.2010	2.5931	3.1058
12	1.7823	2.1788	2.5600	3.0545
13	1.7709	2.1604	2.5326	3.0123
14	1.7613	2.1448	2.5096	2.9768
15	1.7530	2.1315	2.4899	2.9467
16	1.7459	2.1199	2.4729	2.9208
17	1.7396	2.1098	2.4581	2.8982
18	1.7341	2.1009	2.4450	2.8784
19	1.7291	2.0930	2.4334	2.8609
20	1.7247	2.0860	2.4231	2.8453
21	1.7207	2.0796	2.4138	2.8314
22	1.7171	2.0739	2.4055	2.8188
23	1.7139	2.0687	2.3979	2.8073
24	1.7109	2.0639	2.3910	2.7969
25	1.7081	2.0595	2.3846	2.7874
26	1.7056	2.0555	2.3788	2.7787
27	1.7033	2.0518	2.3734	2.7707
28	1.7011	2.0484	2.3685	2.7633
29	1.6991	2.0452	2.3638	2.7564
30	1.6973	2.0423	2.3596	2.7500
40	1.6839	2.0211	2.3289	2.7045
60	1.6707	2.0003	2.2991	2.6603
120	1.6577	1.9799	2.2699	2.6174
∞	1.6449	1.9600	2.2414	2.5758

Source: From Merrington, M., *Biometrika* (Tables of Percentage Points of the t Distribution), 32, 300, 1941.

TABLE A.4: Upper quantiles of an F distribution ($\alpha = 0.05$).

$\nu_2 \backslash \nu_1$	1	2	3	4	5	6	7	8	9
1	161.45	199.50	215.71	224.58	230.16	233.99	236.77	238.88	240.54
2	18.513	19.000	19.164	19.247	19.296	19.330	19.353	19.371	19.385
3	10.128	9.5521	9.2766	9.1172	9.0135	8.9406	8.8868	8.8452	8.8123
4	7.7086	6.9443	6.5914	6.3883	6.2560	6.1631	6.0942	6.0410	5.9988
5	6.6079	5.7861	5.4095	5.1922	5.0503	4.9503	4.8759	4.8183	4.7725
6	5.9874	5.1433	4.7571	4.5337	4.3874	4.2839	4.2066	4.1468	4.0990
7	5.5914	4.7374	4.3468	4.1203	3.9715	3.8660	3.7870	3.7257	3.6767
8	5.3177	4.4590	4.0662	3.8378	3.6875	3.5806	3.5005	3.4381	3.3881
9	5.1174	4.2565	3.8626	3.6331	3.4817	3.3738	3.2927	3.2296	3.1789
10	4.9646	4.1028	3.7083	3.4780	3.3258	3.2172	3.1355	3.0717	3.0204
11	4.8443	3.9823	3.5874	3.3567	3.2039	3.0946	3.0123	2.9480	2.8962
12	4.7472	3.8853	3.4903	3.2592	3.1059	2.9961	2.9134	2.8486	2.7964
13	4.6672	3.8056	3.4105	3.1791	3.0254	2.9153	2.8321	2.7669	2.7144
14	4.6001	3.7389	3.3439	3.1122	2.9582	2.8477	2.7642	2.6987	2.6458
15	4.5431	3.6823	3.2874	3.0556	2.9013	2.7905	2.7066	2.6408	2.5876
16	4.4940	3.6337	3.2389	32.0069	2.8524	2.7413	2.6572	2.5911	2.5377
17	4.4513	3.5915	3.1968	2.9647	2.8100	2.6987	2.6143	2.5480	2.4943
18	4.4139	3.5546	3.1599	2.9277	2.7729	2.6613	2.5767	2.5102	2.4563
19	4.3808	3.5219	3.1274	2.8951	2.7401	2.6283	2.5435	2.4768	2.4227
20	4.3513	3.4928	3.0984	2.8661	2.7109	2.5990	2.5140	2.4471	2.3928
21	4.3248	3.4668	3.0725	2.8401	2.6848	2.5727	2.4876	2.4205	2.3661
22	4.3009	3.4434	3.0491	2.8167	2.6613	2.5491	2.4638	2.3965	2.3419

(*continued*)

TABLE A.4 (continued): Upper quantiles of an F distribution ($\alpha = 0.05$).

$\nu_2 \backslash \nu_1$	1	2	3	4	5	6	7	8	9
23	4.2793	3.4221	3.0280	2.7955	2.6400	2.5277	2.4422	2.3748	2.3201
24	4.2597	3.4028	3.0088	2.7763	2.6207	2.5082	2.4226	2.3551	2.3002
25	4.2417	3.3852	2.9912	2.7587	2.6030	2.4904	2.4047	2.3371	3.2821
26	4.2252	2.3690	2.9751	2.7426	2.5868	2.4741	2.3883	2.3205	2.2655
27	4.2100	3.3541	2.9604	2.7278	2.5719	2.4591	2.3732	2.3053	2.2501
28	4.1960	3.3404	2.9467	2.7141	2.5581	2.4453	2.3593	2.2913	2.2360
29	4.1830	3.3277	2.9340	2.7014	2.5454	2.4324	2.3463	2.2782	2.2229
30	4.1709	3.3158	2.9223	2.6896	2.5336	2.4205	2.3343	2.2662	2.2107
40	4.0848	3.2317	2.8387	2.6060	2.4495	2.3359	2.2490	2.1802	2.1240
60	4.0012	3.1504	2.7581	2.5252	2.3683	2.2540	2.1665	2.0970	2.0401
120	3.9201	3.0718	2.6802	2.4472	2.2900	2.1750	2.0867	2.0164	1.9588
∞	3.8415	2.9957	2.6049	2.3719	2.2141	2.0986	2.0096	1.9384	1.8799

$\nu_2 \backslash \nu_1$	10	12	15	20	24	30	40	60	12	∞
1	241.88	243.91	245.95	248.01	249.05	250.09	251.14	252.20	253.25	254.32
2	19.396	19.413	19.429	19.446	19.454	19.462	19.471	19.479	19.487	19.496
3	8.7855	8.7446	8.7029	8.6602	8.6385	8.6166	8.5944	8.5720	8.5494	8.5265
4	5.9644	5.9117	5.8578	5.8025	5.7744	5.7459	5.7170	5.6878	5.6581	5.6281
5	4.7351	4.6777	4.6188	4.5581	4.5272	4.4957	4.4638	4.4314	4.3984	4.3650
6	4.0600	3.9999	3.9381	3.8742	3.8415	3.8082	3.7743	3.7398	3.7047	3.6688
7	3.6365	3.5747	3.5108	3.4445	3.4105	3.3758	3.3404	3.3043	3.2674	3.2298
8	3.3472	3.2840	3.2184	3.1503	3.1152	3.0794	3.0428	3.0053	2.9669	2.9276
9	3.1373	3.0729	3.0061	2.9365	2.9005	2.8637	2.8259	2.7872	2.7475	2.7067

10	2.9782	2.9130	2.8450	2.7740	2.7372	2.6996	2.6609	2.6211	2.5801	2.5379
11	2.8536	2.7876	2.7186	2.6464	2.6090	2.5705	2.5309	2.4901	2.4480	2.4045
12	2.7534	2.6866	2.6169	2.5436	2.5055	2.4663	2.4259	2.3842	2.3410	2.2962
13	2.6710	2.6037	2.5331	2.4589	2.4202	2.3803	2.3392	2.2966	2.2524	2.2064
14	2.6021	2.5342	2.4630	2.3879	2.3487	2.3082	2.2664	2.2230	2.1778	2.1307
15	2.5437	2.4753	2.4035	2.3275	2.2878	2.2468	2.2043	2.1601	2.1141	2.0658
16	2.4935	2.4247	2.3522	2.2756	2.2354	2.1938	2.1507	2.1058	2.0589	2.0096
17	2.4499	2.3807	2.3077	2.2304	2.1898	2.1477	2.1040	2.0584	2.0107	1.9604
18	2.4117	2.3421	2.2686	2.1906	2.1497	2.1071	2.0629	2.0166	1.9681	1.9168
19	2.3779	2.3080	2.2341	2.1555	2.1141	2.0712	2.0264	1.9796	1.9302	1.8780
20	2.3479	2.2776	2.2033	2.1242	2.0825	2.0391	1.9938	1.9464	1.8963	1.8432
21	2.3210	2.2504	2.1757	2.0960	2.0540	2.0102	1.9645	1.9165	1.8657	1.8117
22	2.2967	2.2258	2.1508	2.0707	2.0283	1.9842	1.9380	1.8895	1.8380	1.7831
23	2.2747	2.2036	2.1282	2.0476	2.0050	1.9605	1.9139	1.8649	1.8128	1.7570
24	2.2547	2.1834	2.1077	2.0267	1.9838	1.9390	1.8920	1.8424	1.7897	1.7331
25	2.2365	2.1649	2.0889	2.0075	1.9643	1.9192	1.8718	1.8217	1.7684	1.7110
26	2.2197	2.1479	2.0716	1.9898	1.9464	1.9010	1.8533	1.8027	1.7488	1.6906
27	2.2043	2.1323	2.0558	1.9736	1.9299	1.8842	1.8361	1.7851	1.7307	1.6717
28	2.1900	2.1179	2.0411	1.9586	1.9147	1.8687	1.8203	1.7689	1.7138	1.6541
29	2.1768	2.1045	2.0275	1.9446	1.9005	1.8543	1.8055	1.7537	1.6981	1.6377
30	2.1646	2.0921	2.1048	1.9317	1.8874	1.8409	1.7918	1.7396	1.6835	1.6223
40	2.0772	2.0035	1.9245	1.8389	1.7929	1.7444	1.6928	1.6373	1.5766	1.5089
60	1.9926	1.9174	1.8364	1.7480	1.7001	1.6491	1.5943	1.5343	1.4673	1.3893
120	1.9105	1.8337	1.7505	1.6587	1.6084	1.5543	1.4952	1.4290	1.3519	1.2539
∞	1.8307	1.7522	1.6664	1.5705	1.5173	1.4591	1.3940	1.3180	1.2214	1.0000

(continued)

TABLE A.4 (continued): Upper quantiles of an F distribution ($\alpha = 0.025$).

$\nu_2 \backslash \nu_1$	1	2	3	4	5	6	7	8	9
1	647.79	799.50	864.16	899.58	921.85	937.11	948.22	956.66	963.28
2	38.506	39.000	39.165	39.248	39.298	39.331	39.355	39.373	39.387
3	17.443	16.044	15.439	15.101	14.885	14.735	14.624	14.540	14.473
4	12.218	10.649	9.9792	9.6045	9.3645	9.1973	9.0741	8.9796	8.9047
5	10.007	8.4336	7.7636	7.3879	7.1464	6.9777	6.8531	6.7572	6.6810
6	8.8131	7.2598	6.5988	6.2272	5.9876	5.8197	5.6955	5.5996	5.5234
7	8.0727	6.5415	5.8898	5.5226	5.2852	5.1186	4.9949	4.8994	4.8232
8	7.5709	6.0595	5.4160	5.0526	4.8173	4.6517	4.5286	4.4332	4.3572
9	7.2093	5.7147	5.0781	4.7181	4.4844	4.3197	4.1971	4.1020	4.0260
10	6.9367	5.4564	4.8256	4.4683	4.2361	4.0721	3.9498	3.8549	3.7790
11	6.7241	5.2559	4.6300	4.2751	4.0440	3.8807	3.7586	3.6638	3.5879
12	6.5538	5.0959	4.4742	4.1212	3.8911	3.7283	3.6065	3.5118	3.4358
13	6.4143	4.9653	4.3472	3.9959	3.7667	3.6043	3.4827	3.3880	3.3120
14	6.2979	4.8567	4.2417	3.8919	3.6634	3.5014	3.3799	3.2853	3.2093
15	6.1995	4.7650	4.1528	3.8043	3.5764	3.4147	3.2934	3.1987	3.1227
16	6.1151	3.6867	4.0768	3.7294	3.5021	3.3406	3.2194	3.1248	3.0488
17	6.0420	4.6189	4.0112	3.6648	3.4379	3.2767	3.1556	3.0610	2.9849
18	5.9781	4.5597	3.9539	3.6083	3.3820	3.2209	3.0999	3.0053	2.9291
19	5.9216	4.5075	3.9034	3.5587	3.3327	3.1718	3.0509	2.9563	2.8800
20	5.8715	4.4613	3.8587	3.5147	3.2891	3.1283	3.0074	2.9128	2.8365
21	5.8266	4.4199	3.8188	3.4754	3.2501	3.0895	2.9686	2.8740	2.7977
22	5.7863	4.3828	3.7829	3.4401	3.2151	3.0546	2.9338	2.8392	2.7628

23	5.7498	4.3492	3.7505	3.4083	3.1835	3.0232	2.9024	2.8077	2.7313
24	5.7167	4.3187	3.7211	3.3794	3.1548	2.9946	2.8738	2.7791	2.7027
25	5.6864	4.2909	3.6943	3.3530	3.1287	2.9685	2.8478	2.7531	2.6766
26	5.6586	4.2655	3.6697	3.3289	3.1048	2.9447	2.8240	2.7293	2.6528
27	5.6331	4.2421	3.6472	3.3067	3.0828	2.9228	2.8021	2.7074	2.6309
28	5.6096	4.2205	3.6264	3.2863	3.0625	2.9027	2.7820	2.6872	2.6106
29	5.5878	4.2006	3.6072	3.2674	3.0438	2.8840	2.7633	2.6686	2.5919
30	5.5675	4.1821	3.5894	3.2499	3.0265	2.8667	2.7460	2.6513	2.5746
40	5.4239	4.0510	3.4633	3.1261	2.9037	2.7444	2.6238	2.5289	2.4519
60	5.2857	3.9253	3.3425	3.0077	2.7863	2.6274	2.5068	2.4117	2.3344
120	5.1524	3.8046	3.2270	2.8943	2.6740	2.5154	2.3948	2.2994	2.2217
∞	5.0239	3.6889	3.1161	2.7858	2.5665	2.4082	2.2875	2.1918	2.1136

$\nu_2 \backslash \nu_1$	**10**	**12**	**15**	**20**	**24**	**30**	**40**	**60**	**120**	**∞**
1	968.63	976.71	984.87	993.10	997.25	1001.4	1005.6	1009.8	1014.0	1018.3
2	39.398	39.415	39.431	39.448	39.456	39.465	39.473	39.481	39.490	39.498
3	14.419	14.337	14.253	14.167	14.124	14.081	14.037	13.992	13.947	13.902
4	8.8439	8.7512	8.6565	8.5599	8.5109	8.4613	8.4111	8.3604	8.3092	8.2573
5	6.6192	6.5246	6.4277	6.3285	6.2780	6.2269	6.1751	6.1225	6.0693	6.0153
6	5.4613	5.3662	5.2687	5.1684	5.1172	5.0652	5.0125	4.9589	4.9045	4.8491
7	4.7611	4.6658	4.5678	4.4667	4.4150	4.3624	4.3089	4.2544	4.1989	4.1423
8	4.2951	4.1997	4.1012	3.9995	3.9472	3.8940	3.8398	3.7844	3.7279	3.6702
9	3.9639	3.8682	3.7694	3.6669	3.6142	3.5604	3.5055	3.4493	3.3918	3.3329
10	3.7168	3.6209	3.5217	3.4186	3.3654	3.3110	3.2554	3.1984	3.1399	3.0798

(*continued*)

TABLE A.4 (continued): Upper quantiles of an F distribution ($\alpha = 0.025$).

$\nu_2 \backslash \nu_1$	10	12	15	20	24	30	40	60	120	∞
11	3.5257	3.4296	3.3299	3.2261	3.1725	3.1176	3.0613	3.0035	2.9441	2.8828
12	3.3736	3.2773	3.1772	3.0728	3.0187	2.9633	2.9063	2.8478	2.7874	2.7249
13	3.2497	3.1532	3.0527	2.9477	2.8932	2.8373	2.7797	2.7204	2.6590	2.5955
14	3.1469	3.0501	2.9493	2.8437	2.7888	2.7324	2.6742	2.6142	2.5519	2.4872
15	3.0602	2.9633	2.8621	2.7559	2.7006	2.6437	2.5850	2.5242	2.4611	2.3953
16	2.9862	2.8890	2.7875	2.6808	2.6252	2.5678	2.5085	2.4471	2.3831	2.3163
17	2.9222	2.8249	2.7230	2.6158	2.5598	2.5021	2.4422	2.3801	2.3153	2.2474
18	2.8664	2.7689	2.6667	2.5590	2.5027	2.4445	2.3842	2.3214	2.2558	2.1869
19	2.8173	2.7196	2.6171	2.5089	2.4523	2.3937	2.3329	2.2695	2.2032	2.1333
20	2.7737	2.6758	2.5731	2.4645	2.4076	2.3486	2.2873	2.2234	2.1562	2.0853
21	2.7348	2.6368	2.5338	2.4247	2.3675	2.3082	2.2465	2.1819	2.1141	2.0422
22	2.6998	2.6017	2.4984	2.3890	2.3315	2.2718	2.2097	2.1446	2.0760	2.0032
23	2.6682	2.5699	2.4665	2.3567	2.2989	2.2389	2.1763	2.1107	2.0415	1.9677
24	2.6396	2.5412	2.4374	2.3273	2.2693	2.2090	2.1460	2.0799	2.0099	1.9353
25	2.6135	2.5149	2.4110	2.3005	2.2422	2.1816	2.1183	2.0517	1.9811	1.9055
26	2.5895	2.4909	2.3867	2.2759	2.2174	2.1565	2.0928	2.0257	1.9545	1.8781
27	2.5676	2.4688	2.3644	2.2533	2.1946	2.1334	2.0693	2.0018	1.9299	1.8527
28	2.5473	2.4484	2.3438	2.2324	2.1735	2.1121	2.0477	1.9796	1.9072	1.8291
29	2.5286	2.4295	2.3248	2.2131	2.1540	2.0923	2.0276	1.9591	1.8861	1.8072
30	2.5112	2.4210	2.3072	2.1952	2.1359	2.0739	2.0089	1.9400	1.8664	1.7867
40	2.3882	2.2882	2.1819	2.0677	2.0069	1.9429	1.8752	1.8028	1.7242	1.6371
60	2.2702	2.1692	2.0613	1.9445	1.8817	1.8152	1.7440	1.6668	1.5810	1.4822
120	2.1570	2.0548	1.9450	1.8249	1.7597	1.6899	1.6141	1.5299	1.4327	1.3104
∞	2.0483	1.9447	1.8326	1.7085	1.6402	1.5660	1.4835	1.3883	1.2684	1.0000

TABLE A.4 (continued): Upper quantiles of an F distribution ($\alpha = 0.010$).

$\nu_2 \backslash \nu_1$	1	2	3	4	5	6	7	8	9
1	4052.2	4999.5	5403.3	5624.6	5763.7	5859.0	5928.3	5981.6	6022.5
2	98.503	99.000	99.166	99.249	99.299	99.332	99.356	99.374	99.388
3	34.116	30.817	29.457	28.710	28.237	27.911	27.672	27.489	27.345
4	21.198	18.000	16.694	15.977	15.522	15.207	14.976	14.799	14.659
5	16.258	13.274	12.060	11.392	10.967	10.672	10.456	10.289	10.158
6	13.745	10.925	9.7795	9.1483	8.7459	8.4661	8.2600	8.1016	7.9761
7	12.246	9.5466	8.4513	7.8467	7.4604	7.1914	6.9928	6.8401	6.7188
8	11.259	8.6491	7.5910	7.0060	6.6318	6.3707	6.1776	6.0289	5.9106
9	10.561	8.0215	6.9919	6.4221	6.0569	5.8018	5.6129	5.4671	5.3511
10	10.044	7.5594	6.5523	5.9943	5.6363	5.3858	5.2001	5.0567	4.9424
11	9.6460	7.2057	6.2167	5.6683	5.3160	5.0692	4.8861	4.7445	4.6315
12	9.3302	6.9266	5.9526	5.4119	5.0643	4.8206	4.6395	4.4994	4.3875
13	9.0738	6.7010	5.7394	5.2053	4.8616	4.6204	4.4410	4.3021	4.1911
14	8.8616	6.5149	5.5639	5.0354	4.6950	4.4558	4.2779	4.1399	4.0297
15	8.6831	6.3589	5.4170	4.8932	4.5556	4.3183	4.1415	4.0045	3.8948
16	8.5310	6.2262	5.2922	4.7726	4.4374	4.2016	4.0259	3.8896	3.7804
17	8.3997	6.1121	5.1850	4.6690	4.3359	4.1015	3.9267	3.7910	3.6822
18	8.2854	6.0129	5.0919	4.5790	4.2479	4.1046	3.8406	3.7054	3.5971
19	8.1850	5.9259	5.0103	4.5003	4.1708	3.9386	3.7653	3.6305	3.5225
20	8.0960	5.8489	4.9382	4.4307	4.1027	3.8714	3.6987	3.5644	3.4567
21	8.0166	5.7804	4.8740	4.3688	4.0421	3.8117	3.6396	3.5056	3.3981
22	7.9454	5.7190	4.8166	4.3134	3.9880	3.7583	3.5867	3.4530	3.3458
23	7.8811	5.6637	4.7649	4.2635	3.9392	3.7102	3.5390	3.4057	3.2986

(*continued*)

TABLE A.4 (continued): Upper quantiles of an F distribution ($\alpha = 0.010$).

$\nu_2 \backslash \nu_1$	1	2	3	4	5	6	7	8	9
24	7.8229	5.6136	4.7181	4.2184	3.8951	3.6667	3.4959	3.3629	3.2560
25	7.7698	5.5680	4.6755	4.1774	3.8550	3.6272	3.4568	3.3239	3.2172
26	7.7213	5.5263	4.6366	4.1400	3.8183	3.5911	3.4210	3.2884	3.1818
27	7.6767	5.4881	4.6009	4.1056	3.7848	3.5580	3.3882	3.2558	3.1494
28	7.6356	5.4529	4.5681	4.0740	3.7539	3.5276	3.3581	3.2259	3.1195
29	7.5976	5.4205	4.5378	4.0449	3.7254	3.4995	3.3302	3.1982	3.0920
30	7.5625	5.3904	4.5097	4.0179	3.6990	3.4735	3.3045	3.1726	3.0665
40	7.3141	5.1785	4.3126	3.8283	3.5138	3.2910	3.1238	2.9930	2.8876
60	7.0771	4.9774	4.1259	3.6491	3.3389	3.1187	2.9530	2.8233	2.7185
120	6.8510	4.7865	3.9493	3.4796	3.1735	2.9559	2.7918	2.6629	2.5586
∞	6.6349	4.6052	3.7816	3.3192	3.0173	2.8020	2.6393	2.5113	2.4073

$\nu_2 \backslash \nu_1$	10	12	15	20	24	30	40	60	120	∞
1	6055.8	6106.3	6157.3	6208.7	6234.6	6260.7	6286.8	6313.0	6339.4	6366.0
2	99.399	99.416	99.432	99.449	99.458	99.466	99.474	99.483	99.491	99.501
3	27.229	27.052	26.872	26.690	26.598	26.505	26.411	26.316	26.221	26.126
4	14.546	14.374	14.198	14.020	13.929	13.838	13.745	13.652	13.558	13.463
5	10.051	9.8883	9.7222	9.5527	9.4665	9.3793	9.2912	9.2020	9.1118	9.0204
6	7.8741	7.7183	7.5590	7.3958	7.3127	7.2285	7.1432	7.0568	6.9690	6.8801
7	6.6201	5.6668	5.5151	5.3591	5.2793	5.1981	5.1156	5.0316	4.9460	4.8588
8	5.8143	5.6668	5.5151	5.3591	5.2793	5.1981	5.1156	5.0316	4.9460	4.8588
9	5.2565	5.1114	4.9621	4.8080	4.7290	4.6486	4.5667	4.4831	4.3978	4.3105
10	4.8492	4.7059	4.5582	4.4054	4.3269	4.2469	4.1653	4.0819	3.9965	3.9090

11	4.5393	4.3974	4.2509	4.0990	4.0209	3.9411	3.8596	3.7761	3.6904	3.6025
12	4.2961	4.1553	4.0096	3.8584	3.7805	3.7008	3.6192	3.5355	3.4494	3.3608
13	4.1003	3.9603	3.8154	3.6646	3.5868	3.5070	3.4253	3.3413	3.2548	3.1654
14	3.9394	3.8001	3.6557	3.5052	3.4274	3.3476	3.2556	3.1813	3.0942	3.0040
15	3.8049	3.6662	3.5222	3.3719	3.2940	3.2141	3.1319	3.0471	2.9595	2.8684
16	3.6909	3.5527	3.4089	3.2588	3.1808	3.1007	3.0182	2.9330	2.8447	2.7528
17	3.5931	3.4552	3.3117	3.1615	3.0835	3.0032	2.9205	2.8348	2.7459	2.6530
18	3.5082	3.3706	3.2273	3.0771	2.9990	2.9185	2.8354	2.7493	2.6597	2.5660
19	3.4338	3.2965	3.1533	3.0031	2.9249	2.8442	2.7608	2.6742	2.5839	2.4893
20	3.3682	3.2311	3.0880	2.9377	2.8594	2.7785	2.6947	2.6077	2.5168	2.4212
21	3.3098	3.1729	3.0299	2.8796	2.8011	2.7200	2.6359	2.5484	2.4568	2.3603
22	3.2576	3.1209	2.9780	2.8274	2.7488	2.6675	2.5831	2.4951	2.4029	2.3055
23	3.2106	3.0740	2.9311	2.7805	2.7017	2.6202	2.5355	2.4471	2.3542	2.2559
24	3.1681	3.0316	2.8887	2.7380	2.6591	2.5773	2.4923	2.4035	2.3099	2.2107
25	3.1294	2.9931	2.8502	2.6993	2.6203	2.5383	2.4530	2.3637	2.2695	2.1694
26	3.0941	2.9579	2.8150	2.6640	2.5848	2.5026	2.4170	2.3273	2.2325	2.1315
27	3.0618	2.9256	2.7827	2.6316	2.5522	2.4699	2.3840	2.2938	2.1984	2.0965
28	3.0320	2.8959	2.7530	2.6017	2.5223	2.4397	2.3535	2.2629	2.1670	2.0642
29	3.0045	2.8685	2.7256	2.5742	2.4946	2.4118	2.3253	2.2344	2.1378	2.0342
30	2.9791	2.8431	2.7002	2.5487	2.4689	2.3860	2.2992	2.2079	2.1107	2.0062
40	2.8005	2.6648	2.5216	2.3689	2.2880	2.2034	2.1142	2.0194	1.9172	1.8047
60	2.6318	2.4961	2.3523	2.1978	2.1154	2.0285	1.9360	1.8363	1.7263	1.6006
120	2.4721	2.3363	2.1915	2.0346	1.9500	1.8600	1.7628	1.6557	1.5330	1.3805
∞	2.3209	2.1848	2.0385	1.8783	1.7908	1.6964	1.5923	1.4730	1.3246	1.0000

(continued)

TABLE A.4 (continued): Upper quantiles of an F distribution ($\alpha = 0.005$).

ν_2 \ ν_1	1	2	3	4	5	6	7	8	9
1	16211	20000	21615	22500	23056	23437	23715	23925	24091
2	198.50	199.00	199.17	199.25	199.30	199.33	199.36	199.37	199.39
3	55.552	49.799	47.467	46.195	45.392	44.838	44.434	44.126	43.882
4	31.333	26.284	24.259	23.155	22.456	21.975	21.622	21.352	21.139
5	22.785	18.314	16.530	15.556	14.940	14.513	14.200	13.961	13.722
6	18.635	14.544	12.917	12.028	11.464	11.073	10.786	10.566	10.391
7	16.236	12.404	10.882	10.050	9.5221	9.1554	8.8854	8.6781	8.5138
8	14.688	11.042	9.5965	8.8051	8.3018	7.9520	7.6942	7.4960	7.3386
9	13.614	10.107	8.7171	7.9559	7.4711	7.1338	6.8849	6.6933	6.5411
10	12.826	9.4270	8.0807	7.3428	6.8723	6.5446	6.3025	6.1159	5.9676
11	12.226	8.9122	7.6004	6.8809	6.4217	6.1015	5.8648	5.6821	5.5368
12	11.754	8.5096	7.2258	6.5211	6.0711	5.7570	5.5245	5.3451	5.2021
13	11.374	8.1865	6.9257	6.2335	5.7910	5.4819	5.2529	5.0761	4.9351
14	11.060	7.9217	6.6803	5.9984	5.5623	5.2574	5.0313	4.8566	4.7173
15	10.798	7.7008	6.4760	5.8029	5.3721	5.0708	4.8473	4.6743	4.5464
16	10.575	7.5138	6.3034	5.6378	5.2117	4.9134	4.6920	4.5207	4.3838
17	10.384	7.3536	6.1556	5.4967	5.0746	4.7789	4.5594	4.3893	4.2535
18	10.218	7.2148	6.0277	5.3746	4.9560	4.6627	4.4448	4.2759	4.1410
19	10.073	7.0935	5.9161	5.2681	4.8526	4.5614	4.3448	4.1770	4.0428
20	9.9439	6.9865	5.8177	5.1743	4.7616	4.4721	4.2569	4.0900	3.9564
21	9.8295	6.8914	5.7304	5.0911	4.6808	4.3931	4.1789	4.0128	3.8799
22	9.7271	6.8064	5.6524	5.0168	4.6088	4.3225	4.1094	3.9440	3.8116
23	9.6348	6.7300	5.5823	4.9500	4.5441	4.2591	4.0469	3.882	3.7502
24	9.5513	6.6610	5.5190	4.8898	4.4857	4.2019	3.9905	3.8264	3.6949

25	9.4753	6.5982	5.4615	4.8351	4.4327	4.1500	3.9394	3.7758	3.6447
26	9.4059	6.5409	5.4091	4.7852	4.3844	4.1027	3.8928	3.7297	3.5989
27	9.3423	6.4885	5.3611	4.7396	4.3402	4.0594	3.8501	3.6875	3.5571
28	9.2838	6.4403	5.3170	4.6977	4.2996	4.0197	3.8110	3.6487	3.5186
29	9.2297	6.3958	5.2764	4.6591	4.2622	3.9830	3.7749	3.6130	3.4832
30	9.1797	6.3547	5.2388	4.6233	4.2276	3.9492	3.7416	3.5801	3.4505
40	8.8278	6.0664	4.9759	4.3738	3.9860	3.7129	3.5088	3.3498	3.2220
60	8.4946	5.7950	4.7290	4.1399	3.7600	3.4918	3.2911	3.1344	3.0083
120	8.1790	5.5393	4.4973	3.9207	3.5482	3.2849	3.0874	2.9330	2.8083
∞	7.8794	5.2983	4.2794	3.7151	3.3499	3.0913	2.8968	2.7444	2.6210

$\nu_2 \backslash \nu_1$	**10**	**12**	**15**	**20**	**24**	**30**	**40**	**60**	**12**	**∞**
1	24224	24426	24630	24836	24940	25044	25148	25253	25359	25465
2	199.40	199.42	199.43	199.45	199.46	199.47	199.47	199.48	199.49	199.51
3	43.686	43.387	43.085	42.778	42.622	42.466	42.308	42.149	41.989	41.829
4	20.967	20.705	20.438	20.167	20.030	19.892	19.752	19.611	19.468	19.325
5	13.618	13.384	13.146	12.903	12.780	12.656	12.530	12.402	12.274	12.144
6	10.250	10.034	9.8140	9.5888	9.4741	9.3583	9.2408	9.1219	9.0015	8.8793
7	8.3803	8.1764	7.9678	7.7540	7.6450	7.5345	7.4225	7.3088	7.1933	7.0760
8	7.2107	7.0149	6.8143	6.6082	6.5029	6.3961	6.2875	6.1772	6.0649	5.9505
9	6.4171	6.2274	6.0325	5.8318	5.7292	5.6248	5.5186	5.4104	5.3001	5.1875
10	5.8467	5.6613	5.4707	5.2740	5.1732	5.0705	4.9659	4.8592	4.7501	4.6385
11	5.4182	5.2363	5.0489	4.8552	4.7557	4.6543	4.5508	4.8592	4.7501	4.6385
12	5.0855	4.9063	4.7214	4.5299	4.4315	4.3309	4.2282	4.1229	4.0149	3.9039
13	4.8199	4.6429	4.4600	4.2703	4.1726	4.0727	3.9704	3.8655	3.7577	3.6465

(*continued*)

TABLE A.4 (continued): Upper quantiles of an F distribution ($\alpha = 0.005$).

$\nu_2 \backslash \nu_1$	10	12	15	20	24	30	40	60	12	∞
14	4.6034	4.4281	4.2468	4.0585	3.9614	3.8619	3.7600	3.6553	3.5473	3.4359
15	4.4236	4.2498	4.0698	3.8826	3.7859	3.6867	3.5850	3.4803	3.3722	3.2602
16	4.2719	4.0994	3.9205	3.7342	3.6378	3.5388	3.4372	3.3324	3.2240	3.1115
17	4.1423	3.9709	3.7929	3.6073	3.5112	3.4124	3.3107	3.2058	3.0971	2.9839
18	4.0305	3.8599	3.6827	3.4977	3.4017	3.3030	3.2014	3.0962	2.9871	2.8732
19	3.9329	3.7631	3.5866	3.4020	3.3062	3.2075	3.1058	3.0004	2.8908	2.7762
20	3.8470	3.6779	3.5020	3.3178	3.2220	3.1234	3.0215	2.9159	2.8058	2.6904
21	3.7709	3.6024	3.4270	3.2431	3.1474	3.0488	2.9467	2.4808	2.7302	2.6140
22	3.7030	3.5350	3.3600	3.1764	3.0807	2.9821	2.8799	2.7736	2.6625	2.5455
23	3.6420	3.4745	3.2999	3.1165	3.0208	2.9221	2.8198	2.7132	2.6016	2.4837
24	2.5870	3.4199	3.2456	3.0624	2.9667	2.8679	2.7654	2.6585	2.5463	2.4276
25	3.5370	3.3704	3.1963	3.0133	2.9176	2.8187	2.7160	2.6088	2.8960	2.3795
26	3.4916	3.3252	3.1515	2.9685	2.8728	2.7738	2.6709	2.5633	2.4501	2.3297
27	3.4499	3.2839	3.1104	2.9275	2.8318	2.7327	2.6296	2.5217	2.4078	2.2867
28	3.4117	3.2460	3.0727	2.8899	2.7941	2.6949	2.5916	2.4834	2.3689	2.2469
29	3.3765	3.2111	3.0379	2.8551	2.7594	2.6601	2.5565	2.4479	2.3330	2.2102
30	3.3440	3.1787	3.0057	2.8230	2.7272	2.6278	2.5241	2.4151	2.2997	2.1760
40	3.1167	2.9531	2.7811	2.5984	2.5020	2.4015	2.2958	2.1838	2.0635	1.9318
60	2.9042	2.7419	2.5705	2.3872	2.2898	2.1874	2.0789	1.9622	1.8341	1.6885
120	2.7052	2.5439	2.3727	2.1881	2.0890	1.9839	1.8709	1.7469	1.6055	1.4311
∞	2.5188	2.3583	2.1868	1.9998	1.8983	1.7891	1.6691	1.5325	1.3637	1.0000

Source: From Merrington, M. and Thompson, C.M., *Biometrika* (Tables of Percentage Points of the Inverted beta (F)-Distribution), 33, 73, 1942.

TABLE A.5: Upper quantiles of the distribution of Wilcoxon–Mann–Whitney statistic.

n_1	α	$n_{23}=2$	3	4	5	6	7	8	9	10	11	12	13	14	15	16	17	18	19	20
	0.001	0	0	0	0	0	0	0	0	0	0	0	0	0	0	0	0	0	0	0
	0.005	0	0	0	0	0	0	0	0	0	0	0	0	0	0	0	0	0	1	1
2	0.01	0	0	0	0	0	0	0	0	0	0	0	1	1	1	1	1	1	2	2
	0.025	0	0	0	0	0	0	1	1	1	1	2	2	2	2	2	3	3	3	3
	0.05	0	0	0	1	1	1	2	2	2	2	3	3	4	4	4	4	5	5	5
	0.10	0	1		2	2	2	3	3	4	4	5	5	5	6	6	7	7	8	8
	0.001	0	0	.0	0	0	0	0	0	0	0	0	0	0	0	0	1	1	1	1
	0.005	0	0	0	0	0	0	0	1	1	1	2	2	2	3	3	3	3	4	4
3	0.01	0	0	0	0	0	1	1	2	2	2	3	3	3	4	4	5	5	5	6
	0.025	0	0	0	1	2	2	3	3	4	4	5	5	6	6	7	7	8	8	9
	0.05	0	1	1	2	3	3	4	5	5	6	6	7	8	8	9	10	10	11	12
	0.10	1	2	2	3	4	5	6	6	7	8	9	10	11	11	12	13	14	15	16
	0.001	0	0	0	0	0	0	0	0	1	1	1	2	2	2	3	3	4	4	4
	0.005	0	0	0	0	1	1	2	2	3	3	4	4	5	6	6	7	7	8	9
4	0.01	0	0	0	1	2	2	3	4	4	5	6	6	7	9	8	9	10	10	11
	0.025	0	0	1	2	3	4	5	5	6	7	8	9	10	11	12	12	13	14	15
	0.05	0	1	2	3	4	5	6	7	8	9	10	11	12	13	15	16	17	18	19
	0.10	1	2	4	5	6	7	8	10	11	12	13	14	16	17	18	19	21	22	23
	0.001	0	0	0	0	0	0	1	2	2	3	3	4	4	5	6	6	7	8	8
	0.005	0	0	0	1	2	2	3	4	5	6	7	8	8	9	10	11	12	13	14
5	0.01	0	0	1	2	3	4	5	6	7	8	9	10	11	12	13	14	15	16	17
	0.025	0	1	2	3	4	6	7	8	9	10	12	13	14	15	16	18	19	20	21
	0.05	1	2	3	5	6	7	9	10	12	13	14	16	17	19	20	21	23	24	26

(*continued*)

TABLE A.5 (continued): Upper quantiles of the distribution of Wilcoxon–Mann–Whitney statistic.

n_1	α	$n_{23}=2$	3	4	5	6	7	8	9	10	11	12	13	14	15	16	17	18	19	20
	0.10	2	3	5	6	8	9	11	13	14	16	18	19	21	23	24	26	28	29	31
	0.001	0	0	0	0	0	0	2	3	4	5	5	6	7	8	9	10	11	12	13
	0.005	0	0	1	2	3	4	5	6	7	8	10	11	12	13	14	16	17	18	19
6	0.01	0	0	2	3	4	5	7	8	9	10	12	13	14	16	17	19	20	21	23
	0.025	0	2	3	4	6	7	9	11	12	14	15	17	18	20	22	23	25	26	28
	0.05	1	3	4	6	8	9	11	13	15	17	18	20	22	24	26	27	29	31	33
	0.10	2	4	6	8	10	12	14	16	18	20	22	24	26	28	30	32	35	37	39
	0.001	0	0	0	0	1	2	3	4	6	7	8	9	10	11	12	14	15	16	17
	0.005	0	0	1	2	4	5	7	8	10	11	13	14	16	17	19	20	22	23	25
7	0.01	0	1	2	4	5	7	8	10	12	13	15	17	18	20	22	24	25	27	29
	0.025	0	2	4	6	7	9	11	13	15	17	19	21	22	25	27	29	31	33	35
	0.05	1	3	5	7	9	12	14	16	18	20	22	25	27	29	31	34	36	38	40
	0.10	2	5	7	9	12	14	17	19	22	24	27	29	32	34	37	39	42	44	47
	0.001	0	0	0	1	2	3	5	6	7	9	10	12	13	15	16	18	19	21	22
	0.005	0	0	2	3	5	7	8	10	12	14	16	18	19	21	23	25	27	29	31
8	0.01	0	1	3	5	7	8	10	12	14	16	18	21	23	25	27	29	31	33	35
	0.025	1	3	5	7	9	11	14	16	18	20	23	25	27	30	32	35	37	39	42
	0.05	2	4	6	9	11	14	16	19	21	24	27	29	32	34	37	40	42	45	48
	0.10	3	6	8	11	14	17	20	23	25	28	31	34	37	40	43	46	49	52	55
	0.001	0	0	0	2	3	4	6	8	9	11	13	15	16	18	20	22	24	26	27
	0.005	0	1	2	4	6	8	10	12	14	17	19	21	23	25	28	30	32	34	37
9	0.01	0	2	4	6	8	10	12	15	17	19	22	24	27	29	32	34	37	39	41
	0.025	1	3	5	8	11	13	16	18	21	24	27	29	32	35	38	40	43	46	49
	0.5	2	5	7	10	13	16	19	22	25	28	31	34	37	40	43	46	49	52	55
	0.10	3	6	10	13	16	19	23	26	29	32	36	39	42	46	49	53	56	59	63

	0.001	0	0	1	2	4	6	7	9	11	13	15	18	20	22	24	26	28	30	33
	0.005	0	1	3	5	7	10	12	14	17	19	22	25	27	30	32	35	38	40	43
10	0.01	0	2	4	7	9	12	14	17	20	23	25	28	31	34	37	39	42	45	48
	0.025	1	4	6	9	12	15	18	21	24	27	30	34	37	40	43	46	49	53	56
	0.05	2	5	8	12	15	18	21	25	28	32	35	38	42	45	49	52	56	59	63
	0.10	4	7	11	14	18	22	25	29	33	37	40	44	48	52	55	59	63	67	71
	0.001	0	0	1	3	5	7	9	11	13	16	18	21	23	25	28	30	33	35	38
	0.005	0	1	3	6	8	11	14	17	19	22	25	28	31	34	37	40	43	46	49
11	0.01	0	2	5	8	10	13	16	19	23	26	29	32	35	38	42	45	48	51	54
	0.025	1	4	7	10	14	17	20	24	27	31	34	38	41	45	48	52	56	59	63
	0.05	2	6	9	13	17	20	24	28	32	35	39	43	47	51	55	58	62	66	70
	0.10	4	8	12	16	20	24	28	32	37	41	45	49	53	58	62	66	70	74	79
	0.001	0	0	1	3	5	8	10	13	15	18	21	24	26	29	32	35	38	41	43
	0.005	0	2	4	7	10	13	16	19	22	25	28	32	35	38	42	45	48	52	55
12	0.01	0	3	6	9	12	15	18	22	25	29	32	36	39	43	47	50	54	57	61
	0.025	2	5	8	12	15	19	23	27	30	34	38	42	46	50	54	58	62	66	70
	0.05	3	6	10	14	18	22	27	31	35	39	43	48	52	56	61	65	69	73	78
	0.10	5	9	13	18	22	27	31	36	40	45	50	54	59	64	68	73	78	82	87
	0.001	0	0	2	4	6	9	12	15	18	21	24	27	30	33	36	39	43	46	49
	0.005	0	2	4	8	11	14	18	21	25	28	32	35	39	43	46	50	54	58	61
13	0.01	1	3	6	10	13	17	21	24	28	32	36	40	44	48	52	56	60	64	68
	0.025	2	5	9	13	17	21	25	29	34	38	42	46	51	55	60	64	68	73	77
	0.05	3	7	11	16	20	25	29	34	38	43	48	52	57	62	66	71	76	81	85
	0.010	5	10	14	19	24	29	34	39	44	49	54	59	64	69	75	80	85	90	95
	0.001	0	0	2	4	7	10	13	16	20	23	26	30	33	37	40	44	47	51	55
	0.005	0	2	5	8	12	16	19	23	27	31	35	39	43	47	51	55	59	64	68

(continued)

TABLE A.5 (continued): Upper quantiles of the distribution of Wilcoxon–Mann–Whitney statistic.

n_1	α	$n_{23}=2$	3	4	5	6	7	8	9	10	11	12	13	14	15	16	17	18	19	20
14	0.01	1	3	7	11	14	18	23	27	31	35	39	44	48	52	57	61	66	70	74
	0.025	2	6	10	14	18	23	27	32	37	41	46	51	56	60	65	70	75	79	84
	0.05	4	8	12	17	22	27	32	37	42	47	52	57	62	67	72	78	83	88	93
	0.10	5	11	16	21	26	32	37	42	48	53	59	64	70	75	81	86	92	98	103
	0.001	0	0	2	5	8	11	15	18	22	25	29	33	37	41	44	48	52	56	60
	0.005	0	3	6	9	13	17	21	25	30	34	38	43	47	52	56	61	65	70	74
15	0.01	1	4	8	12	16	20	25	29	34	38	43	48	52	57	62	67	71	76	81
	0.025	2	6	11	15	20	25	20	35	40	45	50	55	60	65	71	76	81	86	91
	0.05	4	8	13	19	24	29	34	40	45	51	56	62	67	73	78	84	89	95	101
	0.10	6	11	17	23	28	34	40	46	52	58	64	69	75	81	87	93	99	105	111
	0.001	0	0	3	6	9	12	16	20	24	28	32	36	40	44	49	53	57	61	66
	0.005	0	3	6	10	14	19	23	28	32	37	42	46	51	56	61	66	71	75	80
16	0.01	1	4	8	13	17	22	27	32	37	42	47	52	57	62	67	72	77	83	88
	0.025	2	7	12	16	22	27	32	38	43	48	54	60	65	71	76	82	87	93	99
	0.05	4	9	15	20	26	31	37	43	49	55	61	66	72	78	84	90	96	102	108
	0.10	6	12	18	24	30	37	43	49	55	62	68	75	81	87	94	100	107	113	120
	0.001	0	1	3	6	10	14	18	22	26	30	35	39	44	48	53	58	62	67	71
	0.005	0	3	7	11	16	20	25	30	35	40	45	50	55	61	66	71	76	82	87
17	0.01	1	5	9	14	19	24	29	34	39	45	50	56	61	67	72	78	83	89	94
	0.025	3	7	12	18	23	29	35	40	46	52	58	64	70	76	82	88	94	100	106

	0.05	4	10	16	21	27	34	40	46	52	58	65	71	78	84	90	97	103	110	116
	0.10	7	13	19	26	32	39	46	53	59	66	73	80	86	93	100	107	114	121	128
	0.001	0	1	4	7	11	15	19	24	28	33	38	43	47	52	57	62	67	72	77
	0.005	0	3	7	12	17	22	27	32	38	43	48	51	59	65	71	76	82	88	93
18	0.01	1	5	10	15	20	25	31	37	42	48	54	60	66	71	77	83	89	95	101
	0.025	3	8	13	19	25	31	37	43	49	56	62	68	75	81	87	94	100	107	113
	0.05	5	10	17	23	29	36	42	49	56	62	69	76	83	89	96	103	110	117	124
	0.10	7	14	21	28	35	42	49	56	63	70	78	85	92	99	107	114	121	129	136
	0.001	0	1	4	8	12	16	21	26	30	35	41	46	51	56	61	67	72	78	83
	0.005	1	4	8	13	18	23	29	34	40	46	52	58	64	70	75	82	88	94	100
19	0.01	2	5	10	16	21	27	33	39	45	51	57	64	70	76	83	89	95	102	108
	0.025	3	8	14	20	26	33	39	46	53	59	66	73	79	86	93	100	107	114	120
	0.05	5	11	18	24	31	38	45	52	59	66	73	81	88	95	102	110	117	124	131
	0.10	8	15	22	29	37	44	52	59	67	74	82	90	98	105	113	121	129	136	144
	0.001	0	1	4	8	13	17	22	27	33	38	43	49	55	60	66	71	77	83	89
	0.005	1	4	9	14	19	25	31	37	43	49	55	61	68	74	80	87	93	100	106
20	0.01	2	6	11	17	23	29	35	41	48	54	61	68	74	81	88	94	101	108	115
	0.025	3	9	15	21	28	35	42	49	56	63	70	77	84	91	99	106	113	120	128
	0.05	5	12	19	26	33	40	48	55	63	70	78	85	93	101	108	116	124	131	139
	0.10	8	16	23	31	39	47	55	63	71	79	87	95	103	111	120	128	136	144	152

Source: From Verdooren, L.R., *Biometrika* (Table 1 of Extended Tables of Critical Values for Wilcoxon's Test Statistic), 50, 177, 1963.

Appendix B

SAS Programs

B.1 Procedures for Average Bioavailability

Program: BOOKEXAMPLE.SAS

Author: J.P. Liu

Date: June 24, 1991

Description: This program computes the test statistics and confidence intervals based on the methods for a 2×2 crossover design described in Chapter 4 and also examines the assumptions by the methods described in Chapter 8.

Methods: Schuirmann's two one-sided tests procedure
Rodda and Davis's Bayesian procedure
Anderson–Huack's procedure
Mandallaz–Mau's procedure
Nonparametric two one-sided tests procedure
The classical shortest confidence interval
Westlake's symmetric confidence interval
Locke's exact confidence
interval for the ratio by Fieller theorem
Fixed Fieller's confidence interval for the ratio
Nonparametric confidence interval
Normality and independence tests of intrasubject/intersubject
variabilities

Data set: AUC data in Table 3.3 of Chapter 3.

libname out 'XXXXX: [XXXXX.XXXXX]';

Input data and print the raw data.
Sequence = group (=1 and 2)
Subject = subject
Period = period (1=I and 2=II)
Tmt = formulation (1=reference and 2=test)
y = raw AUC

```
data one;
set out.ex361;
proc sort data=one; by group subject tmt;
proc print data=one;

proc means n noprint data=one; by group;
var y;
output out=no n=n;
```

Compute the subject totals.

```
proc means n noprint data=one; by group subject;
var y;
output out=sum sum=ysum;
```

Data set of the number of subjects in each sequence.

```
data no; set no;
n=n/2;

proc sort data=no; by group;

data one; merge one no; by group;

proc sort data=one; by group subject tmt;
```

Perform analysis of variance using the full model with group as carryover effect which is confounded with sequence effect.

```
proc glm data=one;
class tmt period group subject;
model y=group subject (group) period tmt/ss1 ss2 ss3 ss4 solution p;
test h=group e=subject (group)/htype=3 etype=3;
means tmt period group;
lsmeans tmt period/stderr pdiff;
lsmeans group/stderr pdiff e=subject (group);
```

Perform analysis of variance using the reduced model without carryover effect.
Output data set:

tanova – sums of squares and associate degrees of freedom.
lsmean1 – lsmeans of formulation and period means.
pred – intrasubject residuals.

```
proc glm data=one outstat=tanova;
class tmt period subject;
model y=subject period tmt/ss1 ss2 ss3 ss4 solution p;
```

```
output out=pred p=yhat r=resid student=stresid;
means tmt period;
lsmeans tmt period/stderr pdiff out=lsmean1;
proc print data=tanova;
proc print data=lsmean1;
```

Perform analysis of variance on subject totals to obtain the intersubject residuals.

```
proc glm data=sum;
model ysum=group;
output out=predsum p=ysumhat r=residsum student=residsub;

data pred; set pred; if period=1;
```

Obtain the normal scores for intrasubject residuals, plot them versus predicted values and normal scores, and perform Shapiro–Wilk's test for normality.

```
proc rank out=rpred normal=blom data=pred;
var stresid;
ranks rankr;
proc sort data=rpred;

proc plot data=rpred;
plot stresid*yhat;
plot stresid*rankr;

proc univariate normal plot data=pred;
var stresid;
```

Obtain the normal scores for intersubject residuals, plot them versus normal scores, and perform Shapiro–Wilk's test for normality.

```
proc rank out=rpredsum normal=blom data=predsum;
var residsub;
ranks ranksum;
proc sort data=rpredsum; by ranksum;

proc plot data=rpredsum;
plot residsub*ranksum;

proc univariate normal plot data=predsum;
var residsub;
```

Test the assumption of independence between intrasubject and intersubject variabilities.

```
data rpred1; set rpred;
keep subject stresid;
proc sort data=rpred1; by subject;

data rpredsum; set rpredsum;
keep subject residsub;
proc sort data=rpredsum; by subject;

data indep; merge rpred1 rpredsum; by subject;
proc corr pearson spearman data=indep;
var stresid residsub;
```

Create data sets for df, mse, number of subjects, and least squares means of formulation.

```
data error; set tanova; if _SOURCE_='ERROR';
mse=ss/df;
sse=ss;
id=1;
keep id mse sse df;
proc sort data=error; by id;

data no1; set no; if group=1;
n1=n; id=1;
keep n1 id;
proc sort data=no1; by id;

data no2; set no; if group=2;
n2=n; id=1;
keep n2 id;
proc sort data=no2; by id;

data lsmean11; set lsmean1; if tmt=1;
my1=lsmean;
id=1;
keep id my1;
proc sort data=lsmean11; by id;

data lsmean12; set lsmean1; if tmt=2;
my2=lsmean;
id=1;
keep id my2;
proc sort data=lsmean12; by id;
```

Perform Schuirmann's two one-sided tests procedure, compute the 90% classic shortest confidence interval, and conduct Rodda and Bayesian procedure based on the summary statistics extracted from PROC GLM.

t: T-statistics for equality (with p-value = p).
t1: T-statistics for testing that test formulation is not too low (with p-value = p1).
t2: T-statistics for testing that test formulation is not too high (with p-value = p2).
Lower (upper): Lower (upper) 90% confidence limits.
Plower (Pupper): Lower (upper) 90% confidence limits expressed as percentage of the estimated reference mean.
prd: estimated posterior probability between equivalence limits.

```
data twoside; merge lsmean11 lsmean12 no1 no2 error; by id;
spool=mse* (0.5) * ((1/n1) + (1/n2));
se=sqrt (spool);
diff=my2−my1;
t=(my2−my1)/se;
t1=(my2−my1+(0.2*my1))/se;
t2=−((0.2*my1) – (my2−my1))/se;
ct=tinv(0.05, df, 0);
absct=abs (ct);
lower=(my2−my1) – (absct*se);
upper=(my2−my1) + (absct*se);
plower=((lower/my1)+1) * 100;
pupper=((upper/my1)+1) * 100;
p=2*(1−probt (abs (t), df));
p1=1−probt (t1, df);
p2=probt (t2, df);
prd=probt (−t2, df) – probt (−t1, df);
proc print;
var my1 my2 n1 n2 df mse diff t t1 t2 lower upper plower pupper p p1 p2 prd;
```

Perform Anderson–Hauck's procedure based on the summary statistics extracted from PROC GLM.

```
data andhau; merge lsmean11 lsmean12 no1 no2 error; by id;
spool=mse* (0.5) * ((1/n1) + (1/n2));
se=sqrt (spool);
diff=my2−my1;
b11=(−0.2) *my1;
bul=−b11;
t=(my1−my1−(0.5) * (b11+bul))/se;
del=(0.5) * (bul−b11)/se;
u=abs (t) – del;
1=−abs (t) – del;
pu=probt (u, df, 0);
p1=probt (1, df, 0);
p=pu-p1;

proc print;
var my1 my2 n1 n2 df mse diff p;
```

Perform Mandallaz–Mau's procedure based on the summary statistics extracted from PROC GLM.

```
data ManMau; merge lsmean11 lsmean12 no1 no2 error; by id;
spool=mse* (0.5) * ((1/n1) + (1/n2));
se=sqrt (spool);
diff=my2−my1;
meansq1=sqrt (mse* (1+0.8*0.8)/(n1+n2));
meansq2=sqrt (mse* (1+1.2*1.2)/(n1+n2));
t1=(my2−(0.8*my1))/meansq1;
t2=(my2−(1.2*my1))/meansq2;
pu=probt (t1, df, 0);
pl=probt (t2, df, 0);
p=pu−pl;
proc print;
var my1 my2 n1 n2 df mse t1 t2 pl pu p;
```

Compute the Westlake's symmetric 90% confidence interval based on the summary statistics extracted from PROC GLM.
Lower (upper): Lower (upper) 90% confidence limits.
Plower (Pupper): Lower (upper) 90% confidence limits expressed as percentage of the estimated reference mean.

```
data westlake; merge lsmean11 lsmean12 no1 no2 error; by id;
spool=mse*(0.5) * ((1/n1) + (1/n2));
se=sqrt (spool);
diff1=my1−my2;
diff2=diff1;
if diff2=0 then diff2=0.001*my1;
sumk=2*diff2/se;
inc=0.1;
k1=2*sumk;
if sumk > 0 then k1=−2*sumk;
again: k2=sumk−k1;
pr1=probt (k1, df, 0);
pr2=1−probt (k2, df, 0);
prob=pr1+pr2;
if pr1 > 0.1 then k1=2*k1;
if pr1 > 0.1 then goto again;
if pr2 > 0.1 then k1=k1+sumk;
if pr2 > 0.1 then goto again;
start:
k1=k1+inc;
k2=k2−inc;
pr1=probt (k1, df, 0);
pr2=1−probt (k2, df, 0);
```

```
prob=pr1+pr2;
if prob < 0.1 then goto start;
k1=k1-inc;
k2=k2+inc;
inc=inc/5;
if inc < 0.0001 then goto end;
goto start;
end: diff=-diff1;
upper=diff+k1*se;
lower=diff+k1*se;
pupper=100*upper/my1;
plower=100*lower/my1;
proc print;
var my1 my2 n1 n2 df mse diff k1 k2 lower upper plower pupper;
proc sort data=one; by tmt period;
```

Generate the data set of period differences and subject totals.

```
data one1; set one;
if period=1;
y1=y;
drop period y;
data one2; set one;
if period=2;
y2=y;
drop period y;
proc sort data=one1; by group subject;
proc sort data=one2; by group subject;
data work; merge one1 one2; by group subject;
id=1;
proc sort data=work; by id group subject;
data work; merge work lsmean11; by id;
w1=.;
w2=.;
if group=2 then w1=y1;
if group=1 then w1=y2;
if group=2 then w2=y2;
if group=1 then w2=y1;
diffw=w1-w2;
sumw=w1+w2;
d=(y2-y1);
d1=.;
if group=1 then d1=d+(2* (0.2*my1));
if group=2 then d1=d;
d12=d1/2;
d2=.;
```

```
if group=1 then d2=d-(2* (0.2*my1));
if group=2 then d2=d;
d22=d2/2;
t=y1+y2;
p=.;
if group=1 then p=d;
if group=2 then p=-d;
proc print;
proc sort data=work; by group;
```

Obtain STT, STR, and SRR using PROC CORR.

```
proc corr csscp data=work outp=sscp; by group;
var w1 w2;
proc print data=sscp;

data sscp21; set sscp; if group=1;
if _type_='CSSCP' and _name_='W1';
ss22=w1; ss12=w2;
keep group ss22 ss12;
proc sort data=sscp21; by group;
data sscp22; set sscp; if group=1;
if _type_='CSSCP' and _name_='W2';
ss11=w2;
keep group ss11;
proc sort data=sscp22; by group;
data sscp2; merge sscp21 sscp22; by group;

data sscp11; set sscp; if group=2;
if _type_='CSSCP' and _name_='W1';
ss22=w1; ss12=w2;
keep group ss22 ss12;
proc sort data=sscp11; by group;
data sscp12; set sscp; if group=2;
if _type_='CSSCP' and _name_='w2';
ss11=w2;
keep group ss11;
proc sort data=sscp12; by group;
data sscp1; merge sscp11 sscp12; by group;

data sscpf; set sscp1 sscp2;
proc means noprint sum data=sscpf;
var ss11 ss22 ss12;
output out=sscps sum=css11 css22 css12;
data sscps; set sscps; id=1;
proc sort data=sscps; by id;
```

Compute the Locke 90% confidence interval for the ratio based on the summary statistics extracted from PROC GLM and PROC CORR.
flowerp (fupperp): Lower (upper) 90% confidence limits for the ratio by Fieller theorem.
fflowerp (ffupperp): Lower (upper) 90% confidence limits for the ratio by fixed Fieller method.

```
data locke; merge lsmean11 lsmean12 no1 no2 error sscps; by id;
spool=mse* (0.5) * ((1/n1) + (1/n2));
se=sqrt (spool);
ms11=css11/df;
ms12=css12/df;
ms22=css22/df;
r=my2/my1;
ct=tinv (0.05, df, 0);
absct=abs (ct);
w=((1/n1) + (1/n2))/4;
g2=(absct/(my1/sqrt (w*mse))) **2;
g1=(absct**2)/(my1**2)/(w*ms11));
sr1=ms22/ms11;
sr2=ms12/ms11;
k=(r**2) + sr1* (1-g1) + sr2* ((g1*sr2) - (2*r));
flower=.;
fupper=.;
fflower=.;
ffupper=.;
if g1 < 1 and k ge 0 then
flower=((r-(g1*sr2)) - (absct*sqrt (ms11*w)/my1)*sqrt (k))/(1-g1);
if g1 < 1 and k ge 0 then
fupper=((r-(g1*sr2)) + (absct*sqrt (ms11*w)/my1)*sqrt (k))/(1-g1);
k1=r**2+(1-g2);
if g2 < 1 and k1 ge 0 then
fflower=(r-(absct*sqrt (mse*w)/my1)*sqrt (k1))/(1-g2);
if g2 < 1 and k1 ge 0 then
ffupper=(r+(absct*sqrt (mse*w)/my1)*sqrt (k1))/(1-g2);
flowerp=100*flower;
fupperp=100*fupper;
fflowerp=100*fflower;
ffupperp=100*ffupper;
proc print;
var my1 my2 n1 n2 df ms11 ms12 ms22 r flowerp fupperp fflowerp ffupperp;
```

Perform Schuirmann's two one-sided tests procedure based on the period differences.
d: equality of formulation effects.
d12: for hypothesis that the test formulation is not too low.

d22: for hypothesis that the test formulation is not too high.
p: equality of period effects.
t: equality of carryover effect.
The results of d, p, and t should be the same as those from GLM.
The results of d12 and d22 (i.e., p-values) should be the same as those in the data set "twoside."

```
proc ttest data=work;
class group;
var d d12 d22 p t;
```

Perform nonparametric two one-sided tests procedure based on the period differences.
d: equality of formulation effects.
d12: for hypothesis that the test formulation is not too low.
d22: for hypothesis that the test formulation is not too high.
p: equality of period effects.
t: equality of carryover effect.

```
proc npar1way wilcoxon data=work;
class group;
var d d12 d22 p t;
```

Compute nonparametric 90% confidence interval based on all possible differences of the period differences between two sequences.

```
data out1; set work;
if group=1;
d1=d/2;
keep subject d1;
data out2; set work;
if group=2;
d=d/2;
id=subject;
keep id d;
proc sort data=out2; by d;
data out2; set out2;
do subject=1 to 12;
d2=d;
id=id;
output;
end;
keep id subject d2;
proc sort data=out1; by subject;
proc sort data=out2; by subject id;
data diff; merge out1 out2; by subject;
```

```
diff=d1−d2;
index=1;
proc univariate normal plot data=diff;
var diff;
output out=median n=ncom median=median;
data median; set median; index=1;
proc sort data=median; by index;
proc sort data=diff; by index;
data diff; merge diff median; by index;
proc rank out=rdiff data=diff;
var diff;
ranks rdiff;
data rdiff; set rdiff;
w05=43;
w95=144−43+1;
if rdiff=w05 or rdiff=w95;
proc sort data=rdiff; by rdiff;
proc print;
```

B.2 Bayesian Method by Grieve

Program:	BOOKEXGR.SAS
Author:	J.P. Liu
Date:	June 24, 1991
Description:	This program computes the test statistics and estimated posterior probability between equivalence limits by Grieve's Bayesian method for a 2 × 2 crossover design described in Chapter 4.
Methods:	Bayesian method by Grieve.
Data set:	AUC data in Table 3.3 of Chapter 3.

Compute the test statistics and posterior probability in the presence of carryover effects.

Input:	Intersubject/intrasubject sums of squares from the full model with carryover effect, estimates of formulation and carryover effects, estimated reference mean.

```
data one;
sse=3679.43;
ssp=16211.49;
rmean=82.5594;
eqlimit=0.1*rmean;
fhat=−2.2875;
```

```
rhat=-4.7958;
mean=(fhat/2)+(rhat/2);
n1=12; n2=12;
n=n1+n2;
f=(((sse+ssp)**2) * (n-6))/(sse**2+ssp**2);
f=f+4
h=((f-2) * (sse+ssp))/(n-4);
df=f;
m=((1/n1)+(1/n2));
sq=(f*(m*h)/(8*f))/(f-2);
s=sqrt (sq);
df1=(df+1)/2;
df2=df/2;
df3=1/2;
t=abs (tinv (0.05, df, 0));
l=mean-(t*s);
u=mean+(t*s);
12=2*1;
u2=2*u;
tl=(-eqlimit-mean)/s;
tu=(eqlimit-mean)/s;
pu=probt (tu, df, 0);
pl=probt (tl, df, 0);
p=pu-pl;
proc print;
```

Compute the test statistics and posterior probability in the absence of carryover effects.
Input: Intrasubject sum of squares from the reduced model without carryover effect, estimates of formulation effect, estimated reference mean.

```
data two;
sse=3679.43;
rmean=82.5594;
eqlimit=0.1*rmean;
fhat=-2.2875;
mean=(fhat/2);
n1=12; n2=12;
n=n1+n2;
df=n-2;
m=((1/n1)+(1/n2));
sq=df*m*sse/((df-2)*8*(n-2));
s=sqrt (sq);
df1=(df+1)/2;
df2=df/2;
df3=1/2;
t=abs (tinv (0.05, df, 0));
```

```
l=mean−(t*s);
u=mean+(t*s);
12=2*1;
u2=2*u;
tl=(−eqlimit−mean)/s;
tu=(eqlimit−mean)/s;
pu=probt (tu, df, 0);
pl=probt (tl, df, 0);
p=pu−pl;
proc print;
```

B.3 MVUE, MLE, RI, MIR for a 2 × 2 Crossover Design

Program: BOOKLOG.SAS

Author: J.P. Liu

Date: June 25, 1991

Description: This program computes the minimum variance unbiased estimator, maximum likelihood estimator of direct formulation effect on the original scale as well as mean of individual ratios, ratio of least squares means. In addition, this program also calculates the estimated variance of MVUE, estimated bias, mse, variance of MLE and RI by the methods described in Chapter 6.

Methods: MVUE, MLE, RI, MIR for a 2 × 2 crossover design with equal sample size for both sequences. This program can be easily modified for unequal sample sizes.

Data set: Clayton–Leslie AUC data in Table 6.4 of Chapter 6.

```
libname out 'XXXXX: [XXXXX.XXXXX]';
```

Input data and rearrange data so that y11 and y12 represent the responses of two periods for a subject. Do the logarithmic transformation. Compute period differences of log-responses.

```
data book; set out.clayton;
resp=y;
data one1; set book;
if seq=1;
data one11; set one1;
if tmt=2;
y11=resp;
keep subject seq y11;
proc sort data=one11; by subject;
```

```
data one12; set one1;
if tmt=1;
y12=resp;
keep subject seq y12;
proc sort data=one12; by subject;
data one; merge one11 one12;

data one2; set book;
if seq=2;
data one21; set one2;
if tmt=1;
y11=resp;
keep subject seq y11;
proc sort data=one21; by subject;

data one22; set one2;
if tmt=2;
y12=resp;
keep subject seq y12;
proc sort data=one22; by subject;
data two; merge one21 one22;

data work; set one two;
if seq=1 then y=(y11/y12);
if seq=2 then y=(y12/y11);
x11=log (y11);
x12=log (y12);
x=(x11-x12)/2;
id=1;
*proc print;
proc sort data=work; by id seq;
data work1; set work; by id seq;
x1=x;
if seq=2 then x1=-x;
y1=y11;
y2=y12;
```

Compute the formulation effect on the logarithmic scale, mean of individual subject ratios, and ratio of the least squares means.

```
proc univariate noprint normal plot data=work1; by id seq;
var x y y1 y2;
output out=outp n=nx ny ny1 ny2 mean=meanx meany meanry1 meanry2
css=cssx cssy cssy1 cssy2;
data outp; set outp;
n1=ny-1;
```

```
meanx1=meanx;
meany1=meany/2;
if seq=2 then meanx1=-meanx1;
cssx1=cssx;
meanrry1=.;
meanrry2=.;
if seq=1 then meanrry1=meanry1;
if seq=2 then meanrry1=meanry2;
if seq=1 then meanrry2=meanry2;
if seq=2 then meanrry2=meanry1;
drop ny1 ny2 cssy1 cssy2;
proc sort data=outp; by id;
proc means sum noprint data=outp; by id;
var meanx1 meany1 meanrry1 meanrry2 n1 ny cssx1;
output out=out sum=meanx meany meanry1 meanry2 df n cssx;
data out; set out;
meanry1=meanry1/2;
meanry2=meanry2/2;
meanrry=(meanry1)/(meanry2);
n=n/2;
f1=df/2;
a=2/(n);
w=2/n;
a=-a/4;
a1=4*a;
t=abs (tinv (0.95, df, 0));
sq=cssx/df;
sem=sqrt (sq*((1/n) + (1/n)));
tsem=t*sem;
l=meanx-tsem;
u=meanx+tsem;
proc sort data=out; by id;
```

Compute th Phi function in (6.5.2) up to the seventh term and MVUE. Also calculate estimated variance of MVUE, estimated bias, variance, and mse of MLE and MIR.

```
data out; set out; by id;
retain m;
m=0;
m1=0;
do j=0 to 7;
f2=f1+j;
j1=j;
if j le 1 then j1=1;
g1=gamma (f1);
g2=gamma (f2);
```

```
g3=gamma (j1);
m+(g1/(g2*g3)) * ((a*cssx)**j);
m1+(g1/(g2*g3)) * ((a1*cssx)**j);
end;
data out1; set out;
mu=exp (0);
ri=meany;
rm=meanrry;
expx=exp (meanx);
mle=expx;
meanx1=expx*m;
mvue=meanx1;
lmle=exp (l);
umle=exp (u);
vmvue=exp (2*meanx) * ((m**2)-m1);
bmle=expx*((exp((w/2)*sq))-1);
vmle=(exp (2*meanx))*exp (w*sq) * (((exp (w*sq))-1));
msemle=vmle+(bmle**2);
bperiod=(exp (0.14752)+exp (-0.14752));
bri=expx*((exp (2*sq)) * (bperiod)-2)/2;
vr1=(exp ((2*meanx) + (4*sq))) * ((exp (4*sq))-1);
vr2=(1/n) * ((exp (2*0.14752)) + (exp (-2*0.14752)));
vri=(0.25)*vr1*vr2;
mseri=(bri**2) + vri;
drop g1 g2 g3 f1 f2 j1;
proc print;
var mvue mle lmle umle rm ri vmvue bmle vmle msemle bri vri mseri;
```

B.4 Parametric and Nonparametric Versions of Pitman–Morgan Test

Program: BOOKEXVAR.SAS

Author: J.P. Liu

Date: June 27, 1991

Description: This program computes parametric and nonparametric versions of Pitman–Morgan tests based on residuals from sequence-by-period means and test statistics for equivalence in intrasubject variabilities based on Equations 7.38 and 7.39 in this book.

Methods: Parametric and nonparametric versions of Pitman–Morgan test. Parametric and nonparametric versions of the tests for equivalence in intrasubject variabilities.

Data set: AUC data in Table 3.3 of Chapter 3.

Input data set and print the raw data.
Compute the residuals from sequence-by-period means.
Rearrange data so that y11 and y12 represent the two residuals of a subject.
Compute Vik, Uik, Ulik, and Uuik.

```
libname out 'XXXXX: [XXXXX.XXXXX]';

data one;
set out.ex361;
proc sort data=one; by group subject tmt;
proc print data=one;
proc sort data=one; by group period subject;
proc means noprint mean data=one; by group period;
var y;
output out=mean mean=meany;
proc sort data=mean; by group period;
data one; merge one mean; by group period;
resp=y;
y=resp-meany;
data one1; set one;
if period=1;
y1=y;
meany1=meany;
drop period y meany;
data one2; set one;
if period=2;
y2=y;
meany2=meany;
drop period y meany;
proc sort data=one1; by group subject;
proc sort data=one2; by group subject;
data work; merge one1 one2; by group subject;
id=1;
proc sort data=work; by id group subject;
data work; set work;
w1=.; w2=.;
if group=2 then w2=y1;
if group=1 then w2=y2;
if group=2 then w1=y2;
if group=1 then w1=y1;
meanw1=.;
meanw2=.;
if group=2 then meanw2=meany1;
if group=1 then meanw2=meany2;
if group=2 then meanw1=meany2;
if group=1 then meanw1=meany1;
```

```
diffw=w2−w1;
sumw=w1+w2;
11=0.8;
uu=1.2;
sumwl=(11*w1)+w2;
sumwu=(uu*w1)+w2;
proc print;
```

Obtain Pearson and Spearman correlation coefficients by PROC CORR and output sum of squares and cross products of corresponding Vik, Uik, Ulik, and Uuik.

```
proc corr pearson cov data=work;
var w1 w2;
proc corr pearson noprint csscp out=css1 data=work;
var w1 w2;
proc corr pearson cov data=work;
var diffw sumw;
proc corr pearson csscp out=css2 data=work;
var diffw sumw;
proc corr spearman data=work;
var diffw sumw;
proc corr pearson csscp out=css3 data=work;
var diffw sumwl;
proc corr spearman data=work;
var diffw sumwl;
proc corr pearson csscp out=css4 data=work;
var diffw sumwu;
proc corr spearman data=work;
var diffw sumwu;
```

Perform the tests (parametric) mentioned at the introduction of this program by using STT, STR, and SRR.

```
data css11; set css1;
if _type_="CSSCP" and _name_="W1";
ssw11=w1; ssw12=w2;
id=1;
keep id ssw11 ssw12;
proc sort data=css11; by id;
data css12; set css1;
if _type_="CSSCP" and _name_="W2";
ssw22=w2;
id=1;
keep id ssw22;
proc sort data=css12; by id;
data cssraw; merge css11 css12;
```

```
11=0.8;
uu=1.2;
r=ssw12/sqrt (ssw11*ssw22);
f=ssw22/ssw11;
msw11=ssw11/22;
msw12=ssw12/22;
msw22=ssw22/22;
dem=(msw11*msw22) – (msw12**2);
numl=msw22–(ll*msw11) + ((ll–1)*msw12);
numu=msw22–(uu*msw11) + ((uu–1)*msw12);
fl=(21 * (numl**2))/(((ll+1)**2)*dem);
fu=(21 * (numu**2))/(((uu+1)**2)*dem);
fpm=(((f–1)**2)*21)/(4*f*(l–(r**2)));
fp=1–probf (fpm, 1, 21, 0);
t=sqrt (fpm);
tp=2 * (1–probt (abs (t), 21, 0));
tl=sqrt (fl);
tu=sqrt (fu);
if numu lt 0 then tu=–tu;
tpl=1–probt (abs (tl), 21, 0);
tpu=1–probt (abs (tu), 21, 0);
proc print data=cssraw;
var fpm t fp tp fl tl tpl fu tu tpu;
```

Perform the Pitman–Morgan test (parametric) based on the correlation computed from the residuals. The results should be the same as those in data set cssraw.

```
data css21; set css2;
if _type_="CSSCP" and _name_="DIFFW";
ssw11=diffw; ssw12=sumw;
id=1;
keep id ssw11 ssw12;
proc sort data=css21; by id;
data css22; set css2;
if _type_="CSSCP" and _name_"SUMW";
ssw22=sumw;
id=1;
keep id ssw22;
proc sort data=css22; by id;
data csssum; merge css21 css22;
r=ssw12/sqrt (ssw11*ssw22);
msw11=ssw11/22;
msw12=ssw12/22;
msw22=ssw22/22;
f=(21*r**2)/(1–(r**2));
fp=1–probf (f, 1, 21, 0);
```

```
t=sqrt (f);
tp=2* (1-probt (abs (t), 21, 0);
proc print data=csssum;
var r f fp t tp;
```

Perform the test (parametric) for the subhypothesis that the intrasubject variability of the test formulation is not too low, based on the correlation computed from the residuals. The results should be the same as those in data set cssraw.

```
data css31; set css3;
if _type_="CSSCP" and _name_="DIFFW";
ssw11=diffw; ssw12=sumwl;
id=1;
keep id ssw11 ssw12;
proc sort data=css31; by id;
data css32; set css3;
if _type_="CSSCP" and _name_="SUMWL";
ssw22=sumwl;
id=1;
keep id ssw22;
proc sort data=css32; by id;
data csssum1; merge css31 css32; by id;
r=ssw12/sqrt (ssw11*ssw22);
rl=r;
msw11=ssw11/22;
msw12=ssw12/22;
msw22=ssw22/22;
fl=(21*r**2)/(1-(r**2));
tl=r/sqrt ((1-(r**2))/21);
tpl=1-probt (tl, 21, 0);
proc print data=csssum1;
var rl fl tl tpl;
```

Perform the test (parametric) for the subhypothesis that the intrasubject variability of the test formulation is not too high, based on the correlation computed from the residuals. The results should be the same as those in data set cssraw.

```
data css41; set css4;
if _type_="CSSCP" and _name_="DIFFW";
ssw11=diffw; ssw12=sumwu;
id=1;
keep id ssw11 ssw12;
proc sort data=css41; by id;
data css42; set css4;
if _type_="CSSCP" and _name_="SUMWU";
ssw22=sumwu;
```

```
id=1;
keep id ssw22;
proc sort data=css42; by id;
data csssum3; merge css41 css42; by id;
r=ssw12/sqrt (ssw11*ssw22);
ru=r;
msw11=ssw11/22;
msw12=ssw12/22;
msw22=ssw22/22;
fu=(21*r**2)/(1-(r**2));
tu=r/sqrt ((1-(r**2))/21);;
tpu=probt (tu, 21, 0);
proc print data=csssum3;
var ru fu tu tpu;
```

Index

B

C

D

E

F

I

K

L

O

P

Q

R

S

T

U

V

W